Essentials of Orthopedic Surgery

William F. Postma • John N. Delahay
Sam W. Wiesel
Editors

Essentials of Orthopedic Surgery

Fifth Edition

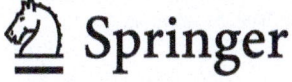 Springer

Editors
William F. Postma
Orthopedic Surgery
MedStar Georgetown University
Hospital
Washington, DC, USA

John N. Delahay
Department of Orthopaedic Surgery
MedStar Georgetown Univeristy
Hospital
Washington, DC, USA

Sam W. Wiesel
Orthopedic Surgery
MedStar Georgetown University
Hospital
Washington, DC, USA

ISBN 978-3-031-66214-0   ISBN 978-3-031-66215-7   (eBook)
https://doi.org/10.1007/978-3-031-66215-7

This Springer imprint is published by the registered company Springer Nature Switzerland AG
The registered company address is: Gewerbestrasse 11, 6330 Cham, Switzerland

If disposing of this product, please recycle the paper.

I would like to dedicate this book to all my teachers and mentors along the way, including my two co-editors. I especially want to dedicate it to my father, Dr. Jan Postma Jr., who instilled in me the work ethic and determination necessary in this profession. He has been an excellent clinician, surgeon, and role model throughout this journey.

—William F. Postma, MD

Preface

The impetus for the 5th edition of this text came from medical students, who requested an update to the 4th edition. They appreciated our approach with *Essentials*, finding it particularly helpful for their education.

The goal of the 5th edition of *Essentials of Orthopaedic Surgery* continues to focus on an up-to-date overview of orthopaedics written expressly for medical students and others who are interested in beginning their study of the musculoskeletal system (including residents in orthopaedic surgery, physiatry, rheumatology, family medicine, and emergency medicine). We have added two new chapters to this book: One in biomechanics and the other in imaging. The remaining chapters have been carefully revised to maintain a standardized format as much as possible.

Every chapter has been authored by a subspecialist in the relevant topic. In updating each section, the authors have tried to eliminate outdated content and focus on providing practical information that is relevant to medical students. Each topic is covered in sufficient depth that when confronted with a specific clinical problem, the student should be able to formulate an initial diagnostic and treatment plan.

We would like to acknowledge several individuals who contributed to this textbook. First, we would like to thank Dr. Bill Oppenheim for supporting the use of figures and illustrations through his generous commitment to the Bill and Patricia Oppenheim Lectureship in Pediatric Surgery at Georgetown. Anna Beaufort produced a number of beautiful original illustrations. We would also like to thank Kristopher Spring from Springer for the guidance in bringing this text to publication. Finally, it has been a truly exciting and stimulating experience to once again work with all the members of the Orthopaedic Department at MedStar Georgetown University Medical Center. Everyone has been enthusiastic, and their contributions were excellent. The editors are deeply appreciative and are very proud of the final text.

Washington, DC, USA   William F. Postma
Washington, DC, USA   Jack N. Delahay
Washington, DC, USA   Sam W. Wiesel
January 5th, 2025

Contents

Contributors

Brock Adams, MD Department of Orthopedics, MedStar Washington Hospital Center, Washington, DC, USA

MedStar Georgetown Orthopedic Institute, Georgetown University School of Medicine, Washington, DC, USA

Nicholas Apseloff, MD Department of Orthopedics, University of Pittsburgh, Pittsburgh, PA, USA

MedStar Georgetown Orthopedic Institute, Georgetown University School of Medicine, Washington, DC, USA

Patrick Burroughs, MD Department of Orthopedics, MedStar Georgetown University Hospital, Washington, DC, USA

MedStar Georgetown Orthopedic Institute, Georgetown University School of Medicine, Washington, DC, USA

Nicholas D. Casscells, MD Department of Orthopedics, MedStar Georgetown University Hospital, Washington, DC, USA

MedStar Georgetown Orthopedic Institute, Georgetown University School of Medicine, Washington, DC, USA

Paul S. Cooper, MD Department of Orthopedics, MedStar Georgetown University Hospital, Washington, DC, USA

MedStar Georgetown Orthopedic Institute, Georgetown University School of Medicine, Washington, DC, USA

R Adams Cowley II, MD Department of Orthopedics, MedStar Georgetown University Hospital, Washington, DC, USA

MedStar Georgetown Orthopedic Institute, Georgetown University School of Medicine, Washington, DC, USA

Jonathan Day, MD Department of Orthopedics, MedStar Georgetown University Hospital, Washington, DC, USA

MedStar Georgetown Orthopedic Institute, Georgetown University School of Medicine, Washington, DC, USA

John N. Delahay, MD Department of Orthopaedic Surgery, MedStar Georgetown Univeristy Hospital, Washington, DC, USA

Brian G. Evans, MD Department of Orthopaedics, MedStar Georgetown Univeristy Hospital, Washington, DC, USA

MedStar Georgetown Orthopedic Institute, Georgetown University School of Medicine, Washington, DC, USA

Edward Fakhre, MD Department of Orthopedics, MedStar Georgetown University Hospital, Washington, DC, USA

Georgetown University School of Medicine, Washington, DC, USA

Joseph L. Ferguson, MD Department of Orthopedics, MedStar Georgetown University Hospital, Washington, DC, USA

Bradley Gelfand, MD Department of Orthopedics, MedStar Georgetown University Hospital, Washington, DC, USA

MedStar Georgetown Orthopedic Institute, Georgetown University School of Medicine, Washington, DC, USA

Robert Golden, MD Department of Orthopedics, MedStar Washington Hospital Center, Washington, DC, USA

MedStar Georgetown Orthopedic Institute, Georgetown University School of Medicine, Washington, DC, USA

Daniel Hampton, MD Department of Orthopedics, MedStar Georgetown University Hospital, Washington, DC, USA

MedStar Georgetown Orthopedic Institute, Georgetown University School of Medicine, Washington, DC, USA

Curtis M. Henn, MD Department of Orthopedics, MedStar Georgetown University Hospital, Washington, DC, USA

Georgetown University School of Medicine, Washington, DC, USA

Evan Jacquez, MD Department of Orthopedics, MedStar Georgetown University Hospital, Washington, DC, USA

MedStar Georgetown Orthopedic Institute, Georgetown University School of Medicine, Washington, DC, USA

Douglass C. Johnson, MD Department of Orthopedics, MedStar Georgetown University Hospital, Washington, DC, USA

John L. Johnson, MD Department of Orthopedics, MedStar Georgetown University Hospital, Washington, DC, USA

MedStar Georgetown Orthopedic Institute, Georgetown University School of Medicine, Washington, DC, USA

Michael J. Kelly, MD Department of Orthopedics, MedStar Georgetown University Hospital, Washington, DC, USA

Department of Orthopedic Surgery, Georgetown University Medical Center, Washington, DC, USA

Michael W. Kessler, MD Department of Orthopedics, MedStar Georgetown University Hospital, Washington, DC, USA

MedStar Georgetown Orthopedic Institute, Georgetown University School of Medicine, Washington, DC, USA

Akhil Jay Khanna, MD Department of Orthopedics, MedStar Georgetown University Hospital, Washington, DC, USA

MedStar Georgetown Orthopedic Institute, Georgetown University School of Medicine, Washington, DC, USA

Denver B. Kraft, MD Department of Orthopaedic Surgery, MedStar Georgetown Univeristy Hospital, Washington, DC, USA

Julia A. McCann, MD Department of Orthopedics, MedStar Georgetown University Hospital, Washington, DC, USA

MedStar Georgetown Orthopedic Institute, Georgetown University School of Medicine, Washington, DC, USA

Evan Michaelson, MD Georgetown University School of Medicine, Washington, DC, USA

MedStar Orthopedic Institue, MedStar Georgetown University Hospital, Washington, DC, USA

Ryan S. Murray, MD Department of Orthopaedic Surgery, MedStar Georgetown Univeristy Hospital, Washington, DC, USA

Kevin W. Park, MD Department of Orthopedics, MedStar Georgetown University Hospital, Washington, DC, USA

MedStar Georgetown Orthopedic Institute, Georgetown University School of Medicine, Washington, DC, USA

Gregory Perraut, MD Department of Orthopedics, MedStar Georgetown University Hospital, Washington, DC, USA

MedStar Georgetown Orthopedic Institute, Georgetown University School of Medicine, Washington, DC, USA

William F. Postma, MD Department of Orthopedic Surgery, MedStar Georgetown University Hospital, Washington, DC, USA

Kenneth M. Vaz, MD Department of Orthopedics, MedStar Georgetown University Hospital, Washington, DC, USA

MedStar Georgetown Orthopedic Institute, Georgetown University School of Medicine, Washington, DC, USA

Brent Wiesel, MD Georgetown University School of Medicine, Washington, DC, USA

MedStar Orthopedic Institue, MedStar Georgetown, University School of Medicine, Washington, DC, USA

Kyle W. Zittel, MD Department of Orthopedics, MedStar Georgetown University Hospital, Washington, DC, USA

MedStar Georgetown Orthopedic Institute, Georgetown University School of Medicine, Washington, DC, USA

Basic Science of Bone and Cartilage Metabolism

Michael J. Kelly and John N. Delahay

Normal Bone Growth and Development

Bone is a biphasic connective tissue consisting of an inorganic mineral phase and an organic matrix phase. The hardness of bone allows it to provide several specialized mechanical functions: the protection of internal organs, the scaffold providing points of attachment for other structural elements, and the levers needed to improve the efficiency of muscle action. In addition, bone serves two biologic functions: a site for hematopoietic activity and a reservoir of minerals needed for metabolic interchange.

Embryology

The major components of the musculoskeletal system originate from the mesoderm layer of the trilaminar embryo. This "middle layer" is populated

M. J. Kelly
Department of Orthopedic Surgery, Georgetown University Medical Center, Washington, DC, USA

Department of Orthopedics, MedStar Georgetown University Hospital, Washington, DC, USA
e-mail: michael.j.kelly@medstar.net

J. N. Delahay (✉)
Department of Orthopaedic Surgery, MedStar Georgetown Univeristy Hospital, Washington, DC, USA
e-mail: delahayj@gunet.georgetown.edu

by mesenchymal cells that are totipotent and capable of differentiating into a number of tissues. The sequence of events important in bone growth and development begins with the appearance of the limb bud at 26 days after fertilization. It is at that time that a tubular condensation of mesenchyme develops centrally in the limb bud. Discrete areas, called interzones, are seen between these condensations and represent the primitive joints, forming in the sixth week of development (Fig. 1.1).

The interzone cells form three lines of cells: chondrogenic cells form articular cartilage, synovial cells form the capsule and synovium, and central cells form the intra-articular structures. Finally, the formation of joints requires repression of chondrogenesis through apoptosis, thus leaving sites of articulation between two surfaces, and allowing for motion.

In the limb bud itself, incredibly complex biochemical interactions occur between the growing tissue and regulatory transcription factors to control its growth. Growth must occur in three planes: longitudinally (proximal to distal), anterior to posterior (ex. radial to ulnar in the hand), and dorsal to ventral (ex. dorsum or palm of the hand) (Fig. 1.2).

Unfortunately, due to the complexity of these developmental processes, the limbs are extremely sensitive to anomalies, accounting for numerous limb deformities seen in the general population.

Also during the sixth week of development, the connective tissue, cartilage, and bone begin to

Fig. 1.1 Appositional growth is seen at the joint surfaces. Note the very high concentration of chondrocyte nuclei near the joint space, corresponding to cellular proliferation. (From Practical Orthopedic Pathology: A Diagnostic Approach, 2015 Elsevier, Deyrup and Siegal, Figure 1-7)

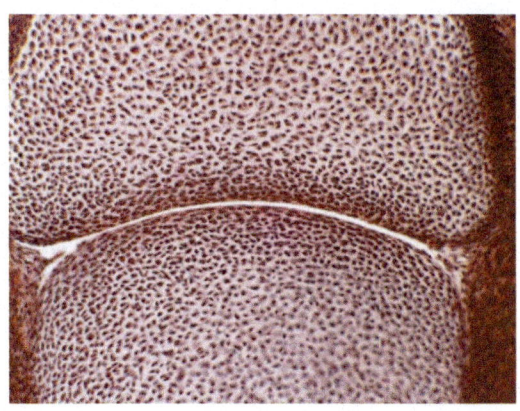

Fig. 1.2 Molecular regulation of limb growth. Through a combination of complex genetics and growth factors, growth of the limb bud mesenchymal tissue is controlled in three planes: (**a**) proximal–distal, (**b**) anterior–posterior, and (**c**) dorsal–ventral. (From Langman's Medical Embryology, 14e, figure 12.9)

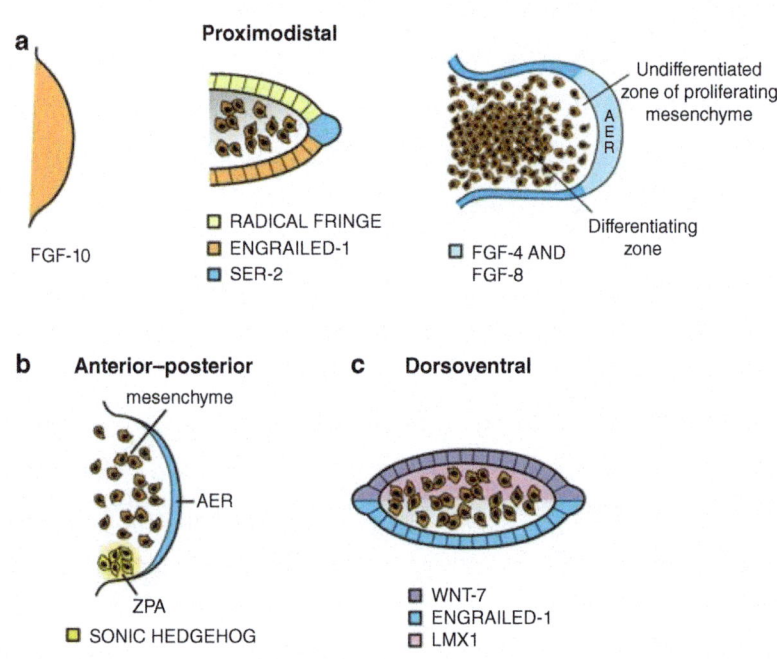

differentiate from the mesenchyme. The center of the limb bud condenses with cells that foretell the skeletal elements, called the chondrogenic core (Fig. 1.3).

With elongation of the limb bud through the processes described above, this tissue progresses distally. In the seventh week, this cartilage core is penetrated by a vascular spindle, bringing a rich vascular supply, occurring coincidentally with the necrosis of the central cartilage cells. Once this vascular spindle is established, nervous and muscle tissue development follows. Finally, the central portion of the model is popu-

lated by osteoblasts, by which matrix is secreted and ossified, immature (woven) bone is formed. Once the central portion of the model is ossified, it is referred to as a primary ossification center, residing within the shaft of the tubular bone (Fig. 1.4).

Further ossification of the skeleton occurs via one of two mechanisms: (1) endochondral ossification and (2) intramembranous ossification. While intramembranous ossification is the result of bone forming directly from primitive fibrous mesenchymal tissue by means of osteoblasts (bone-forming cells), the more common mecha-

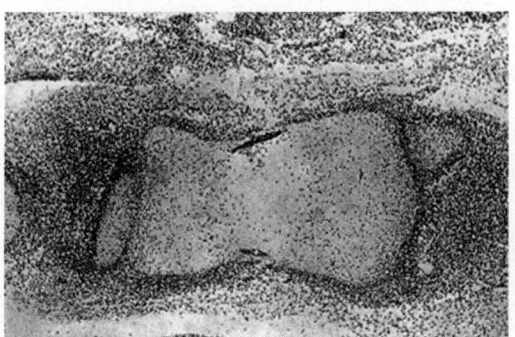

Fig. 1.3 Histologic study of fetus. Here, a sleeve, or collar, of bone begins to surround the outer surface of the chondrogenic core. (From Bogumill GP. Orthopaedic Pathology: A Synopsis with Clinical Radiographic Correlation. Philadelphia, PA: Saunders; 1984. Reprinted with permission)

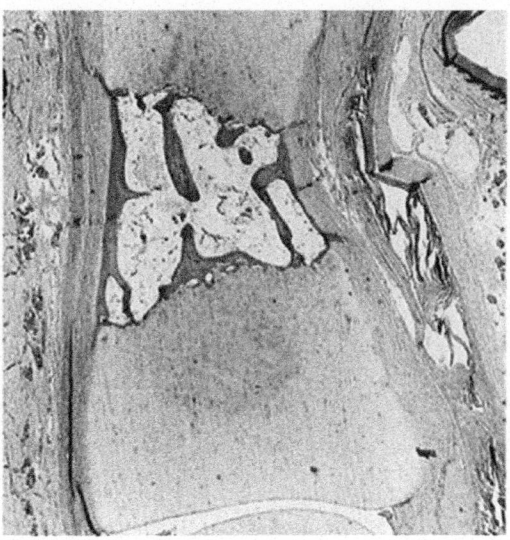

Fig. 1.4 The primary ossification center of a phalanx at approximately 14 weeks gestation, located centrally in the bone. Additionally, early bone marrow contents are being developed. (From Lovell and Winter's Pediatric Orthopaedics—Figure 1-20A)

nism of ossification is endochondral, which uses a cartilage template. In endochondral ossification, the mesenchyme does not form directly into bone-forming cells but in fact produces cartilage forming cells or chondroblasts. After a cartilage model is formed, osteoblasts are brought to the site by blood vessels, which secrete bone matrix and replace the cartilage with bone tissue (Fig. 1.5). Aside from the clavicle and flat bones of the skull (intramembranous ossification), all other bones of the skeleton are formed in this way.

From the second through the sixth embryonic months, progressive changes and remodeling occur in the tubular bones. First, the medullary canal (centrally) cavitates, leaving a hollow tube of bone with a large mass of cartilage persisting at each end (Fig. 1.6).

Within these masses of cartilage, the secondary ossification centers, or epiphyses, will form at both ends (Fig. 1.7).

A cartilage plate (the physis or growth plate) persists between the developing epiphysis and metaphysis and is responsible for growth in length (Fig. 1.8). The covering of the bone, the periosteum, is primarily responsible for growth in girth. In children, the periosteum has two layers—an outer fibrous layer and an inner cambium layer, which is osteogenic.

Fig. 1.5 (a–d) A schematic of endochondral bone formation. This process is contrasted with intramembranous ossification, where bone is formed directly from the mesenchymal tissue without a cartilage intermediary. (From Langman's Medical Embryology, 14e, Figure 12.5)

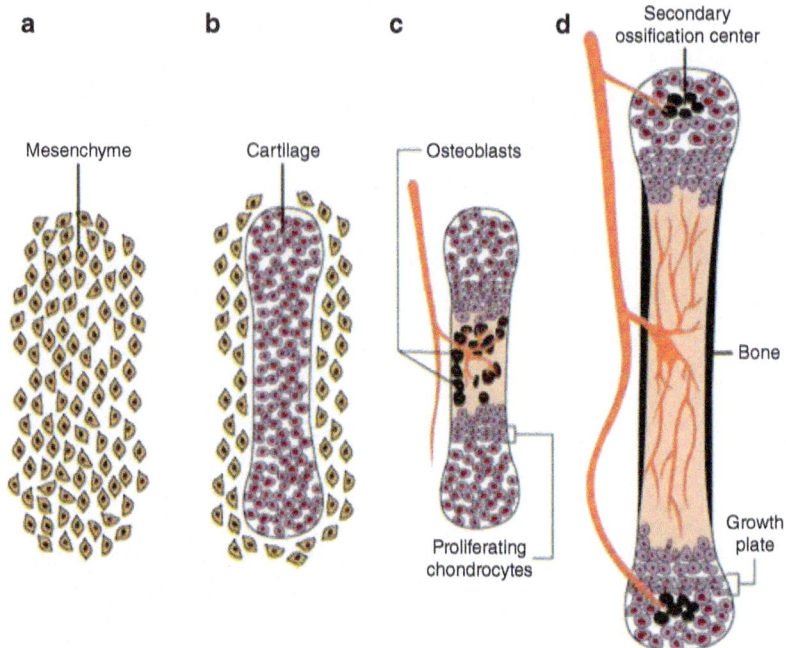

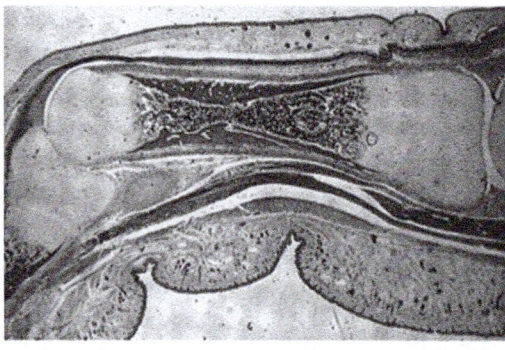

Fig. 1.6 Primary ossification center, near term. There is complete replacement of cartilage in the diaphyseal portion of the cartilage model. The remaining cartilage is confined to both epiphyseal ends of the model. Note the increasing thickness of the cortical portion of bone, which is a result of conversion of periosteum to bone. (From Bogumill GP. Orthopaedic Pathology: A Synopsis with Clinical Radiographic Correlation. Philadelphia, PA: Saunders; 1984. Reprinted with permission)

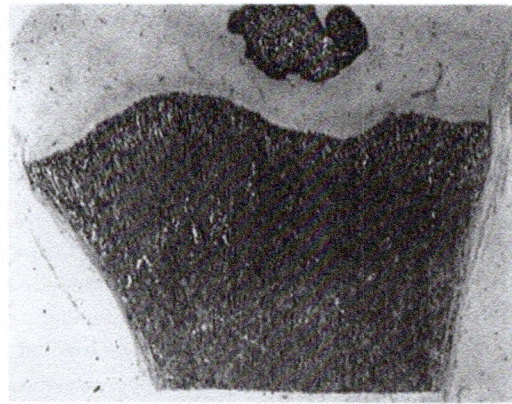

Fig. 1.7 Early secondary ossification center of a mature fetus. The formation of the secondary ossification centers in the lower tibia and upper femur coincides with fetal maturity. The secondary center begins not in the center of the epiphysis but near the growth plate. Expansion, therefore, is eccentric. (From Bogumill GP. Orthopaedic Pathology: A Synopsis with Clinical Radiographic Correlation. Philadelphia, PA: Saunders; 1984. Reprinted with permission)

Fig. 1.8 Anatomy of the growth plate, illustrating the four distinct physeal zones. (From Rockwood and Wilkins, Chapter 2, Figure 2-5)

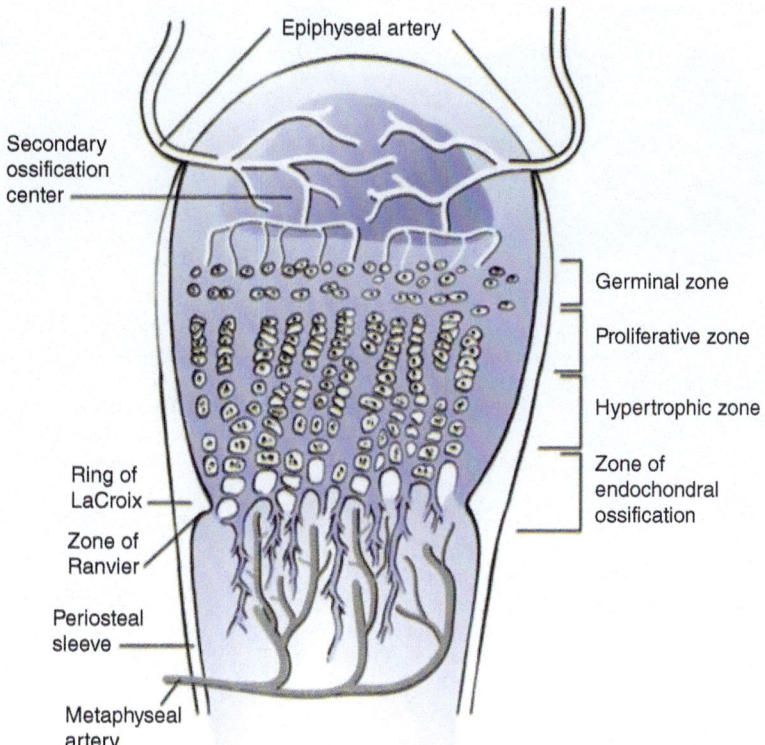

Postnatal Development

The physis and the periosteum continue to function postnatally in the growth and development of the infantile skeleton. Numerous local and systemic factors impact on their activity: vascular, hormonal, and genetic effects all play important roles. In essence, the reworking or remodeling of bone that is already present occurs so that the bone can meet the mechanical and biologic demands placed on it. And this remodeling occurs throughout one's life, with humans displaying triphasic growth—rapid infantile growth, linear childhood growth, and rapid adolescent growth, followed by skeletal maturity.

Bone Tissue

Bone, whether it is immature or mature, consists of cells and a biphasic blend of matrix (organic components) and mineral (inorganic compo-

nent) that coexist in a very exact relationship. The matrix phase consists largely of collagen and glycosaminoglycans (GAGs), which are dimeric disaccharides. Both are products of the osteoblast. Calcium hydroxyapatite—$Ca_{10}(PO_4)_6(OH)_2$ specifically—is the basic mineral crystal in bone, contributing mostly to strength in compression. The bulk of calcium in the skeletal reservoir is bound in the crystals of hydroxyapatite.

Osteoblasts, originating from osteoprogenitor cells, are bone-forming cells that secrete the osteoid matrix components described. As the osteoid matrix is ossified, the osteoblasts become trapped in the matrix they produce and are then referred to as osteocytes, or mature bone cells, which are rather inert. Osteoclasts are multinucleated cells (formed from a fusion of multiple blood monocytes) whose primary function is the degradation and removal of mineralized bone (Fig. 1.9).

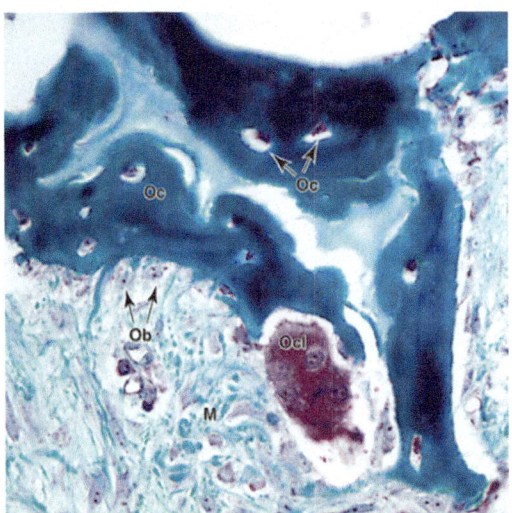

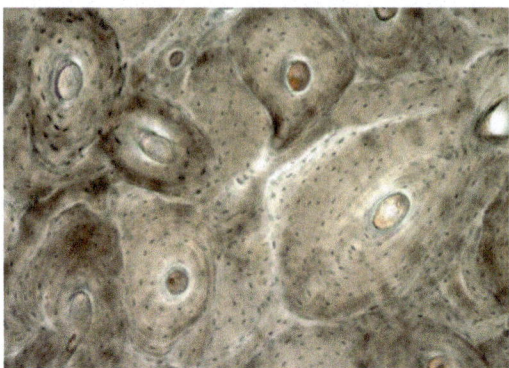

Fig. 1.10 Lamellar bone, or compact bone, showing osteons with concentric lamellae around central canals. (From Junqueira's Basic Histology, Chapter 8, Figure 8-8)

Fig. 1.9 Newly formed bone, composed of mesenchymal tissue (M) containing capillaries, fibroblasts, osteoprogenitor cells, and matrix. The matrix consists of collagen and the three major cell types found in bone tissue, osteoblasts (Ob), osteoclasts (Ocl), and osteocytes (Oc). (From Junqueira's Basic Histology, Chapter 8, Figure 8-2)

Bone Organization

Microscopically, bone is generally described as mature or immature. Mature bone has an ordered lamellar arrangement of Haversian systems and canalicular communications, giving it its classic histologic appearance (Fig. 1.10).

Immature bone, in contrast, has a much more random appearance of collagen fibers dispersed in a matrix of irregularly spaced cells (Fig. 1.11). It is produced rapidly by osteoblasts and "remodeled" by the local cell population, until the mature lamellar pattern is achieved. Immature bone is seen in the adult skeleton only under pathologic conditions (i.e., fracture callus, osteogenic sarcoma, myositis, etc.).

Macroscopically, the lamellar bone is configured either as dense cortical bone or as delicate spicules called trabeculae (Fig. 1.12).

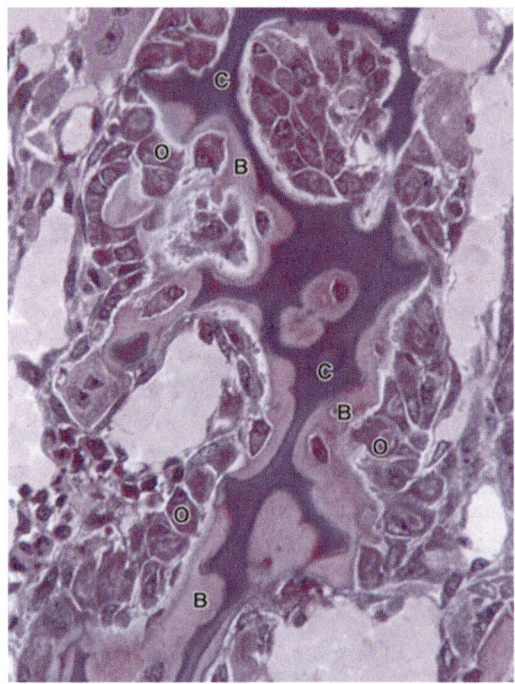

Fig. 1.11 Immature bone, located within a primary ossification center, demonstrating the key features of endochondral ossification, including remnants of calcified cartilage matrix (c) as well as woven bone (b) being actively formed by osteoblasts (o). (From Junqueira's Basic Histology, Chapter 8, Figure 8-15)

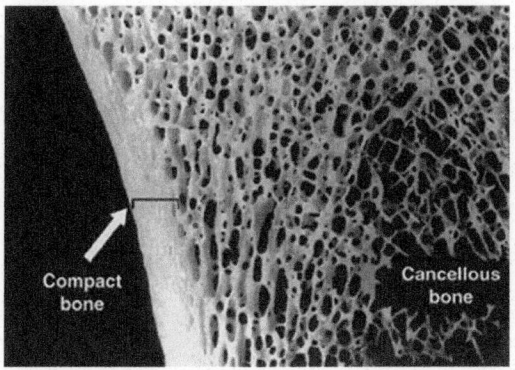

Fig. 1.12 Compact cortical bone peripherally, with a lattice of trabeculae forming cancellous bone at the bone's center. The small trabeculae that make up highly porous cancellous bone serve as supportive struts, collectively providing considerable strength, without greatly increasing the bone's weight. (From Junqueira's Basic Histology, Chapter 8, Figure 8-7). While cortical bone is composed of densely packed Haversian systems, cancellous, or spongy, bone is more loosely organized, giving it room to house the bone marrow

Bone Metabolism

Although the tendency is to think of adult bone as an inert tissue, nothing could be further from the truth. Throughout adult life, there is a constant ebb and flow of bone formation and bone resorption. These two processes are delicately balanced and keep the skeletal mass in a state of equilibrium. A number of factors, systemic and local, affect bone metabolism and hence impact bone turnover and remodeling.

Perhaps the most well-defined factor is mechanical stress, which forms the basis for the classic Wolff's law. Simply stated, trabecular, and to a lesser degree cortical, bone remodels along lines of mechanical stress. Bone forms where it is needed to meet mechanical demands and it is resorbed where the need is less. As a result of the piezoelectric effect, where loaded, that bone functions as a transducer, converting mechanical energy from the applied load into

electrical energy and a voltage gradient is established. In turn, this voltage gradient, that is generated, modulates cellular differentiation (i.e., active osteoblasts in areas of high load, or active osteoclasts in areas where bone is not needed).

Central to the process of bone metabolism, and the actual system in which bone formation and resorption occurs is called the RANK/RANK-ligand/osteoprotegerin (OPG) pathway. RANK (receptor activator of nuclear factor kappa-B) is a receptor residing on the cell surface of the immature, inactive osteoclast. RANK-ligand is a protein secreted by the activated osteoblast, which binds RANK and stimulates maturation of the osteoclast, and affects bone resorption. OPG, on the other hand, while also produced by osteoblasts, functions as a decoy receptor for RANK-ligand. Produced as a means to inhibit bone resorption, OPG binds and sequesters RANK-ligand, inhibiting activation of osteoclasts, and "protecting bone." Thus, as can be inferred, osteoclast function relies on activation from osteoblasts, thus coupling these two processes, and balancing the process of bone metabolism (Fig. 1.13).

Please see the following YouTube link (https://www.youtube.com/watch?v=VwCkyf0lQwo&t=231s) for video explanation of the RANK/RANK-ligand/OPG pathway.

Clinical implications of the RANK-RANK-ligand-OPG system abound. Osteolytic bone metastases, or cancer that has spread to the bones, has been found to be mediated largely by this system, with RANK-ligand production by oncologic cells as the presumed mechanism. In addition, research has indicated that defects in this system play a role in the pathogenesis of many metabolic bone diseases, including osteoporosis (uncontrolled bone resorption), osteopetrosis (absence of bone resorption), and Paget's disease (excessive, coupled bone remodeling producing abnormal quality bone).

Fig. 1.13 The
RANK-RANKL-OPG
system. Osteoclast
function relies on
activation from
osteoblasts, thus
coupling these two
processes, and balancing
the process of bone
metabolism. (From JBJS
Current concepts
Review, A review of
osteocyte function and
the emerging importance
of sclerostin)

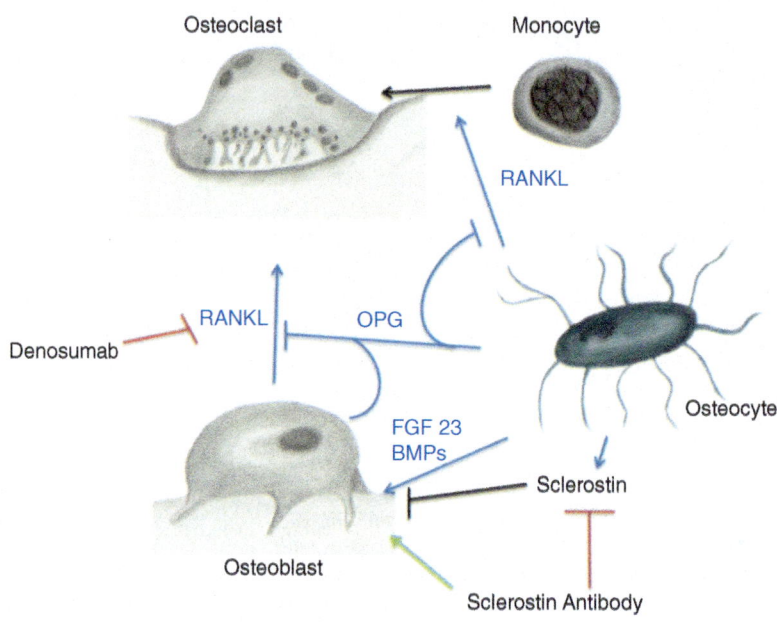

Bone Growth Factors

Much recent research has been aimed at understanding the molecular mechanisms involved in bone growth, and many growth factors have since been described. Bone morphogenic proteins (BMPs), for example, are the bone-forming factors originating from the demineralized bone products used in surgical procedures. BMPs use a complex network of cell receptors to stimulate differentiation of pluripotent mesenchymal stem cells into osteoblasts, and for this reason, have become quite popular in the field of orthopedic surgery. And while BMPs are the most mainstream, they are not alone in their ability to induce osteogenic differentiation—RUNX2 and WNT-Beta Catenin are just a few of the other well-known growth factors affecting bone formation. SOX9, on the other hand, is a chondrogenic growth factor, thus inducing the growth of cartilage. At this time, there remains much to learn about the complex interplay of these growth fac-

tors and both normal growth and pathological states of the musculoskeletal system.

Bone Circulation

Circulation of blood to the bones is critical in normal development as well as in pathological processes and healing of the musculoskeletal system and originates from three sources: (1) nutrient artery system, (2) periosteal system, and (3) metaphyseal-epiphyseal system. The nutrient artery system is referred to as a high-pressure system, fed from direct branches of major named arteries, and entering the medullary canal of the bone through the cortex of the diaphysis of long bones. The periosteal system, in contrast, is a low-pressure system, supplying the outer aspect of the bone (Fig. 1.14). Finally, the metaphyseal-epiphyseal system is a network of arteries surrounding the joints, which also contributes circulation to the growth plate in children via the specially-named perichondral arteries.

Fig. 1.14 Schematic demonstrates the vascular supply to bone, with the main blood supply originating from the nutrient arteries, which penetrate the deeper medullary bone, and the lower-pressure periosteal blood supply, which enables direct perfusion of the more peripheral cortical bone. (From "The Key Role of the Blood Supply to Bone", Bone Research, 2013)

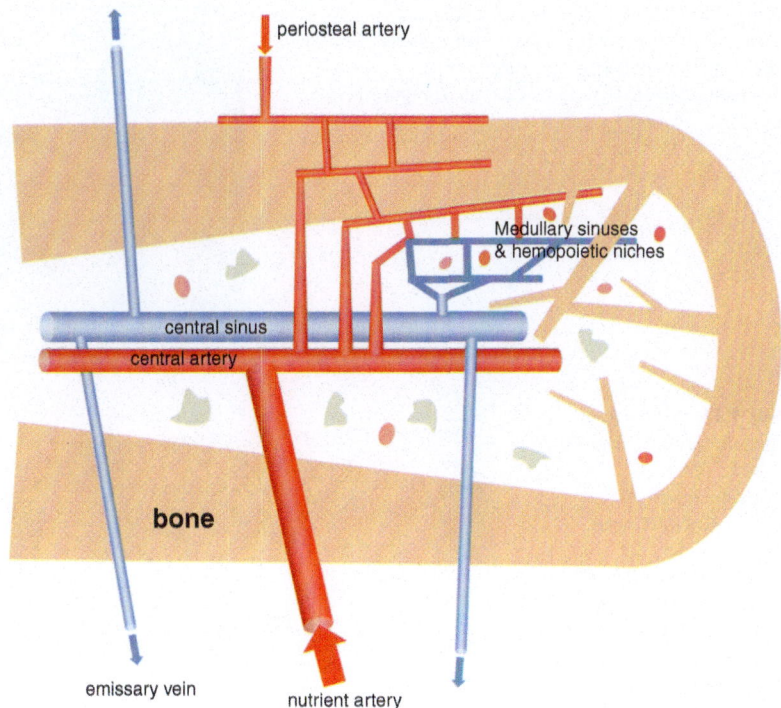

Cartilage

Cartilage, like bone, is a connective tissue. Its histologic organization, however, is far less structured. There exist four histologic types of cartilage, each serving a different function:

1. Hyaline cartilage covers the ends of long bones and provides a smooth, frictionless surface for articulation in a diarthrodial (synovial-lined) joint.
2. Fibrocartilage is typically found in certain non-diarthrodial joints such as the pubic symphysis. It is also located at the margins of certain diarthrodial joints, forming structures such as the glenoid labrum and acetabular labrum. Following injury to hyaline cartilage, repair of the chondral defect is typically accomplished in the form of fibrocartilage.
3. Elastic cartilage is found in certain areas where resilience is important. Examples include the tip of the nose and the ear lobe.
4. Physeal cartilage is found in the physis.

The most important of the four, hyaline cartilage, is a relatively aneural, avascular, and hypocellular connective tissue. By weight, it is 70% water. The remaining 30% is composed of ground substance and cells, known as chondrocytes. The ground substance of hyaline cartilage is composed primarily of type II collagen and GAGs. Collagen endows the cartilage with tensile strength and GAGs are critical for resiliency. Chondrocytes are found in individual lacunae, where they maintain healthy cartilage by actively synthesizing new ground substance components (Fig. 1.15).

The cartilage is grossly organized into multiple layers: tangential (most superficial), transitional, radial, and calcified (Fig. 1.16). Distinguishing these layers is the shape of the chondrocytes, orientation of the collagen fibrils, and percentage of GAGs, with more superficial layers providing tensile strength, and deeper layers accounting for more compressive strength.

The chondral layer receives the bulk of its nutrition not only from the vasculature of the subchondral bone below it, but mostly by diffusion from the synovial fluid it is bathed in.

Fig. 1.15 Chondrocyte cells, with abundant endoplasmic reticulum, necessary for actively secreting their collagen-rich matrix. (From Junqueira's Basic Histology, Chapter 7, Figure 7-7)

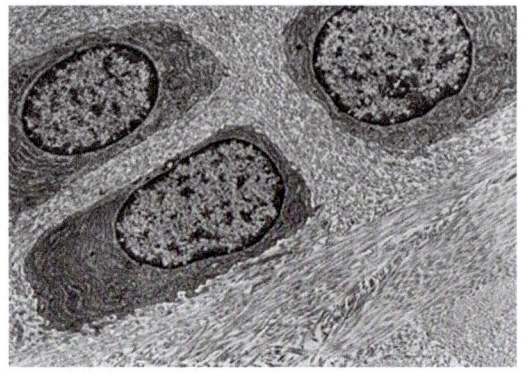

Fig. 1.16 Articular, or hyaline cartilage, caps the end of bones entering diarthrodial joints. As can be seen, collagen fibers run parallel to the articular surface, superficially, gradually changing their orientation with depth to become perpendicular at the junction with the underlying subchondral bone. This specific orientation imparts tension strength superficially, and compressive strength deep. (From Junqueira's Basic Histology, Chapter 8, Figure 8-23)

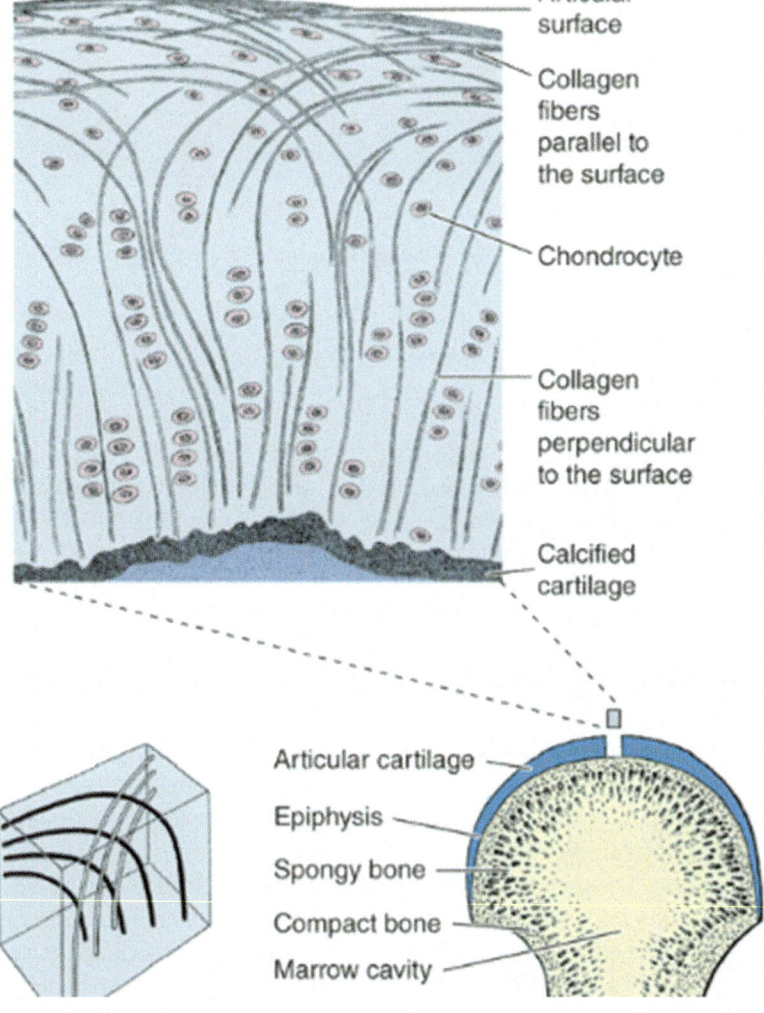

Articular surface

Collagen fibers parallel to the surface

Chondrocyte

Collagen fibers perpendicular to the surface

Calcified cartilage

Articular cartilage

Epiphysis

Spongy bone

Compact bone

Marrow cavity

Proteoglycan aggregates fill the space between the individual collagen fibers in the cartilage tissue, which allows for inflow and outflow of a small amount of water between this space and the synovial fluid. This action produces a biomechanical spring, and with changes in pressure (joint motion and loading), constant movement of water between the tissues results. This provides essential nutrition to the articular cartilage and permits the interchange of oxygen and metabolic waste. Additionally, when healthy, articular cartilage can take on a fully hydrated state, providing an almost frictionless bearing, hence minimizing wear on the articular surface.

Abnormal Bone Development and Metabolism

Most skeletal diseases are the result of disruption of normal bone growth and development, breakdown of bone once it has been normally formed, or alteration of the normal mechanisms of bone formation or bone resorption. The etiologies of the pathologic states, as one would expect, are quite varied, but the final manifestations within the musculoskeletal system frequently show striking similarities.

As one considers the etiology of skeletal disease, it is helpful to first group the possible differential diagnoses by disease category. This permits one to develop a comprehensive list of possible diagnoses that may explain the findings manifested by the skeleton. The seven disease categories are perhaps best organized using the acronym "VITAMIN."

V—vascular
I—infection
T—tumor
A—arthritis
M—metabolic bone disease
I—injury (trauma)
N—neurodevelopmental

The remainder of this chapter will focus on these diagnostic groups and the way in which they affect the skeleton. Specific emphasis will be placed on generalized afflictions of the skeleton. In that light, certain disease categories are more likely to adversely affect the skeleton in a generalized fashion; specifically vascular, metabolic, systemic arthritis, and neurodevelopmental etiologies. The others—infection, injury, and tumor—are more likely to produce localized changes and, therefore, will be highlighted in greater detail in the ensuing chapters.

Metabolic Bone Disease

Disease processes affecting bone often can be understood as a change in the relationship of bone formation and bone resorption. It is therefore important to understand this relationship. By doing so the net effect on the skeleton be appreciated.

The relationship (ratio) of mineral to matrix may be affected in abnormal metabolic states. For example, osteoporosis is a loss of bone mass, but there is an equivalent loss of matrix and mineral; therefore, the ratio remains normal. In contrast, osteomalacia is a relative loss of mineral resulting in a predominance of matrix; thus, a decrease in bone mass is accompanied by a decrease in the ratio of mineral to matrix (Fig. 1.17).

Serum calcium level is rarely representative of skeletal activity. Considering that more than 95% of the body's calcium is stored in bone apatite, it is understandable that the ~180 mg of ionized plasma calcium represents just the "tip of the iceberg." While peripheral sampling of the serum calcium provides only a remote clue to the true content of skeletal apatite, it does provide a convenient way to think about and classify metabolic bone disease.

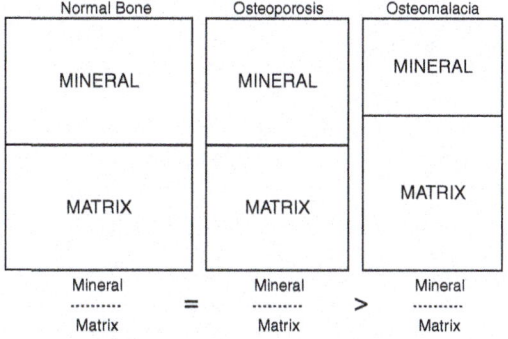

Fig. 1.17 Ratio of mineral to matrix in normal bone and in certain disease states. In osteoporosis, the ratio remains constant and equivalent to normal bone, despite an overall decrease in bone mass. In osteomalacia, there is not only an overall decrease in bone mass, but also a decrease in the ratio of mineral to matrix as a result of skeletal demineralization

Eucalcemic States: Osteoporosis

As mentioned, osteoporosis is a predominance of bone resorption over bone formation, with the net effect being bone loss (Fig. 1.18).

There is a parallel loss of mineral and matrix, so their ratio remains normal. Essentially, osteoporosis is a decrease in bone mass with an increase in cortical porosity and in diaphyseal bone diameter. This latter phenomenon is an attempt by the body to use what limited bone there is to disperse it as far as possible from the neutral axis of the long bone. Mechanically, this increases the torsional rigidity of the bone. Numerous etiologies of osteoporosis have been identified, with the most common causes being postmenopausal, senile, and a long list of secondary causes (endocrinopathies, nutritional deficiencies, side effects of medications including anti-convulsants and glucocorticoids, alcoholism, prolonged immobilization, and more). The most clinically relevant of those listed is the postmenopausal type, which occurs shortly after the withdrawal of estrogen (naturally or surgically), and brings along with it a host of predictable biological changes. This diagnosis is classically referenced against senile osteoporosis, a disease of aging, thus one that affects a slightly older population (Fig. 1.19).

No matter the etiology, the primary pathology remains a quantitative, not qualitative disorder of bone.

With osteoporosis, the new patient will present with a history of pain and/or recurrent fractures. Occasionally, they will complain of early satiety because of abdominal compression resulting from loss of height of the vertebral column (Fig. 1.20).

Similarly, with increasing kyphosis in the thoracic region, they may experience some shortness of breath. On examination, one can find the prominent dowager's hump, barrel chest, protuberant abdomen, and generalized bone pain with percussion tenderness.

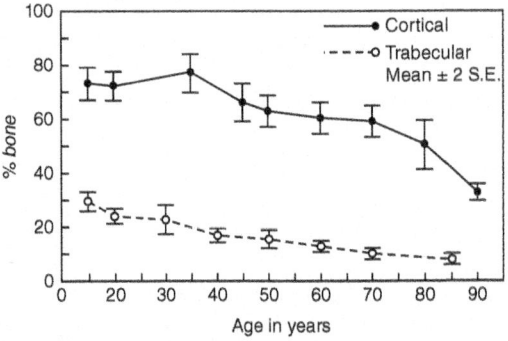

Fig. 1.18 The relative decrease in cortical and trabecular bone with age in apparently normal persons. Note the relatively rapid loss early in life in trabecular bone and comparatively little loss at this age in cortical bone. The situation is reversed after age 55. (From Jowsey J. Metabolic Diseases of Bone. Philadelphia, PA: Saunders; 1977. Reprinted with permission)

Fig. 1.19 Types of involutional osteoporosis. (Source: Modified from Riggs BL, Melton LJ III. Involutional osteoporosis. *N Engl J Med* 1986;314:1676)

	Type 1 (Postmenopausal)	Type 2 (Senile)
Age (years)	50–75	Over 70
Sex ratio (M/F)	1:6	1:2
Type of bone loss	Trabecular	Trabecular and cortical
Fracture site	Vertebrae (crush)	Vertical (multiple wedge)
	Distal radius	Hip
Main causes	Menopause	Aging
Calcium absorption	Decreased	Decreased
(1,25-OH)$_2$-vitamin D synthesis from 25-(OH) Vitamin D	Secondary decrease	Primary decrease
Parathyroid function	Decreased	Increased

Source: Modified from Riggs BL, Melton LJ III. Involutional osteoporosis. *N Engl J Med.* 1986;314:1676

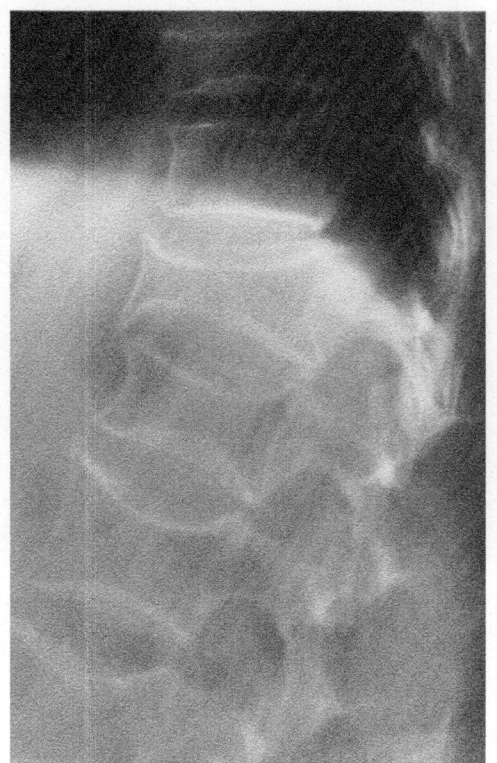

Fig. 1.20 The osteoporotic spine. There exists a relative density of the vertebral body endplates with resorption of the trabeculae of the spongy bone. Anterior wedging and end plate compression are present, due to weakness of the vertebral body end plates. (From Orthopedic Imaging: A Practical Approach. 7E. 2021. Chapter 27, Figure 27.7)

The yearly cost of this disease in dollars, as well as the associated pain and suffering to the patient, is overwhelming. And once fractures start, this condition is associated with a 15–20% increase in mortality, in addition to the aforementioned reduced quality of life related to the associated morbidity. And this is not a rare condition, with recent data suggesting over 1.5 million osteoporotic fractures occurring annually in the USA alone, with compression fractures of the vertebral body, and fractures of the proximal femur, distal radius, and proximal humerus leading the charge. However, until recently, it was quite challenging to quantify bone mass, and thus diagnose this condition reliably.

Typically, a crude estimate of bone density determined by plain radiographs has been used to extrapolate to the amount of bone previously lost.

Classically, once changes are noticeable radiographically, it has been estimated that the bone density has already decreased by 30% or more. Today, however, Dual-energy X-ray absorptiometry (DEXA) scanning allows accurate and reproducible measures of bone mineral density of the spine and the hip. While it requires a minimal amount of radiation to obtain, it remains quite accurate in its goals. Because DEXA has become so mainstream, we now have population-based normal values that allow comparison of an individual's bone density. The difference is expressed as a T score, which represents the number of standard deviations below that of normal, young controls (25–30 year old women, who display peak bone mass). Of note, while the T score is calculated as bone mineral density compared to young controls, the Z score, another used term, is bone mineral density compared to patients of similar age and sex. The definitions based on T scores are as follows:

Normal: 0 to −1
Osteopenia: −1 to −2.5
Osteoporosis: < −2.5

An unfortunate result of mainstream DEXA) scanning has been to adulterate the use of the term "osteopenia." For many years, this term was defined as a generalized decrease in radiographic bone density. As such, it was non pejorative and did not speak to a specific metabolic bone disease. In its present accepted context, the implication of using the term "osteopenia" is to imply a mild form of osteoporosis. This was certainly not the original connotation of the term. Diseases other than osteoporosis, such as hyperthyroidism and multiple myeloma, are characterized by observed generalized decreases in radiographic bone density, hence osteopenia, and are not necessarily just "mild" forms of a different condition.

Once this condition is diagnosed, treatment must ensue, for limitation of bone loss and prevention of fractures is the most prudent approach to patient care. Prophylactic treatment regimens include lifestyle modifications and vitamin supplementation. Regular weight-bearing exercise (walking or jogging, not swimming, which many older patients prefer) and supplemental calcium and vitamin D administration is standard recommendation. Pharmacological treatment is considered for postmenopausal women or men over 50 years old with a history of osteoporotic fracture, or with osteoporosis diagnosed on DEXA scan.

The classic pharmacological agent used in the treatment of postmenopausal osteoporosis was estrogen substitutes. While its efficacy in maintaining skeletal mass is beyond question, its complication profile, including its relation to breast and cervical cancer, heart disease, and venous thromboembolic events (VTE) made its regular use somewhat controversial. In light of this complication profile, other therapeutic regimens were developed and have since been popularized. We will highlight them individually below.

1. Without doubt, the most commonly used agents are the bisphosphonates. Structurally similar to naturally occurring pyrophosphates, they are taken up by osteoclasts, accumulate at sites of bone turnover, and behave as potent inhibitors of bone resorption. It has been said that bisphosphonates are able to "freeze the skeleton" and have been shown to reduce rates of osteoporotic fractures upwards of 50%. While they carry the rare, suspected complications of osteonecrosis of the jaw and atypical subtrochanteric femur fractures in patients on these medications long term, they are clearly first-line treatment for this condition and have been a major pharmacological advancement in the field of orthopedics (Fig. 1.21).

2. Teriparatide is a synthetic form of parathyroid hormone (PTH), which has a direct agonist effect on osteoblasts, thus increasing bone mineral density. Of note, this may at first seem counterintuitive, as the elevated levels of PTH in hyperparathyroidism in fact reduce bone formation in this condition. However, it seems that PTH's effect on bone differs based on dosing and pattern of exposure, and when given as a low-dose, daily subcutaneous injection, it does demonstrate a (paradoxical) effect

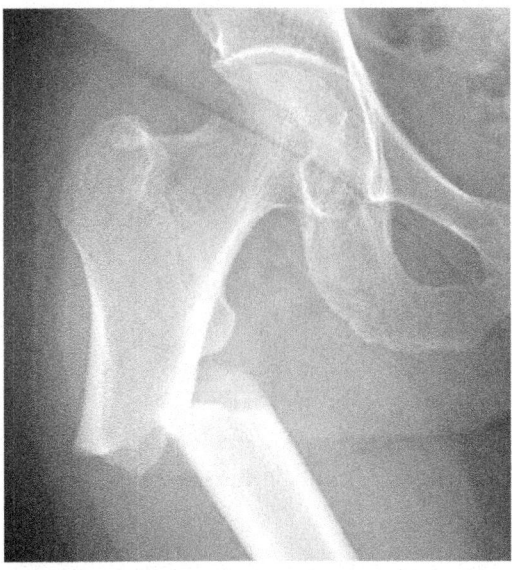

Fig. 1.21 Classic atypical femur fracture in a patient on bisphosphonate medications for extended duration. Note the fracture characteristics, with lateral cortical thickening, and a transverse, non-comminuted fracture line. (From Rockwood and Green's Fractures in Adults, 9e, Tornetta. Chapter 55, Figure 55-1)

as a bone-forming agent. Its niche indication at this time appears to be in preventing junctional kyphosis in those patients undergoing spinal fusion operations.

3. Denosumab is a monoclonal antibody with significant pharmacologic promise. It works against the RANK-ligand molecule in the RANK/RANK-ligand/OPG system, effectively mimicking OPG, and thus protecting the bone.

4. While selective estrogen receptor modulators (SERMs) may be less prescribed now than in the recent past, with the popularization of the bisphosphonate drugs, Raloxifene still has its place in treatment. This drug behaves as an agonist on estrogen receptors in the bone, yet antagonizes estrogen receipts in the breast, thus reducing breast cancer risk, while also improving bone mineral density. Its downsides—hot flashes, and a strict contraindication with a VTE history.

5. Calcitonin is the last pharmacologic option to be discussed. A naturally occurring polypeptide hormone, it acts as a direct inhibitor of

osteoclasts, decreasing bony resorption. Interestingly, it is administered largely in the form of a nasal spray, and its major use now is in decreasing pain associated with vertebral compression fractures.

Hypercalcemic States: Hyperparathyroidism

The effect of PTH on bone is the same whether it is released as a result of a parathyroid adenoma (primary hyperparathyroidism) or by one of several secondary causes. In an attempt to increase serum calcium concentration, PTH stimulates osteoclastic activity, causing an intense resorption of bone. The cavities resulting from this osteoclastic activity fill with vascular fibrous tissue, resulting in the classic "osteitis fibrosa cystica." As the cavities coalesce, they form a single large cyst called a "brown tumor," named for the hemosiderin staining one sees within (Fig. 1.22).

Without doubt, the most common cause of secondary parathyroid hyperplasia in today's world is chronic renal disease, which causes hypovitaminosis D, calcium wasting by way of the kidneys, and a resultant hyperparathyroidism.

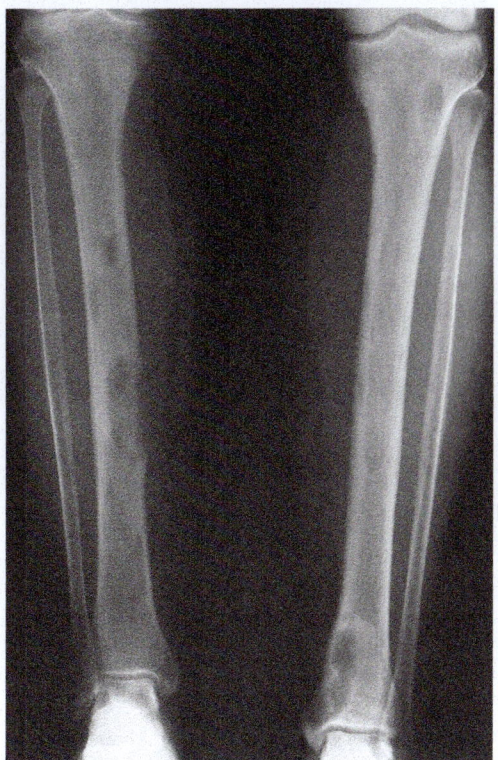

Fig. 1.22 Brown tumors in the bilateral tibiae of a patient with primary hyperparathyroidism. (From Orthopedic Imaging: A Practical Approach. 7E. 2021. Chapter 28, Figure 28.8)

Hypocalcemic States: Rickets and Osteomalacia

The same underlying mechanism accounts for rickets and osteomalacia: faulty mineralization of bone matrix, which results in the presence of unmineralized osteoid about bony trabeculae. The lack of mineral required for adequate mineralization can be due to a number of different etiologies: nutritional deficiencies, malabsorption states, lack of exposure to ultraviolet light, and renal disease are some of the more common.

Notably, if the failure of mineralization impacts the skeleton prior to physeal closure, the result is rickets. The affected patient will demonstrate the characteristic hallmarks of the disease: bowlegs, frontal bossing, ricketic rosary, and knobby joints (Fig. 1.23). All of these findings are due to the presence of large masses of unmin-

eralized osteoid. In addition, abnormalities of the physis and abnormal physeal growth can be anticipated.

If the process impacts the skeleton after physeal closure, the disease that results is osteomalacia. In the adult, these areas of unmineralized osteoid present as radiographic lucent areas in the bone, frequently referred to a Looser's lines (Fig. 1.24). In addition, the bones themselves tend to be somewhat malleable and can bow under load.

Renal Osteodystrophy

Renal osteodystrophy encompasses the skeletal changes that result from long-standing renal disease. These changes are truly a "collage" of the other metabolic bone diseases. To understand the pathogenesis of renal osteodystrophy is to under-

Fig. 1.23 Child with Rickets. (**a**) XR of the hand shows widened growth plates. (**b**) There are irregularly widened physes via the zone of provisional calcification. (From Orthopedic Imaging: A Practical Approach. 7E. 2021. Chapter 27, Figure 27.11)

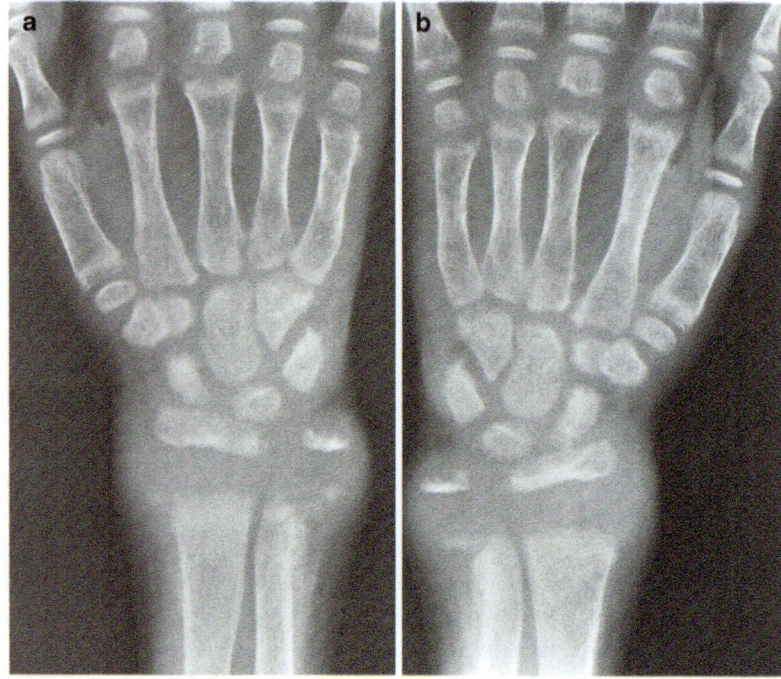

Fig. 1.24 Osteomalacia caused by malabsorption syndrome. Left scapula demonstrates a radiolucent cleft, known as a pseudofracture, or Loosers lines. These lines appear at sites in which stress fractures would occur. In normal individuals, the removed bone in the area of stress fractures is replaced by normal osteons. In persons with osteomalacia, the removed bone is replaced with abnormal osteoid, which fails to mineralize and leaves a linear radiolucency that may persist for years. (From Orthopedic Imaging: A Practical Approach. 7E. 2021. Chapter 27, Figure 27.15)

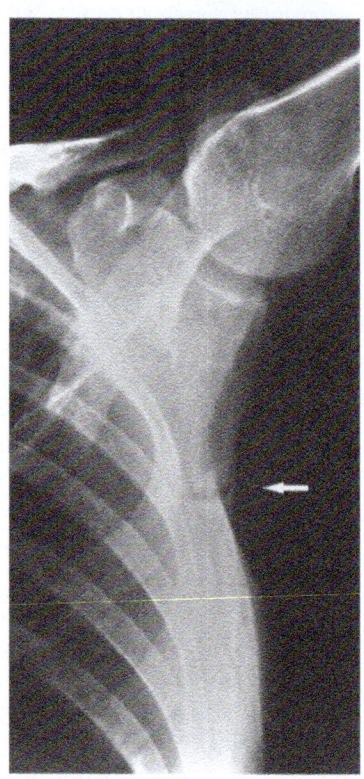

Fig. 1.25 Pathogenesis of renal osteodystrophy

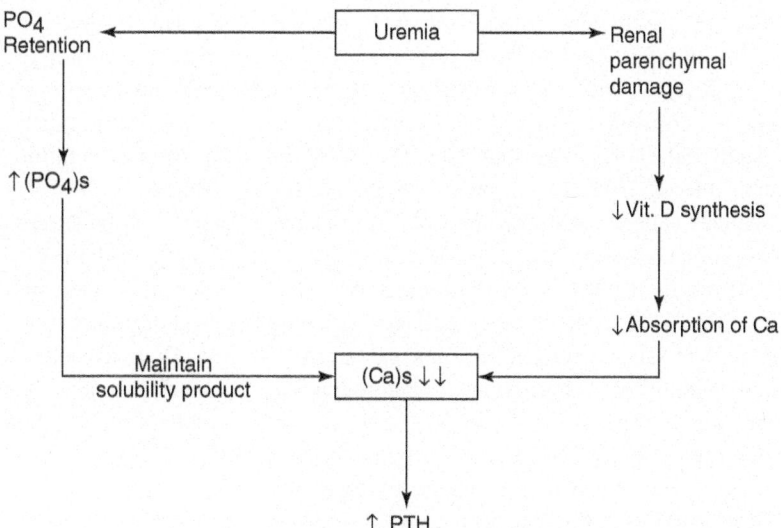

stand the basis of all of the metabolic afflictions of the skeleton (Fig. 1.25).

Chronic uremia allows a two-fold drive to depress the serum calcium. First, the kidney is unable to excrete phosphate; hence the serum phosphate level rises. The serum calcium level is then of necessity driven down to maintain the fixed solubility product. Coincidentally, since the absence of a functional renal parenchyma stops the output of significant amounts of activated vitamin D, intestinal absorption of calcium is retarded, further depressing serum calcium. This dual mechanism profoundly depresses serum calcium, mandating the secondary parathyroid hyperplasia as previously discussed. The changes in the bone reflect the metabolic drives. The vitamin D deficiency is demonstrated by the presence of unmineralized osteoid. And the elevated levels of PTH cause the aforementioned osteitis fibrosis cystica. Unique to this syndrome, hyperphosphatemia results in a diffuse osteosclerosis (Fig. 1.26).

Sick Cell Syndromes

The underlying mechanism seen in these conditions is a qualitative, functional deficit in a specific cell population—despite the fact that the population is quantitatively normal.

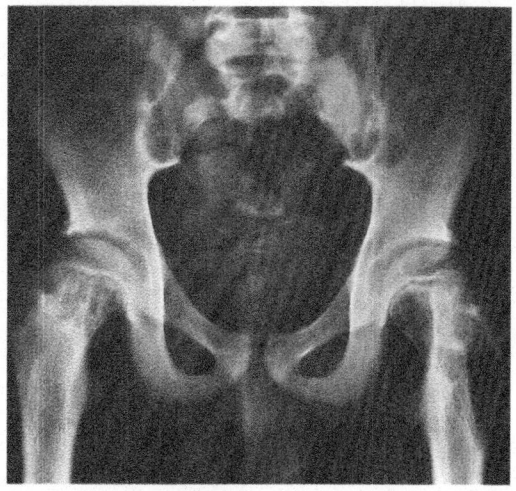

Fig. 1.26 Pelvic radiograph of patient with long-standing renal osteodystrophy due to renal failure in the setting of posterior urethral valves. Sclerotic changes as well as cystic defects in the proximal femora are evident. (From *Orthopedic Imaging: A Practical Approach.* 6E. 2015. Greenspan, Adam, chapter 26, Figure 27.16)

Osteogenesis Imperfecta

Osteogenesis imperfecta (OI), also known as brittle bone disease, is a spectrum of disorders that have a hallmark feature—bone fragility. OI is typified by the impotence of the osteoblasts; they are unable to manufacture and secrete normal collagen. Ossification is, therefore, abnormal (due to insufficient osteoid production) and results in inferior quality bone (Fig. 1.27).

Clinically and radiographically, there is marked cortical thinning and attenuation of the diaphyseal caliber. The long bones, because of their altered anatomy, are at very high risk for fracture, often requiring multiple orthopedic operations by a very young age (Fig. 1.28).

Upwards of 90% of patients with OI have a traceable genetic mutation in collagen (specifically the COL1A1 or COL1A2 genes), and there is significant phenotypic heterogeneity. Individuals can be affected mildly, severely, or even fatally in the perinatal period. In an effort to accommodate the variations in phenotype, the Sillence classification has been adopted by most authors. Four specific types, all transmitted in an autosomal dominant fashion, were described in the original classification.

Type I is the most common form and the mildest clinically. This is the only quantitative disorder in collagen (i.e., not enough made). These patients demonstrate the classic findings of blue sclera, long bone fractures after the age of walking, and a relatively normal life expectancy.

Type II is the lethal form of the disease. A qualitative disorder of collagen similar to types III and IV, these children are usually stillborn or die shortly after birth, usually due to respiratory failure or intracranial hemorrhage.

Type III is the severe nonlethal form, characterized by sclera of normal color, multiple birth fractures, and significant long-term deformity and disability.

Type IV is the intermediate form, with variable manifestations. Notably, it is the least common of the first four types.

The Sillence classification has since been modified to include types five through seven. These three types in fact do not have a type one collagen mutation, but manifest with a similar phenotype and have abnormal bone when viewed microscopically.

Osteopetrosis

Known as a sclerosing bone condition, osteopetrosis results from the failure of the osteoclasts to remove primary spongiosa bone. This latter osseous

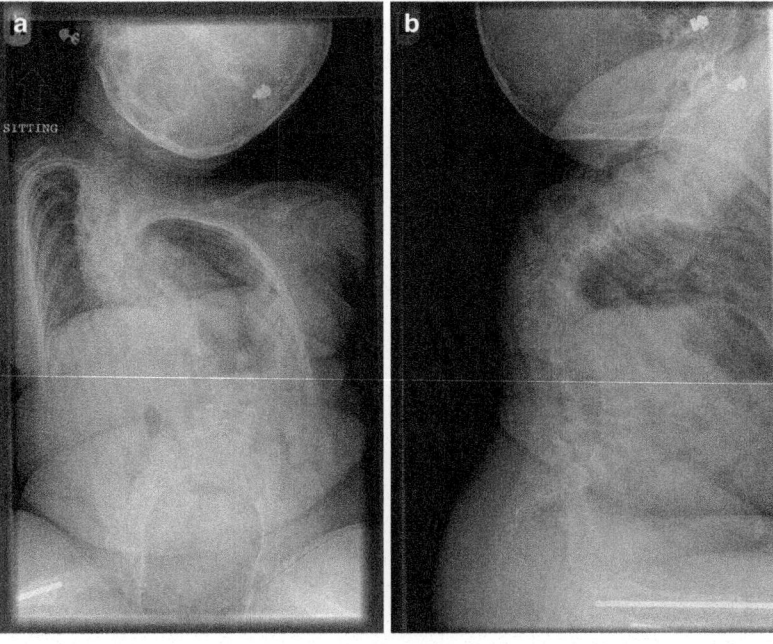

Fig. 1.27 (a, b) Marked degree of spinal deformity in a young patient with severe osteogenesis imperfecta. (From Lovell and Winter's Pediatric Orthopaedics, Chapter 6, Figure 19)

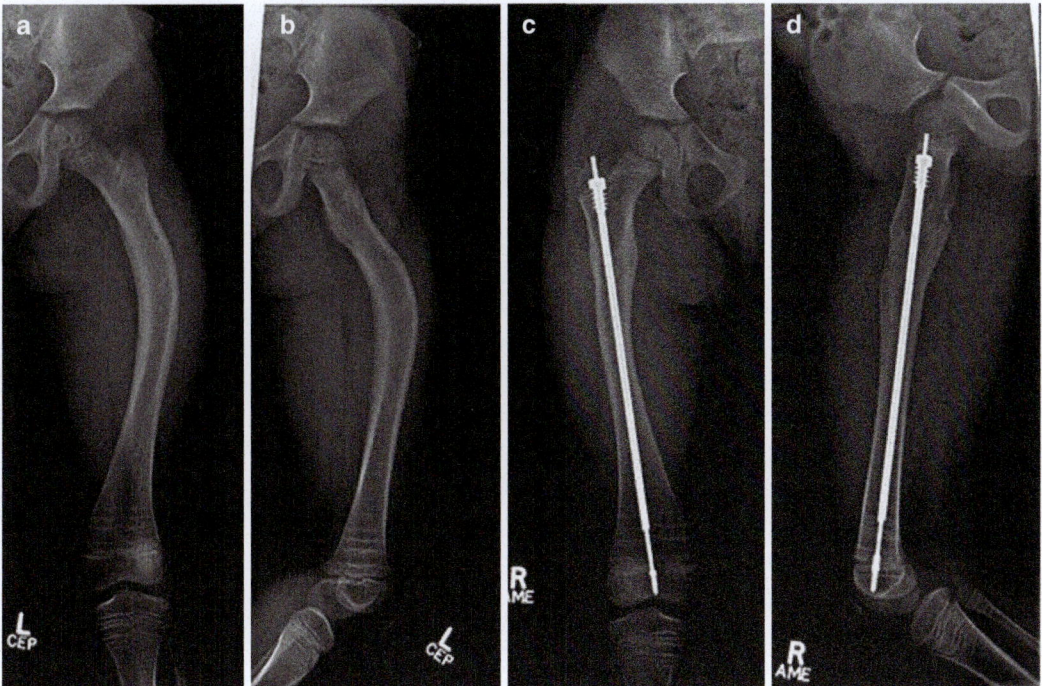

Fig. 1.28 Radiographs demonstrating the deformed femur in a patient with osteogenesis imperfecta. Note the typical slender bones excessively thin cortices (**a**, **b**). Additionally, note the postoperative images after con- trolled osteotomies to realign the bones, (**c**, **d**) stabilized with telescoping intramedullary rods that allow for con- tinued bone growth. (From Lovell and Winter's Pediatric Orthopaedics, Chapter 6, Figure 9)

material then "piles up" in the skeleton, making it appear very dense radiographically (Fig. 1.29).

Despite the fact that the bones look extremely dense and, indeed, lack a medullary canal, they are biomechanically very weak. This results in frequent pathologic fractures. An additional com- plication is the displacement of marrow elements from the long bones. This results in a myelo- phthisic anemia (pancytopenia), and in turn gen- erates extramedullary hematopoiesis. Thus, hepatosplenomegaly as well as a prominent fore- head are usually seen in these patients.

Paget's Disease

Sir James Paget described a syndrome of unknown etiology that bears his name. The initial description referred to the condition as "osteitis deformans," with increased osteoclastic bone resorption contributing to abnormal bone remod- eling (Fig. 1.30). The syndrome is most common in individuals of European descent and in patients typically over the age of 55.

There is strong evidence pointing to a slow virus (paramyxovirus or respiratory syncytial virus) as the cause of Paget's disease. In the set- ting of increased osteoclastic resorption, bone formation and bone resorption dramatically increase. The two processes occur alternately rather than simultaneously in any given bone, with the net effect being bones of increased density with marked trabecular thickening (Fig. 1.31).

The skull, pelvis, spine, tibia, and femur are the favorite targets of this process. Sadly, and not unlike osteopetrosis, the pagetic bones are mechanically weak, making pathologic fracture a frequent complication. Despite the presence of abundant quantities of bone, it is poorly formed and the mineral and matrix are poorly integrated. Bone pain, spinal stenosis, and hearing deficit (resulting from impingement of disorganized, overgrown bone in the skull on the eighth cranial

Fig. 1.29 Osteopetrosis. As can be imagined, when the same pathologic changes of hyperdense bone occur in the long bones (**a**), there is an almost complete absence of marrow cavity (**b**), unsurprisingly contributing to the finding of pancytopenia. (From Lovell and Winter's Pediatric Orthopaedics, Chapter 6, Figure 21A and B)

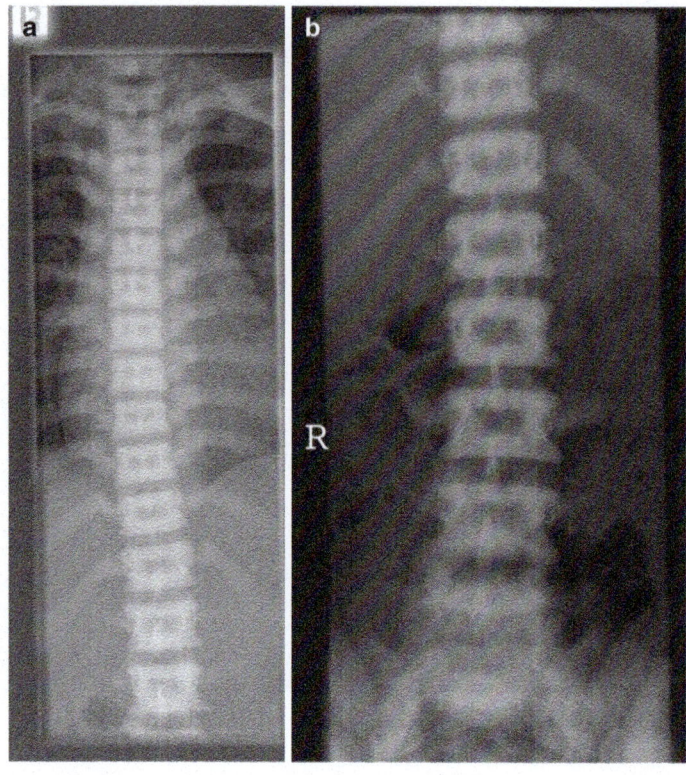

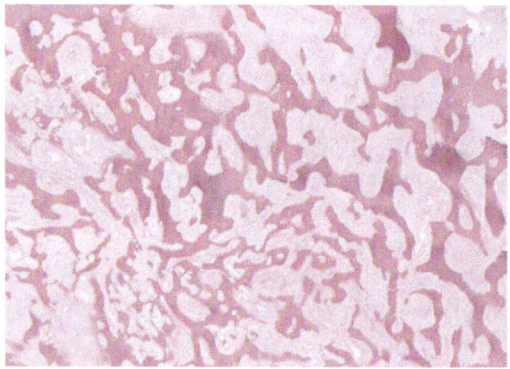

Fig. 1.30 Paget's disease of bone. Microscopic view showing disorganized bony trabeculae with variable thickness and fibrotic bone marrow. (From Practical Orthopedic Pathology: A Diagnostic Approach, 2015 Elsevier, Deyrup and Siegal, Figure 16-8)

nerve) are frequent problems in these patients. Additionally, it is now well described that these patients are at increased risk for secondary Pagetoid osteosarcomas, and while only occurring in less than 1% of Pagetoid patients, the

prognosis associated with this condition is dismal.

Several different therapeutic approaches have been attempted. Currently, bisphosphonates are the frequently employed therapeutic agent. Much like in osteoporosis, they are aimed at osteoclast inhibition, used in an attempt to inhibit bone resorption and also to a lesser degree to block bone mineralization. The rationale again is to "freeze the skeleton," and thereby decrease bone turnover. Cyclic treatment regimens allow new bone to become mineralized while decreasing the osteoclastic activity. The serum alkaline phosphatase level provides a reliable way of monitoring the response to treatment, since it is elevated in the presence of active bone turnover. After bisphosphonates, calcitonin is another treatment alternative, working through its direct effect on osteoclast cells. Of note, teriparatide, a PTH analogue, is actually contraindicated in Paget's disease, due to an associated increased risk of Pagetoid osteosarcoma mentioned above noted in animal studies.

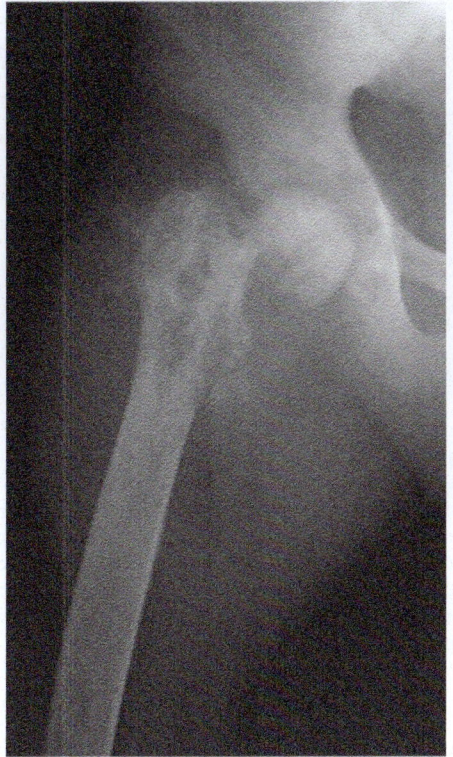

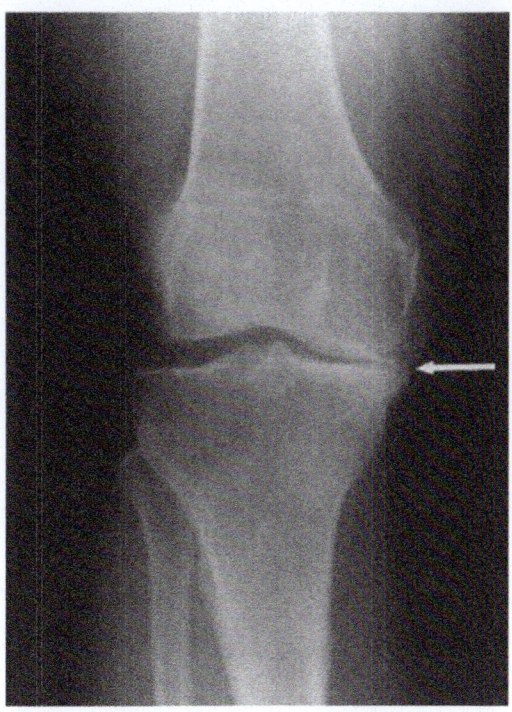

Fig. 1.32 Osteoarthritis of the knee with radiographic evidence of three of the four cardinal findings seen most evidently in the medial femorotibial compartment—narrowing of the joint space, osteophyte formation, and subchondral sclerosis. The fourth findings, cysts, are not clearly seen. (From Orthopedic Surgery: Principles of Diagnosis and Treatment, Figure 18.7)

Fig. 1.31 Paget's disease of bone. X-ray showing dense sclerotic changes with areas of osteolysis. Clearly, through this disease bone, the patient has fractured their hip. (From Practical Orthopedic Pathology: A Diagnostic Approach, 2015 Elsevier, Deyrup and Siegal, Figure 16-7)

Arthritis

It is important to recall that a diarthrodial joint includes three tissues: bone, cartilage, and synovium. Each of the arthritic diseases tends to impact one of these tissues, with changes in the other two resulting as secondary phenomena. The radiographic and microscopic changes encountered represent a composite of the result of the initial injury and the organism's attempt at repair of that injury.

Noninflammatory Arthritis: Osteoarthritis

The most common overall, osteoarthritis can be primary or secondary, if one considers the degenerative joint disease that can follow trauma or other primary events. The process itself targets the articular cartilage. Whether the initial event is mechanical or biochemical remains controversial, however, recent data suggests an increase in proteolytic enzymes and inflammatory cytokines as the primary driving force resulting is progressive damage to the articular surface. The secondary bone changes that occur are reparative in nature. Joint space narrowing, subchondral sclerosis, osteophytes, and subchondral cysts, therefore, are the four classic radiographic changes (Fig. 1.32).

Since this is most typically a disease of weight-bearing joints, the hip and knee are the joints that usually require orthopedic care. That said, with aging of the population, and newer technological advancements, osteoarthritis of the shoulder, elbow, ankle and even wrist have gained more attention. Total joint arthroplasty has

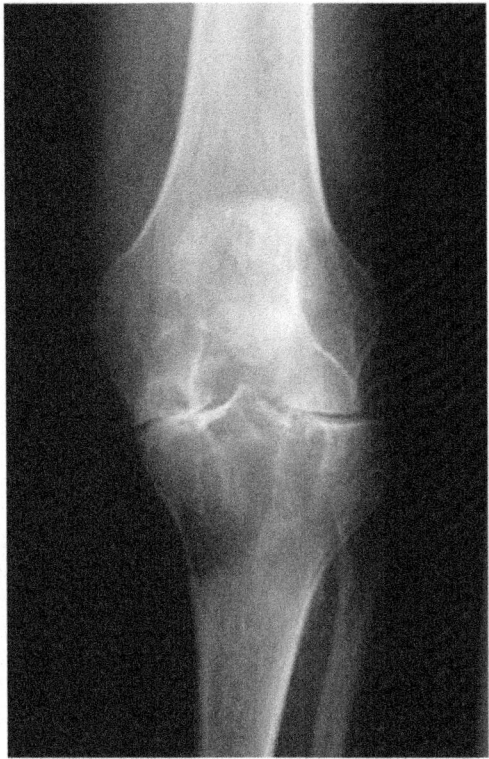

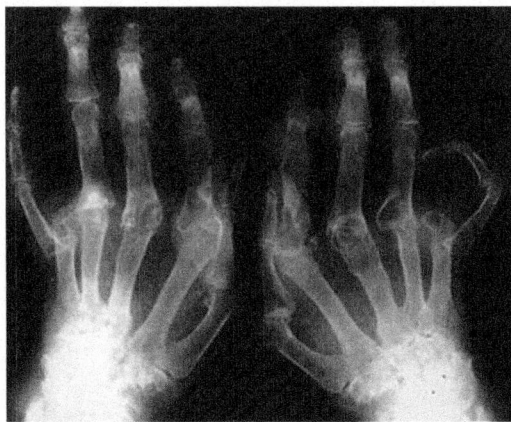

Fig. 1.34 Radiograph of both hands of a patient with long-standing Rheumatoid arthritis. Osteoporosis in all bones is marked. The wrist joints show advanced destruction. There is dislocation of the metacarpophalangeal joints of all fingers. (From Bogumill GP. Orthopaedic Pathology: A Synopsis with Clinical Radiographic Correlation. Philadelphia, PA: Saunders; 1984. Reprinted with permission)

Fig. 1.33 Rheumatoid arthritis in the knee. Note the symmetric joint space narrowing, generalized osteopenia on both sides of the joint, and an absence of osteophytes. (From Orthopedic Surgery: Principles of Diagnosis and Treatment, Figure 18-10)

become the mainstay of surgical management in these patients, producing reliable long-term results.

Inflammatory Arthritis: Rheumatoid Arthritis

Rheumatoid arthritis targets the synovial membrane as the site for the immunologic process that is the root mechanism of this disease. Driven by a cell-mediated immune response, the synovium sees microvascular proliferation, and becomes hyperplastic and hypertrophic. The thickened synovium (now referred to as a pannus) first destroys the articular cartilage by enzymatic degradation, and follows with destruction of the underlying bone by pressure necrosis and erosion. Unlike osteoarthritis, repair changes are, for

the most part, abortive. The radiograph reflects this overall atrophic process. Soft tissue swelling, osteopenia on both sides of the joint (periarticular osteopenia), and bone erosions are the standard findings (Fig. 1.33).

Joint destruction is generally symmetric and much more global than with osteoarthritis, with severe joint space narrowing, erosive changes, and deformity, classically in the hands (Fig. 1.34). While in the recent past extensive alterations in normal anatomy usually necessitated multiple joint arthroplasties over the patient's lifetime, incredible advances in the pharmacologic treatment of rheumatoid arthritis with the disease modifying anti-rheumatic drugs has greatly decreased the need for surgical intervention in this patient population.

Metabolic Arthritides: Crystalline Arthropathy

The common denominator of the metabolic arthritides is the deposition of crystals or metabolic byproducts in or around joints. Destructive changes in these joints necessitate rheumatologic and frequently orthopedic care.

Gout

In gout, monosodium urate crystals are deposited in and around the joints. Finding these crystals in joint fluid is the diagnostic sine qua non of this metabolic imbalance. An intense chemical synovitis and bony erosions can occur. Typically, the first metatarsophalangeal joint is the classic site, but certainly the process can present in any joint, including the spine. The rapid onset and signs of acute inflammation should suggest the diagnosis, which is best confirmed by arthrocentesis. The finding of needle-like, negatively birefringent crystals under polarized light confirms the diagnosis. The treatment is usually medical, typically with anti-inflammatory drugs in the acute setting, or uric acid-reducing medications (allopurinol, colchicine) on a chronic basis.

Pseudogout

Pseudogout is one of the many causes of chondrocalcinosis (simply, calcification of cartilage) and should not be considered synonymous with it. The presence of weakly positively birefringent crystals, rhomboid in shape, attests to the diagnosis. These calcium pyrophosphate dihydrate crystals are radiopaque and, as such, can be viewed on standard radiographs as calcification of fibrocartilage, including the menisci of the knee or the triangular fibrocartilage complex of the wrist (Fig. 1.35).

Similar to gout, treatment frequently revolves around anti-inflammatory drugs, colchicine, or intra-articular steroid injections.

Ochronosis

Ochronosis is a metabolic arthropathy resulting from a rare inborn error of metabolism. The specific metabolic error is an absence of homogentisic acid oxidase, which subsequently results in an accumulation of homogentisic acid intra-articularly. This pathological by-product targets the articular cartilage for its deposition, which gets stiffened and loses its resiliency in its presence. The net result is fissuring and fibrillation of the articular surface, changes that radiographically and pathologically mimic osteoarthritis. The unique feature of this condition is the pigment associated with the by-product that stains the cartilage black, thereby accounting for the blackish tinge of the earlobes and the tips of the nose seen in these patients (Fig. 1.36).

At this time, no primary treatment options for this condition exist, and these patients are treated symptomatically.

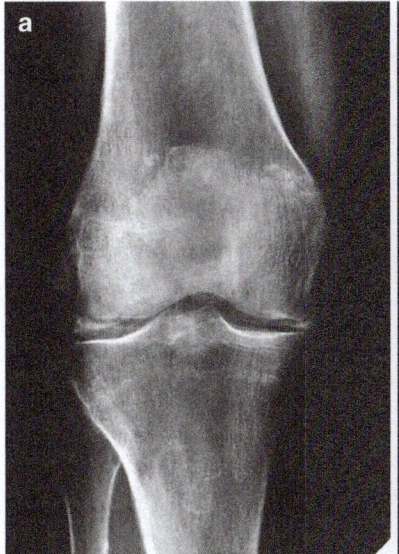 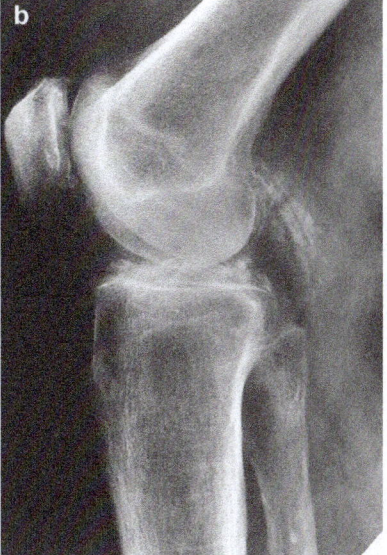

Fig. 1.35 (**a, b**) X-ray of the knee in a patient with pseudogout crystals on aspiration. Note the chondrocalcinosis due to deposition of calcium in the menisci, made of fibrocartilage. (From Orthopedic Imaging: A Practical Approach. 7E. 2021. Chapter 15, Figure 15.44)

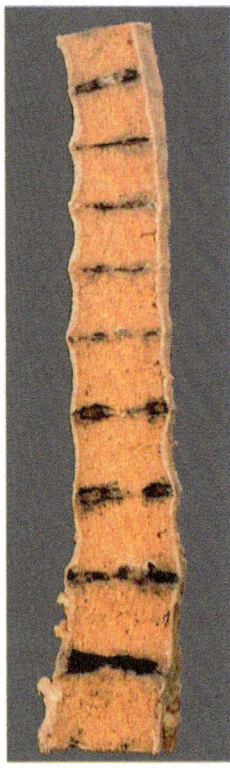

Fig. 1.36 Gross spinal pathology specimen in a patient with ochronosis, showing black pigmentation within the vertebral disc spaces, which are narrowed. (From Orthopedic Imaging: A Practical Approach. 7E. 2021. Chapter 15, Figure 15.60)

Vascular Disease

This diagnostic category is a somewhat diverse grouping of clinical entities that are best considered under this heading lest they be overlooked.

Circulatory Disease: Avascular Necrosis

Afflictions of the vascular tree, especially the arterial side, tend to produce similar lesions in bone, despite the etiology. Bone deprived of a portion of its blood supply becomes necrotic, like all other tissues (Fig. 1.37). This disease process is referred to as osteonecrosis, or avascular necrosis (AVN). Depending on the extent of the vascular involvement, the infarcts can range from small areas of bony necrosis in the metaphysis, which are clinically inconsequential, to extensive involvement at the ends of the long bones, precipitating significant degenerative joint disease (Figs. 1.38 and 1.39).

The radiographic appearance of dead bone is essentially that of sclerosis. In truth, the dead tissue is incapable of changing its density since no viable cells exist. Rather, the viable bone adjacent to the necrotic segment develops a reactive hyper-

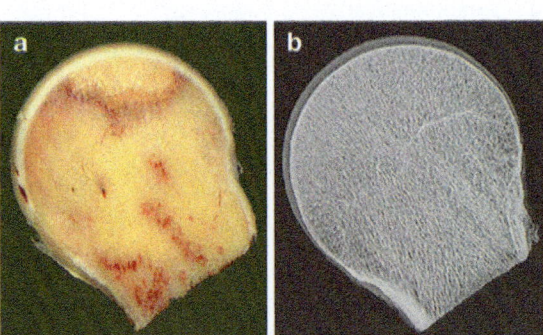

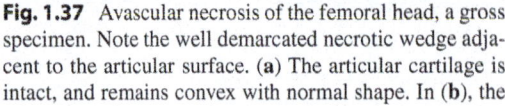

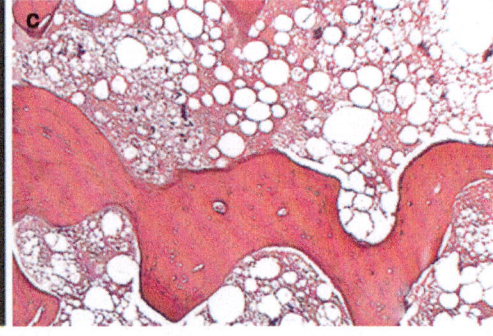

Fig. 1.37 Avascular necrosis of the femoral head, a gross specimen. Note the well demarcated necrotic wedge adjacent to the articular surface. (**a**) The articular cartilage is intact, and remains convex with normal shape. In (**b**), the bony architecture remains intact. The pathology specimen (**c**) shows infarcted, necrotic bone without osteoblastic or osteoclastic activity. (From Orthopedic Imaging: A Practical Approach. 7E. 2021. Chapter 4, Figure 4.86)

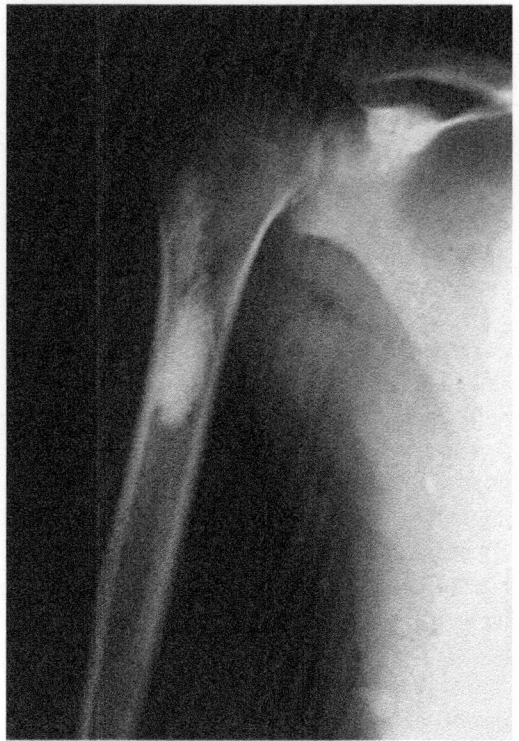

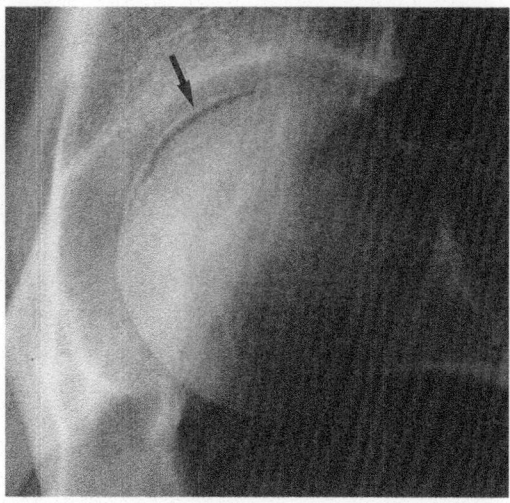

Fig. 1.40 Avascular necrosis of the femoral head in a 45-year-old woman who had sustained a traumatic hip dislocation a few weeks prior. Note the clear crescent sign (black arrow) which depicts a cleft beneath the articular cartilage resulting from compression fractures of dead trabeculae. (From Orthopedic Imaging: A Practical Approach. 7E. 2021. Chapter 4, Figure 4.90)

Fig. 1.38 Radiograph of the proximal humerus in a patient with a history of deep sea diving. The sclerotic area represents infarction of the marrow cavity with the formation of calcium soaps and new bone from the reparative margins. Although apparent radiographically, these lesions were clinically inconsequential. (From Bogumill GP. Orthopaedic Pathology: A Synopsis with Clinical Radiographic Correlation. Philadelphia, PA: Saunders; 1984. Reprinted with permission)

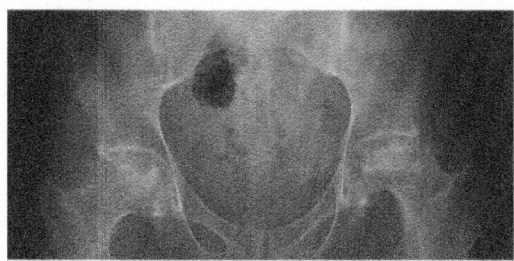

Fig. 1.39 Advanced, severe degenerative joint disease in bilateral hips secondary to avascular necrosis of the femoral heads in a young adult patient with a history of previous bilateral traumatic hip dislocations. (From Orthopedic Imaging: A Practical Approach. 7E. 2021. Chapter 4, Figure 4.93)

emia and resorbs. The area of necrosis then appears to be more dense on the radiograph—so-called relative radiodensity. There is also some compaction of dead trabeculae, as well as marrow necrosis with subsequent saponification and calcification of the dead fat, which additionally explains the sclerotic changes seen on radiographs.

A number of vaso-occlusive phenomena can cause AVN. Although AVN can involve any number of different sites, the femoral head is by far the most typical (Fig. 1.40).

Etiologies of AVN can be grouped by causation:

1. Trauma: damage to vessels supplying the segment of bone in question (i.e., fractures of the femoral neck and scaphoid).
2. Occlusive phenomena:
    (a) Emboli: fat in alcoholism and pancreatitis or nitrogen bubbles in Caisson's disease

(b) Stasis: coagulopathies and hemoglobinopathies
(c) External constriction: vasculitis (i.e., systemic lupus erythematosus), inflammatory bowel disease
(d) External compression: lysosomal storage diseases (i.e., Gaucher's and Fabry's), where stored material compresses intraosseous arterioles
3. Medications: antiretroviral agents for treatment of HIV (i.e., protease inhibitors)
4. Idiopathic (causative factor is unknown): steroid-induced AVN and Chandler's disease

Hematologic Syndromes

The genetic hemoglobinopathies, although not truly circulatory diseases, are best remembered in this group. Sickle cell disease and to a lesser degree thalassemia produce skeletal changes primarily through two mechanisms: myeloid hyperplasia and vaso-occlusive phenomena. Because of the anemia these patients suffer, there is a drive to increase medullary hematopoiesis, and this results in the dilation of bony contours to accommodate a marrow driven to produce more blood. Widening of the diploe of the skull, dilation of the small bones of the hands and feet, and increased trabecular markings are all radiographic hallmarks of this process. The vaso-occlusive effect of these distorted red cells causes bone infarcts similar to those previously discussed. However, in a select group of patients, the infarcts are frequently painful and a component of the "painful crisis." The stasis, sludging, and necrotic bone creates a comfortable environment for bacterial invasion, accounting for the increased incidence of osteomyelitis in these patients.

Hemophilia is a congenital bleeding disorder due to a deficiency in a necessary clotting factor. Hemophilia A is due to a deficiency in antihemophilic factor VII, while hemophilia B is due to a deficiency in plasma thromboplastin, or factor IX. These patients present with excessive bleeding into the joints, most commonly the knee and elbow. These recurrent hemarthroses eventually lead to hemophilic arthropathy, which tends to mimic rheumatoid arthropathy with diffuse, erosive changes (Fig. 1.41).

Separate from the arthritic changes incurred, this disorder carries with it a high risk of developing muscle hematomas, which can precipitate compartment syndrome when occurring in enclosed spaces. When this hemorrhage occurs into the iliopsoas muscle, which resides alongside the femoral nerve in the stout iliopsoas sheath, hip pain with an associated femoral nerve palsy is the result. Administration of the deficient clotting factor is the mainstay of treatment.

Fig. 1.41 Hemophilic arthropathy of the knee and elbow, resulting from recurrent intra-articular bleeding episodes in one's lifetime. (From Orthopedic Imaging: A Practical Approach. 7E. 2021. Chapter 15, Figure 15.72)

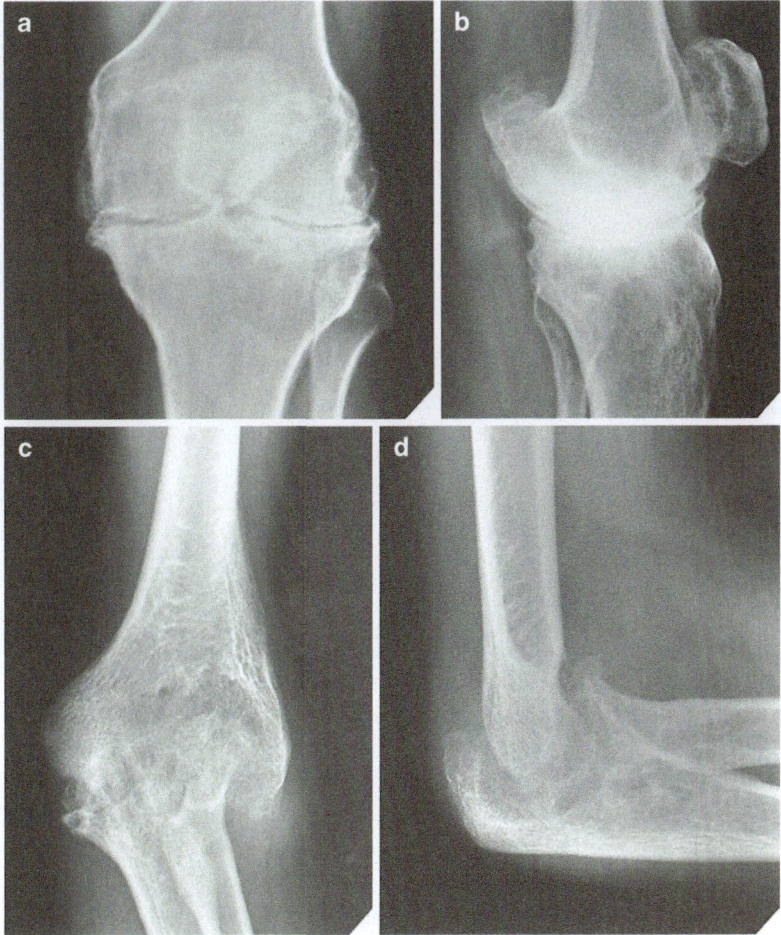

Neurodevelopmental Disorders

The final diagnostic category discussed in this chapter may be the most heterogeneous of all. However, there exists a common theme that ties this eclectic mix of clinical states together—the end result of their pathologies precipitates muscle imbalance and resultant musculoskeletal deformity. An attempt is made to describe them generically and use examples from each category to underscore their impact on the skeleton.

Neurologic Diseases

The deficit produced by neurologic diseases can be either sensory, motor, or central in origin. The level of involvement will determine the skeletal changes.

Central nervous system deficits are typified by cerebral palsy. Most commonly caused by prematurity or prenatal anoxia, resulting damage to the cerebral cortex of the newborn leads to damage to neural tissue that normally inhibits or damps muscular tone. Without normal inhibitory influences, these muscles become spastic. While the associated encephalopathy remains static in nature, muscle spasticity (which on the other hand, is quite dynamic) existing over a protracted period results in muscle imbalance around joints. Ultimately, contractures and chronic joint deformities, such as subluxations and dislocations, will follow. The hip, for example, is of particular concern in the spastic child (Fig. 1.42).

Poliomyelitis is an example of a motor deficit disease. Viral damage to the anterior horn cells of the spinal cord and brainstem results

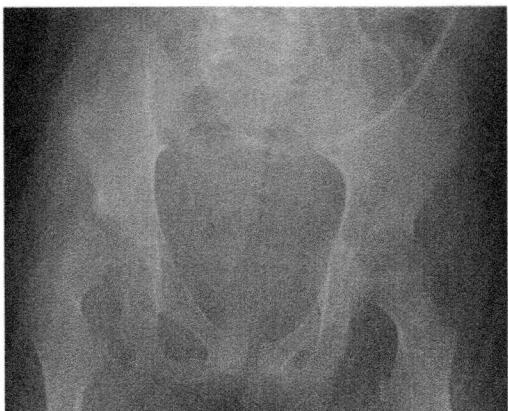

Fig. 1.42 Pelvis X-ray in a child with spastic cerebral palsy. Clearly, the right proximal femur is subluxated from the hip joint, and the femoral head is poorly covered by the malformed acetabulum. (From Orthopedic Surgery: Principles of Diagnosis and Treatment, Figure 11.17)

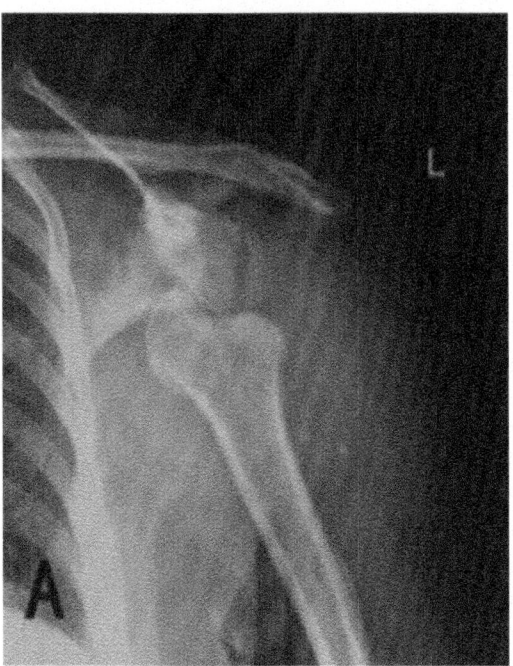

Fig. 1.43 X-ray of the left shoulder in a patient with a cervical syrinx, with destruction, dislocation, periarticular ossification, and partial resorption of the humeral head and glenoid fossa. This is a painless, destroyed joint. (From Neuropathic arthropathy caused by syringomyelia, a Journal of Neurosurgery Clinical Article)

in focal motor weakness in various muscle groups in the extremities. Sensation, however, is maintained. Unfortunately, bone deprived of normal muscle loading tends to become osteopenic. In addition, the variable nature of the involvement causes muscle imbalance around joints, with resultant deformities of bone and joint.

Sensory deficits may result in neuropathic arthritis. Joints deprived of proprioception (a sense of awareness of the position of the body in space) are rapidly destroyed (Fig. 1.43).

The aggressive sequence of microtrauma, recurrent effusions, ligamentous incompetence, articular damage, and severe degenerative joint disease is the fate of patients with tertiary syphilis, diabetes, pernicious anemia, leprosy, and heavy metal intoxications. When occurring in the shoulder, specifically, one must also consider cervical syringomyelia as the primary cause. Although proprioception is the initial sensory component lost, pain fiber deficit usually follows, resulting in destroyed, but painless joints.

Spina bifida, or myelodysplasia, results from the failure of closure of the fetal spinal cord, and results in mixed deficits. This congenital defect combines motor and sensory deficits to produce skeletal changes that parallel both. Osteopenia

and joint deformity culminate in the orthopedic manifestations not limited to long bone fractures, spinal deformity, dysplastic hip joints, knee and foot deformities, and advanced joint destruction. The joints, as expected, are insensate, a fact that only compounds the clinical problems.

Developmental/Congenital Defects

It is important to remember that congenital defects (present at birth) need not be genetic and vice versa. However, any process that impacts on the growing skeleton, whether it be congenital or developmental, can be expected to produce changes. These changes can generally be expected to be alterations in the configuration of the bone itself. Shortening, bowing, or angular deformities may be seen. Changes in bone density may or may not be seen.

Dysplasias

Achondroplasia is the most common skeletal dysplasia and the most common dwarfing syndrome (Fig. 1.44).

It follows an autosomal dominant inheritance pattern, but the majority of cases arise via spontaneous genetic mutations. The genetic mutation lies in the gene encoding fibroblast growth factor (FGF) receptor-3, located on chromosome 4. This genetic defect ultimately disrupts normal endochondral bone growth and, therefore, results in shortening of all bones that depend on this mechanism for their growth. Classic manifestations along with short stature include the following spinal deformities: thoracolumbar kyphosis, foramen magnum stenosis, and lumbar spinal stenosis, as well as a "champagne glass" pelvis—a pelvic outlet wider than it is deep (Fig. 1.45).

Bone dysplasias (intrinsic defects of bone growth) are, as a general rule, genetic in origin despite the fact that some of the milder (tarda) forms may not be apparent until the child begins growing.

Chromosomal Defects

Down syndrome is often characterized by severe ligamentous laxity. This is the basis for the numerous orthopedic conditions that are typical in this group. Atlanto-axial instability, flat feet, patellar subluxation, bunions, and subluxation of the hips all point to the inability of the ligamentous structures to stabilize joints. Many of the chromosomal abnormalities involve defects in mesoderm development, which accounts for the common coincidence of musculoskeletal, genitourinary, and cardiac abnormalities.

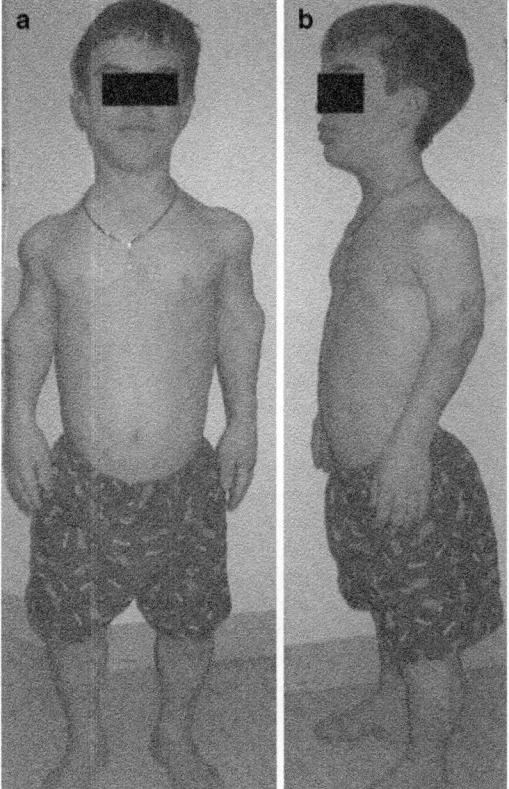

Fig. 1.44 An achondroplastic dwarf. (**a**) Note the proportionately shorter proximal limb segments compared to the distal limb segment, with the hands only racing to the hip region. (**b**) The proximal limb segments are proportionately shorter than the distal, with the hands reaching only to the hip region. The legs are bowed (genu varum) and there is marked lumbar lordosis with prominent buttocks as a result of pelvic tilt. (From Orthopedic Surgery: Principles of Diagnosis and Treatment, Figure 11.57)

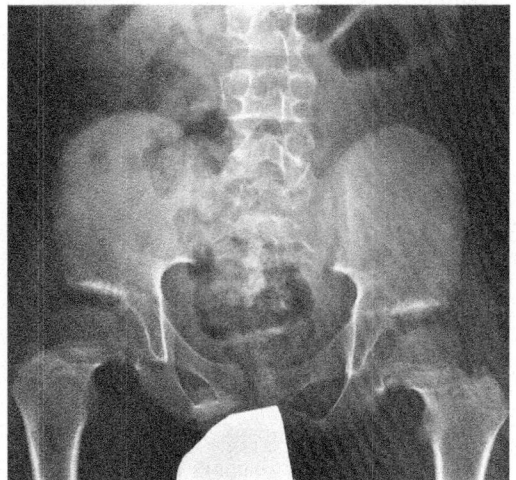

Fig. 1.45 The radiographic appearance of the pelvis of a young boy with achondroplasia. The iliac bones are rounded, and the acetabular roofs are horizontal. The sciatic notch is narrow and the acetabulae broad and flat, resulting from inadequate growth of "Y" cartilage in this region. The shape of the pelvis itself has been described to resemble a champagne glass, wider than it is deep. (From Orthopedic Imaging: A Practical Approach. 7E. 2021. Chapter 15, Figure 33.33)

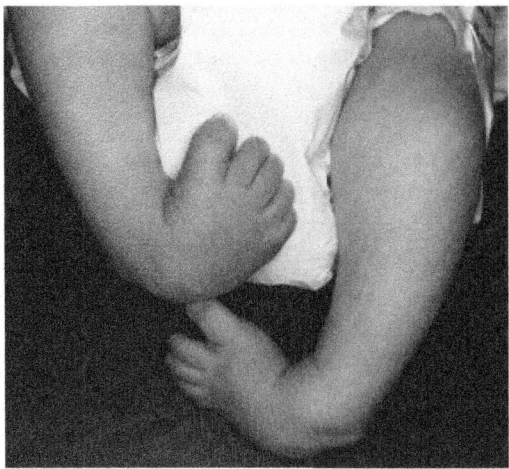

Fig. 1.46 Clubfoot deformity is associated with forefoot supination, deep medial creases, and equinovarus of the hindfoot. (From Orthopedic Surgery: Principles of Diagnosis and Treatment, Figure 11.177)

Congenital Deformity

The clubfoot deformity is the most common musculoskeletal defect with an overall incidence of 1 in 1000 births (Fig. 1.46). A genetic component to this condition is strongly suggested, resulting in muscle contractures contributing to characteristic deformities and ultimately bony malalignment. Usually identified at birth, clubfoot is a generalized dysplasia of the mesenchymal structures (bone, ligament, muscle) of not only the foot but truly the entire leg. In addition to the genetic component, environmental (intra-uterine position) factors have been implicated, but their exact interaction remains unknown.

Miscellaneous

Neurofibromatosis is another relatively common (1 in 3000 live births) condition with multiple classic orthopedic manifestations. Resulting from an autosomal dominant mutation in the neurofibromatosis-1 gene on chromosome 17, extremity deformities, spinal deformities, and classic skin lesions result. Specifically, anterolateral bowing of the tibia, pseudoarthrosis of the bones of the forearm or leg, scoliosis, limb hemi-hypertrophy, skin findings (cafe-au-lait spots and axillary freckling) and the devious presence of malignant nerve sheath tumors are seen.

Summary

Many different pathologic states impact the skeletal system, whether they are primary or secondary. Bone has a limited number of ways of responding to abnormal stimuli whether they are chemical, mechanical, infectious, circulatory, etc. In general, one can expect to see either bone resorption or bone formation, either locally or systemically, dominate the pattern. A working knowledge of the normal usually allows the observer to anticipate the response to many of these pathologic processes.

In this regard, observing the changes that one sees on standard imaging studies will often permit the development of a working differential diagnosis. Using the basic seven disease categories and expanding each into a plausible list of diagnoses should lead, given more data, to a definitive diagnosis and hence appropriate treatment.

Further Reading

Mescher AL, editor. Junqueira's basic histology text and Atlas. 16th ed. McGraw Hill; 2021.

Morcuende JA, Sanders JO. Chapter 1. Embryology and development of the musculoskeletal system. In: Lovell and Winter's pediatric orthopaedics.

Compton JT, Lee FY. A review of osteocyte function and the emerging importance of sclerostin. J Bone Joint Surg Am. 2014;96(19):1659–68. https://doi.org/10.2106/JBJS.M.01096. PMID: 25274791; PMCID: PMC4179450.

Greenspan A. Orthopedic imaging: a practical approach. 7th ed. Wolters Kluwer; 2021.

Deyrup AT, Siegal GP. Practical orthopedic pathology: a diagnostic approach. Elsevier; 2015.

Wiesel et al. Orthopedic surgery: principles of diagnosis and treatment. Springer.

Langman's medical embryology, 14th edn. 2018.

Rockwood and Wilkins fractures in children.

Rockwood and Green's fractures in adults.

Bernstein J, editor. Musculoskeletal medicine. Rosemont, IL: American Academy of Orthopaedic Surgeons; 2003.

Bogumill GP, Schwamm HA. Orthopaedic pathology: a synopsis with clinical and radiographic correlation. Philadelphia, PA: Saunders; 1984.

Buckwalter JA, Einhorn TA, Simon SR, editors. Orthopaedic basic science: biology and biomechanics of the musculoskeletal system. 2nd ed. Rosemont, IL: American Academy of Orthopaedic Surgeons; 2000.

Deng X, Wu L, Yang C, Xu Y. Neuropathic arthropathy caused by syringomyelia. J Neurosurg Spine. 2013;18(3):303–9. https://doi.org/10.3171/2012.11. SPINE12860. Epub 2013 Jan 4. PMID: 23289508.

Marenzana M, Arnett TR. The key role of the blood supply to bone. Bone Res. 2013;1(3):203–15. https://doi.org/10.4248/BR201303001. PMID: 26273504; PMCID: PMC4472103.

Biomechanics and Biomaterials

2

Daniel Hampton and Patrick Burroughs

The topic of biomechanics within orthopedics brings together physics, human biology, and engineering within the musculoskeletal system to describe how forces allow the human body to move and interact with the world. When discussing the orthopedic principles of biomechanics and biomaterials, it is important to first begin with a set of definitions that apply to commonly used terms within this field that are central to all discussions involving physics and engineering.

Scalar and vector are quantities used to describe the state of objects. Both scalar and vectors have magnitude, however, vector quantities differ from scalar quantities because they have both a magnitude and a direction. Mass is a scalar quantity describing the amount of matter within an object. In relation to orthopedics, mass is significant in that it reflects the inertia of an object, and its resistance to acceleration or change in movement. Displacement is a vector quantity that defines the change in position of an object. Velocity is the change in displacement of an object in a direction, measured as distance over time. Velocity has a direction and is therefore a

vector. Acceleration is the change in velocity of an object over time, and is a vector quantity.

Force is the vector quantity that changes an object either in shape or position. Forces have a variety of effects on an object, or body, depending on the composition of the material, the vector of the force, and the relative environment that is interacting with the body. Classically, force is measured and represented as the ability to accelerate an object of known mass.

When determining the effects of a force on a body, it is important to determine the composition of the object, and if it can be considered to behave as a rigid body or deformable body. Within rigid bodies, the particles within the object do not change their position relative to one another while forces are being applied. With deformable bodies, the particles change their position relative to one another [1]. These changes may affect the shape of an object (lengthening a tendon under tension, for example) or its volume. Furthermore, this deformation can be characterized as elastic or plastic.

When materials undergo elastic deformation after a force is applied, it means that the material will return to its original position after the deforming force is removed. When a material undergoes plastic deformation, its shape has changed permanently, and that change in shape will remain after the force is removed. Creep is a specific term to describe plastic deformation that can be observed or measured after a deforming

D. Hampton · P. Burroughs (✉)
MedStar Georgetown Orthopedic Institute,
Georgetown University School of Medicine,
Washington, DC, USA

Department of Orthopedics, MedStar Georgetown
University Hospital, Washington, DC, USA
e-mail: Daniel.m.hampton@gunet.georgetown.edu;
Patrick.J.Burroughs@medstar.net

force is applied over a period of time. The amount of creep an object experiences will increase as time increases [1].

Compression, tension, shear, rotation, or bending are all forces that have specific effects on bones and orthopedic implants and must be considered when discussing biomechanics. Compressive forces act parallel to the surface of a bone or implant and make the matter within that object more compact. When bones fail in compression, resulting fractures include buckle fractures in pediatric patients or a fracture with an associated butterfly fragment. Tension forces also act perpendicular to the surface of an object but act to pull an object apart with collinear forces acting in opposite directions. Bones fail in a transverse pattern when they are under tension. A shear force is an additional external force described in orthopedics that acts on the surface of a bone or object at two points which are eccentrically aligned. Bones are capable of resisting significantly higher compressive forces than shear forces [2, 3].

In addition to the forces already described, moments are vector quantities that cause rotation or bending about a single point, which is the pivot or axis. Moments have an associated moment arm defined by the distance between the axis of rotation or bending of the object and the point at which the force is applied. Moment is closely related to torque, which refers to a specific moment that results in rotation.

Within orthopedics, kinematics describes the motion of joints in the human body. Simple descriptions of these relationships include diagrams of static equilibrium. In order to describe joint kinematics, free body diagrams are drawn, with vectors representing force generated by muscle, moments describing limbs, and weight of objects in motion. When an object is not in motion, or is not undergoing linear or angular acceleration, it can be described as in a state of equilibrium. When objects are in a state of equilibrium, the summation of the separate vectors from forces acting on the object equals zero. Within Biomechanics, statics refers to forces that result in equilibrium, whereas dynamics refers to the study of forces that result in acceleration or rotation of an object.

For the sake of this discussion, Newton's three laws of motion govern the basic principles of mechanics that will be applied to understand biomechanics within orthopedics. Newton's first law states that an object will not change velocity, or will remain at rest, until it is acted upon by an outside force. Newton's second law describes how the motion of a body is affected by an external force, stating that the resulting acceleration of an object as a force is applied is proportional to the sum of the force vectors acting on the object, and inversely proportional to the mass of the object. Newton's third law states that every action, or force, on a body, has an equal and opposite reaction [1, 3].

Now that the basic terms of biomechanics have been covered, they can be applied to the field of orthopedics. In this chapter, we will cover the mechanics of classic mechanical levers with common motions performed by humans in their activities of daily living. To accomplish this, free body diagrams of the limb or motion in focus will be illustrated. In the example of a human hip, as demonstrated in Fig. 2.1, the joint reaction force is demonstrated in the hip and the force of the abductors, mass of body, and relative lengths from the human center of gravity to the femoral head, and from femoral head to greater trochanter must be accounted for. Other forces and measurements within Fig. 2.1 include the weight of the system

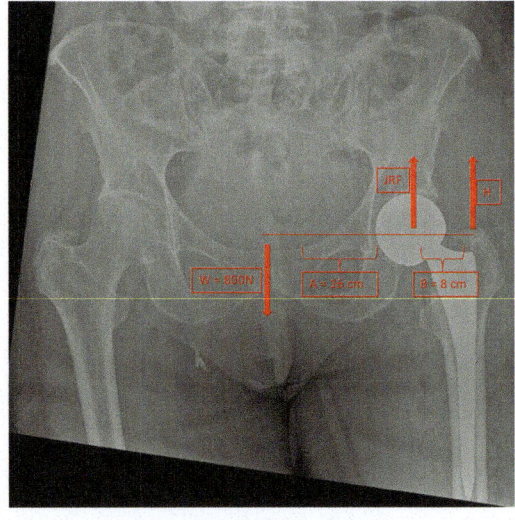

Fig. 2.1 Biomechanics of the human hip

[W] which is equal to the weight of the human body minus the weight of the leg (in this case, the left leg). The force [H] is the force supplied by the abductors of the hip, and [JRF] is the joint reaction force experience within the hip joint. The distance A is measured from the center of rotation of the hip (femoral head) to the insertion of the abductors on the greater trochanter. The distance B is from the center of gravity of the body to the center of rotation of the hip (femoral head). Given these measurements, we can solve for the joint reaction force.

In Fig. 2.1, the weight [W] is 800 N, the distance A is 16 cm (0.16 m), and the distance B is 8 cm (0.08 m). With the system at equilibrium, the force of the hip abductors is equal and opposite to the weight of the body. Therefore, the torque experienced at the center of rotation of the femoral head can be represented with the following equations, which allow us to solve for the force [H] for the abductors.

$$[W] \, (0.16 \, m) - [H] \, (0.08 \, m) = 0$$
$$[800 \, N] \, (0.16 \, m) = [H] \, (0.08 \, m)$$
$$128 \, Nm = [H] \, (0.08 \, m)$$
$$[H] = 1600 \, N$$

In addition, the joint reaction force can be calculated with the following equation:

$$[JRF] - [H] - [W] = 0$$
$$[JRF] - [1600 \, N] - [800 \, N] = 0$$
$$[JRF] = 2400 \, N$$

This means that in the example provided by Fig. 2.1, the joint reaction force at rest is three times the patient's bodyweight.

In Fig. 2.2, a free body diagram is applied to represent the biomechanics of the elbow joint. The elbow is a class 3 lever, and in class 3 levers, the load and the force (effort) are on the same side of the fulcrum, meaning that the force to maintain 90 degrees of flexion at the elbow is between the fulcrum (the radiocapitellar/ulnohumeral joint) and the system weight of the forearm and hand. In addition, the distance from the fulcrum to the effort is always shorter than the distance from the fulcrum to the center of gravity of the forearm. As a result, the force, or effort of the

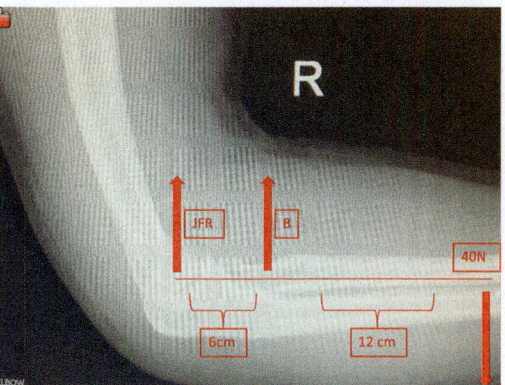

Fig. 2.2 Biomechanics of the human elbow

brachialis to maintain flexion will always be greater than the system weight of the forearm and hand. In Fig. 2.2, the system weight of the forearm and hand is 40 N, with the center of gravity 18 cm (0.18 m) from the elbow joint. The force applied to flex the elbow [B] is directed from the brachialis insertion which is 6 cm (0.06 m) from the elbow joint. In a static system in equilibrium, one can solve for the force applied by the brachialis and the joint reaction force (JRF) experienced at the elbow joint.

$$-([B] \, (0.06 \, m)) + [40 \, N] \, (0.18 \, m) = 0$$
$$[B] \, (0.06) = 7.2 \, Nm$$
$$[B] = 120 \, N$$

When solving for the joint reaction force at the elbow, and assuming a system at equilibrium, the (1) force applied at the joint, the (2) force of the brachialis in maintaining flexion at the elbow, and the (3) weight of the forearm and hand sum to 0.

$$[JRF] + [B] - 40 \, N = 0$$
$$[JFR] = 40 \, N - 120 \, N$$
$$[JFR] = -80 \, N, \text{ this force vector is negative, indi-}$$
cating that it acts in a direction opposite to the weight of the forearm and hand, which is intuitive when looking at the free body diagram.

The topic of biomaterials begins with the fundamental qualities of bones, ligaments, and tendons that make them effective structures to support the human skeleton and permit locomotion. The study of biomaterials within orthopedics also includes other materials, organic and inorganic, that are used to create implants which are commonly used in orthopedic applications. In the same way that biomechanics was reviewed within this chapter, one must first define terms closely related to biomaterials to begin examination of this subject. Each of these materials will be described using a consistent set of terms that effectively describe the qualities of these materials as they apply to orthopedic applications.

Stress is the amount of force applied to an object, divided by the area that the force is applied over. Stress is measured in Newtons per square meter. Strain, on the other hand, is a unitless measure of a distance a material deforms divided by its original length. Young's Modulus of elasticity is a quantitative measure of a material's stiffness and ability to resist deformation when a tensile force is applied to it [2, 3]. A material's Young's modulus is represented by the initial slope of the stress vs. strain curve (Fig. 2.3).

The elasticity of an object refers to the material's ability to return to its original dimensions, length, width, and depth, after a compressive or tensile force causes it to lengthen or shorten (Table 2.1; Fig. 2.4).

The yield strength of an object is the force, represented by the first peak, relative to the Y-axis of the stress vs. strain curve, where a material's properties change from elastic to plastic. After that point, the material is irreversibly deformed and will not return to its original dimensions. For typical metals, the yield strength is reached when a material has undergone a strain of 0.2% [3].

The ultimate strength, sometimes referred to as the tensile strength, is the maximum tensile force that a material can withstand before breaking, and is represented by the highest point on the stress vs. strain curve. The nature of the distance between the yield strength and the ultimate

Table 2.1 Elastic modulus of common orthopedic tissues and biomaterials

Material	Elastic modulus (GPa)
Ceramic	300
Cobalt chrome	230
Stainless steel	200
Titanium	100
Cortical bone	20
Trabecular bone	10
Bone cement	3
Polyethylene	1
Cancellous bone	0.4
Tendon/ligament	0.3
Cartilage	0.02

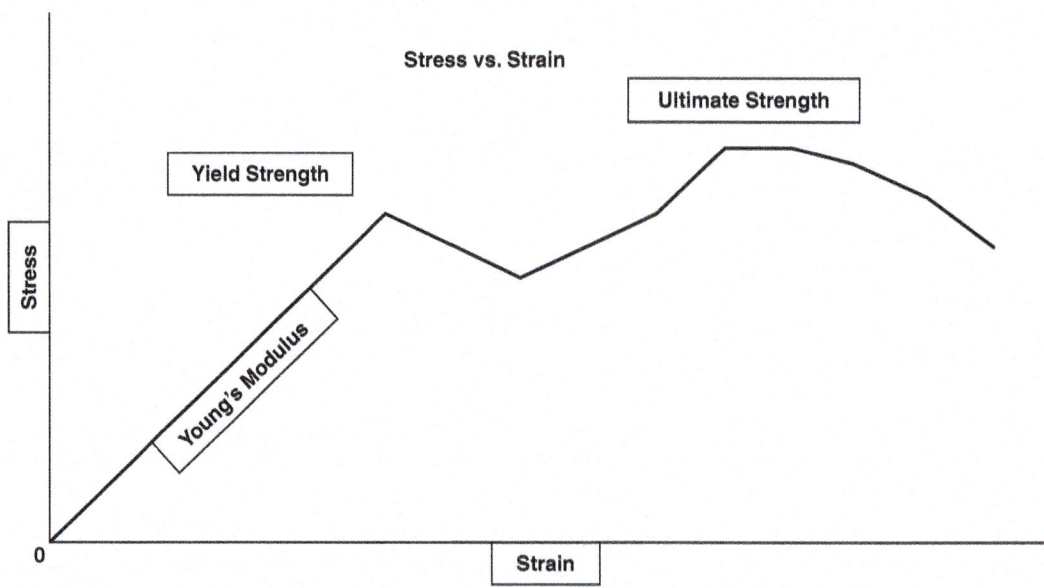

Fig. 2.3 Stress vs. strain curve

Fig. 2.4 Relative values of Young's Modulus. The pneumonic CAST-Bone is helpful to remember the decreasing relative value between ceramic, cobalt chrome (alloy), stainless steel, titanium, and cortical bone [4]

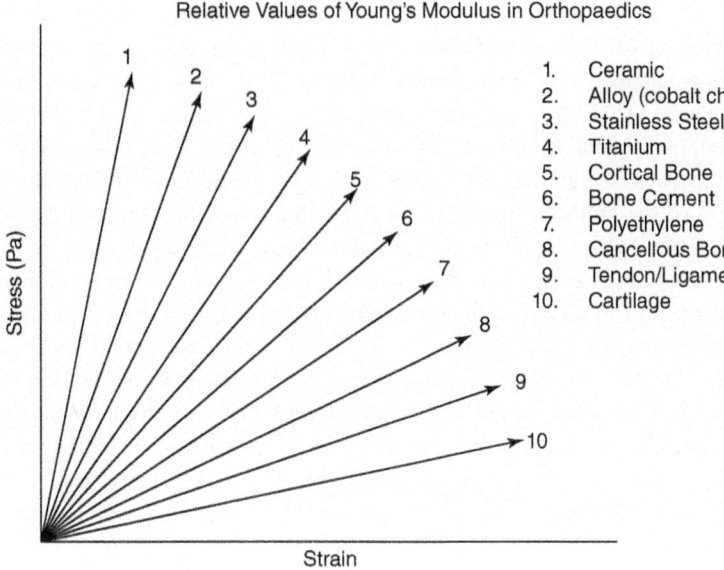

Relative Values of Young's Modulus in Orthopaedics

1. Ceramic
2. Alloy (cobalt chrome)
3. Stainless Steel
4. Titanium
5. Cortical Bone
6. Bone Cement
7. Polyethylene
8. Cancellous Bone
9. Tendon/Ligament
10. Cartilage

strength for two materials can be used to describe an additional material quality, whether they are brittle or ductile. Ductility refers to a material's ability to undergo plastic deformation without failure [5].

When comparing two materials, because the more ductile material can endure more deformation prior to breaking, and therefore tolerate a greater strain, there is a longer distance between yield strength and ultimate strength on the x-axis of the stress vs. strain curve (Fig. 2.3). Conversely a brittle material will deform to a lesser extent, and have a shorter distance between these two points on the x-axis of the stress vs. strain curve. In truly brittle materials, such as polymethyl-methacrylate, the cement used in total joint arthroplasty, the stress strain curve travels directly to the ultimate strength, without a period of plastic deformation.

Aside from ultimate strength, materials often undergo fatigue failure, which refers to fracture, or failure of a material after cyclic loading of a force that is less than the ultimate strength [1].

The toughness of a material is represented as its ability to endure strain and is represented by the area under the stress vs. strain curve. In some materials, including organic materials such as bones, tendons, and ligaments, the rate, or time period over which the tensile force is applied, affects the materials strain behavior in the response to a given stress. Materials with variable stress vs. strain curves depending on the rate of an applied force are referred to as viscoelastic [1, 3].

In addition to the importance of a materials properties, its shape and construction are critical to its performance under load. For example, the bending rigidity of a long object with a rectangular cross-section is calculated differently than the bending rigidity of a cylinder. With a rectangular object, the rigidity is proportional to base of the rectangle multiplied by the height cubed, Rigidity = (base × height^3)/12. In comparison, the bending rigidity of a cylinder is proportional to the radius raised to the fourth power [3]. This is an important concept when considering the difference in rigidity of common orthopedic implants such as intramedullary nails. The bending stiffness of a plate used in a plate and screw construct is proportional to the third power of its thickness.

Material can also be described as isotropic or anisotropic. Isotropic materials behave in the same way when a force, such as compression or tension, is applied, independent of the direction of the force or orientation relative to the material. Metal alloys are generally understood to be isotropic materials. Bone and ligaments, on the other hand, are anisotropic materials. The mechanical properties of anisotropic materials vary as force vectors are applied in different directions through the material [1]. Bones, ligaments, and tendons are composed of collagen fibrils, and the mechanical properties of these tissues depend on the orientation of the collagen fibrils. Wood is another common example of an anisotropic material, due to the mechanical properties of the wood being dependent on the direction of the applied force relative to the grain of the wood.

Organic materials refer to the vast spectrum of matter which is carbon-based and is either found in the natural environment or human-engineered. For this chapter, organic material primarily refers to type one collagen in bone and gives bone its flexibility. Inorganic materials, on the other hand, are not carbon-based, and are not the primary molecules or byproducts of living systems. For this chapter, in reference to biomaterials as it applies to orthopedics and bone composition, inorganic materials are the calcium and phosphate salts that lend bone its stiffness. Inorganic material also refers to the polymer, ceramic, and metal alloys that implants used in orthopedic surgery are composed of.

Polymers are synthetically created chemical compounds composed of identical, repeating units, or "mers", that have a carbon backbone. Polymers are covalently bonded to one another, and the repeating units can be formed into long structures, such as chains or sheets. Polyethylene is a common polymer. Relative to other materials used in orthopedics, such as metal alloys, polymers exhibit increased flexibility and improved resistance to corrosion, however, have decreased strength.

Polymers are commonly used in total joint arthroplasty, reducing friction and improving ear characteristics between the tibial and femoral components in a total knee arthroplasty, or as the portion of the acetabular component in total hip arthroplasty that articulates with the ceramic (or cobalt chromium) femoral head. The polymer chosen for these applications is UHMWPE, Ultra High Molecular Weight Polyethylene, which has been used for decades in total joint arthroplasty. Sheets or rods of UHMWPE are formed into their

desired shape by extrusion or compression molding [6]. At body temperature, UHMWPE is between its glass transition temperature and melting point, allowing it to exist in partially crystalline state and demonstrate desired mechanical properties of high wear resistance, strength as well as resistance to fatigue [6]. UHMWPE is sterilized by various means, including gamma irradiation in air or inert gas, or in ethylene oxide gas [3, 5]. Gamma irradiation is known to increase cross-linking, which enhances resistance to wear while also increasing the brittleness of the polymer and therefore the potential for propagation of fatigue cracks [6].

Brittleness also occurs in UHMWPE due to oxidation, which is a by-product of the irradiation process and generation of free radicals. Currently, there are processes to add Vitamin E to the polymer implants in addition to the cross-linking treatment to potentially mitigate the effects of oxidation and reduce brittleness, but at this time, long-term outcomes of Vitamin E are pending [6, 7]. The other mechanism to improve oxidation in UHMWPE is melting the polymer after irradiation, which effectively reduces free radical levels, but at the same time decreases the crystalline structure of the polymer, which has a detrimental effect on wear properties [7]. Therefore, in polymer processing, there exists a balance between maintaining crystalline structure and removing free radicals. To optimize outcomes in these two domains, UHMWPE undergoes annealing to below melt point, which removes free radicals while having a less deleterious effect on crystalline structure than melting [5, 6].

Ceramic, the next material covered in this text, has been used as an orthopedic implant, and more specifically as a bearing surface for femoral head in total hip arthroplasty, since the 1970s. The design of ceramic implants in total joint arthroplasty has improved in an iterative fashion, and the latest generation of ceramic has several desirable mechanical properties, including hardness, resistance to wear and scratches, wettability, inertness, and biocompatibility [1]. Ceramics are extremely hard but brittle materials; their main drawback as a bearing surface in total joint arthroplasty is that there is a higher risk of fracture when compared to a metal implant. If fracture does occur, the comminution of the ceramic head and subsequent retention of ceramic fragments increases wear, osteolysis, and likelihood of reoperation [3, 5]. When used in combination with a polyethylene liner, there is less wear in ceramic on polyethylene implants when compared to metal on polyethylene [5]. In addition to Alumina (Al_2O_3), zirconia (ZrO_2) is ceramic that was historically used as an orthopedic implant [3]. Zirconia has increased fracture resistance and higher strength when compared to alumina, however, poorer wear properties, roughening of the bearing surface, and manufacturing issues resulted in zirconia being passed over as an implant material [1, 5].

Metals are composed of individual elements aligned in an organized, crystalline structure that provides each particular metal with consistent characteristics with respect to their ductility and strength, as well as their ability to conduct electric current. Two elemental metals used in orthopedics include titanium and tantalum. Titanium is resistant to corrosion due to its ability to readily form a titanium oxide and can be used for fixation of fractures that do not experience high loads. Tantalum is chosen in orthopedic implants for its ability to promote ingrowth of new bone, supporting solid fixation of the implant [1, 3].

In addition to the use of elemental metals, these individual metals may be combined in the form of alloys, allowing their properties to be blended to achieve a desired effect. This is particularly relevant as it applies to surgical implants. This chapter is not all-inclusive but will address several of the more common alloys used within orthopedics.

Stainless steel is a common metal alloy, with varying compositions of iron, carbon, nickel, and chromium. Carbon adds strength to steel at the expense of increased brittleness. Chromium is added to stainless steel to form an oxide that resists corrosion, and nickel increases both the alloys' corrosion resistance, ductility, and its ability to be welded or formed into useful structures [3]. In particular, an alloy of stainless steel—A316L, is used in the field of orthopedics [2, 3]. This alloy is chosen due to its relatively high chromium content and subsequent resistance to corrosion [3].

Titanium is an element of important and common utilization within orthopedics due to its strength, relatively lower density, and resistance to corrosion. Although pure titanium finds limited use within orthopedics [1], titanium alloys that combine varying amounts of aluminum and vanadium have applications in multiple implants, such as intramedullary nails for fractures involving the tibia or femur. In this application, the aluminum and vanadium lend the titanium alloy increased strength and ductility [1, 3].

Alloys of cobalt and chromium are valued for their high strength and longevity. They are common in implants used in total joint arthroplasty. In these use cases, the cobalt chromium alloy is expected to repeatedly resist high loads for several decades. Cobalt alloys may include small amounts of carbon and molybdenum to improve ductility and strength [1].

Corrosion refers to the chemical degradation or dissolving of a material [8]. There are various types of corrosion, and within orthopedics, there are specific instances where these types of corrosion are most prevalent. Corrosion is significant in orthopedics primarily for two reasons. First, there is subsequent weakening of the implant, increasing the risk of failure. In addition, corrosion releases metal ions into both the local environment and systemically within the human body. These ions promote in inflammatory changes that damage tissue and can weaken the interface between the implant and the bone itself [1, 3].

To reduce the incidence of corrosion among metal implants, many have an intentional thin oxide coating that is resistant to further chemical change within the body. However, in instances of pitting corrosion, that oxide has been worn away, and is generally seen in orthopedic implants made of stainless steel, whereas titanium alloy is not prone to pitting corrosion [1, 3, 8].

Galvanic corrosion refers to the degradation that occurs between two different metals when there is an electric potential that exists between them, with one metal acting as an anode and the other a cathode. Galvanic corrosion requires the metals to exist in an electrolyte solution, which describes most environments within the human body. In galvanic corrosion, as electrons flow from the anode to cathode, the anode undergoes corrosion. Within orthopedics, this occurs at the interface of an orthopedic plate made of a titanium alloy that is in contact with stainless steel screws or cerclage wires [8]. Cobalt chromium and stainless steel are known for susceptibility to galvanic corrosion when they come into contact with one another within the body.

Crevice corrosion refers to degradation in metal orthopedic implants that have a crevice geometry. This can be found at the threads of screws, in fatigue cracks, or when implants are brought together with an interference fit [1, 8]. In these situations, the crevice geometry can result in a local pH of 1.0, facilitating corrosion [1].

Fretting corrosion refers to corrosion secondary to micromotion between metals and is often seen at the interface of a tapered stem in the head and neck junction of the implant used in total hip arthroplasty [5].

References

1. Boyer M. AAOS comprehensive orthopaedic review 3. 3rd ed. Wolters Kluwer; 2019.

2. Tornetta P. Rockwood and Green's fractures in adults. Wolters Kluwer;2019.https://go.openathens.net/redirector/georgetown.edu?url=https%3A%2F%2Fotaonline.org%2Fbook%2F2573%2Frockwood-and-greens-fractures-in-adults-9e. Accessed 14 Dec 2022.

3. Miller M, Thompson S. Miller's review of orthopaedics. 7th ed. Elsevier.

4. Rho JY, Ashman RB, Turner CH. Young's modulus of trabecular and cortical bone material: ultrasonic and microtensile measurements. J Biomech. 1993;26(2):111–9. https://doi.org/10.1016/0021-9290(93)90042-d.

5. Jung YL, Kim SY. Alumina-on-polyethylene bearing surfaces in total hip arthroplasty. Open Orthop J. 2010;4:56–60. https://doi.org/10.2174/1874325001004010056.

6. Ansari F, Ries MD, Pruitt L. Effect of processing, sterilization and crosslinking on UHMWPE fatigue fracture and fatigue wear mechanisms in joint arthroplasty. J Mech Behav Biomed Mater. 2016;53:329–40. https://doi.org/10.1016/j.jmbbm.2015.08.026.

7. Oral E, Beckos CAG, Lozynsky AJ, Malhi AS, Muratoglu OK. Improved resistance to wear and fatigue fracture in high pressure crystallized vitamin E-containing ultra-high molecular weight polyethylene. Biomaterials. 2009;30(10):1870–80. https://doi.org/10.1016/j.biomaterials.2008.12.029.

8. Jacobs JJ, Gilbert JL, Urban RM. Corrosion of metal orthopaedic implants. J Bone Joint Surg Am. 1998;80(2):268–82. https://doi.org/10.2106/00004623-199802000-00015.

Musculoskeletal Imaging

3

Akhil Jay Khanna and Bradley Gelfand

Introduction

A proper diagnosis of musculoskeletal pathology by orthopedic surgeons or any musculoskeletal specialist often necessitates both obtaining and analyzing different imaging modalities. Orthopedic surgeons require an understanding of the diagnostic imaging tools available as well as the ability to accurately interpret imaging studies. Historically, conventional radiographs were the only modality available to aid in evaluating musculoskeletal injuries and conditions. Although less technologically advanced than newer techniques, conventional radiographs provide a wealth of information and are readily available. This allowed radiographs to become the workhorse for diagnosing osseous and soft tissue pathology prior to the development of more advanced three dimensional imaging modalities such as computed tomography (CT) and magnetic resonance imaging (MRI). This chapter will provide an overview of imaging in orthopedic surgery including the different modalities and techniques used to evaluate common musculoskeletal manifestations.

Conventional Radiographs

Conventional radiographs are most often the first line diagnostic imaging used to evaluate musculoskeletal pathology. They are relatively inexpensive, readily available, and rapidly obtained. Conventional radiographs are acquired via the use of ionizing irradiation. Through the use of an image intensifier and a cassette, the radiation beam is attenuated by imposing structures. Structures like bone or metal implants will block a larger amount of the radiation beam secondary to their increased density and, thus, leave a region of white on the cassette film. This is opposed to subcutaneous tissue (fat) or air which are less dense and therefore block less of the radiation beam leading to an area of gray or darkness on the receiving film.

Building off of these fundamental principles, it is evident that conventional radiographs are quite important in the evaluation of skeletal trauma when there is concern for a fracture. Radiographs provide a global view of where a fracture is located, the degree of displacement, the presence or absence of comminution as well as any other underlying deformities. When fracture lines are difficult to visualize on conventional radiographs, especially when involving an articular surface, more advanced imaging may be warranted such

A. J. Khanna · B. Gelfand (✉)
MedStar Georgetown Orthopedic Institute, Georgetown University School of Medicine, Washington, DC, USA

Department of Orthopedics, MedStar Georgetown University Hospital, Washington, DC, USA
e-mail: Jay.Khanna@medstar.net;
Bradley.W.Gelfand@medstar.net

© The Author(s), under exclusive license to Springer Nature Switzerland AG 2024
W. F. Postma et al. (eds.), *Essentials of Orthopedic Surgery*,
https://doi.org/10.1007/978-3-031-66215-7_3

as CT which will be discussed later in this chapter. Although conventional radiographs provide a wealth of knowledge regarding the osseous structures, they are less useful in evaluating soft tissues such as ligaments, tendons, and the spinal cord.

When a patient presents to an orthopedic surgeon complaining of pain, a decision must be made as to which bone or joint should be imaged. The following sections will outline the specific radiographic studies that are commonly used to evaluate the most frequent sources of pain or fractures.

Shoulder

Radiographic evaluation of the shoulder generally involves examining the osseous integrity of the proximal humerus, glenoid, and distal clavicle as well as the articulations of the glenohumeral and acromio-clavicular joints, respectively. Specific radiographic views allow for more direct evaluation of various regions of the shoulder based on the respective anatomy. This section will review the most common radiographic views and their clinical applications.

The most basic radiographic views of the shoulder include the **AP (anterior–posterior)** as well as the **True AP (also known as the Grashey View)** (Fig. 3.1). The difference in these two views lies in the coronal orientation of the glenohumeral joint as the joint is angled approximately 40° medial to the coronal plane of the body. Thus, the **AP View** is obtained with the beam perpendicular to the patient's body, while the **True AP/Grashey View** is obtained with the beam perpendicular to the plane of the scapula with the patient rotating their torso to accommodate for the angulation. It is of the utmost importance to understand the difference between these two views as non-orthopedic providers may order an **AP** of the shoulder which does not allow for proper evaluation of the glenohumeral articulation.

To assess the shoulder from a lateral perspective, **a Scapular Y/Neer View** can be obtained by rotating the patient's torso approximately 60°. This will provide a radiograph that is perpendicular to the Grashey view and provides information about the humeral head relative to the glenoid in the anterior–posterior plane.

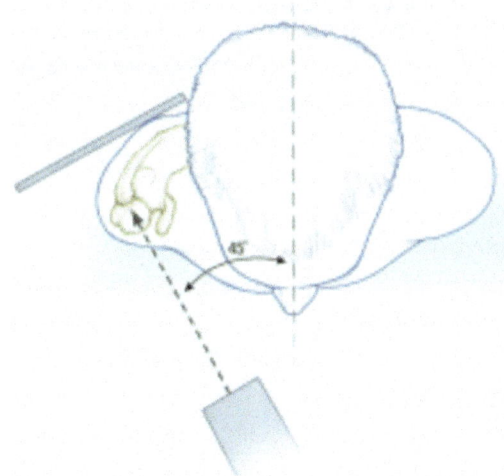

Fig. 3.1 The true AP view of the glenohumeral joint requires the beam to be angled 45° from the sagittal plane

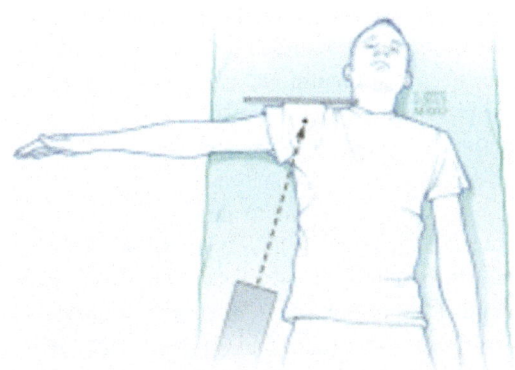

Fig. 3.2 The patient is supine with the arm abducted allowing the X-ray beam to be projected from the axilla to the cassette

The **Axillary View** is the true orthogonal view to the **Grashey View** allowing for assessment of the glenohumeral joint in the axial plane. The axillary view must be obtained when evaluating a shoulder dislocation as it will reveal whether the humeral head is dislocated anteriorly or posteriorly. Although a shoulder may appear dislocated on a True AP, nothing can be concluded about the A-P plane without an orthogonal axillary view. This view is acquired by having the patient abduct their arm to 90° while supine with the radiation beam aimed at the axilla (Fig. 3.2).

In the clinical setting of a dislocated shoulder, an axillary view can be difficult to obtain due to pain. Abducting the shoulder to 90° while dislocated is often quite painful for the patient. A secondary view in the axial orthogonal plane is called the **Velpeau Axillary View**. A **Velpeau** view is obtained by directing the radiation beam in superior to inferior direction over the shoulder while the patient is leaning backwards over a cassette. No manipulation of the extremity is required and this view can be obtained while the patient is in a sling. Radiographic evaluation of a shoulder dislocation is not complete until either an axillary or Velpeau view is seen.

Although the axillary view provides a view of the glenoid, the **West Point View**, provides improved visualization of the anteroinferior glenoid rim which is often fractured (Bony Bankart Lesion) in the setting of a shoulder dislocation. A **West Point View is** obtained by placing the patient prone with their arm abducted to 90°. The radiation beam is then angled approximately 25° cephalad and 25° medial.

As the Shoulder chapter explains, a Hill-Sachs Lesion is often seen after shoulder dislocations. In order to further evaluate the posterolateral humeral head, a **Notch/Stryker View** can be obtained by placing the patient supine, flexing the arm and angling the radiation beam approximately 10° cephalad.

With regard to the clavicle, distal clavicle fractures are often visualized after ordering conventional radiographs of the shoulder. A true AP of the distal clavicle is called a **Zanca View** (**Apical Oblique**), which involves centering the radiograph on the AC Joint with the radiation beam directed approximately 10° cephalad thus removing the profile of the thoracic cage which can obstruct the radiographic view.

Hand/Wrist

The first series of radiographs obtained when evaluating the wrist includes the **PA, Oblique, and Lateral** views. Most commonly, distal radius fractures are evaluated with this series of radiographs. Each view, respectively, allows for proper evaluation of different parameters used to assess the severity of distal radius fractures. The **PA view** visualizes the radial height, defined as the distance

between two lines drawn relative to the radial shaft at the distal ulnar head and the radial styloid. The **PA View** also shows the radial inclination, which is defined as the angle between a line from the DRUJ through radial styloid and a line perpendicular to the radial shaft. Meanwhile, the **Lateral View** will demonstrate the amount of dorsal or volar tilt present. The tilt is measured by an angle between two lines. One line is drawn perpendicular to the radial shaft, while the other connects the volar and dorsal rims of the articular surface of the distal radius. The treating orthopedic surgeon must determine if the lateral view is accurate by assessing the distal pole of the scaphoid. A perfect lateral view will show the distal pole of the scaphoid in line with the hook of the hamate.

Another common injury seen in the wrist is a fracture of the scaphoid. When a patient suffers a fall onto an outstretched hand and complains of wrist pain, the scaphoid must be evaluated with specialized radiographic views. An **Ulnar Deviation** view is performed in the PA projection with the wrist ulnarly deviated to help visualize the waist of the scaphoid. Both **Semi-pronated** and **Semi-supinated views,** which are also known as **Ulnar Oblique** and **Radial Oblique,** respectively, are useful as well. By angling the radiation beam in these various orientations, both the scaphoid waist as well as proximal pole can be visualized.

A **Clenched Fist** view used to assess the relationship between the scaphoid and lunate and any associated widening seen with disruption of the scapho-luante ligament. The patient must clench their fist while supinating and ulnarly deviating relative to the radiation beam.

Lastly, when evaluating the hook of the hamate and the pisiform, a **Carpal Tunnel View** is needed. This view is obtained by hyperextending the hand and directing the radiation beam 30° relative to the horizontal axis.

Pelvis/Hip

Radiographic imaging of the pelvis and hip is used to assess a plethora of orthopedic conditions ranging from osteoarthritis, femoroacetabular impingement, fractures, and more. Understanding the different views available as well as the anatomy of the pelvis allows orthopedic surgeons to properly assess pelvic pathology.

An **AP View** of the Pelvis is always obtained during initial evaluation of the pelvis. Generally taken supine with the patients feet internally rotated 15° to account for the native anteversion of the femoral neck. This helps provide a true coronal view. The **AP View** radiograph demonstrates the hip joints bilaterally and can demonstrate arthritic changes, hip dysplasia, as well as pelvic and acetabular fractures.

The two most common lateral radiographs of the hip are the **Cross Table Lateral** and **Frog Leg Lateral**. A **Frog Leg** lateral is obtained with the patient supine, knee flexed, and hip externally rotated approximately 45°. This is opposed to the **Cross Table Lateral** where the beam is angled from a lateral direction and the contralateral knee and hip are flexed to avoid any overlap on the film.

Every orthopedic surgeon should be familiar with six radiographic anatomical landmarks seen on an **AP View**: iliopectineal line, ilioischial line, the teardrop, roof of the acetabulum as well as both the anterior and posterior rims of the acetabulum. Each of these landmarks represent different anatomic regions of the pelvis. Disruptions of these various lines are discussed further in the trauma chapter.

The **Judet Views** of the pelvis are used to assess the walls and columns of the acetabulum. They are also known as the **Obturator Oblique and Iliac Oblique Views.** These oblique views are obtained by directing the radiation beam 45° oblique in each direction, respectively. The **Obturator Oblique** will profile the anterior column and posterior wall of the acetabulum and will confirm any suspected hip dislocation. The **Iliac Oblique** will profile the posterior column and anterior wall and allows direct visualization of the greater and lesser sciatic notches. A classically tested radiographic finding is the **Spur Sign**, which is indicative of a both column fracture seen on the obturator oblique view.

With regard to the pelvic ring, **Inlet** and **Outlet Views** are needed to fully evaluate the pelvis (Fig. 3.3).

Each view is obtained by angling the radiation beam 20° caudal and cephalad. The **Inlet View**

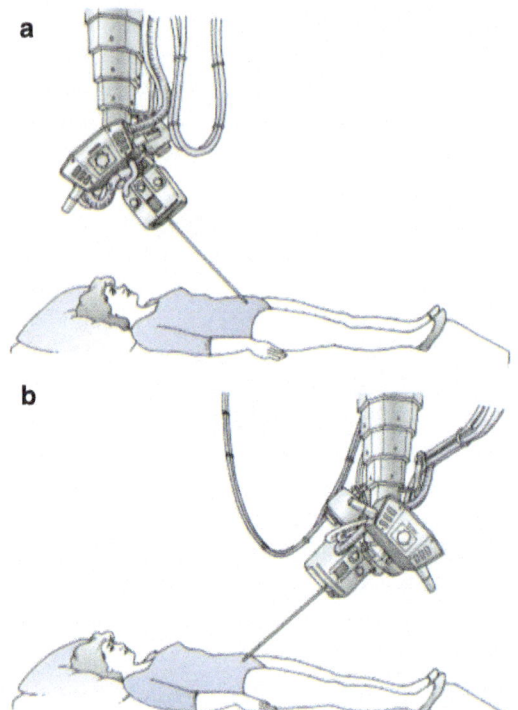

Fig. 3.3 Depiction of X-Ray beam orientation for Inlet (**a**) and Outlet (**b**) views

depicts the amount of anterior–posterior displacement across the ring, while the **Outlet View** will demonstrate superior–inferior displacement. Specifically, these views are crucial when evaluating superior and inferior pubic rami fractures as well as fractures of the sacrum.

The Sacro-Iliac joints sit approximately 30° off plane relative to the remainder of the pelvis, therefore, a **Ferguson View** can be obtained where the radiation beam is angled 30° cephalad relative to the horizontal. This view is optimal when assessing sacro-iliac displacement as well as sacroiliitis in the setting of Ankylosing Spondylitis.

The Knee

Radiographic evaluation of the knee can provide vital diagnostic information in the setting of osteoarthritis, osteochondral lesions, as well as fractures of the tibial plateau and patella. A full series of radiographic evaluation of the knee include an **AP View, Lateral View, and Sunrise View.**

The **AP View** should be obtained with the knee in 30° of flexion while the patient is weight bearing. This allows for more accurate visualization of the knee joint line which is vital when assessing for osteoarthritis and coronal alignment of the knee. Arthroplasty Surgeons must know if a knee is in Varus or Valgus alignment leading up to a Total Knee Arthroplasty.

A common error in knee radiographs is not obtaining an accurate **Lateral View**. An accurate view entails near perfect overlap of the femoral condyles which indicates the radiation beam is truly perpendicular to the knee. If the femoral condyles are not aligned, repeat lateral radiographs should be considered. The **Lateral View** will provide information about the articular surface as well as the height of the patella. The location of the patella relative to the knee joint can help augment a clinical diagnosis of patellar tendon or quadriceps tendon rupture. In the setting of a patellar tendon rupture, the patella will be elevated relative to the joint line secondary to the unopposed pull of the intact quadriceps. Conversely, in the setting of a quadriceps tendon rupture the patella will be sitting inferiorly secondary to the unopposed pull of the intact patellar tendon.

The two views most commonly used to assess the patellofemoral joint are the **Sunrise View** and **Merchant View**. The **Sunrise View** is acquired with the patient prone while flexing their knee greater than 90°. This allows the radiograph to display an axial view of the patella. On the contrary, the **Merchant View** is acquired with the patient supine and the knee flexed to 45°, while the radiation beam is angled 30° from the horizontal. The merchant view will provide information regarding how the patella is sitting within the trochlear groove or detect the presence of patellar subluxation.

Foot and Ankle

Routine radiographic assessment of the ankle begins with three views of the ankle including: **AP View, Mortise View, and a Lateral View**. In order to properly obtain a **Mortise View**, the ankle must be internally rotated approximately 15° to account for the native anatomy of the ankle joint. The medial malleolus sits both anterior and superior relative to the lateral malleolus, therefore internally rotating the extremity will allow the radiograph to capture the ankle joint proper without any overlap from the talus or fibula. More specifically, the **Mortise View** allows for evaluation of the medial clear space of the ankle, represented as the area between the medial aspect of the talus and the medial malleolus. The medial clear space can be widened in the setting of a medial ligamentous injury such as the Deltoid Ligament as well as a syndesmotic injury. In order to determine if the medial aspect of the ankle is unstable, a **Stress View** can be obtained where the examiner manually places an external rotation force on the ankle while stabilizing the tibia to determine if the medial clear space widens on the radiograph.

Routine radiographic assessment of the foot includes **AP, Lateral, Internal, and External Oblique views.** Ideally, foot radiographs are obtained with the patient weight bearing, however, oftentimes this is not tolerated secondary to pain. Specifically, the **internal oblique view** will depict the lateral tarsometatarsal articulations. Both oblique views will also help identify any tarsal coalitions which would be missed on the AP or Lateral.

When discussing imaging of the hindfoot, specific radiographs will provide detailed views of otherwise difficult to visualize landmarks. The **Broden View** allows for visualization of the posterior facet of the calcaneus/subtalar joint. This view is often taken intra-operatively during operative fixation of calcaneus fractures to ensure anatomic reduction. The **Broden View** can be difficult to obtain as the foot/ankle must be in neutral dorsiflexion with the leg internally rotated approximately 30° with the radiation beam centered over the lateral malleolus.

The axial radiograph of the calcaneus is named the **Harris View**. The **Harris View** provides visualization of the middle and posterior facets of the subtalar joint. To obtain a **Harris View**, the ankle is held in dorsiflexion as the radiation beam is directed 45° relative to the horizontal.

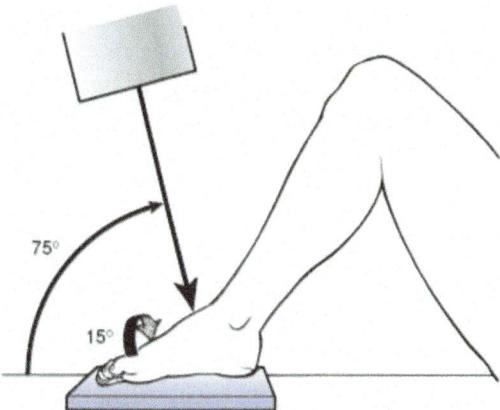

Fig. 3.4 Canale view

Lastly, when assessing fractures of the talus, **Canale and Kelly View** provides a more detailed radiograph of the talar neck. By holding the ankle in equinus and pronating the foot 15°, the **Canale View** can be obtained (Fig. 3.4).

Cervical Spine

Routine radiographic work up of the cervical spine begins with an **AP and Lateral View.** These standard views allow for visualization of the overall alignment of the cervical spine, demonstrating degenerative disease as well as any acute trauma. When obtaining a lateral view, it is important for the patient to be standing upright to the best of their abilities while pulling traction on the shoulders as needed to avoid any interposition or obstruction of the subaxial spine. Due to the natural position of many patient shoulders, a **Swimmers View** can be taken to help visualize the cervico-thoracic junction including the C7-T1 disc space. In order to obtain this image, one arm must be raised, like a swimmer, while the other rests on the patient's side.

In addition to the standard lateral view, flexion-extension views of the c-spine are routinely obtained to evaluate spinal stability. By taking lateral radiographs with the patient actively flexing (chin down) as well as extending (chin up) their neck, images can be compared to analyze any movement or instability. Anatomical landmarks, most often the posterior aspect of the vertebral body, can be compared between the two images to assess for any gross movement indicating instability.

CT

CT, Computed Tomography, is a more advanced imaging technique which builds on the principles of conventional radiographs. A CT Scan generates cross sectional images that are a reconstruction of digital radiographs from multiple planes. This multi-planar high resolution methodology allows for acquisition of a large volume data set in a relatively small amount of time (approximately 10 s). These characteristics make CT scans of utmost value in the trauma setting as a large volume of information about multiple regions of the body can be acquired rapidly.

With more recent advancements in technology, helical CT scanning produces a three-dimensional reconstruction of the osseous structures without additional radiation exposure to the patient. Through retrospective reconstruction of the cross sectional images, the three-dimensional data set can be created. This provides a global evaluation of the structures in addition to the standard **Axial, Sagittal, and Coronal** images that are obtained.

CT imaging, specifically with its application to orthopedic surgery, are most valuable in the assessment of bony injuries as it allows for more detailed evaluation of fracture patterns, severity of fracture displacement, degree of comminution, as well as the articular involvement. Conventional radiographs may fail to reveal an occult fracture or intra-articular extension of a fracture line. Specific examples include osseous evaluation of sacral and pelvic structures, intra-articular joint line depression seen in tibial plateau fractures, distal extension of fracture lines to the plafond in tibial shaft fractures as well as joint depression in calcaneal fractures. In fact, multiple classification systems of specific fractures are based on the CT Scan opposed to conventional radiographs such as the Sanders Classification of Calcaneal fractures (Fig. 3.5).

Fig. 3.5 Roman numerals represent the number of articular fragments while the letters refer to the position of the fracture line

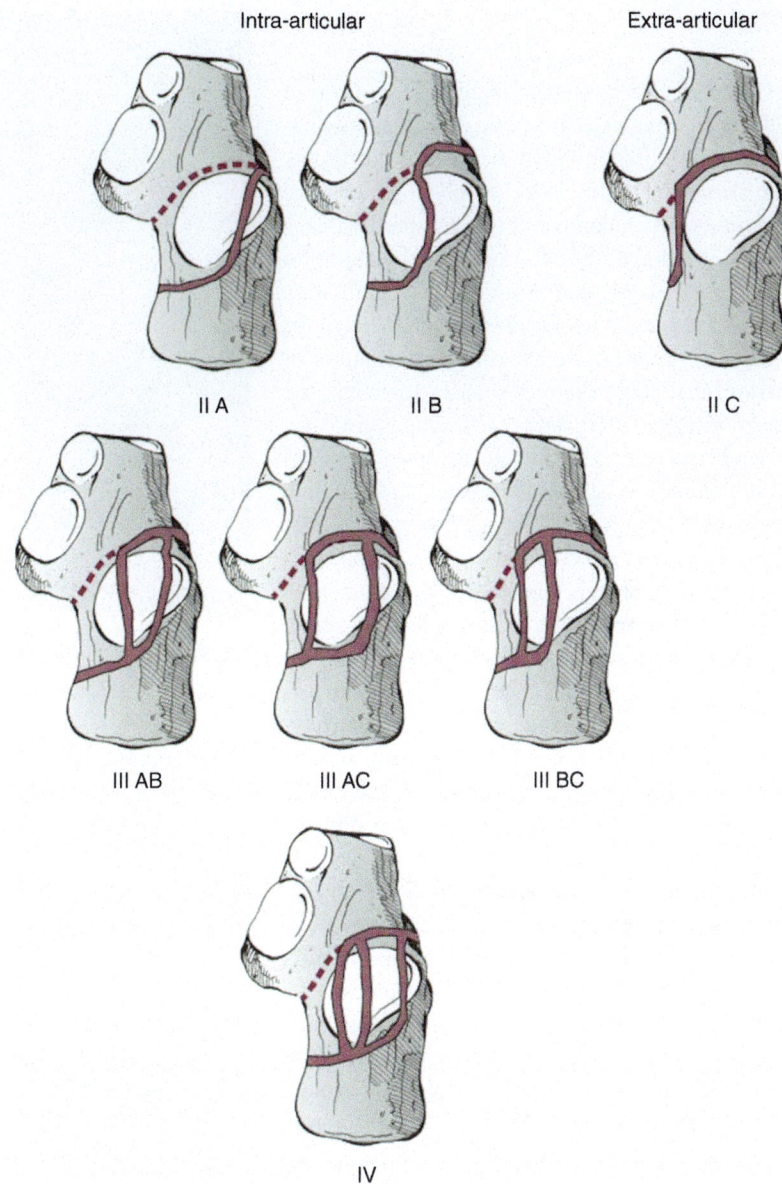

Intra-articular

Extra-articular

II A   II B   II C

III AB   III AC   III BC

IV

Of note, it should be known that CT is most valuable for the assessment of osseous structures opposed to soft tissue (ligaments, menisci, and tendons) or physiologic investigation. There are limited cases where IV or Oral Contrast is used in conjunction with CT scan to evaluate soft tissue; however, this is less common in orthopedic surgery.

In the oncologic setting, CT is vital in characterizing bony lesions. CT imaging will provide information about the extent of cortical bone destruction that otherwise would not have been visualized on conventional radiographs. Understanding lesion mineralization and pattern of bone destruction is essential in the evaluation of osseous tumors, information which otherwise would be unknown without CT. With regard to the soft tissue component of tumors and lesions, CT can demonstrate extension into neurovascular structures; however, this is most often better visualized with other imaging modalities like MRI.

MRI

MRI (magnetic resonance imaging) is a form of advanced imaging that is valuable in the assessment of soft tissues within the realms of orthopedic surgery. Due to its relatively high contrast resolution when compared to other modalities, a major advantage of MRI imaging is its ability to detect soft tissue and bone marrow pathology with great sensitivity. For this reason, MRI is the imaging modality of choice in the evaluation of certain anatomic structures such as ligaments, the menisci, spinal cord, nerve roots, and more.

In broad terms, MRI evaluates the water content in tissues. When tissues are damaged, in both the acute and subacute setting, free extracellular fluid is released which allows MRI to detect this pathology. Based on this principle, tissues with large amounts of water, such as cerebrospinal fluid or synovial fluid, produce bright signals on fluid sensitive MRI Sequences such as T2-weighted images while cortical bone or physeal scar are dark secondary to their low fluid content. Thus, MRI is less useful in evaluating structures with low water content like osseous pathology.

MRI imaging is obtained based on signals detected from hydrogen nuclei as they resonate in a magnetic field. The most common MRI sequences viewed by orthopedic surgeons are T-1 and T-2 weighted images. The T-1 weighted images evaluate the protons species with short relaxation constants (rate at which an excited proton returns to baseline) like adipose tissue opposed to the T-2 images which favor long relaxation constants like water. Thus, fluid like CSF will appear bright on T2 and dark on T1 (Fig. 3.6).

There is a wide range of MRI applications in orthopedic surgery. A good example of MRI clinical application is the evaluation of articular cartilage. Traumatic injuries to cartilage or the subchondral surface, which otherwise would not be visualized on XR or CT, can easily be seen on T2-weighted imaging.

In the setting of a meniscus tear, MRI has demonstrated increased sensitivity and specificity for not only identifying the tear but also high-

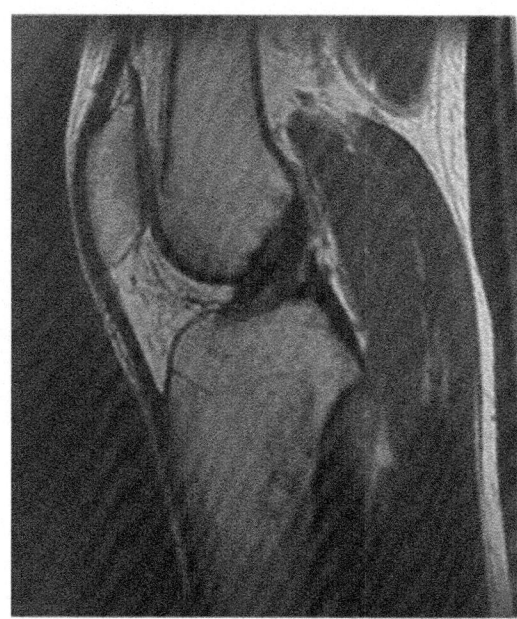

Fig. 3.6 A sagittal T1 image of the knee demonstrating dark ligaments and tendons while the fat appears bright

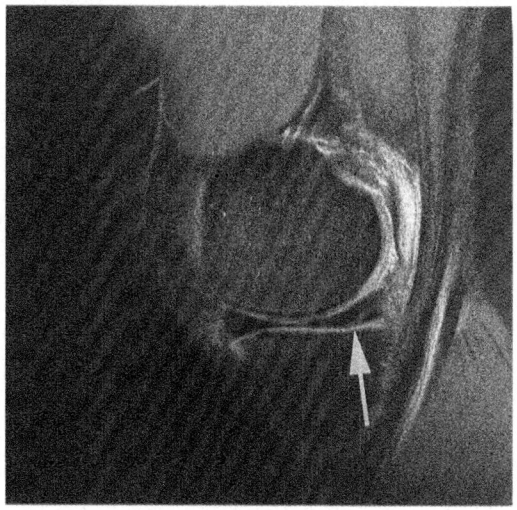

Fig. 3.7 T2 weighted sagittal MRI sequence demonstrated a meniscus tear in the medial compartment of the knee

lighting the precise location as well as orientation of the tear (Fig. 3.7).

A torn ACL is generally easily identifiable on the sagittal MRI of the knee; however, bone bruising patterns may also help diagnose the injury. When a traumatic ACL tear occurs often the posterolateral tibia impacts the femoral condyle. This bruising pattern is seen within the bone marrow on MRI and is termed sulcus terminalis (Fig. 3.8).

Beyond cartilage and the menisci, MRI will help evaluate the fibrocartilaginous labrum in the hip and shoulder. In the hip and shoulder, often a MRI Arthrogram can be helpful where an intra-articular injection of contrast agent helps delineate the joint capsule as well as the integrity of the labrum (Fig. 3.9).

IV Contrast (gadolinium) can be added to MRI studies to further evaluate soft tissue pathology. Gadolinium contrast enhancement will highlight increased blood flow, possible infectious material or demonstrate capillary permeability in an anatomic area of interest when used. This is seen more often in infectious scenarios where there is a clinical concern for abscess formation. Post-gadolinium MR imaging is generally indicated for the evaluation of known or suspected infection and tumors. It can also be indicated for the differentiation of recurrent disc herniation from scar tissue in post-operative spine patients.

With regard to evaluating tendons and muscles, MRI is highly sensitive for detecting injuries. With rotator cuff or extensor mechanism tendon evaluation, MRI is able to identify both partial and full thickness tears. When there is an injury to a muscle, intramuscular fluid collections or hemorrhages will be identified on MRI scans like contusions to the quadriceps or injuries to the hamstrings or hamstring tendon insertions.

This diagnosis of osteomyelitis is discussed throughout the textbook, however, understanding how MRI can aid in diagnosis is of utmost importance. MRI is most useful for identifying marrow and soft tissue edema. Therefore, in the setting of acute infectious etiology within bone, MRI is a sensitive tool, especially within the pediatric population.

Evaluation of spinal pathology relies heavily on MRI. Basic understanding of normal spine anatomy including the intervertebral discs, vertebrae, nerve roots, ligamentum flavum, facet

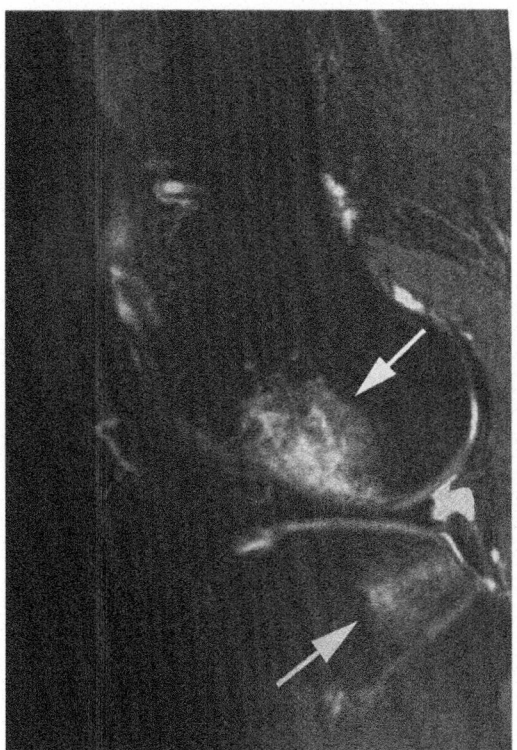

Fig. 3.8 T2 Sagittal MRI shows increased signal in the proximal tibia and distal femur indicating bone contusions in the setting of an ACL tear

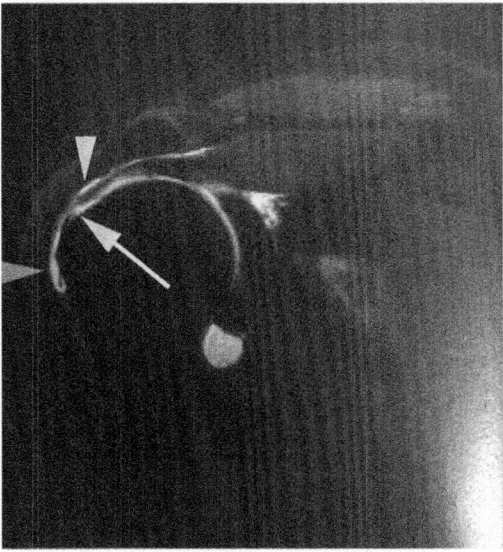

Fig. 3.9 T1 coronal MRI after administration of contrast demonstrating a full thickness tear of the supraspinatus/rotator cuff. Extension of the hyperintense contrast is seen from the defect to the subacromial space

Fig. 3.10 Sagittal and Axial T2 MRI cuts demonstrating a central lumbar disc protrusion

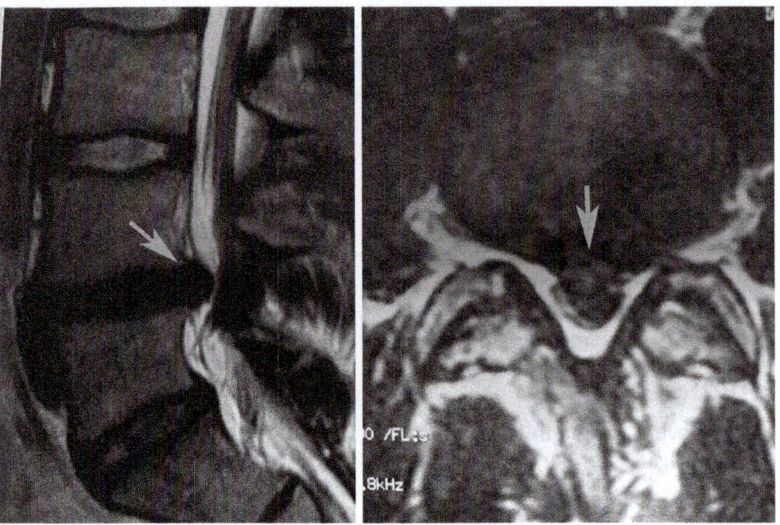

joints, and more will enhance a surgeon's ability to identify pathologic conditions.

The spine is generally composed of 7 cervical vertebrae, 12 thoracic vertebrae, 5 lumbar vertebrae, the sacrum, and the coccyx. The vertebral bodies are separated by intervertebral discs, while the facet joints provide articulations of adjacent vertebrae. Fibrous joints, including the ligamentum flavum, interspinous ligaments, and supraspinous ligaments provide anatomic connections spanning the entire spine.

Disc Herniations represent one of the most common spinal pathologies seen by orthopedic surgeons. Components of the intervertebral disc include the annulus pulposus (outer annulus) and nucleus pulposus (inner annulus). On MRI, discs show intermediate signal on T1 weighted images and high signal on T2 images. The nucleus pulposus, when compared to normal vertebral marrow, appears hyperintense on T2 and hypointense on T1 weighted images. Over time, as patients age and the disc degenerates, T2 signal decreases within the nucleus pulposus and the disc appears dark on all sequences.

When evaluating a sagittal and axial T2 MRI of the spine, analyzing the posterior aspect of the intervertebral disc will demonstrate any herniation or sequestration as well as any other pathology that could be causing nerve root compression (Fig. 3.10).

Bone Scan

In contrast to radiographs, CT and MRI which provide information about the anatomic nature of the structure in question, nuclear scintigraphy or bone scan, provides physiologic information. Bone scan, or more specifically three-phase bone scintigraphy, is a form of nuclear imaging which demonstrates bone turnover.

The fundamentals of acquiring bone scans are based on tissue uptake of radiopharmaceutical agents. When a patient is injected with an agent that emits gamma rays, such as Technetium-99m phosphate, the distribution of the rays can be captured by a gamma (scintillation) camera. The gamma cameras are designed to scan large areas of the body and can rotate to collect from multiple sites of the body. Technetium-99m is the most common radioisotope used given that it is inexpensive, has a half-life of approximately 6 h and its photon energy is easily captured by gamma cameras.

The typical bone scan occurs in a "three-phase" manner: Blood flow phase, soft tissue phase, and delayed/bone phase. Increased uptake is seen in the blood flow phase in areas of mature blood vessels, the soft tissue phase shows increased vascularity in the setting of acute inflammation and bone phase demonstrates sites of bone turnover.

Specific to bone scans, 99m Tc-Methylene diphosphonate (MDP) is often injected as this isotope is sensitive for bony abnormalities. The amount of MDP uptake is based on the osteoblastic activity and vascular nature of bone. Thus, bone scans help provide physiologic information of bone relatively diffusely across the body at the expense of specificity as well as poor spatial and anatomic resolution.

Clinically, bone scan is most useful for evaluating metastatic disease, malignant tumors, metabolic disease, osteomyelitis, as well as stress fractures.

With regard to osteomyelitis, bone scan is a useful tool to help aid in diagnosis especially within the acute form of the infection. Within the first 24 h of infection, radiotracer uptake is generally increased at the site of osteomyelitis. Often, conventional radiographs are unable to detect bony changes early in the infectious course thus proving the usefulness of bone scan. Building off these principles, bone scan is also useful to help differentiate osteomyelitis from another entity like cellulitis or septic arthritis. Increased uptake is seen in all three phases in osteomyelitis compared to increased uptake in the blood flow and soft tissue phase in cellulitis. When compared to MRI, bone scan offers the advantage in that it is able to detect multiple sites of infection compared to the anatomic region scanned during a MRI. This is especially useful in a pediatric patient whose age makes clinical history difficult to obtain while there is a clinical concern for multiple areas of osteomyelitis.

In the setting of metastatic disease, significant bony destruction must occur before conventional radiographs can detect changes thus demonstrating the importance of bone scan in diagnosing disease in the early stages. Although this is a general principle, orthopedic surgeons must be wary as multiple myeloma and purely osteolytic tumors may not produce increased uptake and be viewed as a false negative.

Compared to metastatic disease, bone scan has less use in the setting of primary bone tumors. Although uptake is seen, the area may not be accurate with regard to margins and the amount of soft tissue involvement or extension. Additionally, uptake seen on bone scans cannot distinguish between malignant and benign lesions. Overall, bone scan proves more effective in excluding multifocal disease or metastatic disease opposed to analyzing primary solitary lesions.

The nonspecific nature of uptake seen on bone scans can pose a challenge when interpreting scans in the setting of trauma or persistent pain. Both bony trauma and degenerative osteoarthritis will appear as areas of focal increased uptake. Generally, uptake reaches its peak approximately 7 days after a fracture with return to normal up to 1 year after the initial injury. Stress fractures will demonstrate increased focal uptake.

PET Scan

Positron emission tomography (PET) scan is another modality used to assess the physiologic activity in tissues with the use of glucose metabolism. In contrast to bone scans, in a PET scan, patients are injected with 18-F-labeled 2-fluoro-2-deoxyglucose, which is a marker of glucose metabolism when emitted.

Clinically, PET Scans are most often used in the setting of evaluation of metastatic disease as well as tumor recurrence. Studies have demonstrated increased sensitivity and specificity for differentiating malignant and benign lesions.

In the arthroplasty setting, PET scans have become useful in determining if a patient's pain surrounding an implant is secondary to aseptic loosening as opposed to an indolent infection. It can be difficult to diagnose a chronic prosthetic joint infection if laboratory data is equivocal, thus proving another role for the use of PET scan.

Overall, PET scan is an important diagnostic tool when first line imaging does not yield enough information and a test all orthopedic surgeons should be familiar with.

Further Reading

Domb BG, Tyler W, Ellis S, McCarthy E. Radiographic evaluation of pathological bone lesions: current spectrum of disease and approach to diagnosis. J Bone Joint Surg Am. 2004;86-A(Suppl 2):84–90.

Grissom L, Harcke HT, Thacker M. Imaging in the surgical management of developmental dislocation of the hip. Clin Orthop Relat Res. 2008;466(4):791–801.

Sanders TG, Miller MD. A systematic approach to magnetic resonance imaging interpretation of sports medicine injuries of the knee. Am J Sports Med. 2005;33(1):131–48.

Sanders TG, Morrison WB, Miller MD. Imaging techniques for the evaluation of glenohumeral instability. Am J Sports Med. 2000;28(3):414–34.

Shindle MK, Foo LF, Kelly BT, et al. Magnetic resonance imaging of cartilage in the athlete: current techniques and spectrum of disease. J Bone Joint Surg Am. 2006;88(Suppl 4):27–46.

Court-Brown CM, Tornetta P, McQueen MM, Ricci WM, editors. Rockwood and Green's fractures in adults. 9th ed. Wolters Kluwer Health; 2019.

Fayad LM, Bluemke DA, Fishman EK. Musculoskeletal imaging with computed tomography and magnetic resonance imaging: when is computed tomography the study of choice? Curr Probl Diagn Radiol. 2005;34:220–37.

Genant HK, Wilson JS, Bovill EG, Brunelle FO, Murray WR, Rodrigo JJ. Computed tomography of the musculoskeletal system. J Bone Joint Surg Am. 1980;62:1088–101.

Lee E, Worsley DF. Role of radionuclide imaging in the orthopedic patient. Orthop Clin North Am. 2006;37:485–501.

Abdel-Dayem HM. The role of nuclear medicine in primary bone and soft tissue tumors. Semin Nucl Med. 1997;27:355–63.

Alazraki NP. Radionuclide imaging in the evaluation of infections and inflammatory disease. Radiol Clin North Am. 1993;31:783–94.

Santiago Restrepo C, Giménez CR, McCarthy K. Imaging of osteomyelitis and musculoskeletal soft tissue infections: current concepts. Rheum Dis Clin N Am. 2003;29:89–109.

Delank KS, Schmidt M, Michael JWP, Dietlein M, Schicha H, Eysel P. The implications of 18F-FDG PET for the diagnosis of endoprosthetic loosening and infection in hip and knee arthroplasty: results from a prospective, blinded study. BMC Musculoskelet Disord. 2006;7:20–8.

Wilson JS, Korobkin M, Genant HK, Bovill EG Jr. Computed tomography musculoskeletal disorders. AJR Am J Roentgenol. 1978;131:55–61.

Morgan S, Saifuddin A. MRI of the lumbar intervertebral disc. Clin Radiol. 1999;54(11):703–72.

Skeletal Trauma

4

John L. Johnson and Robert Golden

Introduction

A foundation in orthopedic trauma and fracture care is crucial to understanding the treatment of the musculoskeletal system. Skeletal trauma can be divided into fractures, dislocations, and combinations of these, i.e., fracture/dislocations. A fracture is a disruption in the continuity of cortical and/or cancellous bone. A dislocation is a disruption of the normal articulating anatomy of a joint. Dislocations can be either a complete disruption of the normal anatomy or a partial dislocation, termed as subluxation. A fracture/dislocation is a fracture occurring in or near a joint that results in a subluxation or dislocation of the joint.

J. L. Johnson (✉)
MedStar Georgetown Orthopedic Institute,
Georgetown University School of Medicine,
Washington, DC, USA

Department of Orthopedics, MedStar Georgetown
University Hospital, Washington, DC, USA
e-mail: John.L.Johnson@medstar.net

R. Golden
MedStar Georgetown Orthopedic Institute,
Georgetown University School of Medicine,
Washington, DC, USA

Department of Orthopedics, MedStar Washington
Hospital Center, Washington, DC, USA
e-mail: Robert.D.Golden@medstar.net

Fractures

Initial Evaluation

Initial evaluation of a trauma patient with an extremity injury should begin with a thorough history, physical examination, and radiographic evaluation. Advanced Trauma Life Support (ATLS) principles should be applied prioritizing life over limb.

The history should include the mechanism and timing of injury. The mechanism can yield important information for treatment of the injury in understanding the fracture pattern, risk of associated injuries, and the degree of soft tissue and neurovascular involvement. Important components of the mechanism are blunt vs. penetrating and high vs. low energy. There is a direct correlation between the amount of energy absorbed by the extremity and resulting bone and soft tissue damage. A high energy mechanism such as a motor vehicle collision, or fall from significant height carries more significant risk of injuries to other musculoskeletal structures, head injury, or chest/abdominal injury. Lower energy mechanisms such as a ground level fall are more likely to be isolated injuries with a lower risk of multisystem trauma, and extensive soft tissue damage. However, patients with a pre-existing poor soft tissue envelope such as the elderly may have a significant soft tissue injury despite a relatively low energy mechanism injury. The timing of the injury must also be noted. This is particularly important in the case of a vascular injury and determining the length of time a limb has been ischemic. Ischemia leads to increased risk of infection and tissue loss after 4–6 h of warm ischemia time.

Physical examination of a trauma patient should include the inspection and evaluation of the entire patient to identify any occult injuries as well as a thorough inspection of the affected limb noting any gross deformity and a circumferential examination of the skin. Any open wounds, abrasions, or bruising should be noted. The neurovascular status of the limb should be carefully ascertained and documented. The pulses distal to the injury should be attempted to be palpated. If there is no pulse, this may be due to vascular injury, occlusion due to a displaced fracture or dislocation, vascular spasm, or poor perfusion secondary to shock. A Doppler ultrasound may be used to find the pulse and ABIs (ankle brachial index) documented to better define the vascular status of the limb. Radiographic evaluation should include at a minimum two orthogonal views of any affected bone or joint or any area with any suspicion of an injury, as well as the joint above and below any area of concern.

With a complete history, physical examination, and radiographic evaluation of the affected extremity, the principles described in the remainder of this chapter may be applied to develop a plan for appropriate treatment.

Fracture Descriptors

An adequate grasp of describing fracture patterns is useful both for communication with members of the care team and for appropriate treatment. Though each fracture is different, most of them can be sorted into the following categories. These general descriptors are as follows:

Open versus closed: A closed fracture is one in which the skin is intact over the fracture site. An open fracture is a fracture with a disruption of the skin within the zone of injury of the fracture. Open fractures were colloquially known as "compound fractures." While this term may be useful in discussions with patients, it is not used in orthopedic terminology.

It is important to understand that the clinical and radiographic appearance of a fractured extremity is a snapshot in time. Bones can shift great distances while being fractured; shortening, angulating, and translating. Wounds that appear remote from the resting position of the fracture at the time of patient presentation may in fact have been caused by the bone during the process of it being fractured.

Simple versus comminuted: A simple fracture is one in which there are only two major fragments and one fracture line. A comminuted fracture is one in which there are multiple fragments of bone and multiple fracture lines.

Complete versus incomplete: A complete fracture is one in which the fracture line goes completely across the bone. Incomplete fractures, almost exclusively seen in children, have a fracture line that only crosses one cortex of the bone involved.

Fracture Deformities

A fracture can be deformed in any one of three possible planes. Traditionally, the deformity is described by the relative position of the distal fragment in relation to the proximal fragment. Classic deformations are described as follows:

1. Displacement is the amount of translation of the distal fragment in relation to the proximal fragment in either the anterior/posterior or the medial/lateral planes. Displacement is the opposite of apposition.
2. Angulation occurs when two fracture fragments are not aligned and an angular deformity is present in either the anterior/posterior, the medial/lateral planes, or a combination of both planes. Alignment means that the axes of the proximal and distal fragments are parallel to each other and the joint above and below are in the normal (anatomic) relationship. Angulation is typically described by the direction in which the apex of the angle points— medial, lateral, anterior, posterior, etc.

3. Rotation occurs when there is an axial change between the two fractured fragments in the transverse plane.
4. Shortening or lengthening occurs when the distal fragment is positioned in relation to the proximal fragment to either decrease or increase the overall length of the fractured bone.

Fracture Patterns

A number of basic fracture patterns have been described. They include:

1. Transverse: A pattern where the fracture line is perpendicular to the shaft of a long bone (Fig. 4.1).
2. Spiral: A pattern secondary to a torsional mechanism where the fracture line "wraps around" the bone. This typically results in two sharp diaphyseal spikes on each end of the fracture (Fig. 4.2).

3. Oblique: A pattern where the fracture line crosses the bone at an angle (Fig. 4.3).
4. Impacted or compressed (Fig. 4.4).
5. Avulsion (Fig. 4.5).
6. Complex (Fig. 4.6).
7. Segmental: A pattern where the bone (often the diaphysis) is fractured in more than one location. This pattern is most commonly seen in high energy mechanisms (Fig. 4.7).

Fracture Mode of Loading

The biomechanics that create a fracture can offer some information as to the likely mechanism of injury and clues to other injuries that might have occurred in association with the primary and often more obvious injury. Biomechanical analyses have demonstrated the typical fracture patterns that occur with specific modes of loading:

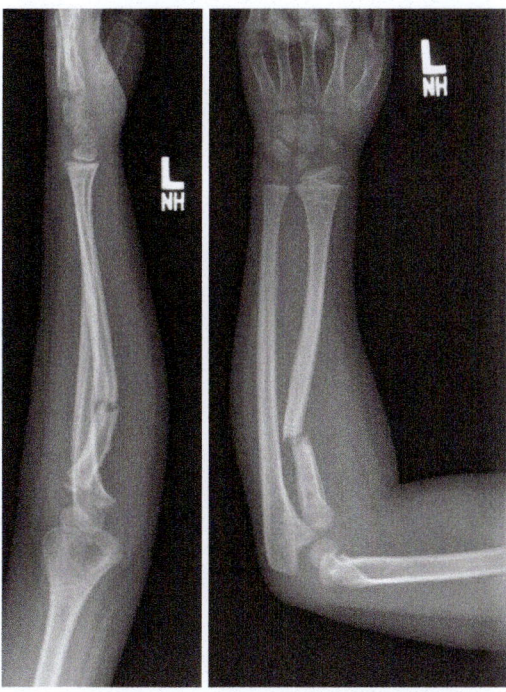

Fig. 4.1 Transverse fracture—a transverse fracture of the radius in a pediatric patient. The fracture line is perpendicular to the shaft

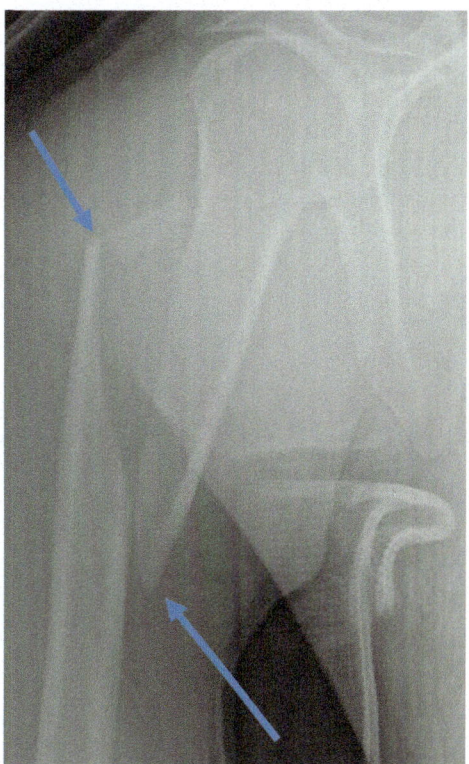

Fig. 4.2 Spiral fracture—a spiral fracture of the humeral shaft. The arrows mark the diaphyseal spikes

Fig. 4.3 Oblique fracture—an oblique radial shaft fracture

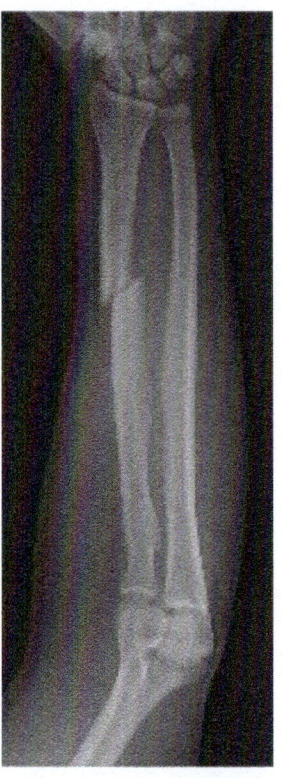

Fig. 4.4 Impacted fracture—a pilon fracture with metaphyseal impaction. The compressed metaphyseal bone is marked by the arrow

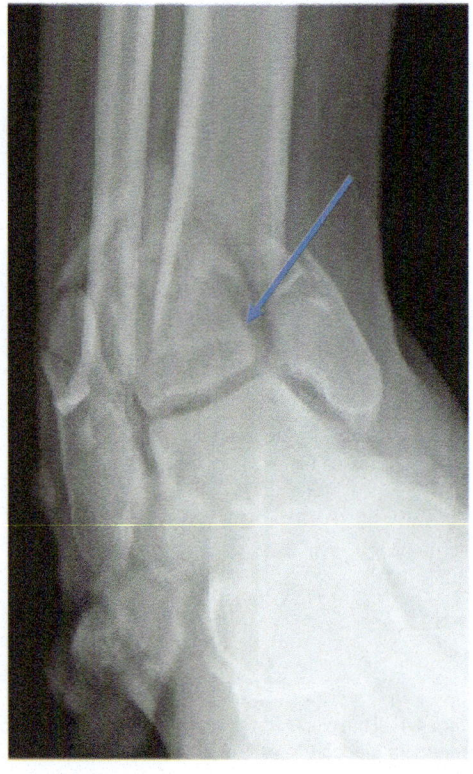

Fig. 4.5 Avulsion fracture—this is a "tongue type" calcaneal fracture. The yellow area denotes the avulsion portion due to the insertion of the achilles

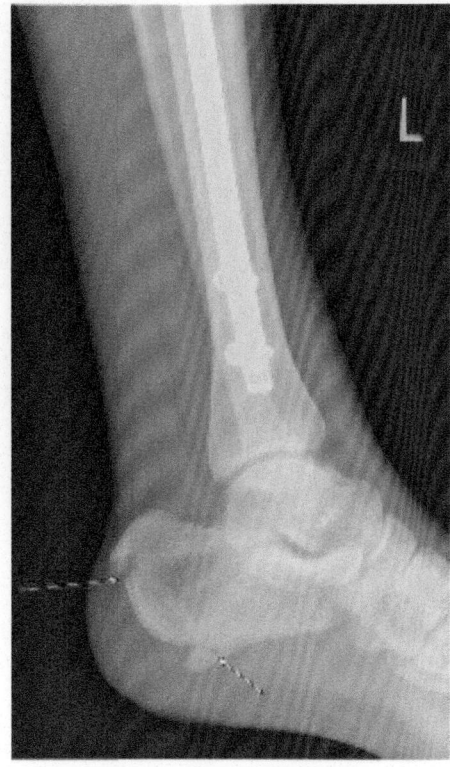

Fig. 4.6 Ballistic humeral shaft fracture—the proximal fragment is severely comminuted; the distal component is oblique

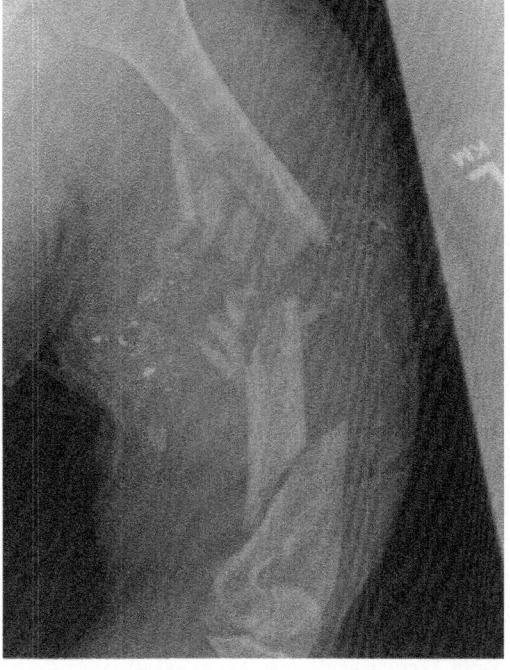

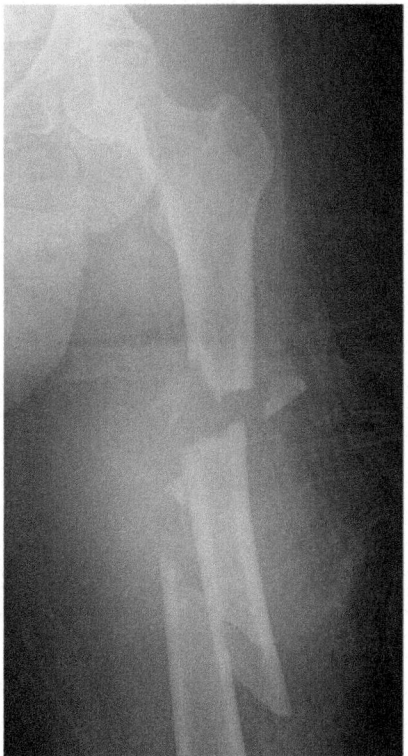

Fig. 4.7 Segmental fracture—a segmental fracture in the femoral shaft

- Bending loading produces a transverse fracture
- Torsional loading produces a spiral fracture
- Axial loading produces a compression or impacted fracture
- Tensile loading produces an avulsion fracture
- Combined loading such as bending and axial loading, which together produce an oblique fracture.

Taken together with the magnitude of fracture displacement and comminution, the fracture pattern suggests the direction and amount of force applied during the injury. From the degree of injury, an extrapolation can be made that predicts the amount of soft tissue damage associated with the fracture.

Soft Tissues

As mentioned above, a number of soft tissues can be damaged. They include the periosteum, blood vessels, nerves, muscles, tendons, and ligaments.

The types of injury involving them are covered in the following sections.

Vascular Injury

Vascular injuries can sometimes be caused by or associated with fractures. When arterial injuries occur, it is always an emergent situation. Vascular/Trauma surgeons should be consulted immediately. Often a combination case in which the orthopedic surgeon temporarily stabilizes the bone and the vascular surgeon restores blood flow is undertaken emergently in order to preserve the limb. Injury to arterial vessels is uncommon because these vessels are elastic and mobile. The vessels can be damaged when they are either inelastic as in atherosclerosis or fixed by soft tissue structures.

One special form of a vascular injury is compartment syndrome. Increased pressure within a fascial compartment can cause muscle necrosis in a relatively short period of time. In the front of the leg, for example, the anterior compartment is bounded by the tibia, the syndesmotic membrane, the fibula, and the fascia overlying the tibialis anterior muscle. Since none of these four boundaries can be stretched, the contents of the compartment—that is, the tibialis anterior muscle among others—will necrose from excess increased pressure occurring after trauma. Muscle necrosis and nerve damage can occur in a relatively short period of time. Early diagnosis is essential. The diagnosis of a compartment syndrome is primarily based on clinical findings although in obtunded patients compartmental pressure monitoring can assist with the diagnosis. The earliest and most reliable diagnostic indicator of compartment syndrome is pain out of proportion on exam, particularly with passive stretch of the muscles in the involved compartment. Once the diagnosis is confirmed, immediate surgical release of the compartment via fasciotomy is required.

Nerve Damage

A nerve can be compressed, contused, or stretched due to a fracture or dislocation. Classic examples include radial nerve injury secondary to fractures of the distal humerus and sciatic nerve injury following posterior fracture dislocations of the hip. The types of neural injuries are as follows:

1. Neuropraxia. Death of the axon does not occur. The most common mechanism is nerve stretch and usually improves by itself in weeks to months. The nerve is anatomically intact and physiologically nonfunctional.
2. Axonotmesis. Axonotmesis is an anatomic disruption of the axon in its sheath. Improvement follows regeneration, the axon growing at a rate of 1 mm a day along the existing axonal sheath.
3. Neurotmesis. This is an anatomic disruption of the nerve including the sheath. Surgical repair is required if recovery is to occur.

Muscle Injury

In any fracture or dislocation, there is always some associated muscle damage. The extent of this damage and the effects vary depending on the direction of force and the amount of energy imparted to the limb during fracture. Rarely complete transection of the muscle belly can occur. More often a partial tear or contusion occurs. Heterotopic ossification is a specific complication of muscle contusion in which heterotopic bone forms within the damaged muscle or in normal muscle after traumatic brain or spinal cord injuries. Certain fractures, such as acetabulum fractures requiring a posterior approach for fixation and distal humerus fractures, are more prone to develop heterotopic ossification than other fractures (Fig. 4.8).

Ligament Tears

Ligaments regulate the movements of bones that form a joint. Damage to these structures are called sprains. Complete disruption can result in a joint dislocation in the acute setting and instability of the joint in the long term.

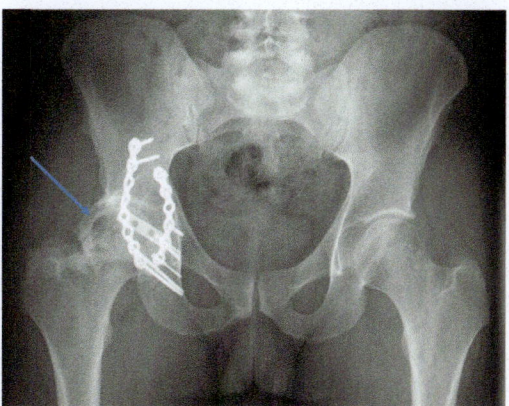

Fig. 4.8 Heterotopic ossification (HO)—the arrow is pointing to an area of HO that occurred following fixation of an acetabular fracture

Age is an important determinant of the injury type that results from the application of a traumatic force. At any given age, the "weak link," or the first structure to fail, varies; it could be bone, ligament, or cartilage growth plates. Once growth plates close, ligaments are the most likely structures to fail in an injury. Ligamentous strength is relatively constant throughout life. With aging, there is a decrease in cancellous bone volume and an increase in cortical bone porosity. With increasing age, therefore, bone becomes weaker; hence, ligament and cartilage injuries are less likely than bone injuries. Thus, the same mode of loading can produce different injury patterns depending on the age of the patient. A lateral force, such as a tackle in football or a blow by an automobile on the outer side of the knee, may cause a fracture through the distal femoral growth plate in a 12-year-old, a tear of the medial and anterior cruciate ligaments in a college football player, and a tibial plateau fracture in a 70-year-old.

Classic Fractures

A number of classic fracture types have been described in the literature. They are defined in the sections below.

Incomplete Fractures

An incomplete fracture, typical in a child, is one that traverses only a portion of the bone. Two variations have been described. A "greenstick" fracture occurs in the diaphyseal portion of a long bone. Separation of the cortex only occurs on the tension side of the bone. The compression side of a greenstick fracture remains intact. The other common type of incomplete fracture is the torus or buckle fracture. This type of fracture occurs in the metaphyseal region of a bone. In a torus fracture, the compression side of bone fails and the tension side remains intact, creating impaction of the cancellous bone. These fractures are almost exclusively seen in the skeletally immature and will be discussed further in the pediatrics chapter.

Stress Fractures

Stress fractures result from repetitive loading. Each load being borne by the bone is below the endurance limit, but through accumulated stress creates a level of force that fatigues the bone to the point of failure. These injuries are commonly seen in the proximal tibia, the second metatarsal, and the femoral neck. They may heal if the cause of the force ceases; that is, if the patient stops the repetitive activity for a period of time. Stress fractures of the femoral neck, especially those located on the tension side of the bone, are predisposed to displacement and are usually treated with surgical stabilization. They usually present as complaints of groin pain in runners. A high index of suspicion in evaluating these patients can avoid catastrophic complications. These fractures are also highly associated with poor nutritional intake and eating disorders. Affected patients should be counseled regarding their exercise and dietary habits.

Pathologic Fracture

These are fractures that occur through abnormal or diseased bone. Among the more common examples are those that occur due to tumors, osteomyelitis, or osteoporosis.

Physeal Fractures

In children, a fracture through the cartilaginous growth plate can occur. The Salter-Harris classification system precisely characterizes these injuries. Physeal fractures heal very rapidly. They may be complicated by complete or incomplete growth arrest, producing shortening or angular deformity of the limb. A complete description and treatment of these fractures can be found in this chapter on pediatric orthopedics.

Intra-articular Fractures

Intra-articular fractures disrupt the joint surface and articular cartilage. Intra-articular fractures can specifically be complicated by joint stiffness and/or the development of posttraumatic arthritis.

Fracture Healing

The biology of fracture healing parallels that of any non-ossified tissue. Fracture healing occurs in three main phases.

1. Vascular phase. This begins at the time of the injury and proceeds through the development of a soft callus. Following an injury, a hematoma forms. The hematoma is infiltrated by cellular elements, which in turn lay down collagen and cause hematoma organization. This is followed by a vascularization, in which the organized hematoma is vascularized by small arterial extensions. The end result of the vascular phase is the development of a soft callus.
2. Metabolic phase. This stage begins about 4–6 weeks after the injury. During this period, the soft callus is reworked by a number of specific cellular elements to produce a firm, hard callus satisfactory for meeting some mechanical demands. There are biochemical changes in pH and oxygen tension during this phase that direct fracture healing.
3. Mechanical phase. This phase begins once a hard callus is present and is then manipulated according to the rules of Wolff's law. Wolff's

law states that bone will remodel according to lines of stress. The result is that bone will be strongest in places where there are more compressive forces. Mechanical stress is required to produce skeletal remodeling during this phase and ultimately to produce a solid, mechanically strong bone.

Evaluation of the Patient with Skeletal Trauma

The complete evaluation of a trauma patient is complex and beyond the scope of this chapter. A number of specific points germane to the orthopedic trauma patient are listed below:

1. History of injury. The mechanism and severity of trauma are important to focus the physical exam and identify commonly associated injuries.
2. Occupation and activity level of the patient. Taking these into account is frequently helpful in determining surgical versus nonsurgical treatment as well as subsequent rehabilitation.
3. Deformity and swelling. These must be carefully evaluated to identify fractures, joint dislocations, or soft tissue injuries.
4. Joint motion. Pain on motion may indicate intra-articular joint involvement.
5. Neurovascular status. It is imperative that the neurovascular status of the extremity be carefully evaluated to document neurologic deficits and to identify surgical emergencies such as compartment syndrome or arterial disruption.
6. Integrity of the skin. Great care needs to be taken to be sure that there is no violation of the skin over the area of the fracture site. An open fracture requires urgent surgical care.

Classifications of Fractures

Fracture classifications are by no means comprehensive or definitive in the description of fractures. Each fracture is different based on the characteristics of the patient, the mechanism, and the overall goals of treatment. An ideal fracture classification has high intraobserver and interobserver reliability, allows for effective communication between members of the care team, and guides treatment. Interobserver reliability is the consistency of the classification between different observers. With a high interobserver reliability, if multiple people read the same imaging, they will reach the same conclusion on the classification of the fracture. Communicability consists of the degree to which the classification can describe the fracture pattern without being able to see the image. How well a classification guide treatment is dependent on how each fracture pattern within the classification can be applied to a treatment algorithm.

Fractures: The Principles of Treatment

All fracture treatments require that two basic goals be accomplished: (1) appropriate reduction of the fracture and (2) maintenance of that reduction. Different techniques may be used for achieving these two goals. Reduction of a fracture can be accomplished by closed manipulation, skeletal traction, or open manipulation. Following reduction, the fracture site must be stabilized so that the fracture will heal in the optimum position. Stabilization can be achieved with external methods such as casts, splints, and external fixators; with internal methods, using various devices such as screws, plates, and intramedullary rods; or through the maintenance of the patient in traction (Fig. 4.9).

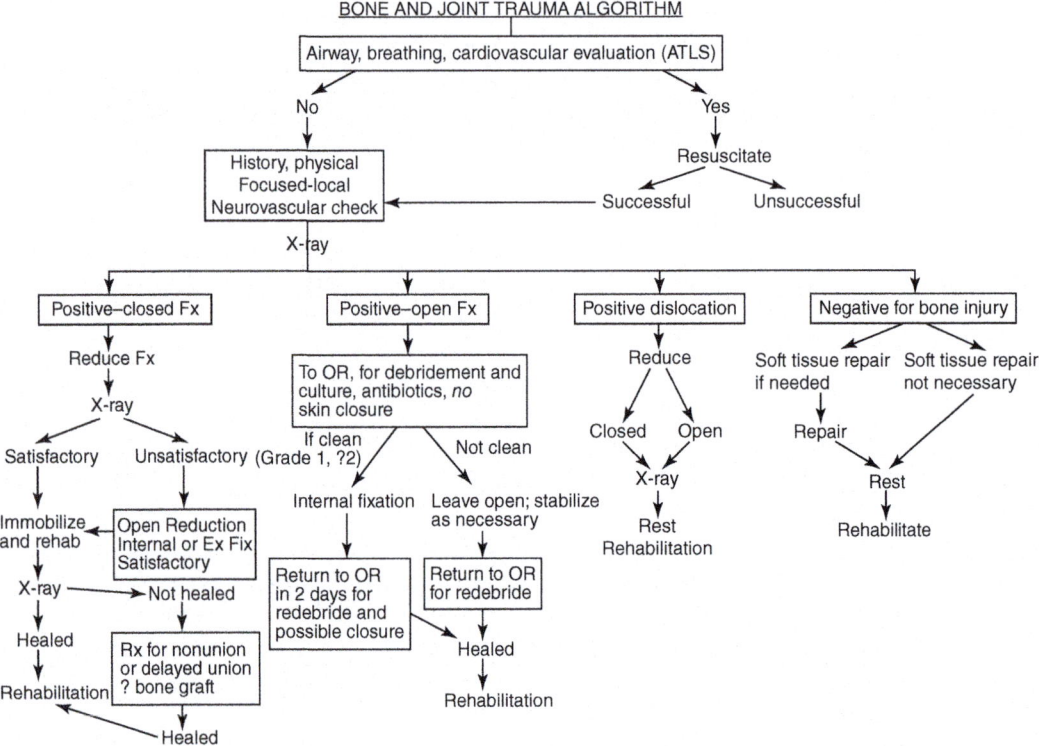

Fig. 4.9 Bone and joint trauma algorithm

Orthopedic Emergencies

There are relatively few orthopedic conditions that require emergent treatment in the operating room. Several conditions may require urgent treatment in the emergency department or trauma bay, though not necessarily emergent surgery. A prominent example is an open fracture. While surgical treatment is nearly always warranted, they can typically be treated and stabilized in the emergency department. One indication for emergent surgery is compartment syndrome which may or may not be associated with skeletal trauma. Another emergency is vascular trauma with a concomitant fracture, which is itself associated with a higher risk of compartment syndrome. Arterial injury must be treated in the operating room as soon as possible to limit warm ischemia time and to preserve the viability of the affected limb. Because an associated fracture will change the natural length of the limb, manipulation of the fractured bone may compromise a

vascular repair. Ideally, such manipulation and stabilization with an external fixator should occur prior to a vascular repair.

Complications of Fractures

There are a number of complications that can occur following fractures and joint dislocations. These include the following:

1. Problems of union.
   (a) Malunion: a bone that heals in poor functional position.
   (b) Delayed union: a fracture that does not heal within the usual time frame.
   (c) Nonunion: a fracture that has not healed and will not heal because it has lost the "biological drive" to heal. In some instances, a pseudarthrosis, or "false joint," develops as a result of a nonunion.

A number of reasons can be found for why fractures do not heal. Excessive motion, infection, steroids, radiation, age, nutritional status, and devascularizaion locally are all causes of delayed healing. Nonunions can be classified as hypertrophic, atrophic, or oligotrophic. Hypertrophic nonunions possess the biology but lack the stability to unite. In contrast, atrophic nonunions lack the biology to heal. Oligotrophic nonunions represent a mixture where minimal callus is seen but it is insufficient to unite the fracture. Recognizing the type of nonunion is important to establish a treatment plan. Hypertrophic nonunions generally require more stable fixation, whereas atrophic nonunions may require bone grafting or other modalities to introduce better biology to the fracture site.

2. Stiffness and loss of motion. These commonly occur following many types of fractures— especially intra-articular fractures, in which arthrofibrosis is known to occur. Additional problems such as bony blocks, loose bodies in the joints, nerve palsies, and posttraumatic arthritis may exacerbate this problem.

3. Infection. Open fractures increase the risk of subsequent infection. Closed fractures treated operatively are also at risk. The use of implants increases the risk of infection simply because they provide a substrate for the microcolonization of certain bacteria. Some bacteria have the unique ability to sequester themselves under a slime-like layer called a glycocalyx, which protects the bacteria from immune attack and antibiotics and makes cultures difficult to obtain. In addition, the presence of necrotic bone contributes to infection risk.

4. Myositis ossificans. This problem, previously mentioned under the heading of muscle injury, is the development of bone in an abnormal location, usually as the result of muscle trauma.

5. Avascular necrosis. This occurs when a portion of the bone loses blood supply and "dies." Certain bones are predisposed to this complication due to a tenuous or retrograde blood supply. The bones most at risk are the head of the femur, the talus, and the scaphoid. If the subchondral bone collapses, the bone changes shape and ultimately arthritis ensues.

6. Implant failure. This is more a complication of treatment rather than of the fracture itself. Placed under enough load or repetitions of load (termed fatigue failure), any implant will eventually fail. Fixation of fractures begins a race between fracture healing and implant failure. Implant failure may lead to a fracture nonunion and frequently leads to revision surgery.

7. Chronic Regional Pain Syndrome (reflex sympathetic dystrophy). This unusual and disastrous complication can be seen after even trivial trauma and causes the development of abnormal sympathetic tone. The mechanism is unknown but may be associated with a partial nerve injury or contusion. The patient develops an exquisitely painful, tender extremity with erythema, bone resorption, and loss of motion. Prognosis depends on early recognition of the syndrome and timely initiation of countermeasures such as sympathetic blocks and aggressive physical therapy. Stellate ganglion blocks are used for involvement of the upper extremity, whereas epidural blocks and lumbar sympathetic blocks are used in the lower extremity.

Principles of Fracture Treatment

The purpose of this section is not to provide an exhaustive list of each fracture. Instead, it is meant to provide a framework of how to stabilize and treat fractures from initial evaluation until fracture union is confirmed clinically and radiographically via surgical or nonsurgical treatment. The goal of treatment for any fracture is to restore length, alignment, and rotation of the bone. This is achieved through fracture reduction. Reduction can be achieved by open (making a surgical incision to visualize the fracture components) or closed (using external manipulation), to approximate the fracture fragments to a more anatomic length, alignment, and rotation. In the case of a fracture dislocation, the primary goal of reduction is to place the joint components into as close to anatomic configuration as possible. Ideally, this allows the joint to remain stable thus minimizing further damage to the articular surface and the surrounding soft tissues. Once a reduction has been achieved, a type of stabilization must be employed in order for the reduction to be maintained.

The most basic means of stabilization include splinting and casting. Casts and splints can be molded with "three points" meaning one point of force is applied above and below the fracture (in the same direction), while another is applied in the opposite direction. This provides a force on either side of the fracture to "hold" the reduction in place via the stiff material of the cast or splint. A splint is a noncircumferential means of stabilization (usually made of fiberglass or plaster) that is used to immobilize fractures. The noncircumferential nature of the splint is meant to accommodate any post-traumatic swelling of the extremity. For this reason, they are most appropriately used to maintain a reduction until a more stable form of immobilization can be applied or until surgery. A cast (also typically made of plaster or fiberglass) is circumferentially applied to the affected extremity. In adult trauma, casts are typically not used as an acute treatment because their circumferential nature does not allow for soft tissue swelling around the fracture. This can increase the risk for

compartment syndrome and compression of neurovascular structures. They can be used for stabilization once swelling has subsided in fractures that are treated nonoperatively to provide greater protection and stabilization than a splint (Fig. 4.10).

Traction is a means of applying longitudinal force to a fracture distal to the fracture site to distract the distal components of the fracture. This employs direct traction on the distal bone segment. With traction applied, ligamentotaxis, the tension across intact soft tissue structures (ligaments) allows for distraction of the fracture fragments. The force applied to the fracture segments via traction and ligamentotaxis then helps realign the fracture and restore length until surgical fixation can be performed. When the structural integrity of a bone is disrupted, it is subject to deforming forces supplied by the now unrestricted pull of the muscles attached to it. The unrestricted pull of these muscles "deforms" or further displaces the fracture segments along the vector of pull as they contract and shorten. In adult trauma this is typically done by means of skeletal traction in the tibia, femur, or calcaneus. A pin is placed through the bone and the skin. Weights are then suspended from either side of the pin to provide a vector of pull to counteract the deforming forces of the fracture.

Fig. 4.10 Distal radius fracture—an example of a well-reduced distal radius fracture with a well-molded splint. Note the dorsal displacement in the injury film (small arrow), and direction of the force used to create the "three point" mold in the reduction film (large arrows)

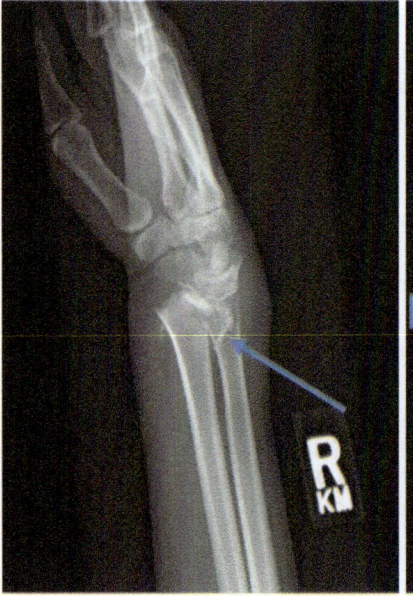
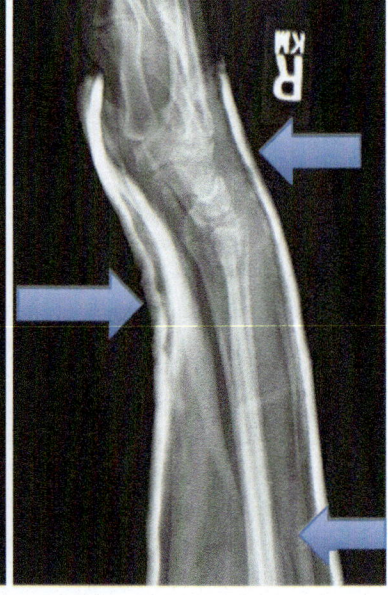

External fixation involves the use of pins placed in the bone along with clamps and rods attached to the external components of the pins to hold the bone in the reduced position. Internal fixation uses orthopedic implants placed on or within the bone to hold the reduced fracture fragment in place. The most commonly used implants include plates, screws, and intramedullary rods or "nails." Each of these methods must be applied surgically and will be described in further detail in the following sections.

Principles of External Fixation, and Damage Control Orthopedics

The term "Damage Control Orthopedics" refers to provisional immobilization or fixation of long bone fractures to minimize the risk of complications such as soft tissue damage, fat embolism, increased inflammatory response or severe hemorrhage. Essentially, the use of less invasive and time-consuming methods of fracture fixation to provide temporary stabilization of fractures to allow time for stabilization of the patient until definitive fixation can be performed. The primary purpose of this is to avoid the "second hit" effect. High energy trauma and shock provoke high levels of inflammation that can progress to a dysregulated immunologic response, the development of organ dysfunction, and ultimately multisystem organ failure. A "second hit" from prolonged surgical intervention may precipitate this process. The goal of damage control orthopedics is to provide stabilization to these injuries when possible while avoiding massive blood loss, prolongation of surgical time, and further aggravation of the patient's inflammatory response. Once adequate resuscitation has been performed and the patient is stable from the perspective of life-threatening sequelae from polytrauma, definitive fixation may then be safely performed.

The primary means of damage control orthopedics is the use of external fixation. External fixation constructs use a combination of pins, clamps, and rods to provide stability to fractures. The pins are placed within the bone at points both proximal and distal to the fracture site to allow for manipulation of each segment. After pins pro-

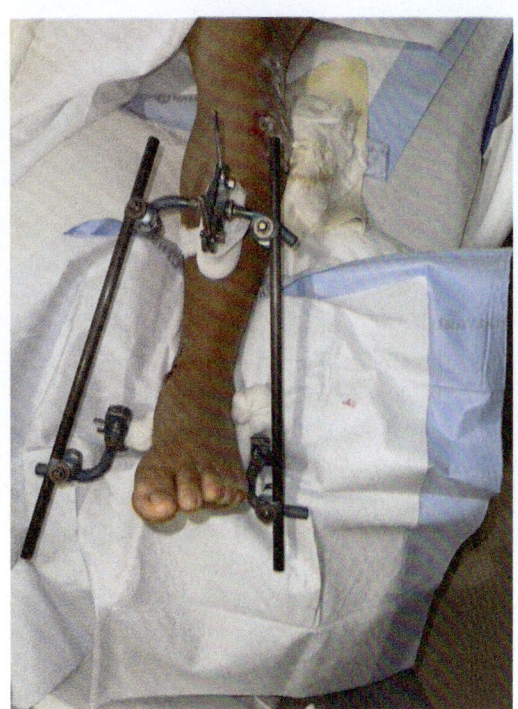

Fig. 4.11 External fixator

vide a direct interface with the bone, a series of clamps and bars allow for manipulation, and ultimately stability of the construct. Clamps can be either simple (one pin to one rod) or modular which allow multiple pins to be connected to a rod. Once the clamps are applied, sidebars, or rods form the link between the proximal and distal bony fragments in the fixation construct. Once the construct is assembled, the proximal and distal fragments can then be manipulated to the appropriate length, alignment, rotation, and joint reduction. Once appropriate reduction is obtained, the clamps can then be tightened to the pins and bars to effectively lock the construct in the desired position (Fig. 4.11).

Principles of Internal Fixation

Open reduction and internal fixation is the most common method of surgical fracture treatment. The core principles of fracture fixation are as follows: Fracture reduction to restore anatomical relationships, fracture fixation providing stability and allowing early motion, and preservation of blood supply to the soft tissues and bone. It is important to understand that fixation devices do not cause the fracture to heal. Rather they provide a stable environment for the bone to heal in an appropriate position through its normal physiology.

With these principles in mind the treating surgeon should consider the type of stability required to treat the fracture and the type of bone healing that the fixation promotes. Absolute and relative stabilities are the two main modes of fracture fixation. Absolute stability limits motion as much as possible to promote primary bone healing. Ideally, this would occur with an anatomic reduction and compression at the fracture site. With this healing mechanism no callus is formed. Instead, the bone uses osteonal cutting cones and remodeling of the compressed bone. Relative stability does not use compression at the fracture site and allows some motion of the fracture components. This promotes healing via callous formation, also known as indirect bone healing. There is a specific amount of motion that will allow bone to heal that can be quantified by the amount of strain present at the fracture site. Both too little and too much motion can result in a nonunion.

Once the fracture pattern, desired type of bone healing, and type of stability have been determined, the next consideration in fracture treatment is the type of fixation that will be used. Plate and screw constructs are one method that can be used to stabilize fractures. Plates can be applied in different ways resulting in different "modes of fixation." Some modes of plating include compression, tension band, bridging, antiglide, buttress, and neutralization.

Compression plating is typically used to treat transverse and oblique fractures. The compression between the plate, bone, and ends of the fracture is generated by screws which engage in the bone. The screw head slides down an inclined plane within the hole, converting the descending movement of the screw into a compressive force at a right angle. Thus tightening the screws onto the plate, and subsequently the bone, compresses the fracture ends together. This mode is a form of absolute stability with the goal of direct bone healing (Fig. 4.12).

Tension band constructs are used in bones that are loaded eccentrically with tension and compression forces and are typically used in periarticular fractures. The plate is applied to the

Fig. 4.12 Radial shaft fracture—this is a radial shaft fracture treated with compression plating. Note the anatomic reduction of the fracture site marked by the arrows

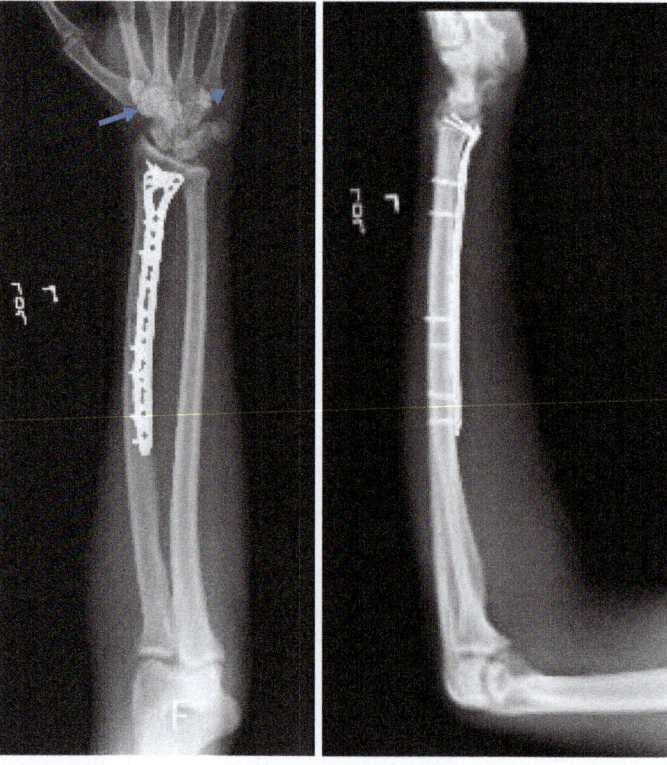

concave (tension) side of the bone. Tensile forces are converted into compression at the fracture site. This mode of fixation is most useful for fractures that have failed in tension such as olecranon and patella fractures. The aim is typically absolute fixation and direct bone healing (Fig. 4.13).

A tension band construct for an olecranon fracture. The tensioned wire (shown by the arrows) converts tensile forces into compression forces across the fracture site.

Neutralization plating is used in conjunction with compression screws known as lag screws typically for oblique or spiral fractures. After an anatomic reduction is made with provisional fixation, lag screws are placed perpendicular to the fracture line to provide compression at the fracture site. The neutralization plate serves to support the lag screws by protecting them by "neutralizing" torsional and bending forces. This is a method of absolute stability with the ultimate goal of direct bone healing (Fig. 4.14).

Buttress and antiglide plating use similar concepts with subtle differences in function to achieve compression at the fracture site. They are placed across vertically oriented partial articular fractures to support or "buttress" the sheared fragment into compression. To accomplish this, an under contoured plate is placed across the proximal and distal components sides of the fragment. With the plate contacting the proximal and distal sides of the fracture, tightening the screws will then buttress the fragment into compression. Antiglide plating uses a similar mechanism but is primarily used to prevent shortening of the metaphyseal or diaphyseal region of the bone rather than an intra-articular fragment. They are combined with lag screws to provide compression. Each mode of fixation provides absolute stability with the ultimate goal of direct bone healing (Fig. 4.15).

A bridge plate is commonly used in comminuted fractures where the individual fracture components are either too small or too complex to be adequately reduced by provisional or definitive fixation. The fracture components are

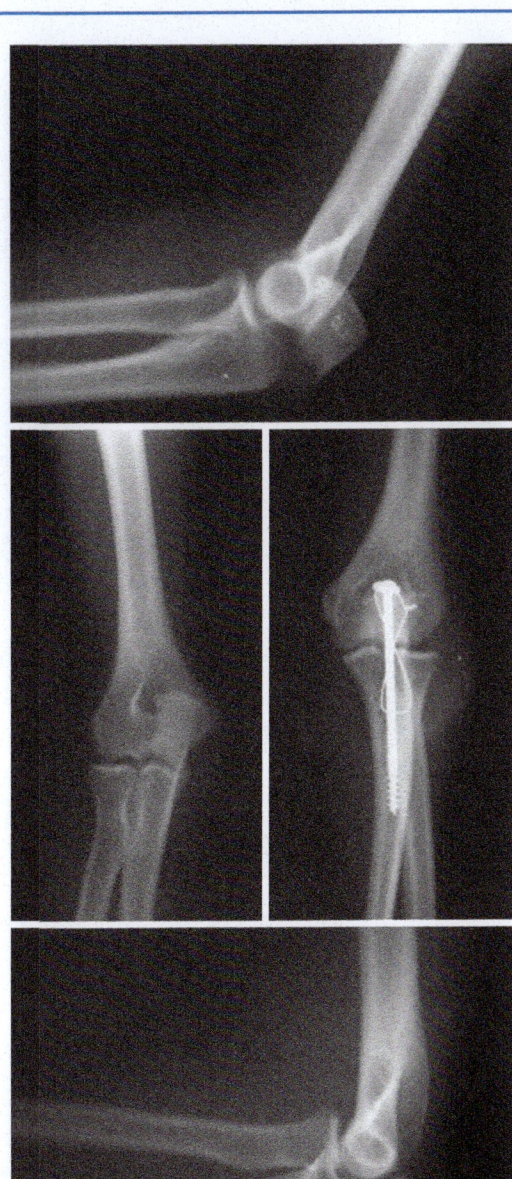

Fig. 4.13 Tension band—this is an example of an olecranon fracture treated with a tension band construct. The wire on the outside of the bone converts tensile forces into compression forces across the fracture site

reduced to appropriate length, alignment, and rotation, and the plate is secured with screws to span or "bridge" the fracture site. This mode of fixation uses relative stability, with the aim of indirect bone healing (Fig. 4.16).

Fig. 4.14 Neutralization plate—a fibula fracture treated with a lag screw and a neutralization plate. The lag screw (marked with the arrow) provides compression across the fracture site, while the plate provides rotational stability

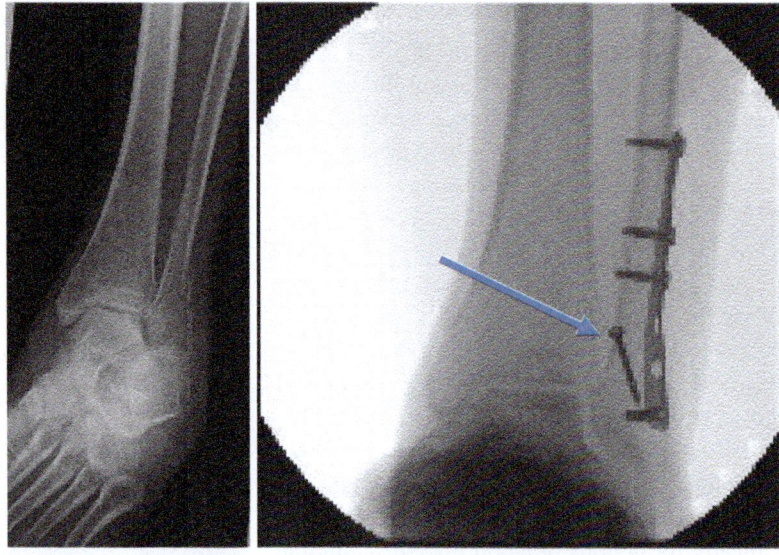

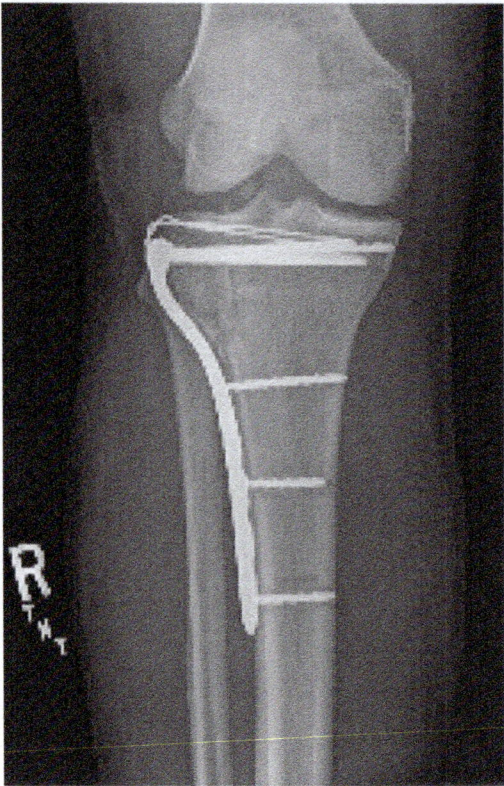

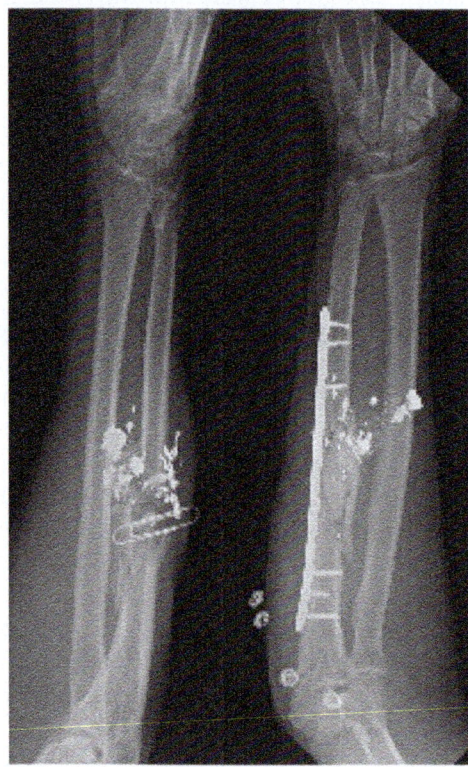

Fig. 4.15 Buttress plate—this is a tibial plateau fracture treated with a buttress plate. The plate pushes, holds up, or "buttresses" the sheared fragment to provide a compressive force across the fracture site

Fig. 4.16 Bridge plating—this plate in this example bridges a comminuted ulna shaft fracture from a ballistic injury

Intramedullary nailing uses similar principles to bridge plating in long bone fractures. Once a nail is positioned across a fracture within the intramedullary canal, the nail is locked in position above and below the fracture site. This provides relative stability, and allows the fracture to heal though indirect bone healing.

Treatment of Long Bone Fractures

Treatment of long bone fractures is centered around providing a favorable environment for the process of bone healing as described earlier in this chapter. The placement of implants via internal fixation is not what "heals" the bone. Implants simply provide the bone with the structural integrity compromised by the fracture to allow fracture healing and remodeling within accepted parameters of length, alignment, and rotation. If each of these parameters can be achieved with nonoperative forms of fracture treatment such as splinting, casting, or bracing, then surgery via internal or external rotation should not be performed.

Treatment of Periarticular Fractures

Successful treatment of periarticular fractures centers around the preservation of the affected cartilage. By preserving as much of the cartilage as possible, the structural integrity of the joint can be maintained to allow smooth articulation of the joint. The basic principles to achieve this are anatomic reduction, stable fixation, early range of motion, and protected weight bearing. Anatomic reduction limits any step offs or gaps in the cartilaginous surface to restore as much of the native joint anatomy as possible. Defects or incongruities in cartilage cause increased permeability, decreased strength, and decreased young's modulus of elasticity of the cartilaginous surface. Reducing the joint as anatomically as possible can never fully prevent these issues, but it can limit the risk of post traumatic arthritis.

Early range of motion serves two essential functions in the postoperative period. First, carti-

lage has a poor blood supply due to its relatively avascular nature and depends on diffusion from synovial fluid for nutrients. Prolonged immobilization of the joint limits diffusion from synovial fluid and leads to atrophy or cartilage degeneration, and decreased proteoglycan/collagen ratio. Range of motion in the postoperative period is thought to mitigate these factors to provide nutrients to the healing cartilage. In addition and just as important, early range of motion limits the degree of stiffness that develops after a fracture has occurred.

Fractures and Dislocations by Region: The Upper Extremity

The treatment of upper extremity fractures follows the same basic principles of anatomic articular reduction, restoration of length, alignment, and rotation. However, the upper extremity has important differences in function, complications, and clinical considerations as compared to lower extremity fractures. The main difference in treatment is that weight bearing is not a primary function of the upper extremity. Rather the primary function of the upper extremity is to be able to position the hand in space. In the context of fracture fixation, and ultimately recovery, the most important of these functions are positioning the hand for activities of daily living. The most basic of these functions are feeding and hygiene. The section below provides an overview of the pathology and treatment of the most common upper extremity fractures.

Fractures of the Clavicle

In adults, fractures of the clavicle typically occur from a fall directly onto the shoulder. Because of the proximity of the subclavian vessel behind the clavicle and the proximity of the brachial plexus, a careful neurovascular evaluation is imperative. There have recently been several large multicenter trials that have helped to define operative indications for clavicle fractures. However, the majority of clavicle fractures can still be treated conservatively with a simple sling. The patient must be told at the time of the fracture that a "bump" or swelling may be noticed after healing has occurred. Not all clavicular fractures heal primarily. If a nonunion develops, it can be treated with internal fixation and bone grafting. Complete healing of a fractured clavicle in the adult will frequently take 3 months or more. Open fractures require operative debridement. Occasionally, the skin is "tented" over a spike of bone and surgical treatment is undertaken to prevent skin compromise. Fractures of the clavicle occurring lateral to the coracoclavicular ligaments may require open reduction and internal fixation if widely displaced due to the high rate of nonunion (Fig. 4.17).

Fractures of the Proximal Humerus

Fractures just distal to the head of the humerus, through the area called the surgical neck, are extremely common in elderly osteoporotic bone. Healing of these fractures, even with some displacement, is rarely a problem. Shoulder stiffness following treatment of this injury may impair function. Recent data suggests that operative and nonoperative treatment have similar functional results. Treatment of this fracture includes early mobilization after a short period of immobilization with a simple sling.

An entirely different injury is seen in the younger patient. Although the fracture pattern may be the same, the mechanism and force vary greatly. The high energy fractures of the proximal humerus seen in younger adults are due to contact sports, motor vehicle accidents, or high-velocity falls. These injuries are often combined with dislocations of the shoulder (described below). Intra-articular fractures of the head of the humerus present a significant problem.

The Neer classification is frequently used to describe these injuries. The classification defines four segments of the proximal humerus: (1) the articular cartilage covered head, (2) the shaft, (3) the greater tuberosity, and (4) the lesser tuberosity. Any fragment separated more than a centimeter or angulated more than 40° is considered as a separate part. Generally speaking, if conservative treatment cannot reduce a two- or three-part fracture, open reduction with internal fixation is performed. A four-part fracture, or one in which the head fragment is split, is often treated by replacement of the humeral head with a prosthesis replacing the broken segments Recently, reverse total shoulder arthroplasty has gained favor over hemiarthroplasty for many patients but is not ideal in the young patient. Inherent to all treatment protocols is an aggressive rehabilitation program to regain shoulder motion. Therefore, fixation must be rigid enough to allow early motion (Fig. 4.18).

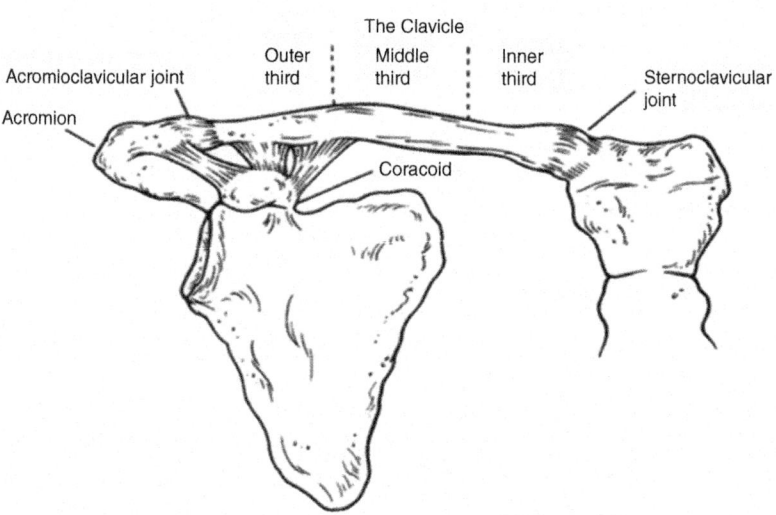

Fig. 4.17 Bony anatomy of the clavicle and scapula

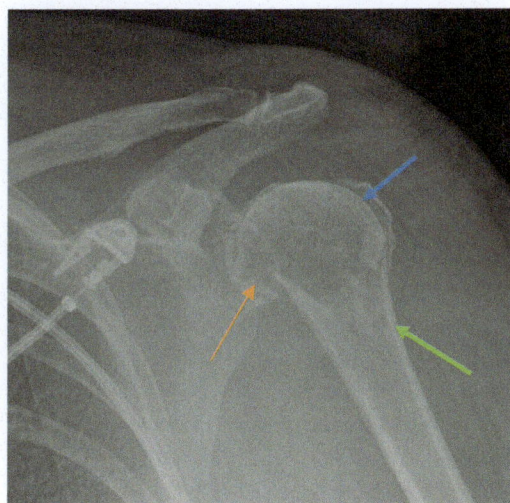

Fig. 4.18 Four part proximal humerus fracture—note the fractures of the lesser tuberosity (orange arrow), greater tuberosity (blue arrow), and shaft (green arrow)

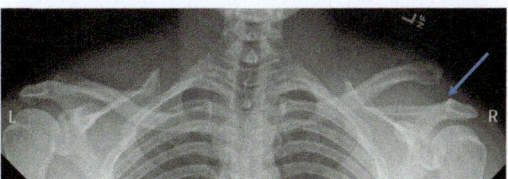

Fig. 4.19 AC separation—note the displacement (marked by the arrow) at the AC joint compared to the contralateral side

Acromioclavicular Separation

An acromioclavicular (AC) separation is a ligamentous injury involving a dislocation between the distal clavicle and the acromion. Such separations are frequently sustained in falls on the "point of the shoulder" and can be divided into six classes. Type I is a sprain of the acromioclavicular ligaments without displacement. There is tenderness in that joint on palpation. A type II injury is a more pronounced deformity of the joint, with some prominence of the distal clavicle felt above the level of the acromion. A complete rupture of the acromioclavicular ligament is present. The X-ray, taken with the patient standing and the arm hanging down with or without weight on it, shows the clavicle to be riding higher, but still in continuity with the acromion. Type III acromioclavicular separations occur with rupture of both the acromioclavicular ligaments and coracoclavicular ligaments (conoid and trapezoid ligaments). The muscles that insert on the clavicle tend to pull it up superiorly, resulting in an obvious deformity. Type IV injuries involve a posterior displacement of the clavicle from the acromion. These injuries are difficult to reduce because they may protrude through the fascia of the trapezius. A type V injury is a dislocation of

the AC joint, with superior displacement of the clavicle greater than twice the normal coracoclavicular distance. Type VI injuries are rare and involve an inferior dislocation of the AC joint. Type I and II injuries are treated conservatively with a sling until pain subsides enough to undergo gentle range of motion exercises and then physical therapy. Treatment of type III injuries remains controversial, with the current trend toward nonoperative treatment. Type IV, V, and VI injuries are almost always treated operatively, with surgical stabilization of the AC joint (Fig. 4.19).

Fractures of the Shaft of the Humerus

Humeral shaft fractures are common, and their patterns vary. Displacement is generally due to eccentric muscular pull with action of the supraspinatus, pectoralis major, and the deltoid determining the displacement of the proximal fragment, The long muscles determine the displacement if the fracture is below the deltoid insertion. Treatment of the humeral shaft fracture has traditionally been nonoperative. Typically, this involves placement of a coaptation plaster splint, followed by a functional brace, as popularized by Sarmiento. The functional brace is a plastic, prefabricated device, usually worn 6–10 weeks. It permits function of the hand while healing progresses.

Radial nerve function must be assessed during the physical examination as radial nerve palsy can occur. Fortunately, most of these nerve injuries are neuropraxias; hence if a radial nerve deficit is present, excellent recovery can be expected although recovery may take many months. The use of plate and screw constructs or intramedullary locked rods for fixation are the primary methods of internal fixation.

Elbow and Forearm

Distal Humeral Fractures in Adults

Intra-articular injuries to the distal humerus are difficult to treat and often result in stiffness and post-traumatic arthritis. Initial treatment is immobilization in a posterior slab splint but the vast majority are treated operatively. Open reduction with anatomic restoration of the articular surfaces and rigid fixation of the fragments to the shaft of the humerus yields the best functional results. The ulnar nerve, because of its location, is at risk during surgery and generally has to be moved from the cubital tunnel during surgical intervention. It is generally agreed that if a traumatized elbow is immobilized for 3 weeks or more a poor result will follow, as the elbow is particularly prone to develop both stiffness and heterotopic ossification. A functional range of elbow motion is approximately 30–110.

Dislocation of the Elbow

A dislocation of the elbow refers to a dislocation of the radiocapitellar joint, the ulnohumeral joint or both. In most cases, the ulna dislocates posterior to the humerus. Reduction of a posterior elbow dislocation is easily accomplished by closed means using manual traction and manipulation. Intravenous sedation and augmentation with local anesthetic injected into the joint is usually adequate for reduction. Radiographs must confirm the reduction. Short-term immobilization for comfort is all that is often required. However, the elbow needs to be examined carefully following reduction to ensure that stability can be maintained. If the elbow remains unstable, ligamentous reconstruction may be required. Following this, active flexion and extension are essential to

regain motion. Any elbow trauma in an adult should be accompanied by a warning that a few degrees of full extension are normally lost, but that this loss will present no functional disability.

Two specific forearm/elbow injuries are often seen. The Monteggia fracture dislocation is a fracture of the proximal ulna with a dislocation of the radial head. It requires not only alignment of the ulna but also reduction of the radial head. While closed reduction is possible in children, in adults the ulna is almost always treated by open reduction and internal fixation with a plate and screws. Radial head position must be assured with X-rays. The Galeazzi fracture dislocation is a fracture of the distal radius with a dislocation of the distal radioulnar joint. This radial fracture is treated by open reduction and internal fixation with plate and screws. The ulnar dislocation may require positioning of the forearm in supination to achieve reduction (Figs. 4.20 and 4.21).

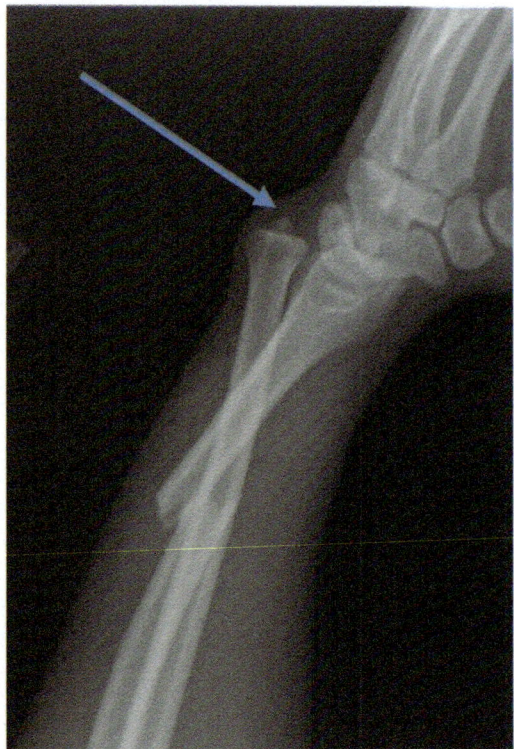

Fig. 4.20 Galeazzi fracture—note the obvious dislocation of the distal radioulnar joint noted with the arrow

Fracture of Both Bones of the Forearm

In children, this fracture is almost always treated nonsurgically by closed reduction and immobilization in a long arm cast. Anatomic reduction is not necessary because of the excellent remodeling potential in children. Six to eight weeks of immobilization is necessary in a child. In adults, because of the concern over loss of pronation and supination and delayed union, operative treatment is indicated. Open reduction of both the radius and the ulna, done through two separate incisions and secured with plates, is the standard treatment.

Fig. 4.21 Monteggia fracture—note the anatomic reduction of the proximal ulna leading to reduction of the radiocapitellar joint

Fractures of the Olecranon

Fractures of the olecranon typically occur secondary to a direct blow. The triceps muscle inserts into the olecranon process, providing extension of the elbow joint. While nondisplaced fractures of the olecranon may be treated closed, displaced fractures are routinely opened and fixed with internal fixation. Early motion is allowed after such a procedure, but lifting must await early bone consolidation, which takes at least 6 weeks (Fig. 4.22).

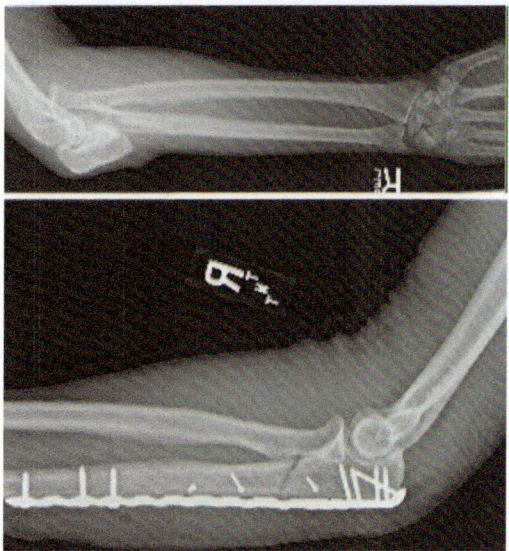

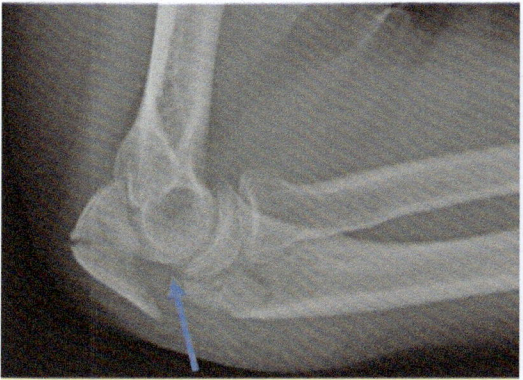 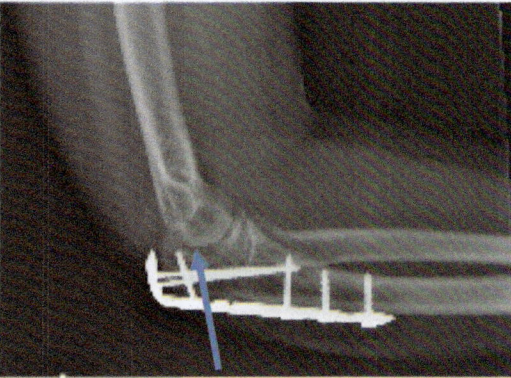

Fig. 4.22 Olecranon fracture—this is a displaced comminuted olecranon fracture treated with ORIF with a plate and screws. The arrows denote the displacement and subsequent reduction of the joint surface

Fracture of the Head of the Radius (Elbow)

This common intra-articular injury usually occurs from a fall on the outstretched hand. When there is little displacement and comminution, and as long as there is no mechanical block to pronation and supination, early active motion is encouraged. For nondisplaced, and minimally displaced injuries, a simple sling can be used for comfort but early range of motion is crucial to prevent stiffness from developing. For fractures with large amounts of displacement and significant comminution, or for those with mechanical blocks to motion, open reduction and internal fixation may be required. For highly comminuted, non-reconstructible radial head fractures, radial head replacement is the best option. Currently, radial head resection alone is not recommended for acute trauma.

A combination of an elbow dislocation, radial head/neck fracture, and a coronoid fracture is known as a "terrible triad" injury. While one should be cautious of using this nomenclature, it is in reference to the challenges, and sequelae of the injury including, pain, stiffness, and instability. The initial treatment is closed reduction and splinting of the elbow but virtually all of these injuries require operative management. This consists of ORIF vs. replacement of the radial head, Coronoid ORIF, and possible reconstruction of the lateral and medial collateral ligaments. To make this determination, the elbow can be brought through range of motion in the operating room under fluoroscopy to determine stability. If the elbow remains unstable after bony fixation, the collateral ligaments should be reconstructed.

Fractures of the Hip and Pelvis

Pelvic Fractures

The unique anatomy of the pelvis presents a challenge in management when it is disrupted. The pelvis is a ring structure of three bones: two innominate bones and the sacrum. They are joined by dense, strong ligamentous structures.

Each innominate bone is formed from three bones: an ilium, an ischium, and the pubis, which fuse at the triradiate cartilage at skeletal maturity. The juncture between the two innominate bones anteriorly is called the symphysis pubis. Posteriorly, the innominate bones join the sacrum through the two sacroiliac joints which are secured by dense sacroiliac ligaments. A pelvis fracture refers to a fracture within the innominate bone, specifically a fracture within the ilium, ischium, or pubis. This is an important distinction with "hip" and acetabular fractures which will be discussed later in the chapter.

The most widely used classification of pelvic ring injuries is the Young-Burgess classification which breaks down the injuries into anterior–posterior compression and lateral compression fracture patterns. The anterior–posterior or lateral compression represents the type of force that was applied to the pelvic ring which ultimately caused the fracture. To classify and treat these injuries appropriately, inlet, outlet, and AP X-ray views of the pelvis must be obtained. The inlet view provides a circumferential view of the pelvic ring and helps to visualize the fracture patterns in the axial plane. The outlet view provides a good view of the sacrum and the vertical orientation of each hemipelvis in relation to the other.

An anterior–posterior compression I injury (APC-I) results in mild diastasis of the pubic symphysis with an intact or minimally displaced SI joint. An APC-II injury has further disruption of the sacrotuberous and sacrospinous ligaments resulting in further diastasis of the pubic symphysis and external rotation of the hemipelvis. However, the posterior SI ligaments remain intact. This is generally defined as a diastasis or widening of over 2.5 cm at the pubic symphysis. An APC-III injury results in disruption of the anterior and posterior ligaments resulting in a completely unstable hemipelvis.

A lateral compression (LC-I) fracture is a fracture of the sacrum and a fracture of the superior ramus, inferior ramus, or both. Often the sacral fracture is minimally displaced but there are cases when extensive displacement of the sacrum occurs. An LC-II fracture is typically a fracture dislocation of the SI joint resulting in a posterior "crescent fracture." An LC-III fracture is a very high energy mechanism resulting in a "windswept" pelvis where one side of the hemipelvis is internally rotated and the contralateral hemipelvis is externally rotated. This creates a lateral compression type pattern on one side with an APC pattern on the other side (Fig. 4.23).

Another type of pattern that can be seen is the vertical shear pattern. This injury pattern is typically from a mechanism such as a fall from height rather than a compression injury. It results in superior displacement of the hemipelvis which can result in a fracture through the innominate bone, disruption of the anterior ring, and SI ligaments, or some combination of each. There are also "combined mechanism" injuries which do not fall cleanly into any of the above patterns but rather represent combinations of them (Fig. 4.24).

APC-I and LC-I injuries are typically lower energy and occur in elderly and osteoporotic patients secondary to minor trauma, such as a fall from a standing position. If this is the only fracture in the pelvic ring, the pelvis is considered stable. Since the overall stability of the pelvic ring is maintained, the treatment is usually early full weight bearing mobilization. The patient usually becomes asymptomatic within a few weeks and fully functional in a matter of 6–8 weeks.

> An outlet view of the pelvis post operatively. Note the view of the cranial aspect of the sacrum, and the SI joints (marked by the arrows) compared to the prior views.

The remainder of the Young-Burgess type fractures predominantly occur following high energy trauma. In these injuries, blood loss is often excessive and should be anticipated. These patients often sustain multiple injuries in addition to their pelvic injury and can present with hemodynamic compromise. Mortality approaches 50% for the most severely injured patients. Initial management consists of maintaining ABCs: airway, breathing, and circulation per standard ATLS protocols. A multidisciplinary approach to care is usually coordinated by the general surgery trauma surgeon when the patient arrives to a trauma center. However, if the patient initially presents to a community emergency department, this care may be coordinated by an emergency room physician or even potentially the orthopedic surgeon, who may have the most experience dealing with traumatic injuries. Early treatment in these severe life-threatening pelvic injuries centers on control of hemor-

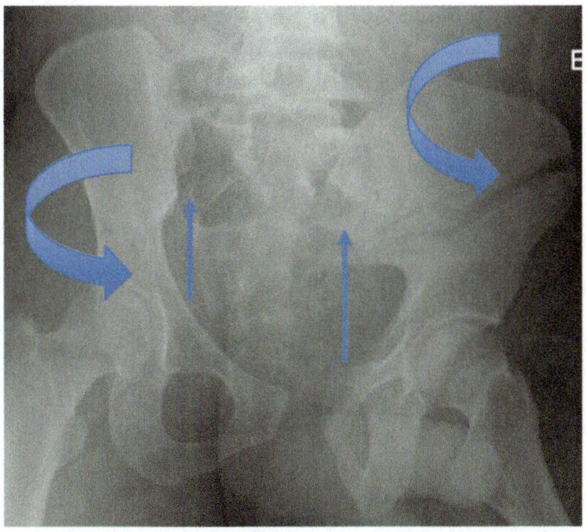

Fig. 4.23 LCIII—example of a "windswept" injury pattern. Note the relative internal rotation of the right hemipelvis and external rotation of the left hemipelvis (curved arrows) and the position of the SI joints (straight arrows)

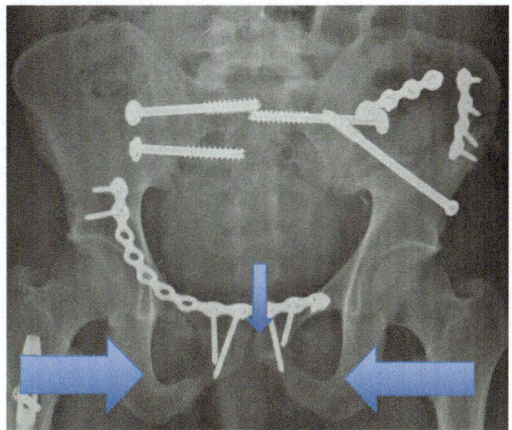

Fig. 4.24 Post-operative reduction—note the symmetry of the obturator foramen (Large arrows) and reduction of the pubic symphysis (small arrow)

rhage, which occurs following disruption of the vast pelvic venous plexus near the posterior aspect of the pelvis. Pelvic binders, circumferential sheets, external fixation, pelvic packing, and angiographic embolization (in cases of arterial laceration) may be employed to decrease pelvic volume, tamponade retroperitoneal bleeding, and coagulate bleeding arteries. Once initial stabilization of the patient has occurred, definitive fixation of the pelvic ring is undertaken once the patient is stable enough for the operation required. This is best performed by a surgeon familiar with the operative treatment of pelvic fractures. Definitive stabilization is achieved through the use of percutaneous screws, open plating, or a combination of both of these methods. Occasionally, an external fixator can also be included in the definitive fixation construct.

Acetabular Fractures and Hip Dislocations

The classic mechanism for a hip dislocation is a "dashboard injury" that occurs from the impact between the dashboard and the knee in a motor vehicle accident, specifically a direct impact to the knee with the hip in flexion, adduction, and internal rotation. This impact drives the hip out posteriorly and can damage the blood supply to the head of the femur as well as the sciatic nerve. The sciatic nerve lies directly posterior to the femoral head. Dislocations of the hip are surgical emergencies. Early reduction decreases the incidence of osteonecrosis of the femoral head. Following reduction, radiographs of the hip and pelvis should be obtained as well as a CT scan of the pelvis. Furthermore, if a fracture is present, the affected leg should be placed in femoral traction.

Fractures of the ilium involving the articular surface of the "socket" of the hip joint are known as acetabular fractures. This results in a disrup-

tion of the articular cartilage of the acetabulum, and disruption of the anterior and/or posterior columns of the pelvis, and the anterior or posterior walls of the acetabulum. These injuries are predominantly high energy in young patients but can be relatively low energy in elderly patients. They can also be associated with a comorbid dislocation of the hip joint. These can occur by a similar mechanism as pure hip dislocations, often as a result of a motor vehicle crash. If a hip dislocation is present, reduction principles as outlined above should be followed. After a reduction is achieved in the case of a fracture dislocation involving the acetabulum, a femoral traction pin should be placed to maintain reduction of the hip joint and immobilize it until the fracture can be treated operatively to avoid pressure on the broken fragments of the joint. A series of Judet films consisting of anterior–posterior, iliac-oblique and obturator oblique X-rays should be obtained. This series of radiographs is used to evaluate the columns and walls of the pelvis and acetabulum, respectively. The Iliac-oblique film is most useful to evaluate the posterior column of the pelvis and the anterior wall of the acetabulum. Conversely, the obturator oblique view is used to evaluate the posterior wall of the acetabulum and the anterior column of the pelvis. Three-dimensional computed tomography is also important to obtain in these fractures to further evaluate the three-dimensional nature of the injury and the anatomy of the surrounding pelvis. Because of the high energy nature of these injuries, they often occur in polytraumatized patients with associated injuries such as rib fractures, closed head injuries, and intra-abdominal injuries. As such, the orthopedic team should work closely with the general trauma team in the care of affected patients and for perioperative planning. As with pelvic ring injuries, the treatment of high energy acetabular fractures is complex and generally performed by orthopedic traumatologists (Fig. 4.25).

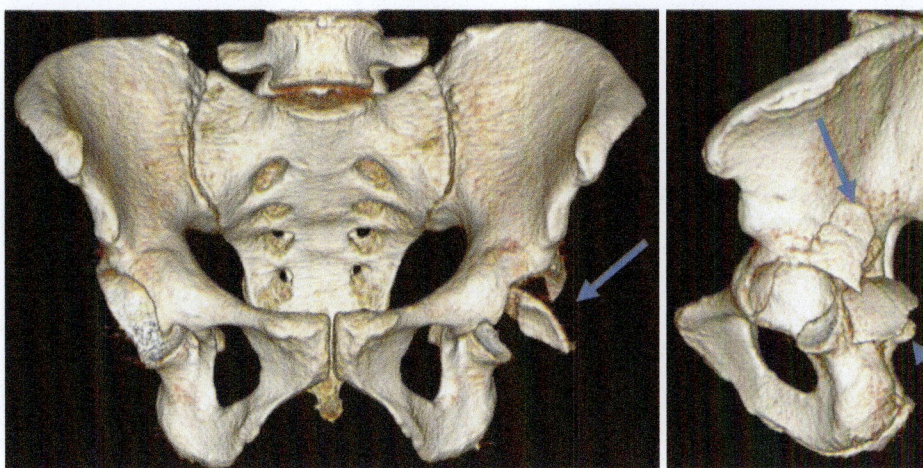

Fig. 4.25 Three-dimensional CT reconstruction—note the posterior wall fracture of the acetabulum (arrows)

Hip Fractures

A "hip fracture" truly refers to a fracture of the proximal femur. The main three hip fractures are femoral neck fractures, intertrochanteric fractures, and subtrochanteric fractures. These are classified based on the region of the proximal femur where the fracture occurs, and treatment varies accordingly.

Femoral Neck Fractures

The neck of the femur is surrounded by the joint capsule. The capsule contains the veins and arteries that are the blood supply to the femoral head. The blood supply to the head is tenuous. It originates from the medial and lateral femoral circumflex arteries at the base of the femoral neck and the extracapsular arterial ring. These vessels nourish the head of the femur. Any disruption of the femoral neck is likely to interfere with the blood supply of the head of the femur. This makes fractures of the femoral neck subject to two problems: avascular necrosis of the femoral head and nonunion. Avascular necrosis occurs in more than one-third of displaced femoral neck fractures. Nonunion is related to the compromised blood supply and the instability of some femoral neck fracture patterns.

Patients with femoral neck fractures present with a shortened, externally rotated limb and have severe pain with log rolling of the limb and with axial loading. Similar to pelvic fractures, femoral neck fractures result from two broad types of injuries: those occurring in young people after high energy trauma and those in elderly patients after simple falls. Femoral neck fractures in young patients should be treated urgently in the operating room. Anatomic reduction and fixation help decrease the likelihood of osteonecrosis. The location and displacement of these fractures help to determine their proper treatment. The goal is to preserve the young patient's native femoral head. Quality of reduction is the most important factor in the prevention of osteonecrosis. However, osteonecrosis, femoral head collapse, and osteoarthritis of the hip joint may still result (Fig. 4.26).

A diagram of the anatomic classification of femoral neck fractures.

Displacement is important to note. In elderly patients, nondisplaced fractures are typically treated with percutaneous screw fixation and protected weight bearing. Displaced fractures are typically treated with hemiarthroplasty or total hip arthroplasty. The indications for total hip arthroplasty in patients with hip fractures include preexisting hip osteoarthritis and an active lifestyle.

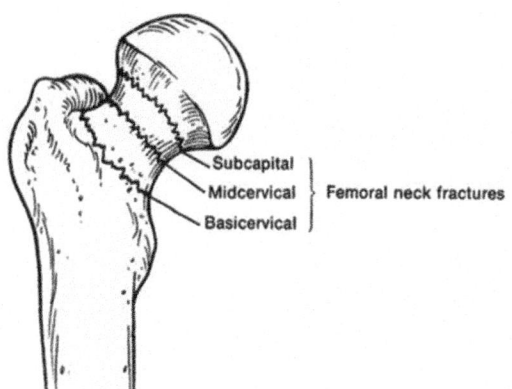

Fig. 4.26 Anatomic location of femoral neck fractures

Nonoperative treatment of femoral neck fractures in elderly patients is reserved for only those special circumstances where the patient is too sick for surgery. Nonoperative treatment carries a 1-year mortality of up to 80% due to the complications of prolonged bed rest including: urinary tract sepsis, pneumonia, deep vein thrombosis, pulmonary embolism, and decubitus ulcers. Even with operative treatment in ideal candidates, in-hospital mortality after femoral neck fracture approaches 3%, and 1-year mortality may reach 20%.

Intertrochanteric Fractures

These femoral fractures occur between the greater and lesser trochanter and lie *outside* the hip joint capsule. The blood supply to the femoral head is therefore not jeopardized by the fracture. On physical examination in the emergency room, these patients, similar to those with displaced femoral neck fractures, will manifest with shortening and external rotation of the limb. Operative fixation is the norm, and multiple options are available. The compression hip screw with side plate and the cephalomedullary nail are the most common devices. Healing of intertrochanteric fractures generally does not suffer from the same issues as femoral neck fractures assuming the overall anatomic alignment is restored as large areas of cancellous bone are loaded in compression by the fracture anatomy and subsequent fixation devices.

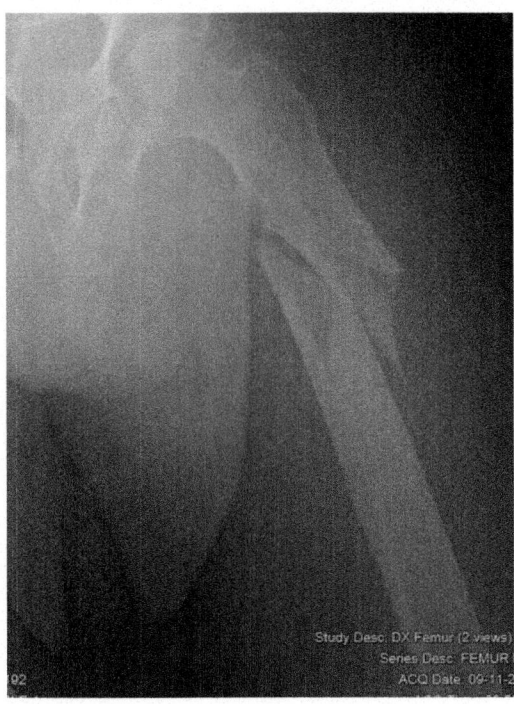

Fig. 4.27 Subtrochanteric femur fracture—this is a displaced subtrochanteric fracture. Note that the relative flexion and abduction of the proximal fragment relative to the distal fragment

Subtrochanteric Fractures

These fractures occur distal to the lesser trochanter. They are characterized by their typical deformation pattern, which includes flexion and abduction of the proximal fragment, with adduction and shortening of the distal fragment. The pull of the iliopsoas and abductors deform the proximal fragment, while the adductors displace the distal fragment. In the younger population, subtrochanteric fractures usually follow the severe trauma of motor vehicle accidents. In the elderly, they are due to osteoporosis or a pathologic process in the subtrochanteric area. With low-energy mechanisms, transverse subtrochanteric fractures should be considered pathologic until proven otherwise. Fixation is generally accomplished using an intramedullary nail with proximal and distal locking screws (Fig. 4.27).

Fig. 4.28 Midshaft Femur Fracture-This comminuted fracture was treated with a femoral nail

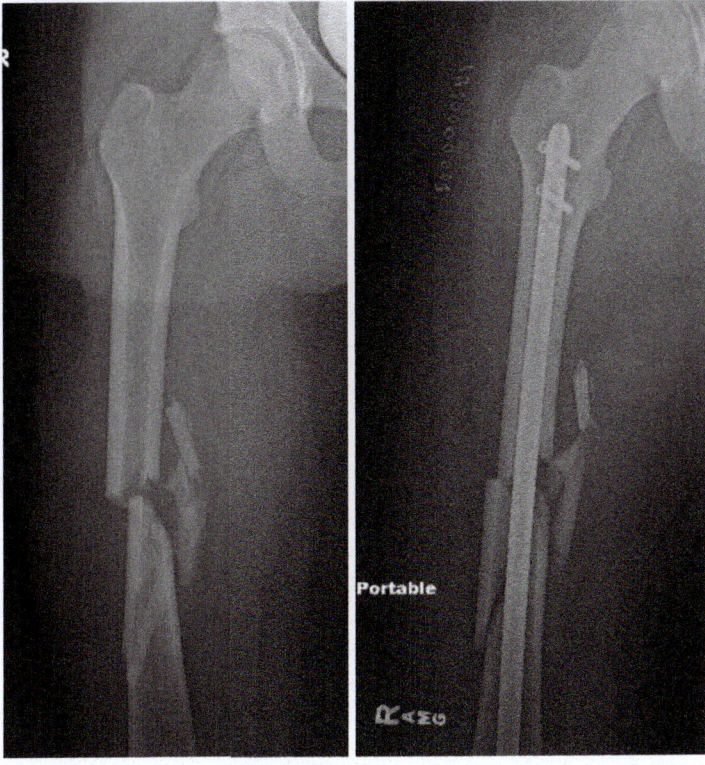

Femoral Shaft Fractures

Femoral shaft fractures most commonly occur secondary to high energy mechanisms. AP and lateral radiographs of the entire femur should be obtained including radiographs of the hip and knee. A common associated injury is an ipsilateral hip fracture. It is critical for this to be ruled out with a standardized protocol often involving a CT scan of the hip or pelvis so that an occult fracture is not missed. In adults, these fractures are almost always treated with intramedullary nails locked proximally and distally to the fracture site. Inserted using minimally open techniques, these devices share load with the bone, thereby stimulating biologic drive for fracture healing and allowing the patient to bear weight as tolerated. Important factors in the intraoperative and postoperative period are evaluating the length, alignment, and rotation of the bone, obtaining fluoroscopic imaging of the ipsilateral hip to evaluate a possible femoral neck fracture, and assessing ligamentous stability of the knee. A comorbid femoral neck fracture should be treated with either open or closed reduction and internal fixation (Fig. 4.28).

Fractures About the Knee

Distal Femoral Fractures

Fractures of the lower end of the femur in the region of the condyles may be supra condylar or Y- or T-shaped, the latter types entering the joint. If displaced, these fractures are treated surgically, with the goal being to obtain an anatomic reduction of the articular surfaces. The reconstructed articular surface is then affixed to the distal femoral shaft. Anatomic restoration is necessary to prevent significant traumatic arthritis of the knee. Rigid fixation is necessary to allow early motion. Weight bearing is delayed for 3 months, but early motion begins within a couple of days of the fixation process. These fractures often encounter difficulty healing and can have a prolonged time course for complete healing.

Fractures of the Tibial Plateau

Tibial plateau fractures involve the intra-articular surface of the proximal aspect of the tibia. They can involve the lateral side in isolation, the medial side in isolation, or a combination of both. Frequently, they are the result of "bumper injuries" after a valgus load when a pedestrian is struck by the bumper of a car. They can result, however, from any type of traumatic loading of the knee joint. A well-established classification system named after the orthopedic surgeon Joseph Schatzker is widely used to describe these fractures. Treatment depends on the degree of displacement and comminution. Nondisplaced fractures may be treated by restricting weight bearing and initiating early motion. Displaced fractures are best treated surgically, including anatomic reduction of the articular surface and stable fixation to the shaft of the tibia.

Early motion is begun after definitive fixation, but full weight bearing should be delayed for 8–12 weeks. The most important distinctions for tibial plateau fractures are whether the fracture is unicondylar or bicondylar, and if the medial aspect of the plateau is affected. Unicondylar plateau fractures typically affect the lateral plateau, are more commonly low energy mechanisms, and often do not require urgent surgical treatment if the knee is otherwise stable. A tibial plateau fracture with a fracture line through the medial plateau is typically due to a higher energy mechanism. These fracture patterns are considered to be a knee dislocation equivalent with higher risk of neurovascular injury and compartment syndrome. If a medial component is seen on imaging, ankle brachial indices should be obtained in the emergency department, and the fracture would be immobilized with an external fixator to allow for soft tissues to become amenable to definitive fixation. After external fixation, a CT scan should be obtained for preoperative planning (Fig. 4.29).

Fractures of the Patella

The patella is a sesamoid bone that gives the quadriceps mechanism a mechanical advantage in knee extension. If the fracture is nondisplaced, or does not affect the extensor mechanism, closed treatment with immobilization for up to 6 weeks can be performed. However, for displaced frac-

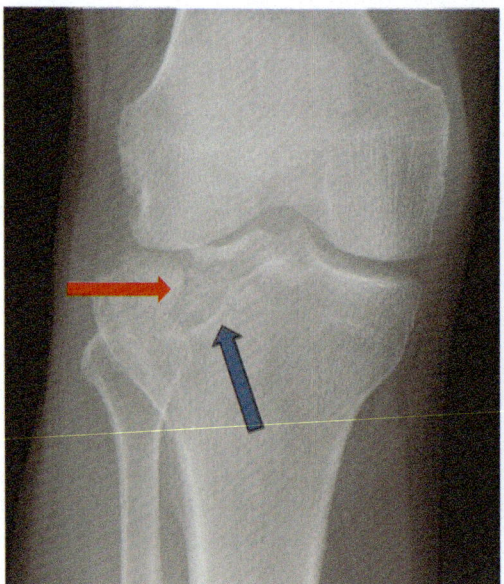
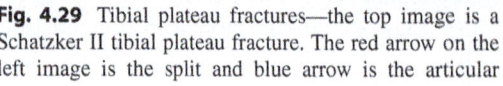
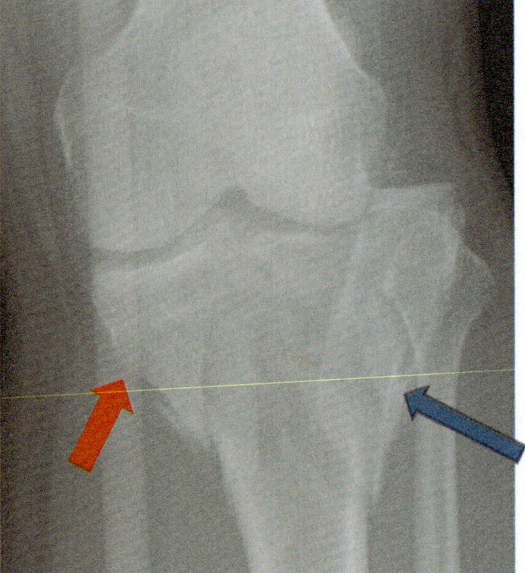

Fig. 4.29 Tibial plateau fractures—the top image is a Schatzker II tibial plateau fracture. The red arrow on the left image is the split and blue arrow is the articular depression. On the right image the red arrow shows the medial piece and the blue shows the lateral piece

tures open reduction and internal fixation is the treatment of choice. As in the fracture of the olecranon, a tension-banding procedure can achieve reliable fixation, but many other constructs involving screws and plates can also be effective. In extremely comminuted fractures, a patellectomy may be the only option to avoid an irregular patellar surface that would result in painful traumatic arthritis of the patellofemoral joint.

Dislocation of the Knee

This injury is often the result of very severe trauma, although can sometimes occur in bariatric patients with otherwise relatively minor falls. When a patient gives a history that the "knee came out of place," the injury is usually not a knee dislocation but rather a patella dislocation or anterior cruciate ligament tear. True dislocation of the knee is a very serious injury notable for a high risk of vascular injury to the popliteal vessels. The popliteal artery is fixed anatomically at the level of the proximal tibia by the interosseous membrane and, therefore, is at great risk when the knee dislocates. Careful physical exam should be performed including a full vascular exam with evaluation of pulses and ABIs. Arteriography can be performed following immediate closed reduction of the dislocation if vascular compromise is suspected. The results of angiography will then determine whether consultation of the vascular surgery team and arterial repair is necessary. If gross instability is present following this injury, an external fixator bridging the knee may be necessary until definitive ligament repair can be performed. Multiple ligament injuries are the norm after knee dislocations. Ligamentous repair/reconstruction is usually necessary after early emergent reduction, external fixation, and vascular management have been accomplished.

Fracture of the Tibial Shaft

Fractures of the tibial shaft are one of the classic fractures in the treatment of long bone injuries and open fractures. Because of its vulnerable location just beneath the skin throughout its length and association with high energy mechanisms, it is prone to open fractures. Because of its tenuous blood supply, open fractures of the tibia are at risk for nonunion. A particular area of concern is at the junction of the middle and distal thirds where a vascular watershed exists, and the muscle envelope is deficient over the anteromedial surface of the bone. The time to fracture union is prolonged, generally taking 16–20 weeks. Nondisplaced or minimally displaced tibial fractures can be treated by the application of a long leg cast. When early healing has occurred, a shorter, the so-called patella tendon bearing cast may be applied. Operative treatment options include percutaneous or open plating, external fixation, and intramedullary nailing. As with long bone fractures in other locations, intramedullary nailing allows relatively early weight bearing and functional return and is generally considered the surgical treatment of choice if the fracture pattern is amenable to its use (Fig. 4.30).

Ankle and Tibial Plafond Fractures

Fractures of the malleoli are termed "ankle" fractures by convention and involve the distal end of the fibula (lateral malleolus), the medial malleolus, and the posterior malleolus of the tibia. The mechanism of injury for these fractures is a torsional force applied to the ankle. Radiographic evaluation of these fractures should include an AP, lateral, and mortise view of the ankle. The mortise view is an oblique view with 15° of internal rotation which provides an en face view of the ankle joint (Fig. 4.31).

A CT scan is typically not required for a simple ankle fracture. A commonly used system for ankle fractures is the Lauge-Hansen classification system which is specific to bi-malleolar fractures of the medial and lateral malleoli. The first word in each category describes the position of foot at the time the force was applied. The second word denotes the anatomic direction of the load (Fig. 4.32).

This system is based on cadaver study and likely does not apply adequately to all fractures. It also has limited value in directing treatment. A

Fig. 4.30 Tibial Shaft
Fracture Treated with an
intramedullary (IM) nail

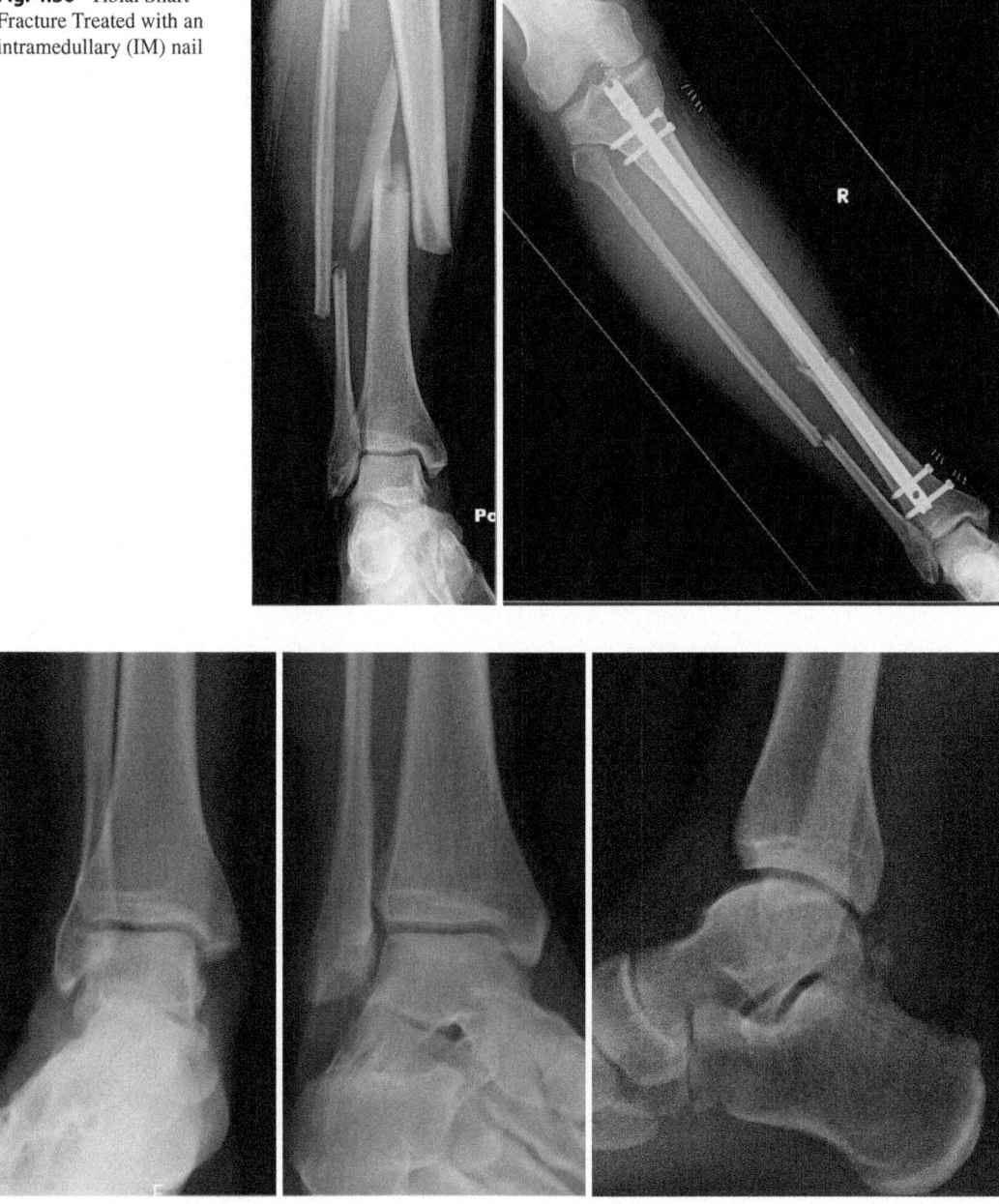

Fig. 4.31 Ankle X-rays-These X-rays are a typical ankle series with a normal appearance. The top left is an AP view, the top right is a mortise view, and the bottom is a lateral view

ubiquitous classification specific to fibula frac-tures is the Weber classification which is strati-fied into A-a fracture distal to the syndesmosis, B-a fracture at the level of the syndesmosis, and C-a fracture proximal to the syndesmosis (Fig. 4.33).

While a nondisplaced fracture of the lateral malleolus with a stable ankle joint may be treated by a simple below-the-knee cast or sometimes a fracture boot, displaced ankle fractures with an unstable ankle joint are typically treated with open reduction and internal fixation. The primary

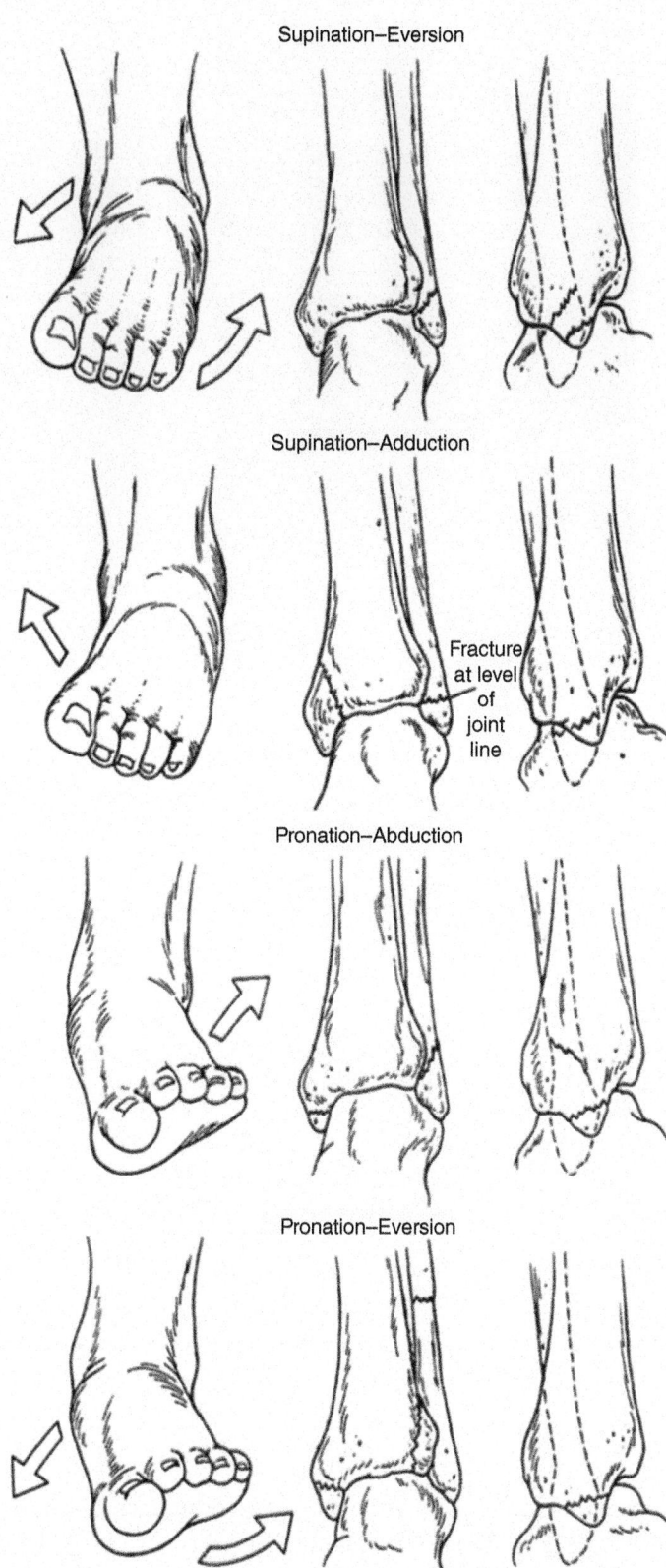

Fig. 4.32 Diagram of the Lauge-Hansen classification of ankle fractures

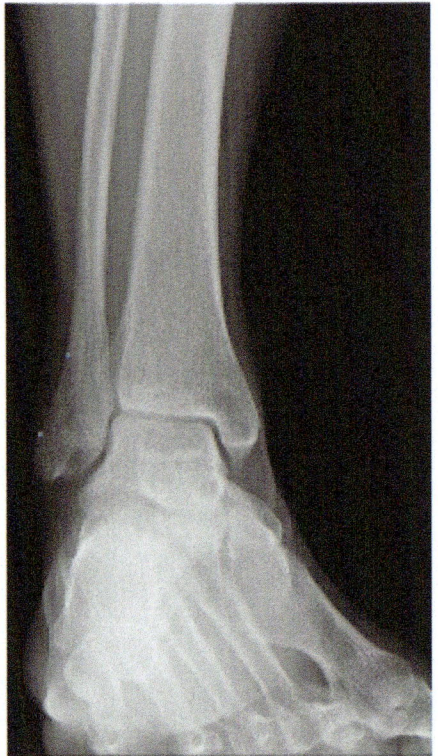

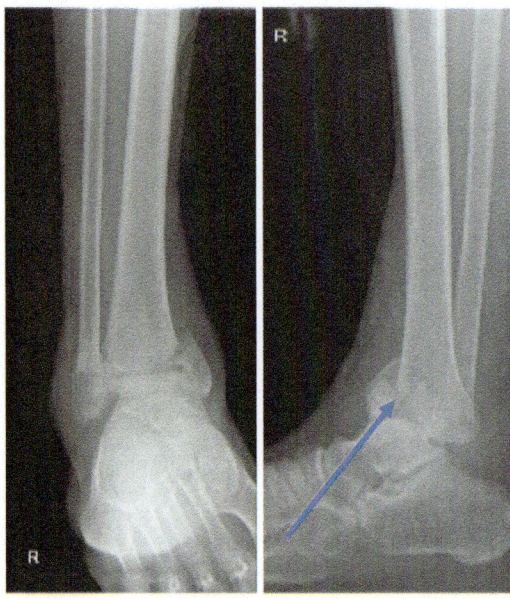

Fig. 4.34 Pilon fracture—a mortise view and lateral view of a pilon fracture. Note the disruption of the tibial plafond marked by the arrow

Fig. 4.33 Weber fracture locations—this is a mortise view of the ankle. The blue dots show the approximate region of the syndesmosis. Fractures below this region are Weber A, fractures within the arrows represent Weber B, and fractures proximal are classified as Weber C

goal of treatment for ankle fractures is anatomic restoration and maintenance of reduction of the mortise of the ankle. Following operative fixation and depending on the fracture pattern, patients may be kept non-weight bearing for 6 weeks, followed by gradual return to weight bearing and initiation of range of motion and strengthening exercises.

Fractures of the distal articular surface of the tibia are categorized separately from common ankle fractures. They typically result from axial loading injuries, as opposed to rotational or torsional forces as with ankle fractures, and involve a significant amount of articular cartilage damage. They are termed pilon (French for "pestle") fractures and represent a difficult management problem. These fractures are often comminuted and length unstable. Furthermore, they have high risk associated with swelling, fracture blisters,

and open fractures. As a result, they are commonly complicated by wound issues and infection. To account for this the typical treatment is restoration of length alignment and rotation with external fixation in the acute setting. After the initial reduction with external fixation, a CT scan should be obtained, and open reduction internal fixation may be performed in a delayed fashion once the soft tissues are amenable. Because of the high energy nature of these fractures and the disruption of the articular cartilage of the tibial plafond, they are frequently complicated by post-traumatic arthritis of the ankle (Fig. 4.34).

Conclusion

Fracture treatment is a foundational aspect of orthopedic care. Understanding the mechanism and timing of the injury combined with a thorough physical and radiographic exam provide the means to develop a clear plan for initial and definitive treatment. The basic tenets involve understanding bone healing principles, types of fixation, and the appropriate application of the mode of fixation that will provide the fracture pattern with stability for the desired type of fracture healing. Successful fracture care applies each of these principles throughout the body and is the basis of each type of fracture surgery.

Further Reading

Augat P, von Rüden C. Evolution of fracture treatment with bone plates. Injury. 2018;49:S2. https://doi.org/10.1016/S0020-1383(18)30294-8.

Bekos A, Sioutis S, Kostroglou A, Saranteas T, Mavrogenis AF. The history of intramedullary nailing. Int Orthop. 2021;45(5):1355. https://doi.org/10.1007/s00264-021-04973-y.

Benders KEM, Leenen LPH. Management of hemodynamically unstable pelvic ring fractures. Front Surg. 2020;7:601321. https://doi.org/10.3389/fsurg.2020.601321.

Bible JE, Mir HR. External fixation: principles and applications. J Am Acad Orthop Surg. 2015;23(11):683. https://doi.org/10.5435/JAAOS-D-14-00281.

Galbiatti JA, Cardoso FL, Ferro JAS, Godoy RCG, Belluci SOB, Palacio EP. Terrible triad of the elbow: evaluation of surgical treatment. Rev Bras Ortop. 2018;53(4):460. https://doi.org/10.1016/j.rbo.2017.05.016.

Guerado E, Bertrand ML, Cano JR, Cerván AM, Galán A. Damage control orthopaedics: state of the art. World J Orthop. 2019;10(1):1. https://doi.org/10.5312/wjo.v10.i1.1.

Hak DJ, Toker S, Yi C, Toreson J. The influence of fracture fixation biomechanics on fracture healing. Orthopedics. 2010;33(10):752. https://doi.org/10.3928/01477447-20100826-20.

Iyer KM, Khan WS. General principles of orthopedics and trauma. 2nd ed. Cham: Springer; 2019. https://doi.org/10.1007/978-3-030-15089-1.

Von Keudell AG, Weaver MJ, Appelton PT, et al. Diagnosis and treatment of acute extremity compartment syndrome. Lancet. 2015;386(10000):1299. https://doi.org/10.1016/S0140-6736(15)00277-9.

Langford JR, Burgess AR, Liporace FA, Haidukewych GJ. Pelvic fractures: part 1. Evaluation, classification, and resuscitation. J Am Acad Orthop Surg. 2013;21(8):448. https://doi.org/10.5435/JAAOS-21-08-448.

Langford JR, Burgess AR, Liporace FA, Haidukewych GJ. Pelvic fractures: part 2. Contemporary indications and techniques for definitive surgical management. J Am Acad Orthop Surg. 2013;21(8):458. https://doi.org/10.5435/JAAOS-21-08-458.

Miller MD, Thompson SR. Miller's review of orthopaedics. J Chem Inf Model. 2016;53(9):53.

Mohanty K, Musso D, Powell JN, Kortbeek JB, Kirkpatrick AW. Emergent management of pelvic ring injuries: an update. Can J Surg. 2005;48(1):49.

Morrey ME, Morrey BF, Sanchez-Sotelo J, Barlow JD, O'Driscoll S. A review of the surgical management of distal humerus fractures and nonunions: from fixation to arthroplasty. J Clin Orthop Trauma. 2021;20:101477. https://doi.org/10.1016/j.jcot.2021.101477.

Seligson D, Mauffrey C, Roberts CS. External fixation in orthopedic traumatology. London: Springer; 2012. https://doi.org/10.1007/978-1-4471-2197-8.

Smith WR, Stahel PF. Management of musculoskeletal injuries in the trauma patient. New York: Springer; 2013. https://doi.org/10.1007/978-1-4614-8551-3.

Tornetta P, Court-Brown CM, Heckman JD, et al. Rockwood, Green, and Wilkins fractures in adults and children, vol. 1–2. 8th ed. Lippincott Williams and Wilkins; 2014.

Watts AC, Singh J, Elvey M, Hamoodi Z. Current concepts in elbow fracture dislocation. Shoulder Elbow. 2021;13(4):451. https://doi.org/10.1177/1758573219884010.

Zalavras CG, Patzakis MJ. Open fractures: evaluation and management. J Am Acad Orthop Surg. 2003;11(3):212. https://doi.org/10.5435/00124635-200305000-00008.

Orthopedic Infections

5

R Adams Cowley II, Kevin W. Park,
and Kenneth M. Vaz

Introduction

When analyzed against common infections, musculoskeletal infections can be challenging to diagnose and thus treat. Unrecognized infections can be both life and limb threatening if not recognized and treated. The most important aspect of caring for patients with a musculoskeletal infection is to come to a timely diagnosis to permit swift appropriate treatment. In these scenarios, most musculoskeletal infections can be effectively treated, decreasing morbidity. Open fractures are an extremely common occurrence in orthopedics, and special attention is given to this topic. While general principles have remained constant, the specific recommendations have evolved. In general, appropriately treated open fractures can typically prevent the establishment of any type of chronic musculoskeletal infection or osteomyelitis.

R. A. Cowley II (✉) · K. W. Park · K. M. Vaz
MedStar Georgetown Orthopedic Institute,
Georgetown University School of Medicine,
Washington, DC, USA

Department of Orthopedics, MedStar Georgetown
University Hospital, Washington, DC, USA
e-mail: RAdams.Cowley@medstar.net;
Kevin.W.Park@medstar.net;
Kenneth.M.Vaz@medstar.net

Pathophysiology of Osteomyelitis

The pathogenesis of osteomyelitis has been well defined; yet the clinical course may vary depending on host, organism, and duration of infection. Thus, osteomyelitis is often classified using these parameters, which aids in determining severity, treatment, and prognosis.

Duration of infections is often divided into either acute or chronic osteomyelitis; this also applies to infections involving the joints such as septic arthritis. Acute osteomyelitis is usually considered to occur within the first 6 weeks following inoculation, with chronic osteomyelitis being greater than 6 weeks.

Bone and joint infections take place via one of two basic mechanisms: exogenous or hematogenous pathways. Exogenous delivery involves direct inoculation of the bone from either trauma, surgery or a contiguous focus of infection. Hematogenous spread is via the vascular system into either osseous or synovial tissue, producing a localized focus of infection. Local tissue compromise (i.e., open fracture) or systemic pathology (i.e., diabetes, immunodeficiency) is often associated with an increased propensity for bone infection by either method.

Two patterns of response occur depending on the infecting organism:

1. Pyogenic organisms: rapidly progressive course of pain, swelling, abscess formation, and aggressive bone destruction
   (a) Example: gram-positive staphylococcus
2. Nonpyogenic: less aggressive insidious granulomatous reaction
   (a) Example: acid-fast bacilli

Age is important in that differences in bone vascular anatomy between adults and children slightly alter the mechanism of hematogenous delivery. In addition, children are susceptible to different organisms depending upon their age.

Exogenous osteomyelitis usually involves a demarcated isolated anatomic site that is inoculated with pyogenic organisms. Typically, these infections are polymicrobial, frequently in association with foreign debris. The bacteria are inoculated into a compromised local environment, with bone and soft tissue disruption providing copious amounts of necrotic and devascularized material favorable for bacterial growth. In addition, tissue devascularization prevents host response mechanisms from reaching bacterial colonies permitting unregulated proliferation.

Once a bone infection is recognized by the host, several steps are unfold:

1. Initial host response to both the injury and infection include activation of inflammatory and immunologic pathways.
   (a) Inflammatory elements serve to destroy bacteria and remove nonviable material.
   (b) Humoral and cellular immunologic mechanisms act to recognize specific bacteria and subsequently confer immunity to prevent further bacterial dissemination.
2. The inflammatory response is initiated with increases in blood flow and vascular permeability, with the delivery of polymorphonuclear leukocytes.
   (a) The leukocytes phagocytize and destroy bacteria and nonviable tissue.
3. Mononuclear cells arrive within 24–48 h and assist in eradication of bacteria and removal

of necrotic bone. As a large number of these cells arrive and die, pus is formed, with an abscess often being clinically appreciable.
4. Granulation tissue surrounds the infected area in an attempt to wall off the infection.
5. Reactive bone formation can occur to further sequester the infection from the host.

Within the infected region, dead bone, the sequestrum, and reactive bone, the involucrum, are appreciated. The treatment of osteomyelitis becomes clear once an understanding of how bacteria gain traction in either damaged tissues or surgical implants. Adhesion to the surface of tissue cells and implants depends on the physical characteristics of the bacteria, the fluid interface, and the substratum.

1. Attachment and Adhesion: anionic surface initially repels anionic bacteria; however, over time, attractive forces (Van der Waals) with hydrophobic molecules on both substrate and bacteria form an irreversible cross link glycoproteinaceous conditioning film.
2. Aggregation: polysaccharide slime layer composed of bacterial extracapsular exopolysaccharides that bind to surfaces, promote cell-to-cell adhesion, microcolony formation, and layering of the microorganisms.
   (a) Additional species of bacteria may attach to the surface of the biofilm.
3. Dispersion: Thriving bacterial colonies may be dispersed by sheer force, enabling a localized colony to establish secondary sites of infection (Fig. 5.1).

These biofilms can lead to antibiotic resistance through decreased metabolic rates and phenotypic changes in surface-adherent bacteria. Therefore, bacteria on surfaces or within microcolonies appear to be physiologically different from free-floating organisms, which may, in part, convey antibiotic resistance.

Treatment of osteomyelitis involves the disruption of these bacterial colonies, which is best achieved with aggressive debridement of nonviable tissues to remove an acceptable bacterial substrate and their associated biofilm. In the

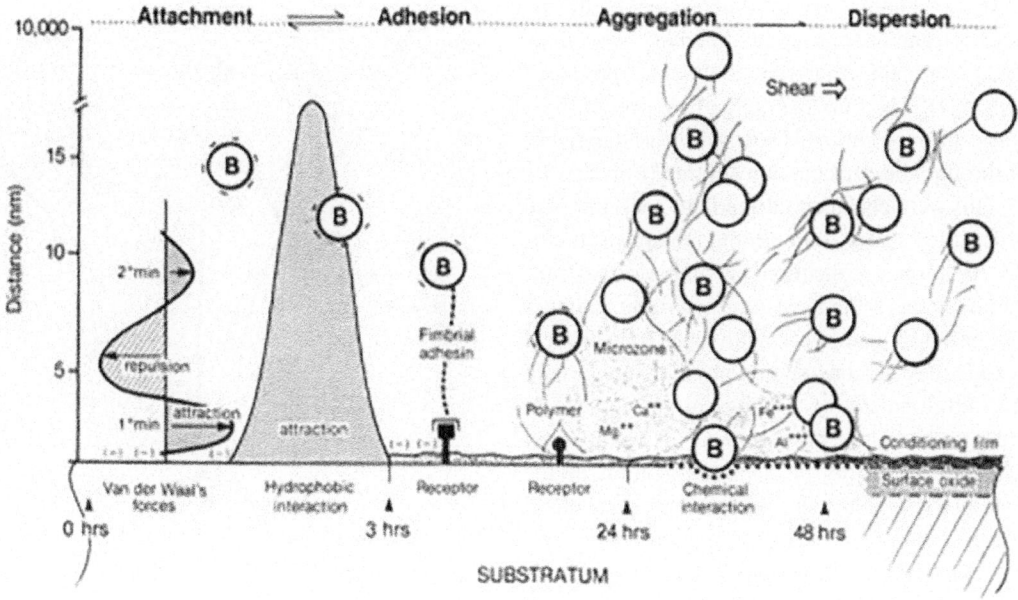

Fig. 5.1 Molecular sequence in bacterial (B) attachment, adhesion, aggregation, and dispersion at substratum surface. A number of possible interactions may occur depending on the specificities of the bacteria or substratum system (graphics, nutrients, contaminants, macromolecules, species, and materials)

case of osteomyelitis involving a prosthesis or fracture implant, it is often necessary to remove either the prosthesis or implant to eradicate the infection.

Pediatric Infections

Acute Hematogenous Osteomyelitis

Hematogenous inoculation represents the most common etiology for acute osteomyelitis. Given the tortuous vascular anatomy of children's long bones, the risk of hematogenous inoculation and proliferation of bacteria is increased.

The nutrient artery of long bones enters through the cortical bone to divide within the medullary canal, ending in small arterioles that ascend toward the physis (Fig. 5.2). Just deep to the physis, these arterioles turn away from the physis and empty into venous pools within the medullary cavity. The acute bend in these arterial loops serve as points of diminished blood velocity, promoting sludging of bacteria directly under

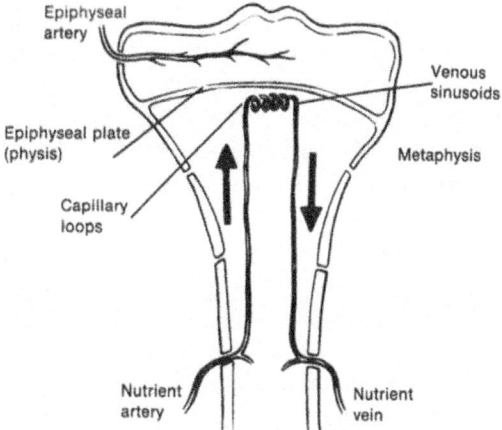

Fig. 5.2 Microcirculation of the metaphysis predisposes it to sludging and infection

the physis. In addition, phagocytic capability and reticuloendothelial function may be depressed in these vascular loops, permitting the establishment of bacterial colonies. Trauma, often associated with the emergence of osteomyelitis in children, may actually promote bacterial seeding and proliferation in metaphyseal sites (Fig. 5.3).

If the immune system fails to eradicate the infection and/or appropriate treatment is not initiated, purulent material will be produced (Fig. 5.4). This pus can spread in one of three ways: through the physis, toward the diaphysis, or through the adjacent bony cortex (Fig. 5.5).

This purulent material tends to seek the path of least resistance, through the metaphyseal cortex, to form a collection of subperiosteal pus. Although this is the most common route, younger children (less than 1 year) with intact transphyseal vessels may demonstrate epiphyseal spread with the development of epiphyseal abscesses. In older children, the development of a subperiosteal abscess results in devascularization of the bone both from thrombosis of the endosteal blood supply and from the stripping away of the overlying periosteum. The periosteum, which is extremely thick and loosely adherent in children, is not easily penetrated. In the devascularization process, it is lifted off the bone, with the inner cambial layer producing a layer of new bone. In this case, the sequestrum and involucrum are formed (Fig. 5.6).

The time frame of diagnosis plays a role in appropriate treatment. The cellulitic phase precedes abscess formation. During this early phase, medical management alone is typically successful to cure the infection. However, once an abscess forms, surgical debridement is necessary for three critical reasons:

1. Remove the nonviable bone
2. Reduce the bacterial population
3. Provide for a vascularized tissue bed for antibiotic delivery

As the majority of pediatric infections emanate via hematogenous seeding from other sites, the specific organisms may differ depending upon the child's age. The vast majority of osteomyelitis in children is secondary to *Staphylococcus aureus* (90%). In neonates, the most common organisms include *Staphylococcus aureus*, group B streptococci, and gram-negative organisms.

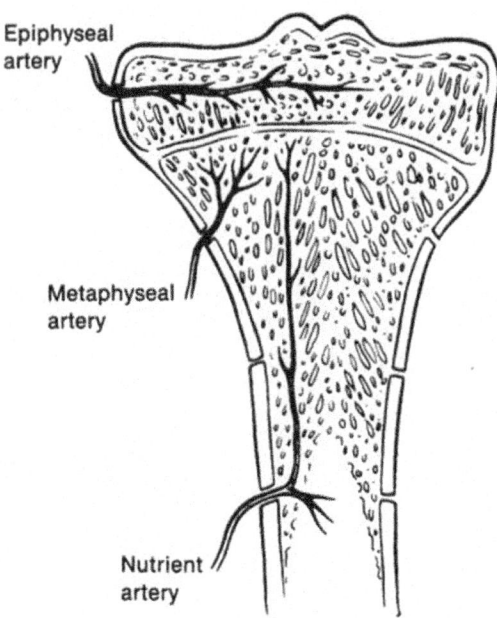

Fig. 5.3 Schematic representation of the blood supply to a long bone

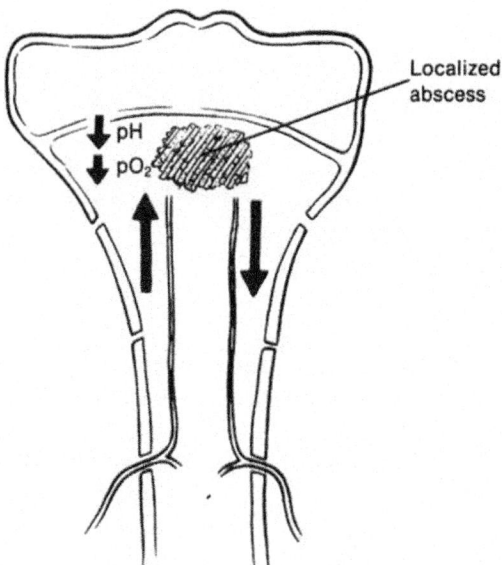

Fig. 5.4 A localized abscess develops, and the microenvironment is altered

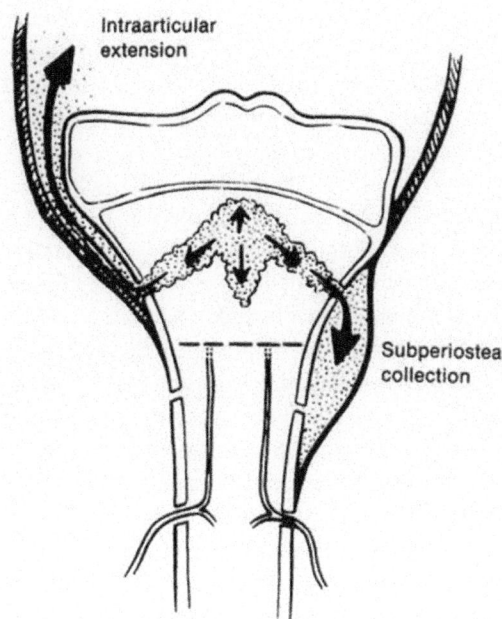

Fig. 5.5 Abscess perforates the metaphyseal cortex and spreads to the subperiosteal space and joint

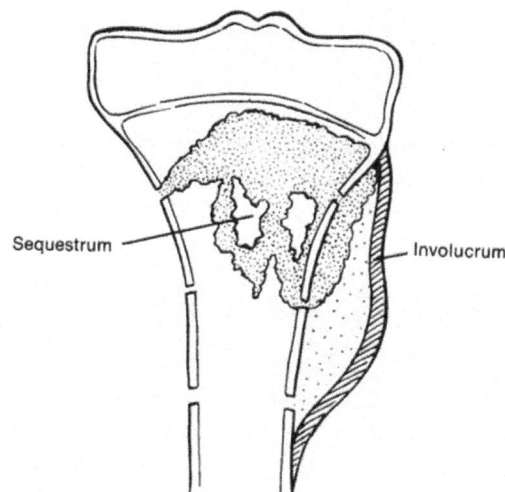

Fig. 5.6 Sequestered fragments of dead bone and periosteal new bone, or involucrum, may be seen on radiographs

Diagnosis and Treatment

Patients present with rapid onset of pain from one to several days in duration limiting the involved extremity's range of motion and weight-bearing. Older patients may be able to assist in localiza-

tion of the pain, although the clinician must be capable of identifying potential sites of referred pain (knee pain for hip osteomyelitis). Children are usually irritable and febrile and often give a history of generalized malaise. Uncovering a potential site of a concomitant infection, such as a recent upper respiratory or ear infection, may provide the clinician with an etiology for hematogenous spread. Physical examination is extremely important, with localized swelling and tenderness often characterizing the physical exam.

Laboratory results are extremely important in diagnosing and treating osteomyelitis; however, they do not replace a complete history and physical examination. A complete blood count with differential, C-reactive protein (CRP) and an erythrocyte sedimentation rate (ESR) are imperative. Adjuvant tests such as serum procalcitonin and interleukin-6 have been shown to provide some utility in pediatric osteomyelitis. While leukocytosis and neutrophilia are typically present, it must be emphasized that not all patients suffering from osteomyelitis present with a classic clinical history, physical findings, and basic laboratory values. Thus, the inflammatory markers convey particular utility in diagnosis. CRP, a direct measure of an inflammatory process, peaks within 48 h, and with appropriate therapy may normalize within 1 week. In comparison, ESR, an indirect measure of inflammation, peaks within 3–5 days and normalizes within several weeks after successful therapy. Thus, CRP has become a useful adjuvant in diagnosis as well as monitoring clinical progression. Of important consideration, diagnosis in neonates may be especially problematic because of the immaturity of their immune system, which may not be able to mount an identifiable host response.

In the acute setting, initial radiographs may be negative, except for soft tissue swelling, because the characteristic changes of osteomyelitis require 10–14 days to be appreciated. Historically, bone scans served as a valuable tool to identify areas of accelerated bone growth; however, magnetic resonance imaging (MRI) with contrast has supplanted all imaging modalities in diagnosis of bone infections. Within the first few days, MRI may demonstrate bone marrow edema as hypointense T1 signal or hyperintense T2 signal (Image 5.1). As the disease progresses, peripheral rim-enhancement may be visible indicating abscess formation.

Bone aspiration is the best means of clinically identifying the presence of a bone infection as well as any organisms associated with it. A large-bore stylet needle (18- or 16-gauge spinal needle) should be used to prevent plugging of soft tissue, bone, or thickened purulent material in the tip. Both subperiosteal and intramedullary sites must be aspirated. In addition, using a second needle, one should consider aspirating the adjacent joint if clinically indicated. Local anesthesia is given, with the needle being easily punched through the soft metaphyseal cortex. If purulent material is obtained, the fluid is sent for immediate Gram stain and culture. The presence of pus necessitates that the patient undergo an operative

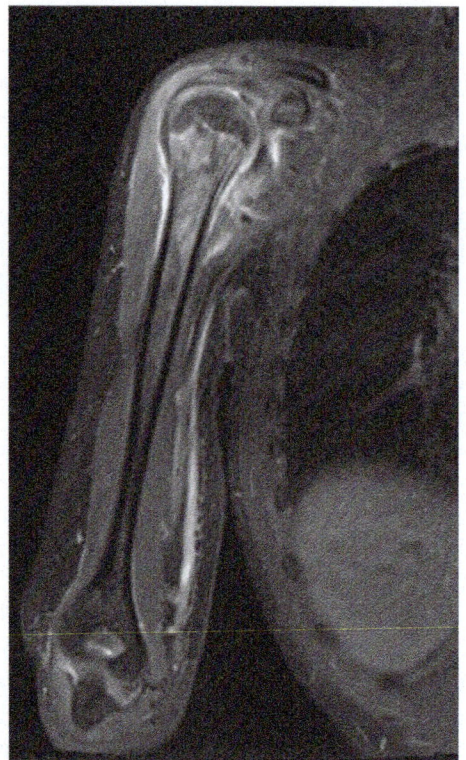

Image 5.1 T1 image marrow changes associated acute osteomyelitis of proximal humerus with notable concerning glenohumeral joint effusion. (Courtesy of Dr. Ryan Murray)

irrigation and debridement. However, antibiotics should be started immediately following aspiration with these initial cultures, serving to direct later modifications to organism-specific antibiotic coverage.

The initial antibiotic choice is often based upon the broad-spectrum approach. In patients who are not allergic to penicillin, a beta-lactamase resistant penicillin derivative should be chosen. Good initial choices include oxacillin or nafcillin, with penicillin-allergic patients often being treated with cefazolin. The optimal length of therapy is still under debate, with a regimen of 3 weeks of IV antibiotics, followed by 3 weeks of oral therapy, often being acceptable. An infectious disease consultation is necessary to help guide antibiotic therapy choice and duration.

In the event that purulent material is not aspirated, sterile saline should be injected, aspirated, and sent for culture in the hopes of identifying an organism. Bacteriostatic saline should not be used as this may inhibit bacterial growth. In cases in which no frank purulent material is aspirated, surgery is usually not indicated, as there is no pus to decompress or necrotic bone to debride. In this setting, the administration of antibiotics is the mainstay of treatment.

Chronic infections are uncommon in children, as patients usually present early in the course of the disease. However, if this scenario occurs, these patients almost invariably require surgical intervention to debride sequestrated tissues. Complications are high in this setting from both the disease process and the surgical procedure, including pathologic fracture and physeal arrest.

Pediatric Septic Arthritis

Acute septic arthritis may develop from hematogenous sources or, more commonly, from extension of an adjacent foci of osteomyelitis into the joint. Susceptible joints are those in which the metaphysis is intra-articular: hip, shoulder, elbow, and ankle (NOT the knee) (Fig. 5.7).

Although relatively uncommon, septic arthritis can rapidly destroy articular surfaces

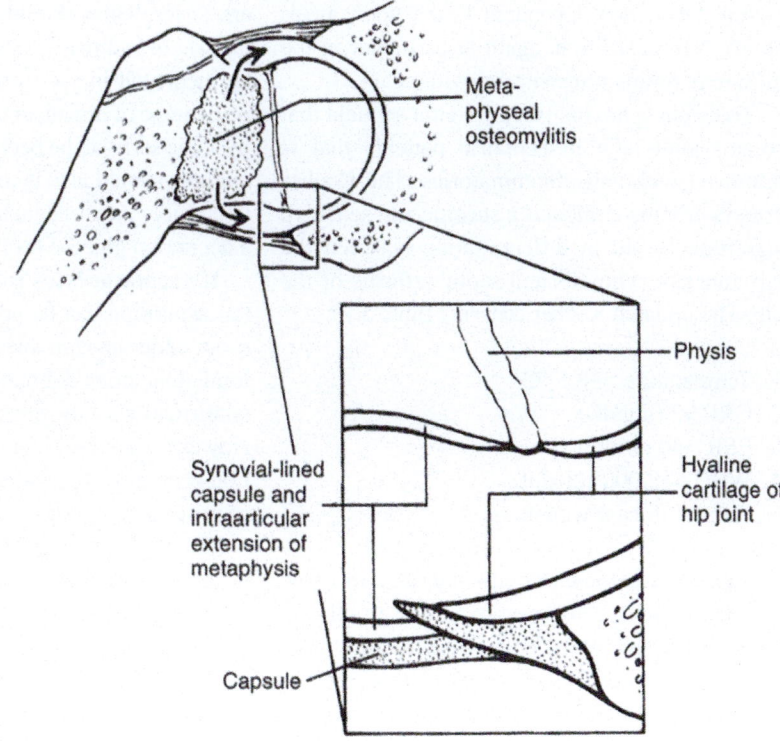

Fig. 5.7 Schematic representation of the immature hip. Metaphyseal osteomyelitis spreads by direct extension into the hip joint

Table 5.1 Common pathogens and recommended treatment for septic arthritis

Age group	Probable organisms	Initial antibiotic choice
Neonate	GBS, *S. aureus*, Gram-negative coliforms	Penicillin, oxacillin, and gentamicin
Infants and children (4 weeks to 4 years)	*S. aureus, H. influenzae*, GBS, GAS, Kingella, Eikenella, Cardiobacterium, Actinobacilus	Cefuroxime
Children (>4 years)	*S. aureus*	Oxacillin or cefazolin
Adolescent	*N. gonorrhoeae*	

via robust enzymatic response of neutrophils and matrix metalloproteinases within 8 h. Concurrently, increased joint pressure leads to osteonecrosis; therefore, septic arthritis must be definitively excluded at symptom onset.

Depending upon the age of the patient, different organisms prevail as likely pathogens (Table 5.1).

Diagnosis and Treatment

Pediatric septic arthritis patients tend to be more toxic than acute osteomyelitis with higher temperatures, more pain, and notably elevated inflammatory markers. Understandably, these children are extremely reluctant to move the involved extremity or infected joint. With increased fluid in the affected joint, patients tend to position their joints to maximize joint capsule space. For example, the hip, this is usually flexion abduction and external rotation. For the knee, this tends to be roughly 30 degrees of flexion. Radiographs may demonstrate a joint effusion and associated soft tissue swelling.

As mentioned previously, the window for treatment for septic arthritis is 8 h before irreversible damage to the cartilage via enzymatic reactions of the inflammatory cells occurs. Thus, a septic joint is considered a surgical emergency.

Given low cost and wide-spread availability, ultrasound has become the mainstay for evaluation. In particular for hips, bilateral imaging is recommended for comparison and because contralateral disease has been described. MRI is an option, but center-dependent based upon availability. Septic arthritis, again in particular in the hips, may mimic transient synovitis.

Transient synovitis is a post-viral sequela that creates joint pain in pediatric patients that is improved with anti-inflammatories. The Kocher criteria provide clinicians a specific and sensitive algorithm to aid in differentiating between the hip transient synovitis and septic arthritis of the hip. The updated Kocher criteria (Table 5.2):

1. Temperature >38.5 °C
2. CRP >2 (mg/dL)
3. ESR >40 mm/h
4. WBC >12,000 cells/µL
5. Refusal to bear weight

Some have extrapolated this algorithm from the hip to other joints. However, regardless of clinical suspicion, a joint aspiration is mandatory for diagnosis. Ultrasound or fluoroscopy may be used to aid in retrieval of fluid especially in less accessible joints such as the hip. An arthrogram for the hip may be added as well to confirm appropriate location. Usually, a form of sedation is required for children as they simply will not tolerate the aspiration. The fluid should be analyzed for gram stain, culture, cell count with differential, and for the presence of crystals. In the majority of cases the joint aspiration will demonstrate a WBC count greater than 50,000; this may often exceed 100,000 in severe cases. The white blood cell population is usually composed of polymorphonuclear leukocytes, comprising as much as 90–95% of the cells in fulminant cases. On occasion, circumstances may require the clinician to inform the laboratory of the possible organism as special techniques may be necessary. For lyme endemic

areas, serologies should be sent. As *Haemophilus influenzae* is difficult to culture, the specimen must be incubated in a CO_2 environment. Because the percentage of organism retrieval has been reported by some series to be between 70% and 85%, blood cultures should also be obtained. Additional clues to possible infection include an elevated protein or a decreased glucose level in the joint aspirate.

If a septic arthritis is highly suspected, the initial aspiration can be performed in the operating room under general anesthesia, to be followed by immediate open debridement and irrigation upon confirmation of the presence of pus or organisms. However, having a diagnosis prior to the operation is prudent to avoid unnecessary consumption of hospital resources.

The goals of an irrigation and debridement are decompression of all purulent material, irrigation of both bacteria and host lysozymes from the joint, and debridement of nonviable tissues.

Reexamination of the joint is necessary following surgery or aspiration to be assured a purulent material has not reaccumulated.

Intravenous antibiotics are initiated immediately following acquisition of joint fluid. Again, antibiotic choice is based upon the suspected pathogens with the assistance of an infectious disease consultation. Compared to treatment of osteomyelitis, the antibiotic course for septic arthritis is usually shorter (4 weeks), with 2 weeks of IV antibiotics followed by an additional 2 weeks of oral therapy.

Adult Osteomyelitis

For adult osteomyelitis, the management involves determining the level of infection and consideration of several patient variables to create an appropriate treatment plan:

1. Physiology of patient
   (a) Malnutrition, immune deficiency, malignancy, diabetes, chronic lymphedema, venous stasis, major vessel disease, extensive scarring, other
2. Anatomic site
3. Psychosocial factors

Table 5.2 Number of positive Kocher criteria finds correlated with percent probability of hip septic arthritis

Number of factors	% Probability of septic arthritis
0	17
1	36
2	62
3	83
4	93
5	98

In conjunction with an infectious disease consultation, the goal of treatment should be determined: suppressive or curative.

The Cierny–Mader classification of Osteomyelitis assists surgeons in determining the prognosis of available treatment modalities through anatomic location and host factors: (Fig. 5.8).

Location
Stage I: Medullary
Stage II: Superficial
Stage III: Localized
Stage IV: Diffuse

Host
Type A: Normal
Type BL: Locally compromised
Type BS: Systemically compromised
Type C: Treatment is worse to patient than infection

Stage I medullary osteomyelitis is completely endosteal and does not require bone stabilization following debridement. Stage II superficial osteomyelitis only involves the outer cortex and again, which does not require bone reconstruction following local excision of infected material. Stage III localized osteomyelitis combines types I and II, therefore requires full thickness cortical resection to effectively debride the bone. Although this does not confer segmental instability, eventual bone grafting techniques may need to be employed to reestablish continuity. Stage IV osteomyelitis results in wide-spread cortical and endosteal infection, with segmental resection being required to eradicate the infection. Diffuse osteomyelitis is mechanically unstable both before and after debridement; thus, stabilization and eventual bone reconstruction is required.

Fig. 5.8 The Cierny classification of chronic osteomyelitis: type I, medullary; type II, superficial; type III, localized full thickness; type IV, diffuse

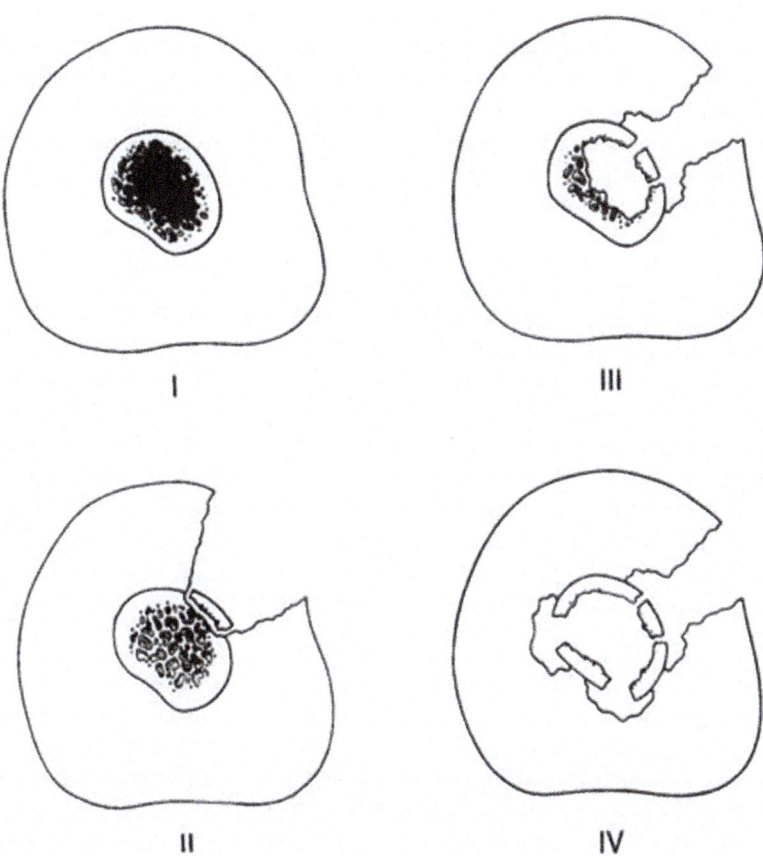

Surgical treatment of osteomyelitis involves three main facets:

1. Extensive debridement
2. Vascular soft tissue coverage
3. Bone stabilization

An aggressive debridement of nonviable tissues to healthy bleeding tissue is crucial to achieving successful eradication of osteomyelitis by preventing residual bacteria from persistently reinfecting the bone.

Multiple cultures of all debrided material should be obtained before the initiation of antibiotic therapy to aid in guiding cultures specific antibiotic selection. Often the patient may require several debridements until the wound is considered to be clean prior to addressing soft tissue coverage. Basic soft tissue flap coverage options include:

1. Simple skin graft
2. Local transpositional muscle graft
3. Vascularized free flap

Muscle transposition and free flaps provide a fresh bed of vascularized tissue to assist in bone healing and antibiotic delivery.

Finally, bone stability must be considered. This step remains last as placing a graft into an incompletely resolved infection provides a nutrient rich environment for infection to proliferate. Cancellous and cortical autografts may be used. The Masquelet technique (MT) and the Ilizarov bone transport (IBT) technique are the two prominent methods that address significant segmental bony defects.

MT is a two-stage procedure. In the first stage, anti-microbial cement is placed in the defect. This cement is left for 6–8 weeks to permit the formation of a self-induced periosteal membrane. Once this membrane is formed, the second stage is performed to remove the cement and place cancellous bone graft.

IBT is technically demanding and requires a longer treatment duration. IBT consists of application of a small pin (Ilizarov) or half-pin external fixator with gradual distraction. After a latency period of approximately 7–10 days, distraction begins at a rate of 0.75–1 mm per day. As distraction is carried out, the soft tissues regenerate along with the bone to cover the newly generated tissue.

The comparison of these two techniques have generated a large volume of research with comparable results.

Adult Septic Arthritis

As with children, septic arthritis in adults can develop from hematogenous sources, direct inoculation, contiguous soft tissue infection, or peri-articular osteomyelitis. Several patient factors predispose patients such as IV drug abuse, immunosuppressants, systemic corticosteroid use, and pre-existing arthritis. Similar to children, *Staphylococcus aureus* is the most common pathogen isolated from infected adult joints (44%). Neisseria gonorrhoeae is another common adult pathogen, with a reported incidence of 11%. The joints most commonly involved are the knee (40–50%), hip (20–25%), and shoulder and ankle (10–15%). In IV drug abusers, the sternoclavicular, sacroiliac, and manubriosternal joints are common sites, with Pseudomonas aeruginosa often being isolated.

Presentation and diagnosis do not differ greatly between adults and children. Adult patients present with pain, swelling, and a decreased range of motion of the affected joint. Evaluation involves routine laboratory tests (CBC, CRP, ESR), blood cultures, and joint aspirations. The appearance of the synovial fluid (straw, cloudy, or purulent) as well as the WBC count, the percentage of polymorphonuclear cells, and cultures can assist in the diagnosis. In adults, crystal analysis is even more critical as crystal-induced arthropathy can appear quite similar to a septic arthritis (Table 5.3).

Treatment of an adult with a septic arthritis requires aggressive irrigation and debridement utilizing either arthroscopic techniques or an open arthrotomy. Infectious disease consultation is often obtained to determine antibiotic choice, route of administration, and duration.

Table 5.3 Synovial fluid

Examination	Normal	Noninflammatory	Inflammatory	Septic
Appearance	Transparent	Transparent	Opaque translucent	Opaque, cloudy, purulent
Viscosity	High	High	Low	Variable
WBC/mm^3	<200	<200	5000–75,000	>50,000
PMN (%)	<25%	<25%	>50%	>75%
Culture	–	–	–	Often positive
Associated conditions	–	Degenerative joint disease Trauma Neuropathic PVNS SLE Acute rheumatic fever	Rheumatoid arthritis Crystalline-induced arthritis Seronegative arthritis SLE Acute Rheumatic fever	Bacterial infection Compromised immunity

Esterhai JL, Gelb I: Adult septic arthritis. Orthop Clin North Am 18:503–514, 1991; reprinted with permission

Open Fractures

An open fracture involves exposure of fractured bone to the outside environment. This exposure increases the risk of bone contamination from foreign debris and inoculation with bacteria. Concomitantly, open fractures are often associated with severe soft tissue damage, devascularization, and devitalization of bone fragments facilitating an even more favorable environment for bacterial growth.

While many grading systems have been created, perhaps the most widely used classification of open fractures comes from Gustilo–Anderson. This classification considers energy, wound size, soft tissues damage, level of contamination, fracture comminution, periosteal stripping, skin coverage, and presence of neurovascular injury. From the classification system, an antibiotic has been developed providing utility in initial management (Table 5.4).

While the Gustilo-Anderson system affords ease of applicability, particularly size of wound, the zone of injury may be much larger than the wound. Thus, this system can be misleading in its categorization.

The most critical aspect of care for open fracture occurs in the emergency department. Time to antibiotics has been shown to be vital in preventing catastrophic infections. A tetanus booster is commonly given as well.

Formerly, open fractures were taken for operative debridement within 6 h of injury as the status of the patient permitted. The standard of care has shifted based on several landmark studies demonstrating no difference in outcomes between debridement with 6 and 24 h. Open fractures are still considered operative emergencies and need to be taken to the operating room as soon as the patient is considered medically stable enough to tolerate surgery but now within 24 h.

After ensuring administration of antibiotics, gentle wound irrigation and application of a sterile dressing should be performed. Depending on the fracture, a reduction and splint immobilization may be indicated just as with any closed injury. Cultures in the emergency department are frequently contaminated providing minimal, if any, therapeutic value and are thus not recommended. The general principles regarding antibiotic therapy is that first-generation cephalosporins are given regardless of grade. For Gustilo type III, the addition of an aminoglycoside has been traditionally recommended; however, controversy regarding this addition is present. For any farm injuries or those associated with bowel contamination, the addition of an aminoglycoside and penicillin are recommended.

In the operative suite, assessment of the extent of injury and aggressive debridement should be undertaken in the operating room in an emergent manner. As with any debridement, the removal of any devitalized tissues is critical to prevent proliferation of bacterial growth. As mentioned previously, the zone of injury is often greater than the wound. Determining this zone of injuries

Table 5.4 Gustilo-Anderson classification

	I	II	IIIA	IIIB	IIIC
Energy	Low	Moderate	High	High	High
Wound size	<1 cm	1–10 cm	Usually >10 cm	Usually >10 cm	Usually >10 cm
Soft tissue damage	Minimal	Moderate	Extensive	Extensive	Extensive
Contamination	Clean	Moderate	Extensive	Extensive	Extensive
Fracture comminution	Minimal	Moderate	Severe	Severe	Severe
Periosteal stripping	No	No	Yes	Yes	Yes
Skin coverage	Local	Local	Local	Free or rotational flap	Free or rotational flap
Neurovascular injury	None	None	None	None	Vascular injury requiring repair

allows for a more comprehensive debridement. Often this determination can be challenging during the index procedure; thus, many advocate for a second look procedure 48–72 h prior to wound closure especially for higher energy injuries. If a wound is not closed primarily during the index procedure, wound vacuums are applied and remain until eventual closure providing three critical benefits: decreasing wound tension, removal of fluid accumulation, and protection from the outside environment.

Presence of Morel Lavellée lesion, a closed shearing injury separating the fascia and subcutaneous skin, requires special attention. These shearing lesions create a deep space that provides an unwanted hospitable environment for bacterial proliferation. A surgical drain to compression may be placed to close down this dead space and minimize risk of infection.

Fracture stabilization is a pertinent facet of the operative intervention. While disagreement exists on the manner, a general consensus is that there needs to be some form of stabilization for soft tissue healing, early mobility, and pain control. For grossly contaminated wounds, temporizing measures may be employed including splinting or external fixation. External fixation can represent a definitive treatment; however, intramedullary nailing or plate/screw fixation are commonly employed for definitive fixation once the site is sufficiently debrided.

A delayed primary closure may be all that is required in grade I and grade II fractures, whereas skin grafting or soft tissue transfers may be necessary for grade III fractures. Options for soft tissue coverage should be individualized for the patient and the degree of injury. For more complex soft tissue defects, a plastic surgeon consultation may be recommended.

Nutritional status plays a vital role in wound healing especially considering the increased metabolic demand of polytraumatized patients. Systemic parameters that have been shown to impede soft tissue healing include a serum albumin less than 3.5 mg/dL, prealbumin <16 mg/dL, transferrin <212 mg/dL, or a total lymphocyte count less than 1500 cells/mL. For those with diabetes, tight glycemic control is pertinent to reduce the risk of infection. As such, nutritional resuscitation and blood glucose management become vital in the perioperative setting.

If an infection such as wound dehiscence, abscess formation or osteomyelitis develops following an open fracture, then the same principles of debridement apply with one important exception—the retention of implants for fixation of the fracture. In patients who present with an infection surrounding an intramedullary nail or plate, the wound should be aggressively debrided and the implant maintained if fracture stability is being achieved. Loose implants should be removed and either replaced or substituted by another implant type (i.e., an external fixator replacing a loose plate and screws). Intravenous antibiotics should be administered and directed toward isolated organisms for at least 6 weeks. Once a fracture has healed, the implant can be removed and further debridement performed as necessary. This approach reduces the complexity of treatment from an infected nonunion to an infected united bone with a better prognosis for successful healing and eradication of the infection.

Prosthetic Joint Infections (PJI)

The presence of a foreign substrate such as an arthroplasty can provide bacteria with an excellent site for binding and colonization. Unfortunately, the diagnosis of a PJI remains challenging. The onset of symptoms in relation to the time of surgery plays a role in the diagnosis. Acute infections are defined within 3–6 weeks of surgery and chronic infections are considered greater than 3–6 weeks.

Obvious findings like wound dehiscence, drainage, erythema, and effusions with systemic symptoms (fevers, chills, malaise) immediately warrant work up and likely intervention. However, some may present with indolent subclinical symptoms that could easily be overlooked; thus, a high level of clinical suspicion is required.

Plain films are the main imaging modalities utilized for PJI for comparison to prior films. Profound bone resorption surrounding implants may also be suggestive of infection; however, similar changes can be seen with aseptic loosening without an associated infection (Image 5.2).

Laboratory values, although often abnormal, are also not specific for infection. Bone scans using technetium 99m and indium-111 help detect inflammation and leukocytes, respectively, with great sensitivity (99%), however, suboptimal specificity; thus, these scans are uncommonly used. Similarly, positron emission tomography (PET) scans have been described to identify areas of high metabolic activity with a high sensitivity and specificity; however, due to cost restrictions and availability, PET scans are not frequently utilized.

Obtaining basic laboratory values are standard of care including a CBC as well as inflammatory markers. The WBC count is rarely elevated except in a fulminant infection. The inflamma-

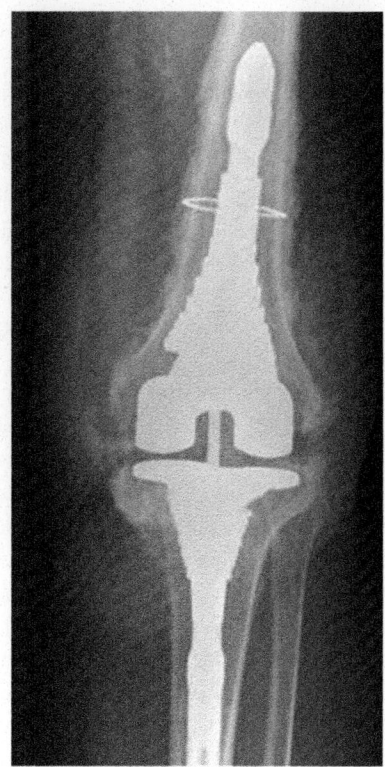

Image 5.2 Anterior posterior plain radiograph demonstrating a hinge total knee replacement with distal femur cerclage and notable bony resorption associated with prosthetic joint infection. (Courtesy of Dr. Kenneth Vaz)

tory markers, ESR and CRP, are generally elevated. While not commonly utilized, serum interleukin-6 (IL-6) has been shown to have the highest correlation with periprosthetic joint infection with a sensitivity of 100% and specificity of 95%.

An aspiration still remains the best single test to identify a subclinical infection, with a sensitivity of 90%, specificity of 80%, and an accuracy of 78%. For more confined joints such as the hip, fluoroscopy or ultrasound should be used to confirm needle localization within the joint. These samples should be sent for the same tests as native septic joints (cell count, culture, gram stain, crystal). Traditionally, a chronic PJI is suspected if there are greater than 3000 WBCs/μL. Higher thresholds for acute PJIs remain controversial. Other synovial tests may be sent as well, which provide particular diagnostic value in the culture negative specimens including synovial CRP. The addition of alpha-defensin immunoassay, a peptide release by neutrophils, may aid clinicians as this is 100% sensitive and 98% specific for PJI. Another benefit for alpha-defensin is the sensitivity is not affected by previous antibiotic administration. Similar to urinalysis, leukocyte esterase colorimetric strips may be performed on the synovial samples to demonstrate neutrophil activity. With recent awareness of more fastidious organisms such as Cutibacterium acnes (formerly Propionibacterium acnes), some centers have begun to hold specimens for 3–4 weeks to allow for their possible identification. With the advent of next generation sequencing, uncovering a microbial source through this polymerase chain reaction (PCR) test and other nucleic acid amplification tests (NAATs) may be feasible for previous culture negative samples. Implementing this technique into the standard workup has yet to manifest as cost and availability remain a few of the barriers.

In 2011, the Musculoskeletal Infection Society (MSIS) and Infectious Disease Society developed criteria in hopes of standardizing and improving diagnostic accuracy. Subsequently, this criteria was updated in 2018 by Dr. Jared Parvizi to address the limitations of the initial algorithm. This criteria is divided into major and minor criteria boosting a 98% sensitivity and 99.5% specificity for diagnosis of PJI.

Major Criteria: (PJI if 1 major criteria exists)
1. Sinus tract communicating with the prosthesis
2. Pathogen isolated by culture from 2 separate tissue or fluid samples

Minor Criteria (PJI ≥6, inconclusive 5–2, no infection 1–0)
1. Elevated synovial WBC (>3000 cells/μL) or Leukocyte Esterase—3 points
2. Positive synovial alpha-defensin—3 points
3. Elevated synovial PMN (>80%)—2 points
4. Elevated synovial CRP (>6.9 mg/L)—1 point

While the 2018 MSIS criteria has aided in standardizing care, the inconclusive zone forces the surgeon to utilize their own clinical judgment.

Treatment of PJI should account for the patient's ability to tolerate surgery and chronicity of infection. For those unfit for surgery, chronic suppressive antibiotic therapy may be the only option. While this option may provide symptomatic relief, success of complete eradication is limited; thus, this therapy typically is reserved for palliative patients. For acute infections, some propose the biofilm has not been developed; therefore, an aggressive debridement and polyethylene liner exchange with component retention may be sufficient. Some surgeons argue a one-stage complete component exchange and debridement can be a suitable option in appropriate patients who are otherwise healthy and are infected by low-virulent organisms. However, currently, the gold standard treatment remains a two-stage revision arthroplasty. The first stage entails complete removal of all components with placement of an antibiotic spacer. The second reimplantation stage occurs in delayed fashion with >6 weeks intervals demonstrating greater overall success. In all circumstances, an infectious disease consultation is recommended as these patients require extended antibiotic regimens. Salvage options are available including resection arthroplasty, arthrodesis, and amputation. These options should be matched with appropriate candidates based upon their issue and preference.

Summary and Conclusions

The prompt diagnosis of a musculoskeletal infection is the most vital aspect in the appropriate management of these conditions. Though the diagnosis may at times prove difficult due to a variety of mitigating circumstances, the prudent use of laboratory data, imaging studies and sound clinical acumen should minimize delay or missed diagnosis. Acute treatment of an infection is substantially more straightforward than management of chronic musculoskeletal infections and their unfortunate sequelae.

Further Reading

Perry KI, Hanssen AD. Orthopaedic infection: prevention and diagnosis. JAAOS J Am Acad Orthop Surg. 2017;25:S4–6.

Chen AF, et al. What's new in musculoskeletal infection: update across orthopaedic subspecialties. JBJS. 2017;99(14):1232–43.

Kocher MS, Zurakowski D, Kasser JR. Differentiating between septic arthritis and transient synovitis of the hip in children: an evidence-based clinical prediction algorithm. J Bone Joint Surg Am. 1999;81(12):1662–70. https://doi.org/10.2106/00004623-199912000-00002. PMID: 10608376.

Olsen MA, et al. Risk factors for surgical site infection following orthopaedic spinal operations. JBJS. 2008;90(1):62–9.

Rasouli MR, et al. Risk factors for surgical site infection following total joint arthroplasty. JBJS. 2014;96(18):e158.

Connell MC. In: Wiesel SW, Delahay JN, editors. Essentials of orthopedic surgery, vol. 615. New York: Springer; 2007.

Flow Investigators. A trial of wound irrigation in the initial management of open fracture wounds. N Engl J Med. 2015;373(27):2629–41.

Tumors of the Musculoskeletal System

6

Jonathan Day and Brock Adams

Background

Both benign and malignant tumors can arise from mesenchymal soft tissue or bone of the extremities and axial skeleton. All tumors of the musculoskeletal system arise from one of the following histological tissues: bone (osteoid forming tumors), cartilage (chondroid forming tumors), muscle, or fibrous connective tissue. In addition, tumors can rarely arise from arteries or nerves.

The vast majority of tumors are benign. Malignant tumors of the musculoskeletal system are termed sarcomas, which comprise about 80 different types arising from mesenchymal or connective tissues [1]. It is estimated that roughly 16,000 new cases and 6000 deaths are attributed to sarcomas annually in the USA. Still, this accounts for less than 1% of all malignant cancer diagnoses [2].

Contrary to most malignant diagnoses that occur in the later decades of life, most bone sarcomas (osteosarcoma and Ewing's sarcoma) occur during childhood or adolescence. Soft tissue sarcomas tend to be found starting in the third decade of life and become more common as age increases. Bone tumors typically present with pain, while soft tissue tumors tend to present as a painless mass.

It is fundamental for orthopedic surgeons to have a sound understanding of musculoskeletal tumors. This includes an understanding of the general workup and to the ability to determine which patients should be referred to a subspecialized orthopedic oncologist. Early detection, combined with proper techniques of diagnosis and treatment, can dramatically improve the chances of achieving functional limb salvage and minimizing morbidity. Advances in imaging, chemotherapy, and radiation therapy, coupled with a better understanding of the biological behavior of mesenchymal neoplasms, have led to a rational basis for diagnosis, staging, and treatment.

The aim of this chapter is to provide an up-to-date, comprehensive review of the most common benign and malignant tumors of the musculoskeletal system, as well as the general workup, diagnosis, treatment options, and prognosis.

J. Day
MedStar Georgetown Orthopedic Institute, Georgetown University School of Medicine, Washington, DC, USA

Department of Orthopedics, MedStar Georgetown University Hospital, Washington, DC, USA

B. Adams (✉)
MedStar Georgetown Orthopedic Institute, Georgetown University School of Medicine, Washington, DC, USA

Department of Orthopedics, MedStar Washington Hospital Center, Washington, DC, USA
e-mail: Brock.W.Adams@gunet.georgetown.edu

Natural History of Bone and Soft Tissue Tumors

Mesenchymal tumors have characteristic patterns of behavior and growth that help distinguish it from other tumors. These unique features form the basis for tumor staging and treatment.

Biology and Growth

Sarcomas grow in a centrifugal fashion with the youngest and most viable cells toward the periphery. They tend to push the normal tissue away as they expand as opposed to many carcinomas, which infiltrate and invade the surrounding tissue. In contrast to benign lesions that often are surrounded by a true capsule, malignant lesions are surrounded by a pseudocapsule formed by compressing the normal tissue surrounding the lesion as it grows. This is composed of a fibrovascular zone of reactive tissue that contains some tumor cells within it. The thickness of this layer can vary by degree of malignancy and histologic subtype.

High-grade sarcomas characteristically have poorly defined reactive zones. In addition, tumor nodules that are not in continuity with the main tumor may be present in tissue that appears normal. Low-grade sarcomas rarely form tumor nodules beyond the reactive zone.

Local anatomy influences the growth of sarcomas by setting natural boundaries to extension. In general, sarcomas take the path of least resistance. Fascial boundaries such as the periosteum, compartmental fascia, or a vascular sheath form effective barriers. Bone tumors grow via three mechanisms: compression of normal tissue, resorption of bone by reactive osteoclasts, and direct destruction of normal tissue. Benign bone tumors grow and expand via the first two mechanisms, whereas malignant ones expand via direct tissue destruction. In addition, benign tumors are usually unicompartmental, meaning they remain confined to and may expand the bone in which they reside. In contrast, malignant bone tumors are often bicompartmental, meaning they destroy the overlying cortex and push directly into the adjacent soft tissue. With this concept in mind, soft tissue tumors may start in one compartment (intracompartmental) or between compartments (extracompartmental). This determination of anatomic compartments is especially important when considering limb-preservation surgery.

Five Patterns of Tumor Behavior

On the basis of biologic considerations and natural history, all bone and soft tissue tumors, benign and malignant, may be classified into five categories, each of which shares certain clinical characteristics and radiographic patterns. Treatment of tumors is also similar for tumors in each group. The five categories are as follows:

1. *Benign/Latent*

    These lesions grow slowly during the normal development of the individual. As the growth of the individual stops, the growth of the lesion stops and sometimes resolves spontaneously. These lesions are typically not symptomatic and as a general rule do not progress to malignancy. Observation is the most common course of treatment. Examples include lipomas and fibrous cortical defects.

2. *Benign/Active*

    These lesions exhibit progressive growth and bone lesions are often symptomatic. Treatment is with excision for soft tissue lesions or curettage for bone lesions. It is not necessary to remove the reactive zone. Chondroblastoma and osteoid osteoma are examples.

3. *Benign/Aggressive*

    These lesions are locally aggressive but do not metastasize (with the notable exception below). Tumor can extend beyond the capsule and into the reactive zone. Treatment aims to remove the reactive zone by resecting a cuff of normal tissue for soft tissue tumors. For bone lesions this is approximated by removing the reactive zone with a high-speed burr and using a physical or chemical adjuvant to kill remaining tumor cells. Giant cell tumor of bone (benign but can metastasize) and fibromatosis are in this group (Fig. 6.1).

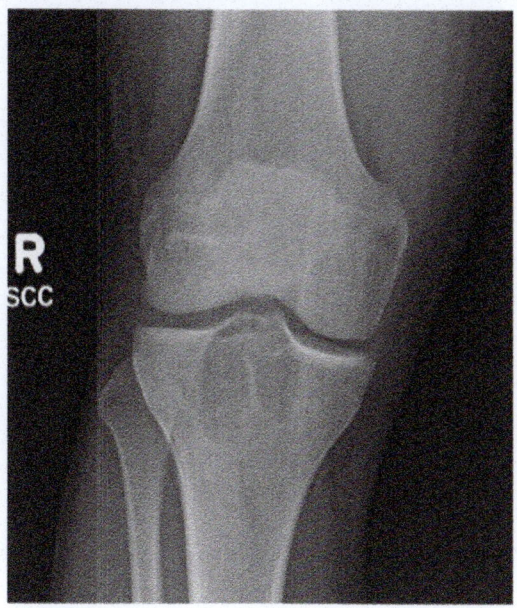

Fig. 6.1 A giant cell tumor of bone with a secondary aneurysmal bone cyst. This represents an aggressive benign lesion. Note the easily recognizable sharply defined border. Plain radiographs are the most important study in the diagnosis of bone tumors

4. *Malignant, Low Grade*

These lesions have the ability to metastasize but do so at a low rate. Tumor can expand beyond the compartment and tumors cells are present in the reactive zone. Treatment involves removal of the lesion with a cuff of normal tissue, but no adjuvant therapy is necessary. Examples are parosteal osteosarcoma and low-grade soft tissue sarcomas.

5. *Malignant, High Grade*

These lesions grow rapidly and metastasize early and at a high rate. These tumors may have a poorly defined pseudocapsule and tumor nodules can extend beyond the reactive zone into the normal tissue. Excision with a cuff of normal tissue is necessary for surgical treatment. Chemotherapy is required for bone tumors and some soft tissue tumors to lessen the rate of metastasis. Radiation is required for soft tissue tumors to reduce the chance of local recurrence. Classic intramedullary osteosarcoma and undifferentiated pleomorphic sarcoma (UPS) are in this category.

Mechanisms of Tumor Spread

Unlike carcinomas, bone and soft tissue sarcomas disseminate almost exclusively hematogenously. Because of this, the lungs are by far the most common site of metastatic spread with 80–90% of metastases found in the lungs. Bone is the next most common site of metastasis. Both bone and soft tissue sarcomas can spread via the lymphatic system to regional lymph nodes. The rate of lymphatic spread varies by disease entity, but in general is just under 5%.

The histologic hallmark of malignant sarcomas is their potential to break through the pseudocapsule to form satellite lesions. Discontinuous tumor, commonly referred to as a skip metastasis, is a tumor nodule located in the same bone or compartment as the primary tumor but is not contiguous with it.

The mechanism of spread and common sites of metastatic spread are important to keep in mind when evaluating a patient with a sarcoma and guide the choice of imaging studies necessary to determine the stage of disease.

Clinical and Radiographic Evaluation

Clinical Evaluation

It is often said that the importance of the clinical history and physical examination should not be overlooked, and this is certainly true in the evaluation of musculoskeletal tumors. The location of a tumor, the rate at which it is growing, pain, or any history of trauma are all key points to obtain from the history. On examination it is important to note the size of the mass, its relation to surrounding structures, whether it appears to be superficial or deep, tenderness, the appearance of the overlying skin, and whether it is firm or soft. While mesenchymal tumors spread hematogenously for the most part, an examination of the regional lymph nodes should be included.

Special attention should be paid to the characteristics of pain. In bone tumors, pain is an important feature distinguishing aggressive or malignant tumors from more latent lesions. Pain that arises from a bone lesion typically is described as a dull aching type pain. It is often present at rest as well as with activity and classically wakes the patient up at night. This is in contrast to more common musculoskeletal sources of pain which are typically worse with certain types of activity and improve with rest. A lesion in the proximal humerus of a patient presenting with vague, dull pain waking them up at night and full range of motion of the shoulder is worrisome. A lesion in the proximal humerus of a patient presenting with pain with overhead activity after an injury is not worrisome. Interestingly, the same does not hold true for soft tissue tumors. The most common presentation of a soft tissue sarcoma is a painless, enlarging mass. While there are more painful benign soft tissue tumors than malignant ones, both benign and malignant soft tissue tumors may present as painless or painful masses.

Radiographic Evaluation

X-Rays

Conventional anteroposterior (AP) and lateral radiographs remain essential in the initial characterization and diagnosis of musculoskeletal tumors. Further advanced imaging is often dictated by initial plain radiographic findings. Proper interpretation of a lesion on X-rays can be guided by answering four classic questions proposed by Dr. William F. Enneking:

1. What is the anatomic location and extent of the lesion?
2. What is the lesion doing to the bone?
3. What is the bone doing to the lesion?
4. What is the tissue type of the lesion?

Distinctions between benign, aggressive, and frankly malignant lesions can be made on the basis of this analysis. Benign lesions have well-defined borders often with a surrounding rim of sclerotic bone and do not penetrate the cortex. In contrast, malignant lesions have poorly defined sometimes permeative borders and can destroy the cortex. Many bone lesions in particular have a characteristic appearance on X-ray and a diagnosis can often be made based off the X-ray along. In general, plain radiographs are the most important imaging study when determining the type of bone tumor (Fig. 6.2).

Computed Tomography

Computed tomography (CT) allows high-resolution cross-sectional imaging of bone. While it can be used to evaluate soft tissue structures, soft tissue tumors, and the extent of a tumor both in the intramedullary space and in the soft tissue, CT is most helpful looking at the calcified portions of the bone. Thinning or scalloping of the cortex and subtle periosteal reaction are best seen on CT. Similarly, faint matrix production may be difficult to discern on plain X-ray, but relatively easy to see on CT. CT can also be helpful for preoperative planning purposes, especially in more complex structures such as the pelvis. A CT of the chest is often used for staging purposes.

Magnetic Resonance Imaging

Magnetic resonance imaging (MRI) provides detailed multiplanar information of both bone and soft tissue. It gives great visualization of anatomic compartments, vessels, other soft tissues, and bone. MRI shows the extent of the tumor in both the bone and soft tissue and its relation to the surrounding structures in great detail. It is valuable for preoperative planning. While MRI can be helpful from a diagnostic standpoint, diagnosis typically cannot be made on the basis of the MRI characteristics alone. An MRI done to evaluate a tumor should include a true T1 sequence, a T2 sequence with fat suppression, and a T1 post-contrast image with fat suppression (Fig. 6.3).

Nuclear Medicine

Bone scintigraphy can be helpful in assessing the primary lesion and to screen for distant metastasis. The delayed phase of a technetium-99 scan is used most commonly. While

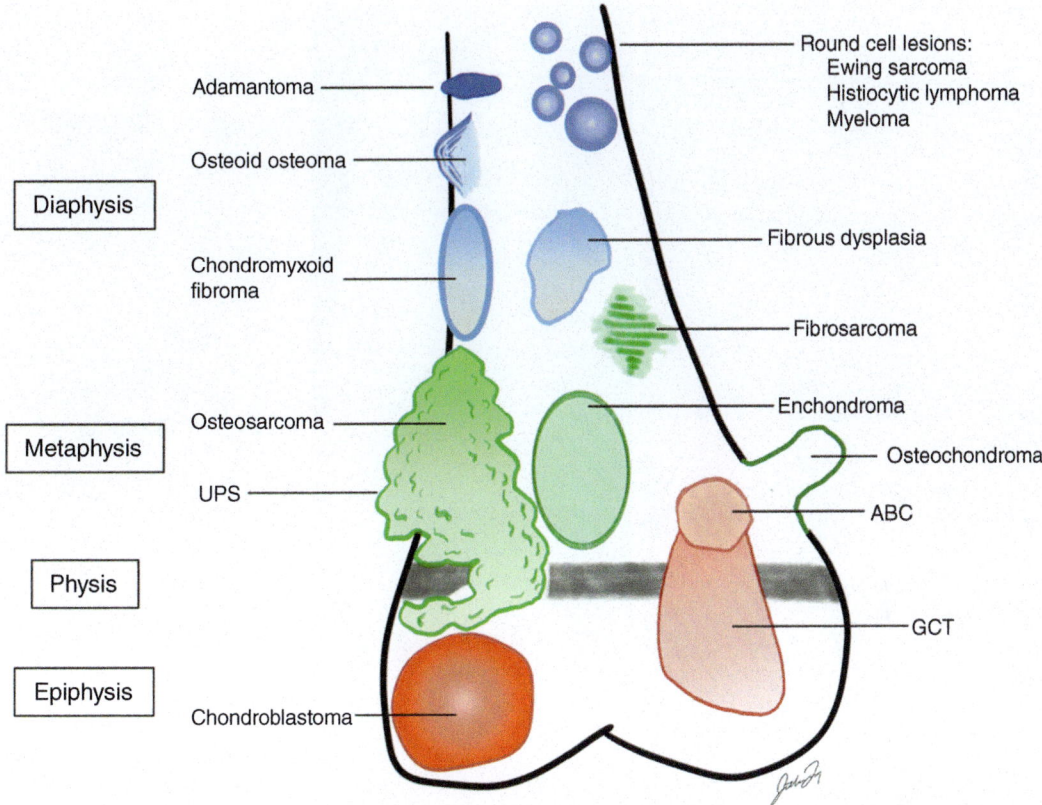

Fig. 6.2 Schematic of typical locations of common bone tumors. The anatomic location, whether diaphyseal, metaphyseal, or epiphyseal, is one of the most important determinants of tumor type. Cortical, medullary, or eccentric location is also important. One should always pay special attention to the presence of matrix formation

the level of uptake compared to the surrounding bone can be used to distinguish between latent and more aggressive lesions, the level of discrimination is relatively low. Because of this, bone scan is used primarily to screen for metastatic disease.

Positron Emission Tomography (PET) is used to measure the metabolic activity of a lesion. F-18 flouro-2-deoxy-D-glucose (FDG) is most commonly used. Similar to bone scan, there is a correlation between uptake on PET and how aggressive the tumor is. It can be used to assess treatment response. PET is used less frequently for staging in sarcoma than some other malignancies, owing to the relatively predictable pattern of spread, but use of PET for sarcoma is becoming more widespread.

Ultrasound

Ultrasound can be used to evaluate soft tissue tumors. While it is operator dependent, it can often be obtained more quickly than axial imaging. Using Doppler, it can be used to assess the vascularity of the lesion. Ultrasound can also be used to guide needle placement for biopsy.

Angiography

While the need for true angiography has decreased as the image quality and availability of MRI has improved, it is sometimes still the best way to assess the vascularity or intravascular involvement of a tumor. Preoperative embolization of highly vascularized tumors prior to surgical resection can significantly reduce blood loss and intraoperative morbidity.

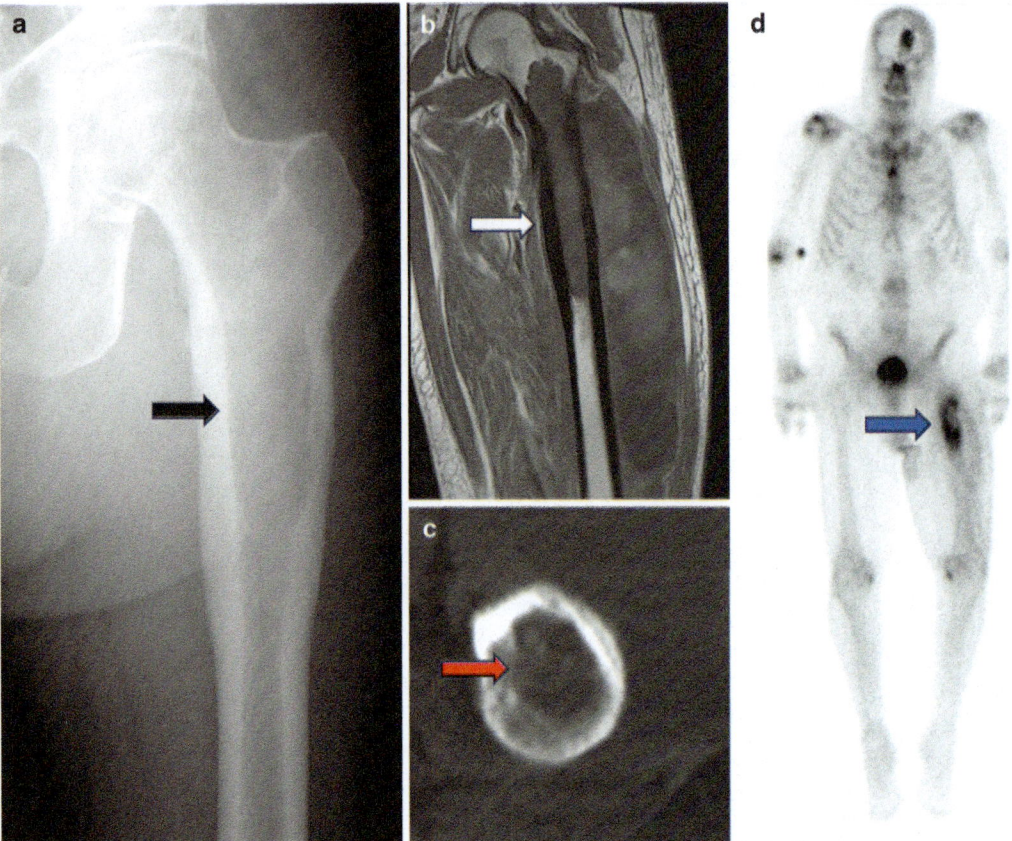

Fig. 6.3 Radiographic (**a**), T1 weighted coronal MRI (**b**), axial CT (**c**), and whole body technetium bone scan (**d**) of a patient with a grade-2 chondrosarcoma. While the plain radiograph is most important diagnostically (black arrow), MRI shows the tumor extent in the bone and soft tissue (white arrows), CT shows the faint chondroid matrix and abnormal cortex (red arrow), while bone scan shows increased uptake at the lesion and screens for additional lesions (blue arrow)

Staging

Staging of a bone or soft tissue sarcoma is the process of determining the local extent of the tumor and any potential sites of distant metastasis. If there is clinical or radiographic suspicion of an aggressive or malignant tumor, staging studies should be performed prior to biopsy. Staging can guide proper location and method of biopsy. X-rays should always be a part of the local imaging. Beyond this, initial staging typically includes MRI of the entire bone or region affected, CT of the chest, and a technicium-99 whole body bone scan.

Staging Systems

The purpose of a surgical staging system is to organize patients into groups that correlate with overall outcome and survival. This has prognostic value and can guide treatment decisions for both physicians and patients. There are two widely used staging systems in orthopedic oncology. Historically, the most widely used system is the Musculoskeletal Tumor Society (MSTS) system based on the system proposed by William Enneking [3]. The system from the American Joint Committee on Cancer (AJCC) is the other widely used system and is the most common system used in specialties outside of orthopedics. Stage in both systems correlates with overall survival with higher stage having a worse prognosis.

The MSTS system takes three factors into account. i.e., the tumor grade, local extent, and the presence or absence of metastatic disease. The same system is used for both bone and soft tissue sarcomas.

1. *Surgical Grade*

The histological grade of a lesion correlates with its growth rate or aggressiveness. Tumors are divided into two groups—low grade versus intermediate and high-grade. Low-grade lesions are malignancies with low potential to metastasize.

2. *Surgical Site*

Anatomic site is either intracompartmental or extracompartmental. A compartment is defined as an anatomic space bound by natural barriers to tumor extension such as a single bone. More aggressive tumors tend to expand outside of their original compartment.

3. *Metastatic Disease*

The presence of metastatic disease is a poor prognostic factor. The 8th edition of the AJCC staging system is slightly different for bone and soft tissue sarcomas [4]. It uses grade, tumor size, the presence of discontinuous tumor (for bone sarcomas), and the presence of lymph node or distant metastasis (Tables 6.1 and 6.2). Recent literature has proposed alternative staging systems which con-

Table 6.1 AJCC (*8th edition*) staging system for soft tissue sarcomas

G, *Histologic grade*	G1	Well-differentiated, low grade
	G2	Moderately differentiated, high grade
	G3	Poorly differentiated, high grade
T, *Primary tumor*	T1	≤5 cm in greatest dimension
	T2	>5 cm and ≤10 cm in greatest dimension
	T3	>10 cm and ≤15 cm in greatest dimension
	T4	Tumor >15 cm in greatest dimension
N, *Regional node*	N0	No regional lymph node metastasis
	N1	Regional lymph node metastasis
M, *Distant metastasis*	M0	No distant metastasis
	M1	Distant metastasis
Stage groups	IA	G1, T1, N0, M0
	IB	G1, T2/3/4, N0, M0
	II	G2/3, T1, N0, M0
	IIIA	G2/3, T2, N0, M0
	IIIB	G2/3, T3/4, N0, M0
	IV	Any G, Any T, N1, M0
		Any G, Any T, Any N, M1

Table 6.2 AJCC (*8th edition*) staging system for bone sarcomas

G, *Histologic grade*	G1	Well-differentiated, low grade
	G2	Moderately differentiated, high grade
	G3	Poorly differentiated, high grade
T, *Primary tumor*	T1	≤8 cm in greatest dimension
	T2	>8 cm in greatest dimension
	T3	Discontinuous tumor in primary bone site
N, *Regional node*	N0	No regional lymph node metastasis
	N1	Regional lymph node metastasis
M, *Distant metastasis*	M0	No distant metastasis
	M1a	Distant metastasis—lung
	M1b	Distant metastasis—other sites
Stage groups	IA	G1, T1, N0, M0
	IB	G1, T2/3, N0, M0
	IIA	G2/3, T1, N0, M0
	IIB	G2/3, T2, N0, M0
	III	G2/3, T3, N0, M0
	IVA	Any G, Any T, N0, M1a
	IVB	Any G, Any T, Any N, M1b

sider other factors such as histologic grade, tumor size, and anatomic depth [5].

Biopsy

Biopsy Techniques

The planning and technique of a biopsy are very important. Biopsies should be performed after staging studies are obtained [6]. Biopsy should be done in the plane of eventual tumor resection and should be closely coordinated by the treating physician. Biopsy should be taken from the periphery of the lesion where the most viable tissue and immature cells are found. In a bone lesion, the soft tissue component should be biopsied if present. Care should be taken not to contaminate potential tissue planes or flaps that will compromise the management of the lesion. A poorly planned biopsy can result in delayed diagnosis, larger definitive procedures, increased need for flap coverage, and higher rate of amputation [7].

Core-Needle Biopsy
To minimize contamination and morbidity, core-needle biopsy of soft tissue and bone sarcomas is generally recommended over incisional biopsy (Fig. 6.4). Core-needle biopsy provides adequate tissue for diagnosis with accuracy similar to open

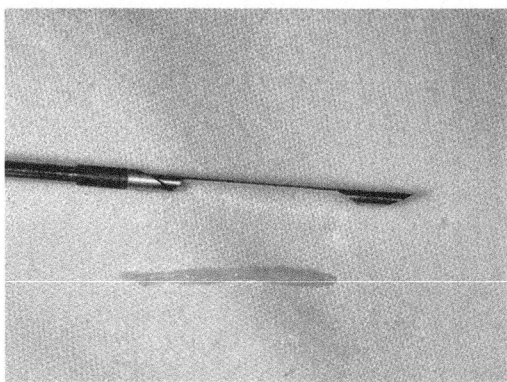

Fig. 6.4 Clinical photograph of core-needle and specimen. Multiple specimens from different portions of the tumor can be obtained through one biopsy site. The orthopedic oncologist should either perform or oversee placement of the needle

biopsy. The risk of seeding the biopsy tract is lower [8]. In contrast to fine-needle aspiration, core-needle biopsy preserves the intercellular architecture in addition to the cellular appearance, which is important in the histologic diagnosis of mesenchymal neoplasms.

Imaging should be performed prior to biopsy. Image guidance with either CT or ultrasound can be used as needed and can be useful in tumors in close proximity to neurovascular structures, areas of complex anatomy, or when significant heterogeneity or evidence of necrosis is present on imaging.

Incisional Biopsy
While a core-needle biopsy is sufficient in the majority of cases, an open, or incisional, biopsy may still be indicated when core-needle biopsy is not diagnostic or a high volume of tissue is necessary. This requires proper technique to minimize contamination. While the biopsy should always be done in the plane of eventual resection, this is most important in an open biopsy. A tourniquet is generally advised to help facilitate visualization of tumor and meticulous hemostasis should be maintained. Tissue dissection should be minimized, and dissection of neurovascular structures should be avoided.

Excisional Biopsy
Some small, superficial lesions may be removed as an excisional biopsy. This involves excising the lesion with a wide margin or a cuff of normal tissue. Criteria to consider excisional biopsy include small size, superficial location or relatively close to the fascia, minimal morbidity, and neoadjuvant therapy would not change surgical approach or outcomes.

Overview of Surgical Procedures

Surgical removal—including curettage, resection, and amputation—is the mainstay of treating musculoskeletal tumors (Fig. 6.5). The extent of the surgical procedure necessary is determined by both tumor type and the local anatomy. A classification scheme of surgical procedures based on

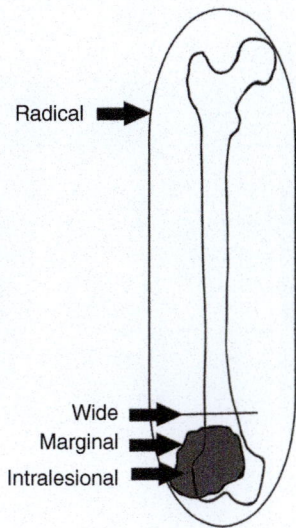

Fig. 6.5 Schematic diagram illustrating different resection types

the surgical plane as well as method of resection is summarized below. This provides a standardized terminology when discussing surgical treatment of both bone and soft tissue tumors and is widely used in clinical practice as well as the published literature.

1. **Intralesional** procedures involve opening the pseudocapsule and removing the tumor in piecemeal fashion. Biopsies are by definition intralesional. Most benign bone tumors are treated with an intralesional procedure or curettage.
2. **Marginal** procedures involve opening the pseudocapsule and removing the mass in a single piece. This leaves the pseudocapsule behind. Marginal resections are not used for sarcomas since tumor cells are known to reside in the pseudocapsule. Low-grade lipomatous soft tissue masses are typically removed with a marginal resection.
3. **Wide** **(intracompartmental)** procedures, also referred to as *en bloc* resections, involve resecting the entire lesion including the surrounding pseudocapsule and a cuff of normal tissue. There is no specific thickness of normal tissue necessary to perform a wide resection. As opposed to carcinomas, which often require a specific margin measured in

centimeters, a wide margin in sarcoma is defined as at least single layer of cells.
4. **Radical (extracompartmental)** procedures involve resection of the entire compartment (or compartments) involved by the tumor. Although this term still appears in the literature, it most often is used because of differences in terminology and billing codes and does not reflect a true radical resection. A true radical resection at this point is primarily historical in nature and is not necessary unless done to achieve a wide margin as described above.

It is important to note that all the above can be performed via a limb-sparing approach or via amputation. Amputation does not automatically provide a wide margin. Both the local tumor extent and the local anatomy dictates how a particular margin can be obtained.

In general, benign bone tumors can be adequately treated with either intralesional procedure (curettage) or a marginal excision. For benign bone lesions, this typically involves making a cortical window and using curets to remove the lesional material. A high-speed burr is then used to remove the reactive zone. An adjuvant is then often used to kill any remaining tumor cells. This may be a cryoablation to freeze the tumor cavity, use of an argon beam, or a chemical adjuvant such as phenol. Removing the reactive zone and use of an adjuvant are important in reducing the recurrence rate, which can be as high as 50% for some tumors after a simple curettage (Fig. 6.6).

Malignant tumors as a rule should be excised with a wide margin. Most tumors, 90–95%, can be excised with a limb-sparing operation, but if a wide margin cannot be safely obtained, amputation should be considered. As mentioned above, there is no specific thickness of normal tissue that must be maintained around the tumor to achieve a wide margin. That being said, the biology of the individual tumor type and its propensity for local recurrence and the effectiveness of adjuvant treatment in the form or radiation or chemotherapy should be taken into account when deciding how aggressively to pursue limb salvage.

Fig. 6.6 Giant cell tumor of the distal femur (**a**). Radiograph after intralesional curettage, removal of the reactive zone with a high-speed burr, and cryoablation. Reconstruction consisted of iliac crest bone graft along the articular surface, cementation, and a locking plate (**b**). This represents the common surgical treatment for benign but aggressive tumors

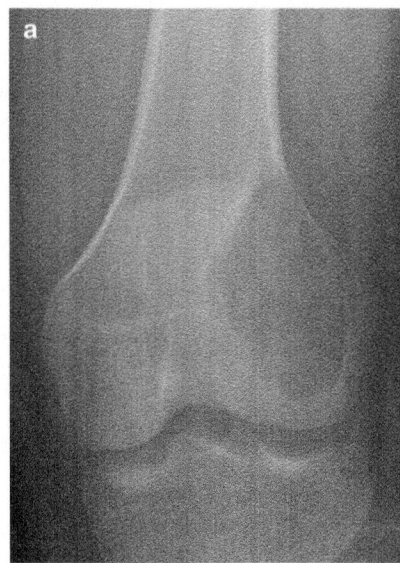
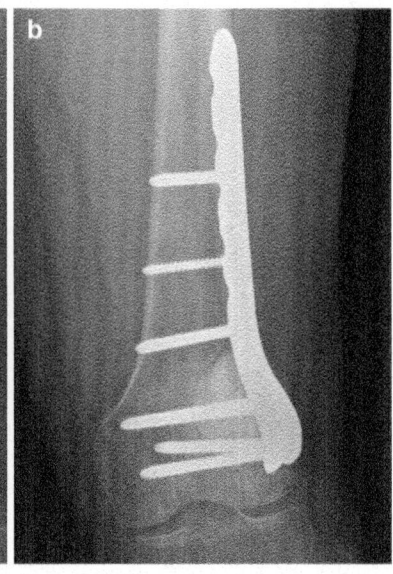

Principles of Limb-Sparing Surgery for Bone and Soft Tissue Sarcomas

Successful limb-sparing surgery involves three key phases: tumor resection, skeletal reconstruction, and soft tissue coverage. Firstly, proper resection of the tumor, including the margin of surrounding bone and/or soft tissue should follow these four principles:

1. Major neurovascular bundle should be tumor-free and protected.
2. Wide resection of tumor with a normal muscle cuff circumferentially.
3. En bloc resection of all previous biopsy sites and potentially contaminated sites.
4. Bone resection should be planned based on tumor extent as seen on MRI.

After resection of bone tumors, attention is turned to skeletal reconstruction (Fig. 6.7). Reconstructive options include an endoprosthesis, bulk allograft, allograft prosthetic composite, structural autograft, and distraction osteogenesis. The degree of resection, the limb involved, the age and health of the patient, and patient preference should all be taken into account. Endoprosthetic reconstruction is commonly used in skeletally mature individuals. It offers reliable results particularly in resections involving a joint.

Modularity in implant design provides flexibility to meet varying needs. Another advantage is immediate fixation which in turn facilitates early mobilization and rehabilitation. Prostheses are available that allow noninvasive expansion of the prosthesis to facilitate limb salvage in skeletally immature patients. Allograft is another commonly employed option. While osteoarticular allografts are sometimes used, allografts are most often used in intercalary fashion when the closest joint and/or physis can be spared.

Finally, soft tissue and muscle transfers are indicated to cover and close the defect as well as restore motor function if possible. Local muscle transfers also serve to protect exposed neurovascular bundles and bone. Adequate soft tissue coverage is mandatory to maximize patient functional outcomes. Additionally, all dead space should be closed, often with placement of surgical drains to allow adequate postoperative drainage and prevent hematomas.

Amputation

Although the majority of tumors can be removed with limb-sparing techniques, about 5–10% of patients with musculoskeletal tumors require amputation. Indications for amputation include neurovascular involvement by the tumor, inade-

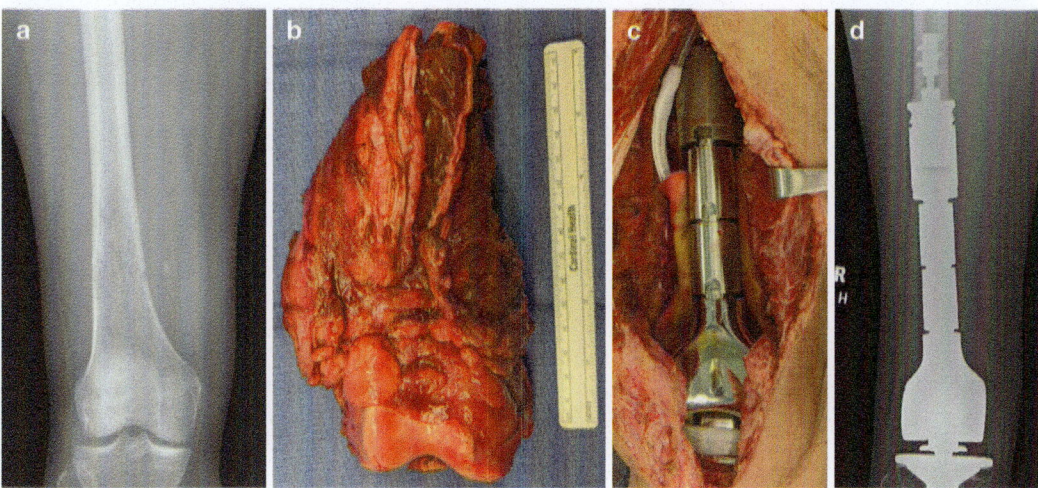

Fig. 6.7 An undifferentiated pleomorphic osteosarcoma of the distal femur treated with a wide resection and endoprosthetic reconstruction. (**a**) Preoperative radiograph, (**b**) Gross specimen, (**c**) Modular prosthesis, (**d**) Postoperative radiograph

quate soft tissue for coverage or function, and lack of a good skeletal reconstructive option. The response of the tumor to adjuvant treatment also affects the decision for limb salvage versus amputation. Infection is a common late indication for amputation after a limb salvage procedure. Soft tissue contamination from a poorly planned biopsy or treatment of a fracture through an unrecognized primary bone tumor may also lead to amputation. Although a pathologic fracture through a sarcoma is a poor prognostic indicator, the overall survival for patients treated with amputation versus limb salvage is similar, so this alone does not necessitate amputation.

Surgical Treatment of Metastatic Disease to the Bone

The goal of surgical treatment of carcinoma that has metastasized to the bone is different than that of treating a primary bone tumor. The aim is to minimize pain and maximize function by preventing fractures and stabilizing fractures that have already occurred. There is no need to resect the lesion unless it is necessary to improve stabilization. Resecting metastatic lesions does not affect the overall survival of the patient but can

increase the morbidity of surgery. There are exceptions to this rule, such as oligometastatic renal cell carcinoma, where resection can improve overall survival. The approach to metastatic disease to the bone can be found later in this section.

Malignant Bone Tumors

Primary malignances of bone originate from mesenchymal cells (sarcoma) or bone marrow cells (myeloma and lymphoma). Bone is also a common site of metastasis from a variety of carcinomas. This section will review the most common malignant bone tumors, as well as their characteristic patient demographics, clinical exam, radiographic and histologic findings, treatment options, and outcomes in the literature (Table 6.3).

Classic Intramedullary Osteosarcoma

Osteosarcoma is a high-grade malignant spindle cell tumor arising from bone. Characteristically, it features osteoid, or immature bone, formed by a malignant spindle cell stroma. Osteosarcoma provides the model for which treatment of all

Table 6.3 Overview of musculoskeletal tumors

Histologic type	Benign	Malignant
Chondrogenic	Osteochondroma Chondroma Chondroblastoma Chondromyxoid fibroma	Chondrosarcomas
Osteogenic	Osteoid osteoma Osteoblastoma	Osteosarcoma Parosteal osteosarcoma Ewing's sarcoma Malignant giant cell tumor Adamantinoma
Fibrogenic	Fibroma Fibrous histiocytoma	Fibrosarcoma
Neurogenic		Chordoma
Vascular	Hemangioma	Hemangiopericytoma
Lipogenic	Lipoma	Liposarcoma

other bone sarcomas is based. Through the use of multiagent chemotherapy overall survival improved from around 15% to over 70% in the 1970s. At the same time, advances in reconstructive surgery allowed for limb-sparing surgery to take the place of amputation as the standard surgical treatment. Since this significant shift, interestingly, the treatment and overall survival of osteosarcoma patients has remained relatively static.

Clinical Presentation

Osteosarcoma occurs most commonly in childhood and adolescence; however, it can occur at any age. There is a second peak in incidence over the age of 60. This is due primarily to disease associated with conditions such as Paget's disease or prior radiation.

Osteosarcoma most commonly affects the bones of the knee joint (50%) and proximal humerus (25%). The axial skeleton is affected less often. Laboratory findings are usually not helpful in diagnosis, but alkaline phosphatase can be elevated. Elevated serum alkaline phosphatase is not specific as it is often elevated in other skeletal pathologies such as hyperparathyroidism, fibrous dysplasia, and Paget's, but a high alkaline phosphatase in a patient with osteosarcoma is a poor prognostic factor.

Pain in the affected extremity is often the presenting symptom. Physical exam often discloses a firm, soft tissue mass fixed to the underlying bone. Systemic symptoms are rare. Patients may

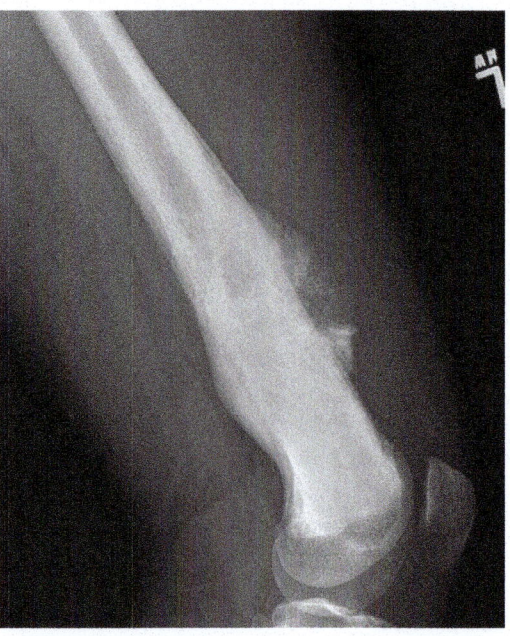

Fig. 6.8 An osteogenic osteosarcoma with dense intramedullary bone formation and a sunburst pattern of periosteal reaction

present with pathologic fracture. This no longer is seen as an absolute indication for immediate amputation but is a poor prognostic factor [9].

Radiographic Findings

Plain radiographs of the involved bone reveal a characteristic pattern of increased intramedullary sclerosis with areas of radiolucency (Fig. 6.8). Borders are poorly defined with cortical destruction. Tumors typically arise in the metaphyseal

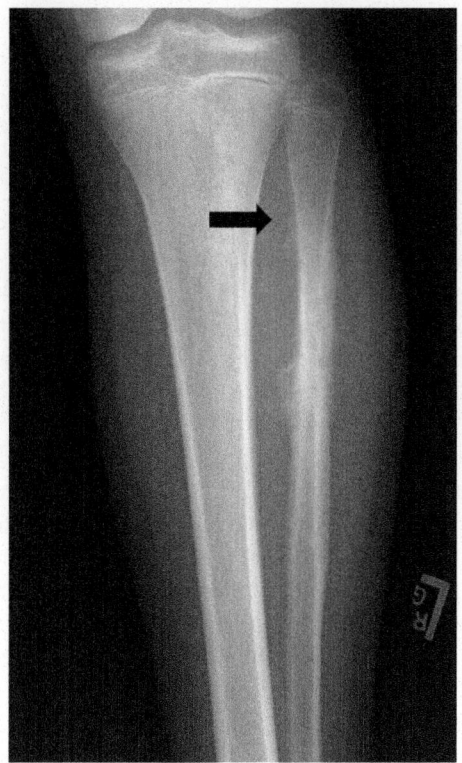

Fig. 6.9 An osteosarcoma of the fibula. Note the triangular area of periosteal bone formation, or Codman's triangle (arrow)

portion of the bone. There may be periosteal reaction, such as a Codman's triangle, formed as the tumor extends into the soft tissue and lifts the periosteum off the cortex (Fig. 6.9). A soft tissue shadow or bone formation in the soft tissue may also be evident. Osteosarcomas may be primarily sclerotic, lytic, or a mixed appearance. While the appearance does not infer prognostic value, it is important to recognize these patterns. Purely lytic osteosarcomas can be more difficult to recognize than the other patterns and may be mistaken for other entities, such as a giant cell tumor, aneurysmal bone cyst, or metastatic carcinoma.

Histologic Characteristics

The diagnosis of osteosarcoma is based on the identification of a malignant stroma that produces unequivocal osteoid matrix. The stroma consists of a disorganized cluster of highly atypical cells. These pleomorphic cells contain hyperchromatic, irregular nuclei. Intercellularly, there is a lace-like immature osteoid. An osteosarcoma may be made up predominantly of cells producing osteoid or other elements such as cartilage producing cells or fibroblasts. These are referred to as osteogenic, chondrogenic, and fibrogenic osteosarcomas respectively. Even if the vast majority of the tumor is composed of other elements, if there is a small component with osteoid producing cells, it is treated as an osteosarcoma.

Treatment Strategy

Treatment of osteosarcoma involves a combination of chemotherapy and surgery in the form of a wide resection [10]. Wide resection is most often achieved with a limb-sparing approach with skeletal reconstruction. First line chemotherapy most often involves a combination of high dose methotrexate, doxorubicin, and cisplatin, although, in adults, methotrexate is often omitted. Many other agents and regimens have been used, both as initial treatment and for those with a poor response to initial chemotherapy, but none to date have yielded better results than the above combination. Most often patients will receive preoperative chemotherapy followed by surgery followed by postoperative chemotherapy. This order of treatment has the potential benefits of allowing for the manufacturing of a custom prosthesis, a reduction in size of the soft tissue component, although this is uncommon, and allows for an assessment of the effectiveness of chemotherapy through examination of the surgical specimen. The order of surgery and chemotherapy does not have an effect on the overall outcome however and in some instances, immediate surgery followed by adjuvant chemotherapy may be best.

For patients with metastatic disease, the same initial treatment algorithm is used. The primary tumor is typically still resected as this offers a survival benefit. Likewise, in patients with a relatively small number of metastatic lesions (oligometastatic disease), surgical resection of the metastatic lesions can offer a survival benefit.

Outcomes

After the significant improvement in outcomes in the 1970s associated with the use of multiagent chemotherapy, the overall survival rates have been relatively steady [11]. The 5-year overall survival for patients with an isolated osteosarcoma is 76%. For patients with metastatic disease it is between 20% and 25%. Patients treated with surgery only have a 5-years survival of 15–20% owing to the high rate of micrometastatic disease present on presentation that goes untreated without the use of chemotherapy [11].

Variants of Osteosarcoma

There are a number of variants of osteosarcoma. In addition to the intramedullary (or classic) type discussed above, the most commonly referred to subtypes are parosteal, periosteal, and telangiectatic osteosarcoma. The first two of these arise from the surface of the bone and predictably are referred to as surface-based lesions. The third is a purely lytic lesion.

Parosteal osteosarcoma is a low-grade surface-based lesion. It most commonly presents around the ages of 30–40. It arises from the metaphysis of the bone, with 60–70% of lesions found at the distal femur. Radiographically, it is distinguished by a densely ossified mass that appears to be "stuck onto" the surface of the bone (Fig. 6.10). Some involvement of the marrow cavity is commonly seen on axial imaging, but the majority of the marrow should be normal. Histology reveals relatively hypocellular stroma with mature appearing

bony trabeculae and can be mistaken for normal bone by the pathologist without a clinical history. Due to the low-grade nature, metastatic disease is rare. Treatment is wide excision alone without chemotherapy. The long-term survival is very good at about 95%.

Periosteal osteosarcoma is an intermediate-grade surface-based lesion. It often presents in adolescence and early adulthood. Radiographically, it tends be a broad-based lesion often with saucerization of the cortex and a sunburst pattern of periosteal reaction. It typically involves 50% of the cortex or less. While most commonly found in the metaphysis, it can be found in the diaphyseal portion of the bone more commonly than other types of osteosarcoma. Histologically, periosteal osteosarcomas tend to have a predominant chondrogenic component. Surgical treatment is a wide resection with this often being possible with a hemicortical resection. The role for chemotherapy is less well established in periosteal osteosarcoma than other variants. The same chemotherapy regimen as intramedullary osteosarcoma has typically been used, but smaller, more peripheral lesions appear to have similar outcomes with or without chemotherapy [12]. Overall outcome is somewhat better than intramedullary osteosarcoma.

Telangiectatic osteosarcoma is a rare high-grade lesion seen at similar ages and locations as intramedullary osteosarcoma. On plain radiographs, it is

Fig. 6.10 Plain radiograph (**a**) and axial CT (**b**) of a distal femoral parosteal osteosarcoma. Although the tumor wraps around 50% of the cortex, the medullary space is essentially normal

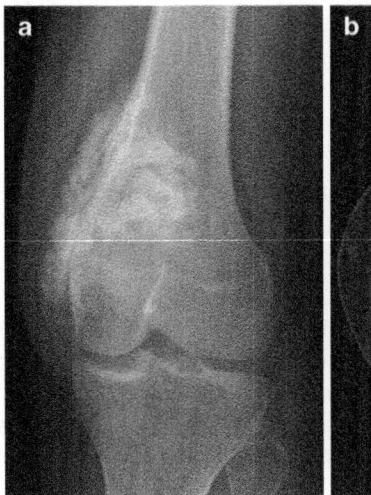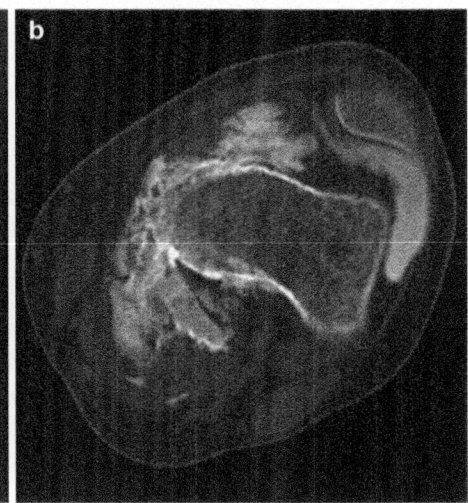

a purely lytic lesion arising from the metaphysis of the bone that often has an expansile component. On MRI, fluid-fluid levels are often seen demonstrating the blood-filled cystic components. The appearance can closely resemble an aneurysmal bone cyst. It is important to consider a telangiectatic osteosarcoma on the differential whenever treating the much more common aneurysmal bone cyst. Treatment and outcomes for telangiectatic osteosarcoma are the same as for the classic intramedullary type.

Chondrosarcoma

Chondrosarcoma is the second most common primary malignant spindle cell tumor. In contrast to osteosarcoma, the primary neoplastic tissue is cartilaginous without evidence of primary osteoid formation. There are a wide variety of chondrosarcomas ranging from atypical cartilaginous tumors of the extremity with little to no metastatic potential to dedifferentiated chondrosarcoma with an aggressive course and poor overall prognosis. The majority of tumors are primary, but secondary chondrosarcomas comprise 20–25% of tumors [13]. More rare variants include clear cell and mesenchymal chondrosarcomas.

Clinical Presentation
While chondrosarcoma can occur in a wide age range, it is primarily a tumor of adulthood. In an adolescent with a malignant chondrogenic tumor, a diagnosis of chondrosarcoma should be viewed with suspicion as chondroblastic osteosarcoma is much more common in this age group. In patients in the fifth decade of life and later, distinction between metastatic carcinoma and chondrosarcoma must often be made. The majority of lesions are found centrally or in the proximal extremities.

Pain is the most common presenting symptom although an enlarging mass is sometimes the most prominent symptom. Even intermediate-grade tumors can sometimes develop a large soft tissue mass. Lesions in the spine or pelvis may present with referred pain. In a patient with an osteochondroma, growth of the lesion or a new onset of nonactivity related pain heralds a malignant transformation.

Secondary chondrosarcomas arise most commonly from osteochondromas with enchondromas being the next most common underlying lesion. Solitary osteochondromas and enchondromas have a relatively low risk of malignant transformation of around 1%. Patients with multiple hereditary exostosis have between a 6% and 10% lifetime risk of malignant transformation. Patients with multiple enchondromas, or Ollier's disease, have a 25–30% risk of malignant transformation. Patients with multiple enchondromas and angiomas, or Maffucci's syndrome, are thought to have an even higher lifetime risk of malignancy, including chondrosarcoma.

Radiographic Findings
In general, chondrosarcomas are aggressive appearing lesions with radiographic evidence of a characteristic ring and arc or punctate calcification chondroid matrix. Low-grade lesions often have relatively well-defined borders and look similar to enchondromas but have significant endosteal scalloping and potentially mild expansile remodeling of the cortex (Fig. 6.11). Radiographic change over time in an otherwise benign appearing lesion is another sign of malignancy. High-grade lesions are less well-defined and, in addition to endosteal scalloping, can also have additional features including expansile remodeling of the cortex, periosteal reaction, complete break in the cortex, and soft tissue extension (Fig. 6.12).

Location of the tumor makes a significant difference in the radiographic interpretation. Benign enchondromas in the small bones of the hand or foot can have significant endosteal scalloping and cortical expansion or remodeling that would be consistent with a chondrosarcoma in a different region of the body. Conversely, benign appearing chondroid lesions located centrally such as the pelvis can behave aggressively.

Histologic Characteristics
In general, there is tremendous histologic variability. High-grade examples can be easily identified, whereas certain low-grade tumors are more difficult to distinguish from enchondromas. Low-grade chondrosarcomas are characterized by an

Fig. 6.11 Low-grade chondrosarcoma or atypical cartilaginous tumor of the distal femur. Plain radiograph (**a**) appears similar to an enchondroma. CT (**b**) shows significant endosteal scalloping (arrow). Patient had longstanding activity related pain from osteoarthritis of the knee and a new onset of pain at night

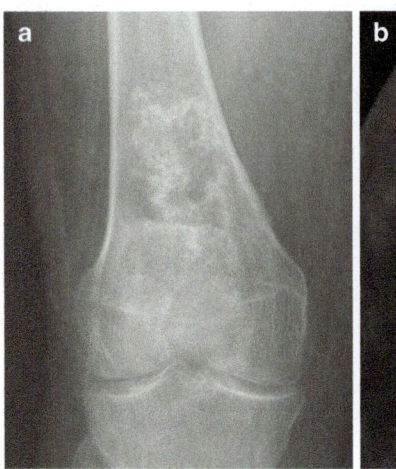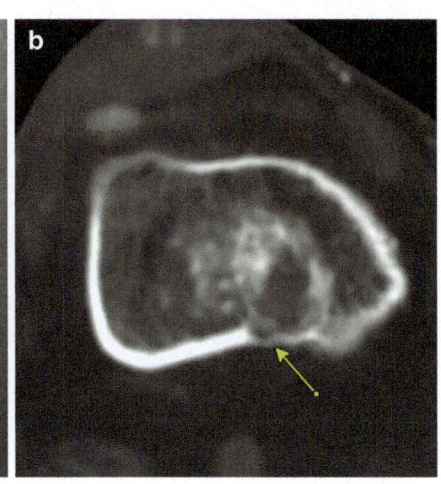

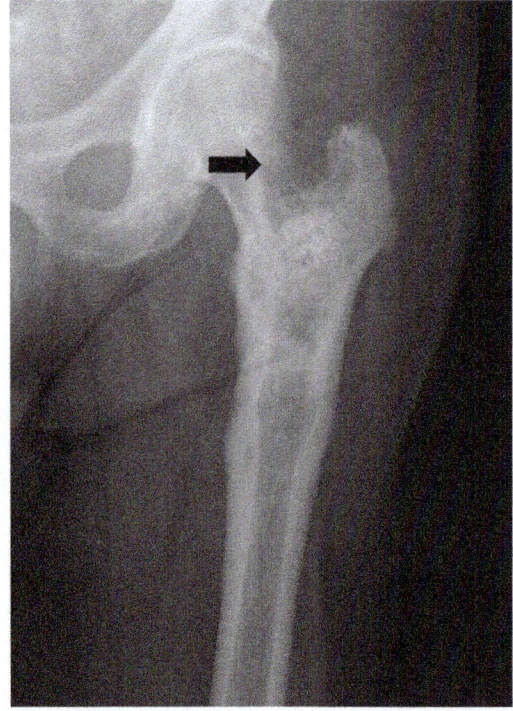

Fig. 6.12 Intermediate-grade chondrosarcoma with high-grade dedifferentiated component. The tumor has expanded and thickened the cortex. The high-grade component corresponds to the more lytic area indicated by the arrow

chondrosarcomas. The pathologist should consult with the radiologist or treating surgeon when developing a histologic diagnosis. Because of the difficulty of histologic diagnosis, preoperative biopsy is often not utilized, with the primary indication for biopsy being to distinguish cartilage lesions from other tissue types such as chondroblastic osteosarcoma or metastatic carcinoma.

Treatment Strategy

Chondrosarcomas are generally not responsive to either chemotherapy or radiation. Because of this, surgery is the mainstay of treatment. Low-grade lesions, particularly in the extremity, can be treated with an intralesional procedure usually followed by a local adjuvant such as cryosurgery [14]. Intralesional procedures are more controversial in the pelvis, and many orthopedic oncologists recommend wide excision of even grade 1 chondrosarcomas in this area. Intermediate and high-grade lesions, regardless of location, are treated with wide resection and appropriate reconstruction.

Outcomes

Outcome is highly dependent on grade. An atypical cartilaginous tumor in the extremity has close to 100% long-term survival. A typical intermediate-grade chondrosarcoma has a 5-year survival of 60–70%. Dedifferentiated chondrosarcoma has a 5-year survival of less than 10%.

increased number of chondrocytes within a chondroid matrix. Higher grade lesions have proportionally increased cellularity with marked variation in cell size. Nuclear atypia with binuclear cells are more often seen in higher grade

Centrally located lesions have a worse prognosis than more distal lesions.

Variants of Chondrosarcoma

There are a number of variants of chondrosarcoma. Some notable ones are discussed below.

Clear Cell Chondrosarcoma

Clear cell chondrosarcoma is a rare subtype of chondrosarcoma. It is a low-grade tumor that is most notable for its epiphyseal location. Early recognition can be difficult as it is often mistaken for chondroblastoma. Metastatic disease is somewhat infrequent and often occurs after local recurrence. Primary treatment is wide excision.

Mesenchymal Chondrosarcoma

A rare and aggressive variant, mesenchymal chondrosarcoma has a predilection for flat bones as opposed to long tubular bones. It typically presents in a younger age group and has high metastatic potential. It is characterized histologically by small, compact cells intermixed with islands of cartilaginous matrix. Preferred treatment is wide resection with adjuvant chemotherapy, although because of the rarity of the tumor, there is no good data to show chemotherapy improves overall outcomes. The 10-year survival rate is reportedly 28% [15].

Dedifferentiated Chondrosarcoma

Roughly 10% of chondrosarcomas may dedifferentiate into either a fibrosarcoma or osteosarcoma. Dedifferentiation usually occurs in older individuals and carries a dismal prognosis. Surgical treatment remains wide resection. Adjuvant chemotherapy is typically given but may not significantly affect the poor overall outcome.

Ewing Sarcoma

Ewing sarcoma, a round cell sarcoma of bone, is the second most common pediatric bone sarcoma, behind osteosarcoma. The lesion is char-acterized by poorly differentiated, small, round cells with marked homogeneity. The histologic appearance is evident in both the clinical and radiographic presentation. Although historically associated with a high mortality, outcomes have improved significantly. Standard treatment for both local control and systemic therapy continues to evolve [16].

Clinical Presentation

Ewing sarcoma, similar to osteosarcoma, has a peak incidence in the second decade of life. The average patient with Ewing sarcoma is slightly younger than the average osteosarcoma patient. The majority of patients present in the first two decades of life and it is unusual for a patient to present after the age of 40. Common sites of disease include the femur, tibia, humerus, and flat bones including the pelvis. As with all bone sarcomas, pain is the most common presenting symptom with a palpable mass often present. About 25% of patients have metastatic disease on presentation. After the lungs, bone, and notably bone marrow are the most common sites for metastasis. Because of this, a bone marrow biopsy is required in addition to the standard staging workup in Ewing sarcoma. Alternatively, PET has been shown to have a similar sensitivity as bone marrow biopsy detecting bone marrow metastasis and can also screen for other sites of disease.

Unique to Ewing sarcoma are the systemic signs of illness, including fever, anorexia, weight loss, leukocytosis, and anemia. The lactate dehydrogenase level may be elevated in addition to mild increase in inflammatory markers. Physical exam can reveal a tender mass with overlying erythema and induration. Because of this, it can sometimes be difficult to distinguish between Ewing sarcoma and osteomyelitis without a biopsy.

Radiographic Findings

The radiographic appearance of Ewing sarcoma shares many characteristics with other round blue cell tumors. Lesions most often arise from the metaphysis but can extend to or arise from the diaphysis. Tumors have a permeative lytic appearance (Fig. 6.13). There can be a relatively large, often circumferential, soft tissue component with relative sparing of the cortex. As the soft tissue mass lifts the periosteum, the reactive new bone formation often forms in layers creating the classic "onion skin" appearance.

Histologic Characteristics

Ewing sarcoma is classically characterized by large nests and sheets of uniform round cells with round nuclei. The sheets are often compartmentalized by intersecting collagenous trabeculae. Nucleoli are uncommon and mitotic activity is usually minimal. Histologically, Ewing sarcoma must be differentiated from osteomyelitis and Langerhans cell histiocytosis in addition to neuroblastoma in very young patients and lymphoma in older patients. The immunostain CD99 is sensitive for Ewing sarcoma, although not specific. The vast majority of Ewing sarcomas have a spe-

cific genetic mutation with the presence of one of these being essentially diagnostic. The most common translocation is t(11:22) producing the fusion protein EWS-FLI1.

Treatment Strategy

Historically, Ewing sarcoma was treated with external beam radiation. Currently, surgery, chemotherapy, and radiation are all used in the treatment of Ewing sarcoma. Treatment can be thought of as chemotherapy for systemic disease plus local control using surgery and/or radiation. While radiation previously was the primary mode of local control, it has fallen out of favor because of short- and long-term side effects. Outcomes appear to be worse than in patients treated with surgery, although this is confounded by inherent selection bias. Radiation continues to be widely used in tumors that are either unresectable or where surgery is associated with unacceptable morbidity. Surgical treatment involves wide resection with standard reconstruction options. More recently, postoperative radiation has been shown to been useful in cases where adequate surgical margins could not be obtained.

The most common chemotherapy regimen involves a combination of five drugs: vincristine, doxorubicin, cyclophosphamide, ifosfamide, and etoposide. Compressed dose schedules have been shown to be more effective.

Outcomes

Currently, the 5-year overall survival for patients with isolated disease ranges from 65% to 83%. The 5-year survival for patients with metastatic disease is 25–40% [17]. Poor prognostic indicators other than metastatic disease at presentation include large tumor size, more centrally located tumors, and older age at presentation.

Undifferentiated Pleomorphic Sarcoma

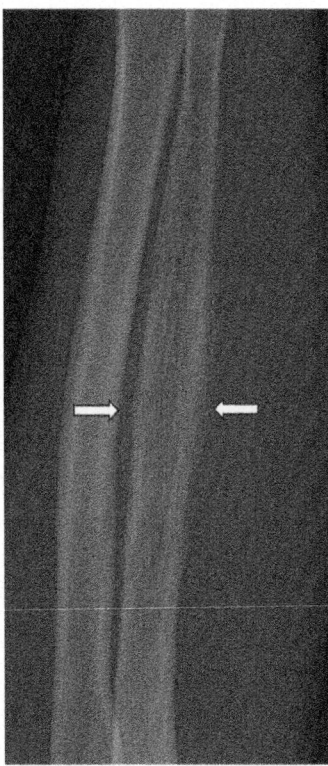

Fig. 6.13 Permeative lesion of the ulna with "onion skin" periosteal reaction, typical of Ewing sarcoma and other round blue cell tumors of bone (arrows)

Undifferentiated pleomorphic sarcoma (UPS), formerly known as malignant fibrous histiocytoma (MFH) of bone, is a high-grade malignant tumor that is histologically similar to its soft tissue counterpart. It is primarily a disease of adulthood, with the most common sites being metaphyseal long bones, particularly around the knee. Presentation is similar to that of osteosarcoma although the incidence of pathologic fracture may be higher.

Imaging is not specific and consists of a poorly defined lytic lesion with cortical destruction and a soft tissue mass. Histologically, the lack of osteoid distinguishes UPS of bone from osteosarcoma.

Treatment is the same as for osteosarcoma with chemotherapy using an osteosarcoma protocol and surgery in the form of wide resection. Outcomes are slightly worse than for osteosarcoma with a 5-year overall survival of about 60%.

Benign Bone Tumors

Benign bone tumors are more common than malignant ones, and usually first appear during childhood or adolescence. Treatment ranges from observation to wide excision. Many benign tumors are treated with intralesional curettage often with a local adjuvant. Some lesions can be treated percutaneously with minimal morbidity. Treatment is largely dictated by the natural history of the specific entity, with preservation of function as the main goal of treatment. In general, preoperative staging studies are accurate and the correct diagnosis can often be made on the basis of plain radiographs alone.

Enchondroma

Enchondromas may be solitary or multiple (Ollier's disease), with occurrences reported in most bones. The rate of malignant transformation is difficult to determine for solitary lesions but is thought to be approximately 1% and 30% in patients with Ollier's disease. Patients with Maffucci's syndrome (multiple enchondromas and angiomas) have a high lifetime risk for both chondrosarcoma and other malignancies. Biologic potential varies by site. Enchondromas

in the hand and foot behave indolently despite aggressive features on both radiographs and histology (Fig. 6.14). Enchondromas in the pelvis and other flat bones occur rarely and even benign appearing lesions often need to be treated as chondrosarcomas.

Enchondromas are most often found incidentally. They are rarely painful unless a pathologic fracture exists. If patients do present with pain, careful workup should be performed as this is likely a sign of local aggressiveness and possible malignancy.

Plain radiographs are often diagnostic. A geographic lesion with the ring and arc or stippled calcifications of chondroid matrix is present with little or no endosteal scalloping. Some enchondromas, frequently in the hand and foot, are purely lytic; these can often be distinguished by their lobular appearance on MRI. Enchondromas are distinguished from low-grade chondrosarcomas, or atypical cartilaginous tumors in the extremity, primarily by their lack of significant endosteal scalloping.

Histologically, enchondromas are relatively hypocellular and consist of bland, small chondrocytes within lacunar spaces surrounded by chon-

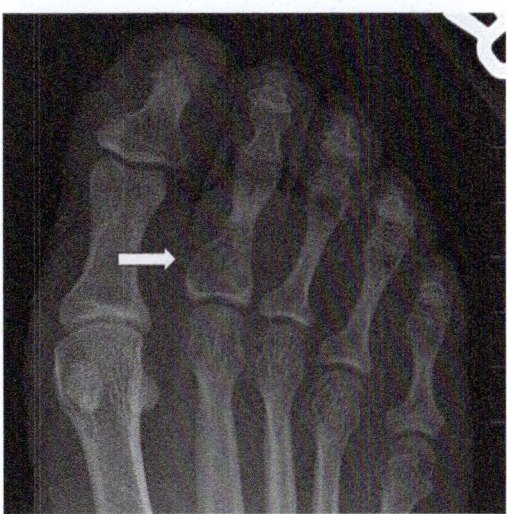

Fig. 6.14 Enchondroma of the second toe proximal phalanx. Note the stippled calcifications of chondroid matrix (arrow). While significant expansion and endosteal scalloping signals a more aggressive lesion in the long bones, this is consistent with an enchondroma in the small bones of the hand and foot

droid matrix. Histologic features vary considerably by location and as previously mentioned, it is difficult to distinguish between enchondroma and low-grade chondrosarcoma by histology alone.

Enchondromas rarely require treatment. When treatment is necessary, a simple curettage is often curative. If atypical cartilaginous tumor is a possibility, a local adjuvant such as cryosurgery should be added to reduce the chance of local recurrence.

Osteochondroma (Exostosis)

Osteochondromas are the most common benign bone tumor. They typically grow along with the individual until skeletal maturity is reached. They are characteristically sessile or pedunculated, arising from the cortex of long tubular bones adjacent to the physis. Osteochondromas are usually solitary but can be multiple in multiple hereditary exostosis (MHE). MHE is caused by an autosomal dominant germline mutation in tumor suppressor genes EXT1, EXT2, or EXT3. Mutation in the EXT1 gene has a more severe phenotype with more osteochondromas, greater deformity, and a higher chance of malignant transformation (Fig. 6.15). Solitary osteochondromas frequently have somatic mutations in the EXT1 gene. Solitary osteochondromas have a 1% chance of malignant transformation, while MHE patients have a 6–10% chance of malignant transformation with the risk

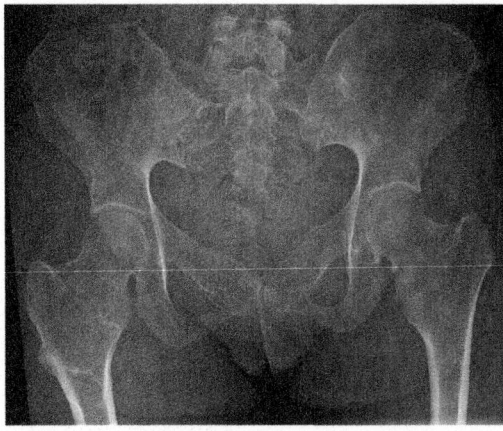

Fig. 6.15 Multiple hereditary exostosis. There is flaring of the proximal femoral metaphysis in addition to multiple osteochondromas (arrows)

varying by the underlying genetic mutation as noted above. Osteochondromas of the pelvis may be at higher risk for malignant transformation than other lesions.

Plain radiographs are usually diagnostic, with no further tests required. Radiographs show an exostosis with continuity of the cortex and medullary bone between normal bone and the lesion. Sessile osteochondromas, of note, may prove to be a diagnostic challenge as they must be differentiated from a parosteal osteosarcoma. CT can be helpful in assessing the cortex in either sessile lesions or larger lesions that may wrap around the bone. MRI is useful to assess for a soft tissue component when there is a question of malignant transformation. MRI can also be used to assess the thickness of the cartilage cap. The thickness of the cartilage cap may be an unreliable indicator for malignancy, but a cap of over 2 cm thick in an adult is worrisome for malignancy.

In general, surgical removal is recommended only for symptomatic osteochondromas. For a patient with a newly symptomatic osteochondroma, the clinician should first distinguish between mechanical type symptoms and pain arising from the tumor itself. Tumor type pain or growth after skeletal maturity should prompt an evaluation for a secondary chondrosarcoma. If symptomatic osteochondromas do not respond to conservative treatment, surgical treatment involves a marginal excision involving the entirety of the cartilage cap. Disruption of the cartilage cap can result in an unnecessarily high risk of local recurrence.

Osteoid Osteoma

Osteoid osteomas are benign lesions, with a characteristic pain pattern. The most common anatomic sites are the femur and tibia; however, they can occur in virtually any bone. Pain can precede the appearance of radiographic abnormalities and lesions can be quite small, so there is often a lag time in proper diagnosis.

The hallmark clinical finding of an osteoid osteoma is severe, well-localized aching type pain. Pain is relieved with nonsteroidal anti-inflammatories

(NSAIDs). The extent of pain relief is often dramatic with pain relief within 30 min, and a history of pain relief with NSAIDs is essential for diagnosis. Patients commonly come to the office having taken NSAIDs on a regular basis for a year or more. Periarticular lesions are associated with pain and swelling that often mimic monoarticular arthritis. Lesions involving the spine can present as painful scoliosis.

Osteoid osteomas can be found in any portion of the bone. Therefore, the position of the lesion relative to the cortex, periosteum, and spongiosa determine the radiographic appearance. The most common site is intracortical, with plain radiographs demonstrating a characteristic radiolucent nidus surrounded by dense, reactive bone. When the tumor is intramedullary, the sclerotic response is less dramatic. Osteoid osteomas are often only a few millimeters in diameter making them difficult to see on plain radiographs. CT is often the best way to localize these lesions. The most obvious feature on MRI is often the surrounding marrow edema.

Traditionally, surgical treatment required simple curettage of the lytic nidus. Given the small size of the nidus and the surrounding sclerotic bone, this can prove difficult. Using a burr down technique to slowly remove sclerotic bone until visualizing the bright red nidus, which can then be curetted, is a helpful method to do this. The majority of lesions are currently treated using CT-guided radiofrequency ablation. MRI guided

high intensity focused ultrasound (HIFU) has also been used. Both ablation options are effective, but their use is limited in areas such as the spine or tibia if the lesion is too close to a nerve root or the skin respectively.

Aneurysmal Bone Cysts

Aneurysmal bone cysts (ABC) are benign tumors that are most common prior to skeletal maturity. They also have no potential for malignancy. ABCs are usually found in the metaphyseal region of long bones or the posterior elements of the vertebrae. They can be primary or secondary lesions. Primary lesions are more common in skeletally immature patients and are associated with a genetic translocation that upregulates ubiquitin-specific protease 6 (USP6). Secondary lesions may arise from almost any bone tumor, with giant cell tumor of bone the most common. ABCs seen in adulthood are more likely to be secondary lesions.

Radiographically, ABCs are eccentric, purely lytic, and expansile. They can thin the cortex significantly to the point it is only visible on CT. Fluid-fluid levels, indicating blood-filled cysts, are seen on MRI. A soft tissue component can also be seen on MRI. Histology shows benign spindle cells surrounding blood-filled spaces (Fig. 6.16). Telangiectatic osteosarcoma should always be on the differential and biopsy is indi-

Fig. 6.16 Aneurysmal bone cyst in a 14 year male. Plain radiographs (**a**) and MRI showing fluid-fluid levels (**b**)

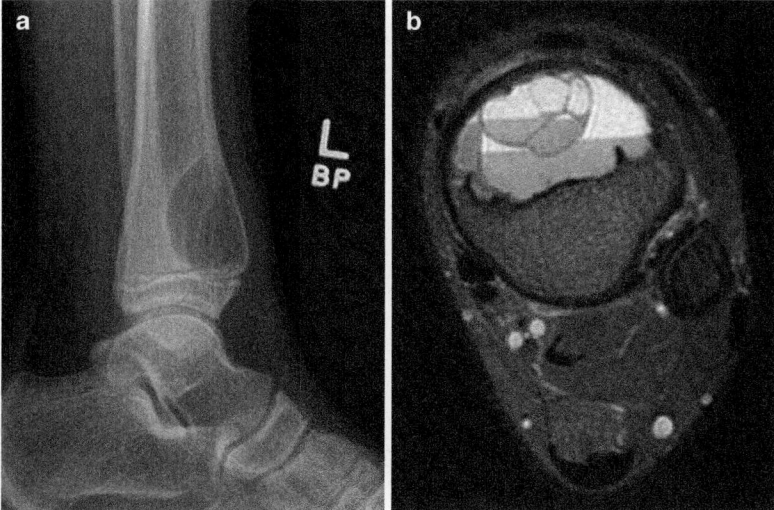

cated for lesions with more aggressive features, such as a soft tissue component.

The most common treatment is a standard intralesional procedure with open curettage with the use of a local adjuvant. When the lesion abuts an open physis, consideration should be given to accepting a higher local recurrence rate in order to avoid injury to the physis. Another treatment option gaining acceptance is the use of doxycycline. Percutaneous doxycycline mixed with albumin was first used in the spine but is now being used elsewhere. This has the obvious advantage of avoiding the morbidity of open surgery. A number of technical variations have been used, but results are promising [18].

Unicameral Bone Cysts

Unicameral bone cysts (UBCs), or simple bone cysts, are non-neoplastic lesions that occur during skeletal growth (Fig. 6.17). They are usually found in the metaphysis and/or diaphysis of long bones. The majority of lesions occur in the proximal humerus with the proximal femur being the next most common site.

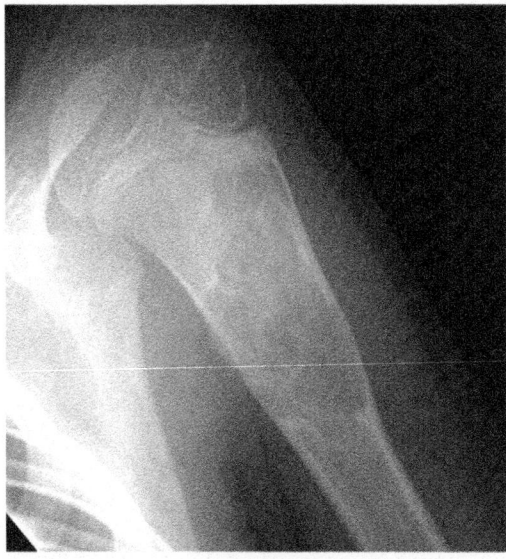

Fig. 6.17 A unicameral bone cyst of the proximal humerus in the skeletally immature patient

The lesions themselves are usually painless although patients commonly have pain at presentation. Pain is indicative of either a fracture or the micromotion from an impending fracture.

UBCs appear as a geographic expansile lytic lesion on plain radiographs. In contrast to an ABC, they typically expand the bone symmetrically and do not expand beyond the width of the physis. If a fracture has occurred, a fragment of the cortex can be seen within the cyst cavity; this is known as the "fallen leaf" sign. Due to this characteristic, non-aggressive appearance, they can usually be diagnosed with plain films alone, and are rarely confused with other benign or malignant tumors. Therefore, further staging studies are usually not indicated.

UBCs have been treated with a wide variety of percutaneous strategies. The outcomes for these strategies are similar and the need for multiple treatments is common. Good outcomes have been obtained with injection of methylprednisolone and bone graft after aspiration of the lesion. Pathologic fractures are allowed to heal. Ten to fifteen percent of lesions resolve after fracture and fracture healing facilitates percutaneous treatment in those lesions that do not resolve. Internal fixation is only necessary for lesions in the proximal femur.

Giant Cell Tumor of Bone

Giant cell tumor of bone is the prototypical benign but aggressive tumor of bone. It is a locally aggressive tumor starting in the metaphysis of long bones extending up to the subchondral surface. They are most commonly found about the knee but can be found in any bone with the distal radius and sacrum being other notable locations. Lesions are more common in females than males. They most commonly occur between the third and fifth decades of life. Giant cell tumors also have the notable distinction of being benign and having a 2–5% chance of metastatic spread to the lungs. Pain both at rest and at night is the predominant symptom at presentation.

Giant cell tumor of bone has a readily recognizable appearance on plain radiograph when located in the long bones (*Refer to Figs. 6.1 and 6.6*). They have a razor-sharp margin but typically lack a sclerotic rim. The lesion is usually eccentrically located and extends to the subchondral bone. Local advanced imaging is usually not necessary for lesions in the appendicular skeleton, but MRI and/or CT can be helpful for lesions in the pelvis or spine. CT scan of the chest should be included to screen for the presence of pulmonary metastasis. Preoperative biopsy is warranted for lesions in the pelvis and spine and in more aggressive appearing lesions to rule out malignant tumors.

Two basic cell types constitute typical giant cell tumor of bone. The stroma is characterized by polygonal to somewhat spindled cells containing central round nuclei. Scattered diffusely throughout the stroma are benign, multinucleated giant cells.

Treatment is most commonly an intralesional procedure with the procedure providing a model for the treatment of other benign tumors. A cortical window is made with a high-speed burr. Curets are then used to remove all visible lesional material; the initial portion can be sent for frozen section to confirm the diagnosis. The high-speed burr is then used to remove the reactive zone around the lesion. A local adjuvant is then used to kill any remaining tumor cells. Cryosurgery is typically used at our institution. Reconstruction involves filling the cavity with polymethyl methacrylate after placing bone graft along the subchondral surface. A locking plate or intraosseous rush rods are usually placed prior to cementation to increase torsional stability.

Not all giant cell tumors are best treated with an intralesional procedure. If sufficient cortical destruction has occurred or an expendable bone is involved, wide resection is the treatment of choice. Radiation has been used, particularly in sacral lesions not amenable to surgery, but its use should be avoided for the most part due to a significant risk of malignant transformation. Tumor osteolysis occurs through the receptor activator of nuclear factor kappa beta (RANK) pathway. Denosumab acts on this pathway and has a role in the treatment of giant cell tumor. Denosumab is used primarily to treat unresectable tumors or patients with metastatic disease. It can also be used in the preoperative setting to allow for an intralesional procedure of a tumor that would otherwise require wide resection. This should be done with caution as high-recurrence rates have been reported when adequate curettage of the surrounding reactive bone is not performed.

Eosinophilic Granuloma

Eosinophilic granuloma is the term used for an isolated lesion of Langerhans cell histiocytosis (LCH). LCH can affect many different organ systems and the extent of disease varies widely. Young children are most commonly affected. Presenting symptoms for patients with skeletal involvement includes pain, but may also include local swelling and malaise, fever, or even leukocytosis.

The skull is the most location with the pelvis and proximal long bones also commonly affected. In the long bones, lesions arise in the diaphysis or metadiaphysis. Lesions may appear well-circumscribed with a sclerotic rim or may have a more permeative appearance with significant endosteal scalloping or periosteal reaction. Eosinophilic granuloma is known as "the great mimicker" due to its variable appearance that can be similar to a wide variety of lesions. Because of this, biopsy is necessary.

Isolated eosinophilic granulomas often resolve without treatment or after needle biopsy alone. Lesions can be successfully treated with intralesional steroid injection or with curettage and bone grafting for lesions with more significant cortical involvement. Patients with multisystem disease are treated with chemotherapy.

Metastatic Bone Disease, Myeloma, Lymphoma, and Pathologic Fractures

Natural History

With an aging population and advances in the treatment of many cancers, the overall number of people living with cancer continues to increase.

While the rate differs by primary tumor, bone is the third most common site of metastatic disease. Estimates of the prevalence of patients with metastatic disease range from 300,000 to 600,000 people in the USA. Bones in the axial skeleton and proximal extremities are most often affected. Within the spine, certain regions are more commonly affected than others. Metastatic spread more frequently impacts the lumbar, thoracic, than cervical spine. Batson's venous plexus provides the anatomic basis for differences in bony locations primarily impacted by metastatic disease spread [19]. Batson's venous plexus describes the paravertebral venous system that connects the basivertebral veins and the pelvic and thoracic veins.

A patient presenting with a bone lesion is more likely to have metastatic disease than a primary bone tumor if they are over the age of 40 [19]. The most common primary tumors to metastasize to bone are breast, prostate, lung, renal, thyroid, and gastrointestinal cancers. Although multiple myeloma arises from the bone marrow, from the treatment perspective of an orthopedic surgeon, it can be approached in the same fashion as metastatic disease to the bone. Orthopedic surgeons are frequently involved in the care of these patients, so they must be able to identify and treat patients with metastatic bony disease.

Clinical Characteristics and Physical Examination

Pain is the most coming symptom for patients presenting with metastatic disease to the bone. Pain arising from the tumor itself is typical of most bone tumors and is commonly described as a dull, aching pain present at rest and pain that wakes the patient up at night. Mechanical pain that is worse with weight bearing is indicative of strain from an impending fracture. Pathologic fracture is another common initial presentation. Tumors in the spine may cause neurologic symptoms as well. Differentiating between pain arising from the tumor, mechanical pain, and standard musculoskeletal pain is an important factor in

deciding treatment. Pain from a bone lesion or pathologic fracture is often the first sign of cancer. In patients with a known primary cancer, lesions are often seen on staging workup. While these lesions are less likely to need orthopedic treatment as they are often asymptomatic, attention should be paid to high-risk areas such as the spine and proximal femur.

Radiographic Findings

Most metastatic disease to the bone appears as a lytic lesion with cortical destruction. Appearance ranges from a relatively well-defined punched out lesion to a more permeative appearance. Most lesions start in the medullary space, although lung metastases can arise from the cortex. Breast cancer metastases classically have a mixed lytic and blastic appearance, with a lytic lesion with some areas of bone formation in and around the lesion. Most prostate cancer lesions are blastic with dense sclerotic bone formation.

CT is helpful to assess the degree of cortical involvement of the lesion. It is the most accurate way to assess for fracture risk. CT also offers a view of the intramedullary extent of a lesion. In a patient with an unusual fracture mechanism, a CT of the involved bone offers a quick way to screen for cortical thinning or a marrow replacing lesion that would be indicative of a pathologic fracture.

MRI is certainly the most sensitive way to screen for metastatic disease to the bone. It offers the best view of the intramedullary extent of a lesion. Significant soft tissue extension is relatively rare in metastatic disease, but MRI is the best way to characterize this. MRI is not helpful in assessing fracture risk.

A technetium bone scan assesses for osteoblastic activity. It is most helpful to screen for other skeletal disease. Purely lytic lesions will not have significant uptake on a bone scan, so a skeletal survey is typically used to screen for skeletal disease in myeloma. A bone scan is frequently recommended to assess if an incidentally found lesion is "active" and requires further workup or not. While bone scan may be helpful, its sensitivity and specificity differentiating benign from malignant lesions is low.

Staging and Biopsy

When a patient presents either with a new bone lesion or a pathologic fracture with suspected metastatic disease, biopsy and basic staging should be done prior to any surgical treatment. Imaging and lab work should typically be done prior to biopsy. Standard imaging after local radiographs includes a CT of the chest, abdomen, and pelvis and a whole body technetium bone scan. Laboratory work includes a complete blood count, complete metabolic panel with calcium level, and serum protein electrophoresis. Additional laboratory values may be obtained but tend to be low yield from a diagnostic standpoint.

As noted above, a tissue diagnosis is necessary before any treatment is started. This step should not be skipped or abbreviated in an effort expedite care. In a patient with no prior history of cancer or a patient with previously localized cancer who present with an isolated bone lesion, biopsy should be done as a separate procedure. This allows for a final pathologic diagnosis rather than relying on intraoperative frozen section. The reliability of frozen section relies on a number of factors, including the underlying histology, but the overall accuracy compared to final diagnosis is estimated to be 90–95% [20]. Core-needle biopsy is most commonly done and is often performed under image guidance. In a patient with a known primary cancer and multiple bone lesions or wide spread metastatic disease, biopsy at the time of surgery is sufficient as the effect on treatment decisions is less. In general, patients with previously biopsy proven metastatic disease do not require additional biopsy unless there is a suspicion for a second primary tumor.

Treatment Strategy

Patients with metastatic bone disease should always be treated in the setting of a multidisciplinary team. In addition to administering chemotherapy, medical oncologists can help assess overall prognosis to guide treatment decisions. Most patients with bone lesions should also receive either a bisphosphonate or denosumab to lessen the chance of additional skeletal disease. External beam radiation can be used to palliate pain from bone lesions and slow the local progression of disease. This can be done in isolation or after surgical fixation. Radiologists can assist with biopsy or preoperative embolization of bone lesions.

The orthopedic goals of treatment for patients with metastatic disease differ from those targeted toward patients with primary bone tumors. Resecting the bone lesion does not affect outcome, so orthopedic treatment is aimed pain reduction, fracture prevention, ambulation, and preventing additional neurological sequelae. There are exceptions to this rule with the most obvious being patients with renal cell carcinoma and isolated metastatic lesions. There is a survival benefit to resection of the metastatic lesion in this case.

Fracture prevention is an important part of the orthopedic care of patients with metastatic disease (Fig. 6.18). Patients who undergo prophylactic fixation of a lesion have shorter hospital stays, faster return to activity, fewer complications, and better overall survival when compared to those who require surgery to fix a pathologic fracture. Pain is the most important indicator of fracture risk. A patient with functional pain (pain with weight bearing) and a lytic lesion is at high risk of fracture (Fig. 6.19). Beyond this, CT is the most accurate was to assess the cortical involvement of a lesion. Although not as accurate as CT, a readily available way to assess fracture risk is with plain radiographs and Mirel's criteria [21]. The criteria used are the site of the lesion, pain characteristics, the type of lesion, and the size as judged on the plain radiograph. A score of greater than 8 suggests prophylactic fixation (Table 6.4).

While surgical treatment should be tailored to the individual patient, a number of general treatment strategies are frequently employed. Treatment should allow immediate weightbearing whenever possible. Extensive surgical procedures should be avoided when possible.

Fig. 6.18 Patient with multiple myeloma and multiple impending fractures including the distal femur and proximal tibia. Preoperative radiograph (**a**) and postoperative radiograph (**b**) after curettage, cementation, and locking plate application

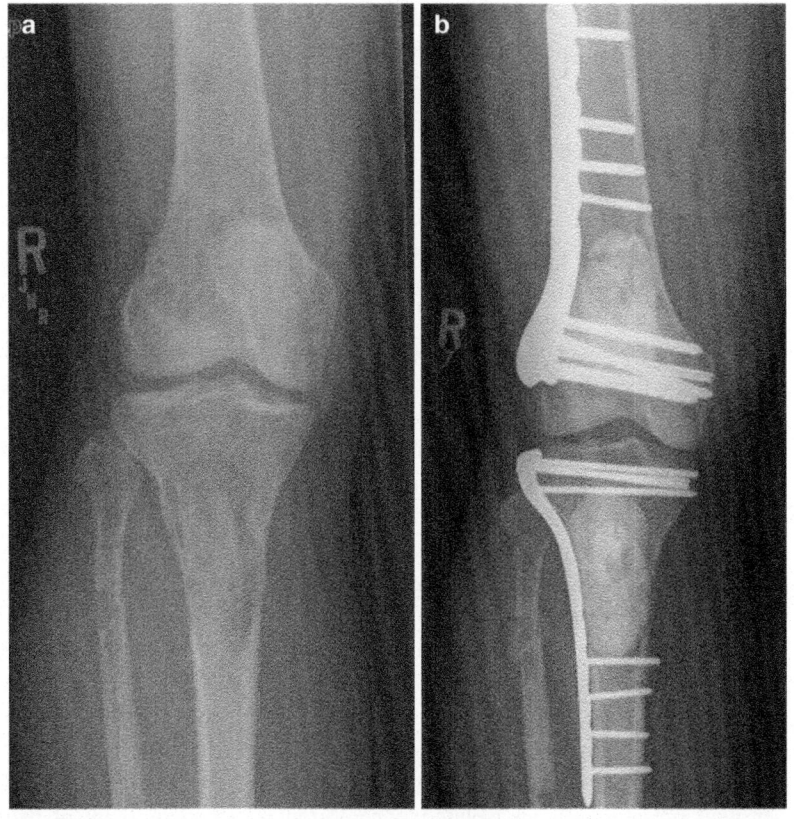

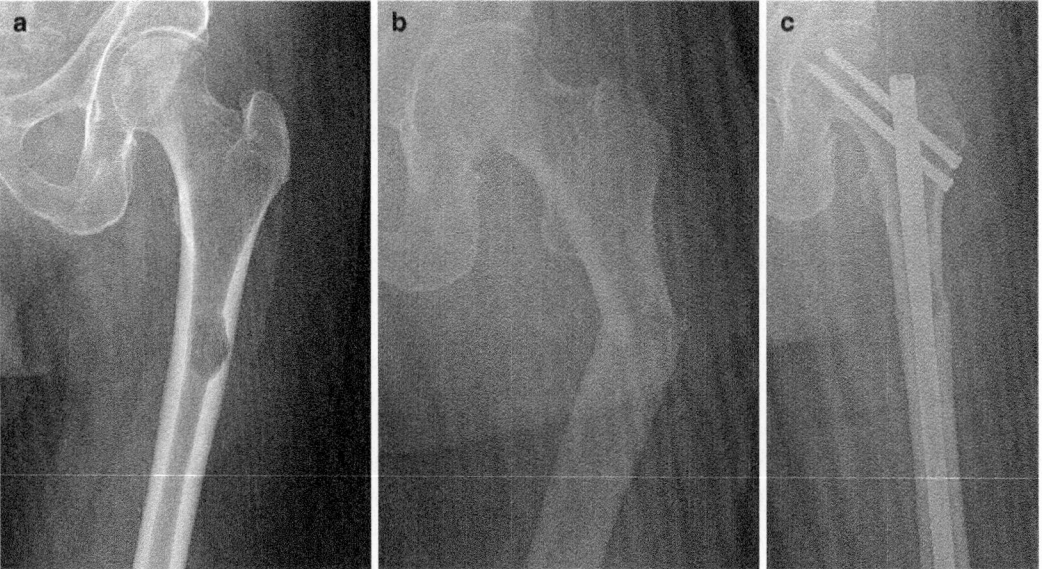

Fig. 6.19 Proximal femur lesion from multiple myeloma (**a**). Patient had functional pain and unfortunately fractured prior to prophylactic fixation (**b**). He was treated with an intramedullary nail (**c**)

Fig. 6.20 Patient with oligometastatic renal cell carcinoma involving proximal humerus (**a**) Patient was treated with resection and endoprosthetic reconstruction after preoperative embolization (**b**)

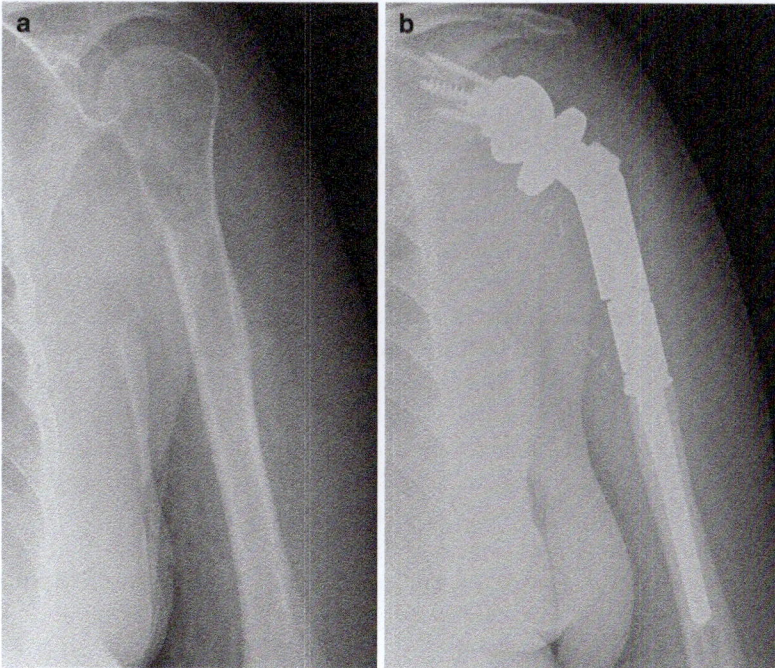

Table 6.4 Mirel's criteria for prophylactic fixation

Score	1	2	3
Site	Upper limb	Lower limb	Peritrochanteric
Pain	Mild	Moderate	Functional
Lesion	Blastic	Mixed	Lytic
Size	<1/3	1/3 to 2/3	>2/3

A score > 8 suggests prophylactic fixation

1. Long bone lesions not immediately adjacent to a joint are treated with intramedullary fixation. This can be supplemented with cementation as needed.
2. Metaphyseal lesions not amenable to intramedullary fixation can be treated with curettage, cementation, and locking plate fixation.
3. Periarticular lesions are best treated with endoprosthetic reconstruction when possible (Fig. 6.20).
4. Lesions in the pelvis most often do not require surgical fixation. Periacetabular lesions that remain symptomatic after radiation can be treated percutaneously after ablation. More extensive lesions involving the acetabulum are best treated with arthroplasty often augmented with cement, screws, or metal augments.

Soft Tissue Sarcomas

Soft tissue sarcomas (STS) are malignant tumors arising from or within the soft tissue. There are over 50 types of soft tissue sarcomas. This heterogeneous group of tumors arise specifically from the supporting extraskeletal mesenchymal tissues of the body, that is, muscle, fascia, connective tissues, fibrous tissues, and fat. Although they are rare, accounting for less than 1% of malignancies, they are about three times as common as bone sarcomas. The tendency for growth, recurrence rate, rate and pattern of metastatic spread, and responsiveness to radiation and chemotherapy all differ by tumor type. Although treatment is becoming more specific to tumor type over time, the same basic approach to treatment strategy can be used for all soft tissue sarcomas.

Clinical Presentation

While some soft tissue sarcomas are more common in children and young adults, soft tissue sarcomas as a whole become more common as age increases. Soft tissue sarcomas can occur though out the body, with about half occurring in the extremities. The lower extremity is more commonly involved than the upper extremity.

Most soft tissue sarcomas present as a painless enlarging mass. They can be firm or soft. If they are located superficial to the fascia, they may be mobile. While only about 1% of superficial masses are sarcomas, half of all sarcomas are superficial. Systemic signs, such as fever, malaise, and weight loss, and laboratory changes are rare. The nonspecific presentation is the cause of frequent missed diagnosis and unplanned excisions. A degree of clinical suspicion should be maintained when approaching any soft tissue mass, and a large, deep mass should be presumed to be a sarcoma until proven otherwise.

Radiographic Findings

Plain radiographs often show a soft tissue shadow corresponding to the mass. They can be useful to look for calcifications within the mass.

Plain radiographs can also assess for any secondary involvement of the bone. MRI is the most useful imaging modality to assess soft tissue sarcomas. The multiplanar images give a detailed view of the extent of the mass and its relationship to the surrounding muscular compartments and neurovascular structures (Fig. 6.21). MRI is relatively unhelpful from a diagnostic standpoint, however. The imaging characteristics of a soft tissue sarcoma are nonspecific on MRI. In general, the mass is heterogeneous in nature and relatively dark, or isointense to muscle, on the T1 weighted images and bright on the T2 weighted images. Postcontrast imaging reveals variable enhancement.

Biopsy and Staging

Once imaging is completed, biopsy is necessary. Biopsy is typically done as a needle biopsy. This can be done in the clinic for superficial masses that can be easily palpated. For masses that are deep, close to major nerves or vessels, or appear to be largely necrotic on MRI, biopsy can be done under ultrasound or CT guidance. Small, superficial lesions can often be removed as an excisional biopsy. Biopsy should be guided by the treating surgeon.

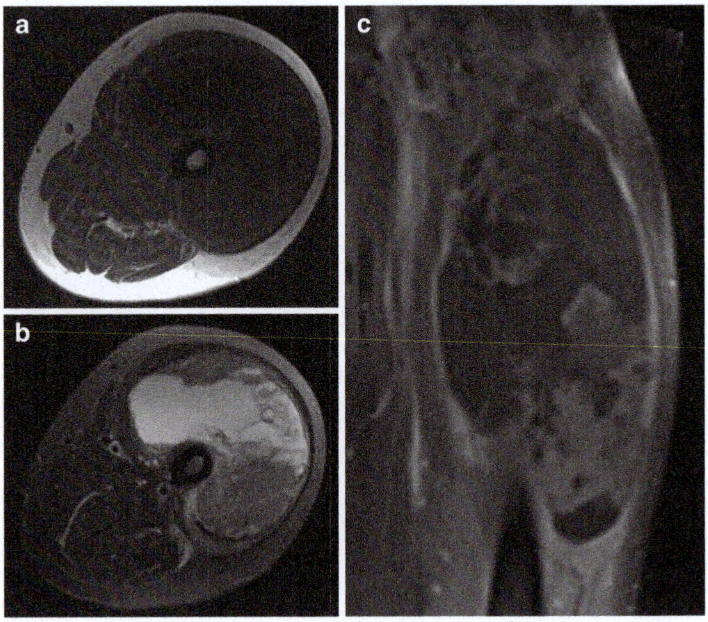

Fig. 6.21 High-grade undifferentiated pleomorphic sarcoma of the anterior thigh. The tumor is heterogenous and relatively dark on the T1 weighted sequence (**a**), bright on the T2 weighted sequence (**b**), and has nodular enhancement after contrast administration (**c**). This is the classic appearance of a soft tissue sarcoma and is not specific to subtype

Soft tissue sarcomas have a similar pattern of spread as bone sarcomas. Because of this staging involves an MRI of the tumor and surrounding compartments, CT of the chest, and a bone scan.

Treatment

Treatment for soft tissue sarcoma involves wide resection of the mass. For many low-grade lesions, no other treatment is necessary (Fig. 6.22). High-grade lesions and those with a propensity for local recurrence require the addition of either radiation or chemotherapy. The most widely accepted treatment for large, high-grade soft tissue sarcomas is a combination of wide resection and external beam radiation [22].

Radiation can be given in the preoperative or postoperative setting. Standard dosing is 50–65 Gy delivered over 25–30 fractions. While the sequence of radiation and surgery does not affect overall survival, there are advantages and disadvantages to each. Preoperative radiation allows for a lower overall dose and slightly shorter treatment interval. It can make the pseudocapsule easier to dissect from the surrounding tissue and potentially make the tumor smaller. The major disadvantage to preoperative radiation is an increase in the wound complication rate to about 30% [23]. Postoperative operative radiation has the advantage of a lower wound complication rate. Disadvantages stem from the higher overall dose and larger treatment area that is necessary. These include increased fibrosis, risk of fracture, and potentially a higher rate of radiation induced sarcoma. Pre- or postoperative radiation reduces the chance of local recurrence to less than 10% [23].

Chemotherapy in the treatment of soft tissue sarcoma remains controversial. It is routinely used in patients with metastatic disease. In isolated disease, its use is less widespread. Data on overall survival has shown variable effectiveness. This is probably due at least in part to the wide heterogeneity of diseases and their variable responsiveness to chemotherapy [24]. A large meta-analysis of randomized controlled trials showed a 11% improvement in overall survival in patients treated with a regimen including both doxorubicin and ifosfamide for large, deep, high-grade soft tissue sarcomas of the extremity [24]. Chemotherapy for isolated tumors is typically given in the preoperative setting and most often is used in conjunction with either pre- or postoperative radiation therapy.

Patients receiving unplanned surgery for soft tissue sarcoma remain persistently common. These patients have a 50% chance of having residual disease after the initial surgery. Treatment for these patients is effectively the same as for an

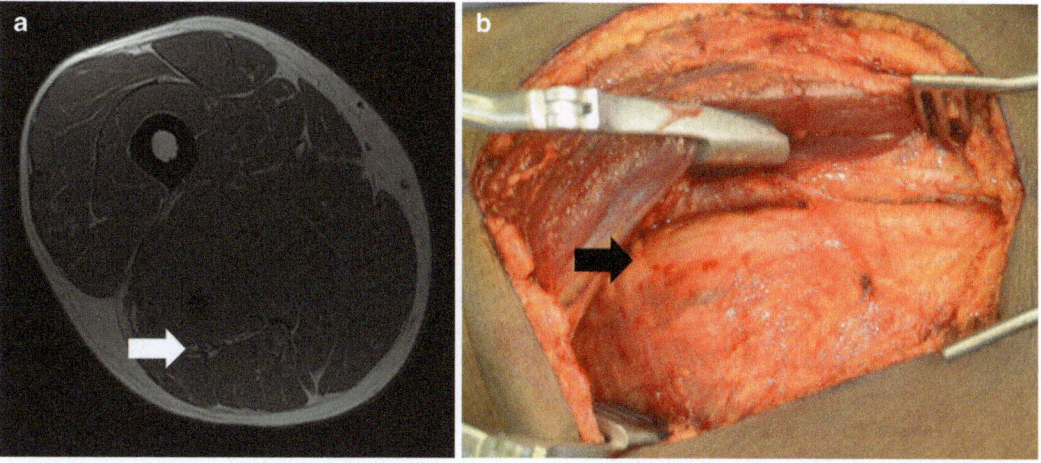

Fig. 6.22 Low-grade fibromyxoid sarcoma (**a**). The sciatic nerve is immediately adjacent to the mass (arrows). The nerve was freed from the mass leaving the surrounding adventitial tissue as the margin (**b**)

untreated tumor with wide resection of the entire surgical bed in conjunction with radiation and possibly chemotherapy depending on the underlying histologic subtype.

Outcomes

Outcomes for soft tissue sarcomas vary by subtype. Poor prognostic factors include large size, high-grade tumors, deep tumors, and metastatic disease. Patients receiving an unplanned excision have increased local morbidity including additional surgical procedures, a greater need for plastic surgery reconstruction, and a higher rate of amputation. Notably, an adverse effect on survival has not been shown.

Undifferentiated Pleomorphic Sarcoma (UPS)

Undifferentiated pleomorphic sarcoma (UPS), formerly known as malignant fibrous histiocytoma (MFH), is the most common soft tissue sarcoma in adults. It is a high-grade tumor that lacks differentiation into a more specific subtype. Histologically, it is composed of pleomorphic spindle cells arranged in a storiform pattern with frequent mitosis. It follows the typical pattern of presentation of a painless mass in the lower extremity. Other common sites include the upper extremity and then the retroperitoneum.

Prognosis depends on the factors listed above. The 5-year overall survival is approximately 60%.

Liposarcoma

Liposarcoma is the second most common soft tissue sarcoma and comprises a wide range of malignant potential dependent on the individual grade of the tumor. Tumors range from well-differentiated liposarcoma (termed atypical lipomatous tumor in the extremities) with essentially no metastatic potential to a pleomorphic liposarcoma that has a similar outcome to UPS. The common feature among all liposarcomas is the presence of immature lipoblasts seen on histology. Fat can be easily seen on MRI in low-grade lesions, while high-grade lesions share the typical appearance of a high-grade sarcoma. Atypical lipomatous tumors are sometimes indistinguishable from benign lipomas on imaging with diagnosis made by the presence of MDM2 staining.

Myxoid Liposarcoma

Myxoid liposarcoma is the most common subtype of liposarcoma and has some notable features. They are typically low-grade but can be high-grade lesions which are usually associated with a large round cell component. Myxoid liposarcoma is associated with translocation t(12;16). Radiographically, it contains components that are relatively dark on T1 sequences and bright on T2 sequences owing to the high myxoid component. Myxoid liposarcoma has an unusual pattern of spread for a sarcoma. In addition to the lungs and bone, it can spread to sites including the retroperitoneum and liver. Bone lesions are difficult to detect by CT, technetium bone scan, or PET, making whole body MRI the imaging modality of choice to screen for extrapulmonary disease. Myxoid liposarcoma is also notable for its significant response to radiation, even with relatively low doses.

Leiomyosarcoma

As its name suggests, leiomyosarcoma classically arises from smooth muscle cells, particularly from those of the abdominopelvic organs. They occur most commonly in the uterus and are therefore more common in females. They also occur in the extremities and comprise about 10–15% of all extremity-associated sarcomas, with the thigh being the most common location [25]. In the extremities, lesions most often arise from a vessel wall. Histologically, leiomyosarcoma is characterized by intersecting fascicles of spindle cells containing elongated nuclei within an abundance of eosinophilic cytoplasm [26].

While treatment is similar to other soft tissue sarcomas, leiomyosarcoma is considered to be more sensitive the chemotherapy than other sarcomas. Overall survival at 5 years is close to 70% [27].

Fibrosarcoma

Fibrosarcoma is a malignant soft tissue tumor composed of fibroblasts with varying amounts of collagen fibers organized in a classic "herringbone" pattern [28]. While commonly discussed, fibrosarcoma is not a particularly common type of soft tissue sarcoma [29]. It is most commonly a disease of older age, and often occurs as a dedifferentiated component of a lower grade tumor. Treatment and prognosis are similar to other high-grade soft tissue sarcomas [30].

Synovial Sarcoma

Synovial sarcoma is a soft tissue sarcoma that usually occurs in young adults. It has a characteristic translocation t(X;18) producing a fusion protein SYT-SSX1, 2, or 4. Patients with the SYT:SSX1 fusion protein have a worse prognosis. Contrary to what the name would suggest, synovial sarcoma does not arise from the synovium or a synovial cell. The cell of origin is unknown. Synovial sarcoma can be found throughout the body but is the most common soft tissue sarcoma of the foot.

MRI appearance of synovial sarcoma is similar to other soft tissue sarcomas. It does have a high rate of calcification that can be seen on X-ray. Synovial sarcoma classically has a biphasic appearance histologically with both spindle cell and epithelial cell components.

Metastatic disease develops in up to 50% of patients with synovial sarcoma. Synovial sarcoma has long been thought to have a higher incidence of lymph node metastasis, although more recent data would suggest the incidence is similar to other soft tissue sarcomas. Chemotherapy, particularly regimens containing ifosfamide, has been shown to improve overall survival. Overall survival remains poor with 50% 5-year survival.

Epithelioid Sarcoma

Epithelioid sarcoma is a low-grade sarcoma that occurs most commonly in the upper extremity. It is the most common soft tissue sarcoma in the hand and occurs more commonly in males than females. Clinically, masses often appear similar to a hypertrophic scar and because of this and their slow growth, diagnosis is often delayed. Epithelioid sarcomas are also histologically challenging to diagnose, and they are often mistaken for necrotizing granulomas. The lungs are the most common site of metastasis, but epithelioid sarcoma has a high rate of lymph node metastasis [31]. Regional metastasis in addition to other atypical sites of metastatic disease are also relatively common. Because of this, a sentinel node biopsy and a PET scan should be included in staging. The disease course is characterized by a high rate of late local recurrence and regional metastasis. Five-year survival is close to 80%, but it is not uncommon for patients to have multiple metastatic lesions removed in an extremity before eventually developing pulmonary disease [32].

Benign Soft Tissue Tumors

All mesenchymal tissue can give rise to benign lesions. They may occasionally be confused with malignant lesions, or they may become symptomatic because of their size, anatomic location, or both. Benign lesions are much more common than their malignant counterparts. Imaging features are often similar. It is important to differentiate between benign and malignant lesions to avoid over- and undertreating, respectively.

Lipomas

Lipomas are the most commonly occurring mesenchymal tumor, and primarily form in adults. They can occur essentially anywhere in the body. The majority are in the subcutaneous tissue, but lipomas also occur deep to the fascia. While most lipomas are solitary occurrences, approximately

5–10% of patients with lipomas will have multiple lesions. Intramuscular lipomas can grow quite large with masses in the thigh reaching 40 cm. This large size does not infer malignancy, although a large lipoma may be mistaken for a sarcoma prior to imaging (Fig. 6.23). Lipomas develop from histologically normal fat cells and consist of monotonous sheets of mature fat cells that are ovoid to round and usually contain a single fat droplet that compresses the nucleus. Occasionally myxoid changes, dense trabeculae, and interdigitating capillary vessels can be seen on histological examination. Lipomas probably have no potential of malignant transformation. MRI is diagnostic in the vast majority of cases. A tumor with signal equal to the subcutaneous fat on all sequences with an internal complexity equal to or less than the complexity of the subcutaneous fat is a lipoma. No biopsy is necessary in this instance. Treatment for most lipomas is observation. Large intramuscular lipomas are often removed as they become symptomatic,

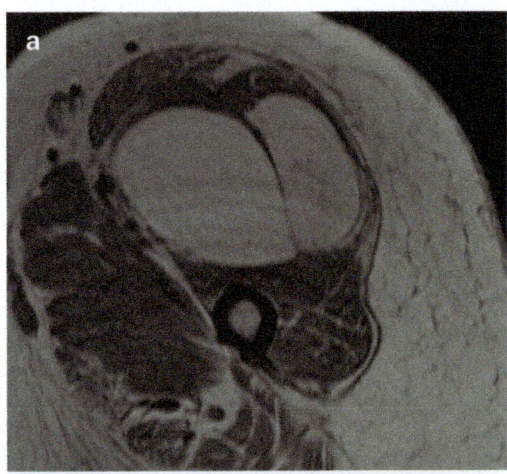
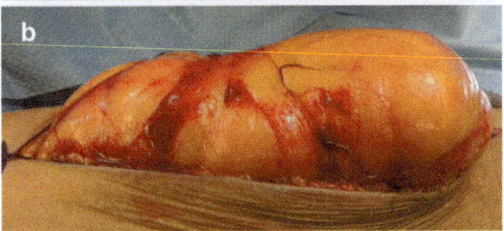

Fig. 6.23 T1 weight MRI (**a**) and clinical picture (**b**) of an intramuscular lipoma of the thigh

while superficial lesions typically are removed only for cosmetic reasons.

Benign Tumors of Peripheral Nerves

Schwannoma

Schwannomas, or neurilemmomas, are benign tumors of the peripheral nerve sheath. Their progenitor cells are Schwann cells, giving rise to the name. They are encapsulated—which is a defining feature when compared to the other predominant benign peripheral nerve tumor, neurofibromas, which are unencapsulated. On histological examination, schwannomas are comprised of Antoni A (cellular) and Antoni B (loose myxoid) components. They typically occur in isolation but may occur with other peripheral lesions (Schwannomatosis) or in conjunction with lesions in the vestibular nerves (Neurofibromatosis type 2). Schwannomas can be painful or present with paresthesias, but often are asymptomatic. Imaging shows a fusiform lesion that is bright on T2 sequence sometimes a string sign is evident (Fig. 6.24). Surgical treatment involves simple excision of the mass after splitting the nerve fibers and opening the capsule.

Neurofibroma

Neurofibromas are another common benign tumor of peripheral nerves. They can be solitary or multiple. Lesions may be cutaneous, subcutaneous, or plexiform. Most lesions are asymptomatic, but plexiform lesions may be painful. On histological examination, neurofibromas are comprised of Schwann cells associated with collagen fibrils and myxoid material. Imaging can be similar to schwannoma. A target sign may be seen on an axial view of the lesion, a thin rim of normal intermuscular fat often surrounds the lesion (a split fat sign). Neurofibromas can be part of neurofibromatosis type 1 (NF1), which can have a constellation of additional symptoms including Café-au-lait spots, axillary and inguinal freckling, optic gliomas, and Lisch nodules. Plexiform neurofibromas

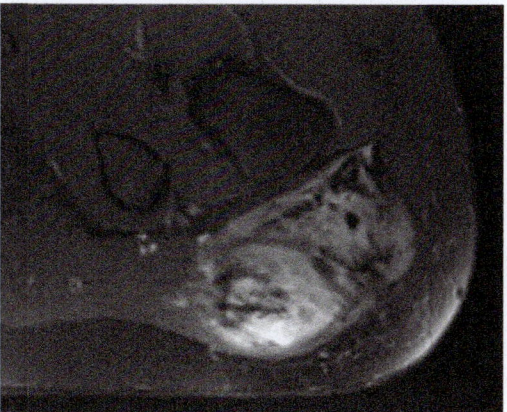

Fig. 6.25 Fibromatosis involving the gluteus maximus. Fibromatosis often has an infiltrative border as seen on the medial aspect of the mass as well as areas of dark signal on all sequences because of dense fibrous tissue

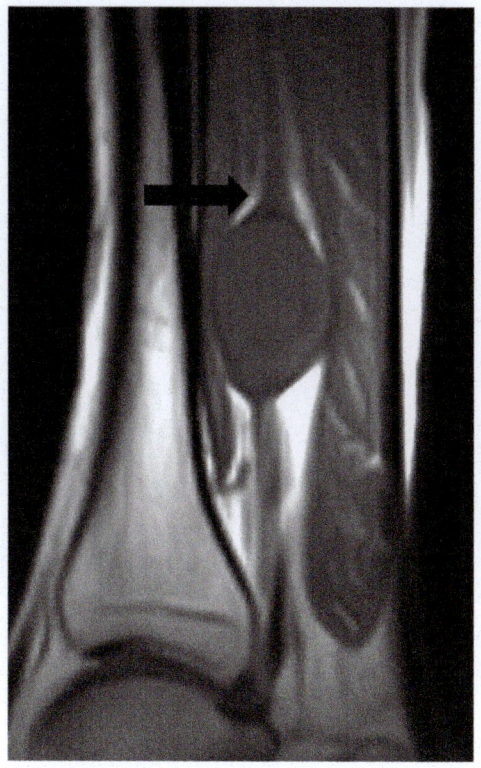

Fig. 6.24 Schwannoma arising from the tibial nerve with nerve evident along mass or string sign (arrow)

carry a risk for malignant transformation into a malignant peripheral nerve sheath tumor (MPNST), which is heralded by an enlarging mass and change in pain. Patients with NF1 have an approximately 10% risk of malignant transformation. Treatment for a neurofibroma is typically observation. Lesions can be removed, but excision of a lesion from a large nerve can result in loss of function. Treatment of MPNST is the same as other soft tissue sarcomas.

Fibromatosis

Fibromatosis, also known as a desmoid tumor, is a benign fibrous tumor that can be very locally aggressive. Fibromatosis can be associated with familial adenomatous polyposis (FAP). Tumors are "rock hard" on examination and may be tender. The tumor has an infiltrative border allowing it to invade beyond its easily recognized boundar-

ies into multiple anatomic compartments. Signs of this infiltrative irregular border can be seen on MRI. The other defining imaging feature is areas of dark signal on both T1 and T2 sequences because of the dense fibrous tissue (Fig. 6.25). Treatment historically has been wide excision. Because of the infiltrative border, recurrence rates are as high as 50%. This can lead to multiple surgeries and in the retroperitoneum can lead to death. Multiple treatment modalities including NSAIDs, tamoxifen, low-dose chemotherapy, and radiation have all been used in the treatment of fibromatosis. When left untreated, many tumors stop growing approximately 1 year after presentation. This, along with the poor outcomes of active treatment strategies, has led to observation with serial MRIs being the preferred initial treatment strategy.

Benign Vascular Lesions

Vascular malformations can be categorized in a number of ways and include capillary, cavernous, venous, or arteriovenous lesions (Fig. 6.26). While there is differing terminology, a hemangioma is commonly viewed as a type of vascular malformation. Capillary hemangiomas are the most common subtype. Vascular malformations or hemangiomas are not neoplastic. Patients

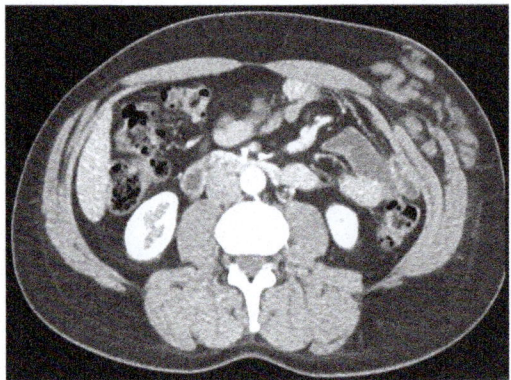

Fig. 6.26 CT of the abdomen showing a vascular malformation of the left flank extending into the abdominal wall musculature

often present with a mass that fluctuates in size and may be painful. On MRI, serpiginous vessels that are bright on T2 sequences are intermixed with areas of normal looking fat. Well-defined calcifications, called phleboliths, may be seen on plain radiographs. When classic imaging features are present, no biopsy is necessary. Treatment is typically observation with symptomatic management. Symptomatic lesions can be treated with sclerotherapy or excision, although the recurrence rate is high.

Tumors Originating from the Joint

The list of tumors that arise from the synovium or occur intraarticularly is short. While a malignancy can arise intraarticularly, this is exceedingly rare. In general, treatment decisions can be made from clinical examination and imaging without biopsy. The primary differential for intraarticular lesions is typically inflammatory arthropathies.

Tenosynovial Giant Cell Tumor

Tenosynovial giant cell tumor (TSGCT) can occur both intra- and extraarticularly. Intraarticular disease is more commonly known as pigmented villonodular synovitis (PVNS) and has a nodular and diffuse form. The nodular, or

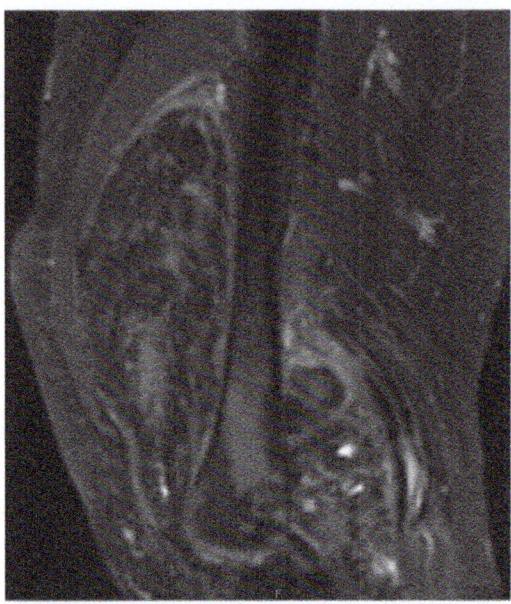

Fig. 6.27 Diffuse tenosynovial giant cell tumor with extensive involvement of anterior and posterior knee. There are many areas of low signal within the lesion on this T2 weighted sequence corresponding to hemosiderin deposition. Patient was treated with staged anterior and posterior synovectomy followed by low-dose external beam radiation

localized, form has an indolent course with symptoms caused primarily by mass effect. Diffuse TSGCT is an aggressive disease of synovium characterized by prominent synovial proliferation with formation of villi and nodules caused by overexpression of colony stimulating factor 1 (CSF1). The knee joint is classically involved in a majority of cases, followed by hip and ankle joints.

Diffuse TSGCT commonly occurs between the second and fifth decades of life. Patients complain of pain, joint swelling, and recurrent effusion. Arthrocentesis of the involved joint reveals bloody or brownish synovial fluid. MRI shows nodular thickening of the synovium that enhances with contrast administration. Masses can extend outside of the joint capsule. There are typically punctate areas that are dark on both T1 and T2 sequences corresponding to areas of hemosiderin deposition (Fig. 6.27). Histological findings are nonspecific, and usually reveal a heterogeneous population of cells within the synovium, including histiocytes, xanthoma cells, hemosiderin-laden macrophages, and multinucleated giant cells.

Treatment for nodular or localized disease is simple excision. Diffuse disease requires complete synovectomy. Postoperative radiation of 30–35 Gy reduces the risk of local recurrence. In patients with extensive or recurrent disease a CSF1 inhibitor is available, although its role in the treatment of TSGCT is not well-defined at this time.

Ganglia

Ganglia, or ganglion cysts, are cystic structures arising from the joint lining or tendon sheath and are common. They are very common in the hand and wrist and predominantly affect women in the second to fifth decade of life. Ganglia most often form in the wrist, but other sites include the metatarsophalangeal joints, ankle, and knee. Ganglia are not neoplastic, but the etiology of their formation remains uncertain; two predominant theories include the extrusion of synovial fluid from a capsule and degeneration of connective tissue secondary to repetitive injury. MRI reveals a homogenous lesion that is dark on T1 sequences and bright on T2 sequences that communicates with a joint or tendon sheath. Biopsy is typically not indicated. Histopathologic examination should demonstrate mucin-filled synovial cell lined sac. Treatment is based on severity of symptoms, and options include observation, aspiration, and excision. Notably, care should be taken with apparent ganglia that have an unusual appearance or are distant from any joint or tendon sheath. These, along with apparent atraumatic hematomas, are common sources of misdiagnosis for soft tissue sarcomas.

References

1. Gage MM, Nagarajan N, Ruck JM, et al. Sarcomas in the United States: recent trends and a call for improved staging. Oncotarget. 2019;10(25):2462.
2. Siegel RL, Miller KD, Jemal A. Cancer statistics, 2018. CA Cancer J Clin. 2018;68(1):7–30.
3. Enneking WF, Spanier SS, Goodman MA. A system for the surgical staging of musculoskeletal sarcoma. Clin Orthop Relat Res. 1980;153:106–20.
4. Amin MB, Edge SB, Greene FL, et al. AJCC cancer staging manual, vol. 1024. New York: Springer; 2017.
5. Cates JM. The AJCC 8th edition staging system for soft tissue sarcoma of the extremities or trunk: a cohort study of the SEER database. J Natl Compr Cancer Netw. 2018;16(2):144–52.
6. Dahlin DC. Bone tumors: general aspects and data on 6,221 cases. Springfield, IL: Charles C. Thomas Publisher; 1978.
7. Vodanovich DA, Choong PF. Soft-tissue sarcomas. Indian J Orthop. 2018;52:35–44.
8. Gerrand CH, Rankin K. The hazards of biopsy in patients with malignant primary bone and soft-tissue tumors. In: Classic papers in orthopaedics. London: Springer; 2013. p. 491–3.
9. Damron TA, Morgan H, Prakash D, Grant W, Aronowitz J, Heiner J. Critical evaluation of Mirels' rating system for impending pathologic fractures. Clin Orthop Relat Res. 2003;415:S201–7.
10. Lin PP, Patel S. Osteosarcoma. In: Bone sarcoma. New York: Springer; 2012. p. 75–97.
11. Kager L, Zoubek A, Pötschger U, et al. Primary metastatic osteosarcoma: presentation and outcome of patients treated on neoadjuvant Cooperative Osteosarcoma Study Group protocols. J Clin Oncol. 2003;21(10):2011–8.
12. Assi T, Kattan J, Nassereddine H, et al. Chemotherapy in the management of periosteal osteosarcoma: a narrative review. J Bone Oncol. 2021;30:100389.
13. Wells ME, Childs BR, Eckhoff MD, Rajani R, Potter BK, Polfer EM. Atypical cartilaginous tumors: trends in management. JAAOS Glob Res Rev. 2021;5(12):e21.00277.
14. Marcove RC. Chondrosarcoma: diagnosis and treatment. Orthop Clin N Am. 1977;8(4):811–20.
15. Stiller C, Trama A, Serraino D, et al. Descriptive epidemiology of sarcomas in Europe: report from the RARECARE project. Eur J Cancer. 2013;49(3):684–95.
16. Iwamoto Y. Diagnosis and treatment of Ewing's sarcoma. Jpn J Clin Oncol. 2007;37(2):79–89.
17. Womer RB, West DC, Krailo MD, et al. Randomized controlled trial of interval-compressed chemotherapy for the treatment of localized Ewing sarcoma: a report from the Children's Oncology Group. J Clin Oncol. 2012;30(33):4148.
18. Woon JT, Hoon D, Graydon A, Flint M, Doyle AJ. Aneurysmal bone cyst treated with percutaneous doxycycline: is a single treatment sufficient? Skeletal Radiol. 2019;48:765–71.
19. DiCaprio MR, Murtaza H, Palmer B, Evangelist M. Narrative review of the epidemiology, economic burden, and societal impact of metastatic bone disease. Breast. 2022;279:65–75.
20. Bhaker P, Mohan H, Handa U, Kumar S. Role of intraoperative pathology consultation in skeletal tumors and tumor-like lesions. Sarcoma. 2014;2014:902104.

21. Mirels H. The classic: metastatic disease in long bones. A proposed scoring system for diagnosing impending pathologic fractures. Clin Orthop Relat Res. 2003;415:S4–13.

22. Grimer R, Judson I, Peake D, Seddon B. Guidelines for the management of soft tissue sarcomas. Sarcoma. 2010;2010:506182.

23. O'Sullivan B, Davis AM, Turcotte R, et al. Preoperative versus postoperative radiotherapy in soft-tissue sarcoma of the limbs: a randomised trial. Lancet. 2002;359(9325):2235–41.

24. Pervaiz N, Colterjohn N, Farrokhyar F, Tozer R, Figueredo A, Ghert M. A systematic meta-analysis of randomized controlled trials of adjuvant chemotherapy for localized resectable soft-tissue sarcoma. Cancer. 2008;113(3):573–81.

25. Mangla A, Yadav U. Leiomyosarcoma. 2019.

26. Crew AJ, Clark J, Fisher C, et al. Fusion of SYT to two genes, SSX1 and SSX2, encoding proteins with homology to the Kruppel-associated box in human synovial sarcoma. EMBO J. 1995;14(10):2333–40.

27. Serrano C, George S. Leiomyosarcoma. Hematol Oncol Clin. 2013;27(5):957–74.

28. Davis DD, Shah SJ, Kane SM. Fibrosarcoma. In: StatPearls. Treasure Island, FL: StatPearls Publishing; 2022.

29. Angiero F, Rizzuti T, Crippa R, Stefani M. Fibrosarcoma of the jaws: two cases of primary tumors with intraosseous growth. Anticancer Res. 2007;27(4C):2573–81.

30. Augsburger D, Nelson PJ, Kalinski T, et al. Current diagnostics and treatment of fibrosarcoma–perspectives for future therapeutic targets and strategies. Oncotarget. 2017;8(61):104638.

31. de Visscher SA, van Ginkel RJ, Wobbes T, et al. Epithelioid sarcoma: still an only surgically curable disease. Cancer. 2006;107(3):606–12.

32. Enzinger F, Epithelioid sarcoma. A sarcoma simulating a granuloma or a carcinoma. Cancer. 1970;26(5):1029–41.

Pediatric Orthopedics

7

Denver B. Kraft, John N. Delahay, and Ryan S. Murray

Biological Differences

Growth

As mentioned, the fact that the child's skeleton is growing, both longitudinally and latitudinally, positions it uniquely for damage from the adverse effects of trauma and disease. The extent of this damage is a reflection of the rate of growth and the immaturity of the skeleton. Hence, an insult will have a greater impact, if applied at the time of more rapid growth (a growth spurt) or when the skeleton is very young (neonate).

Remodeling

The immature skeleton can remodel to a much greater degree than that of the adult. Due to the presence and activity of multiple cell populations, damage to the skeleton can be repaired more extensively than one should anticipate in

the adult. The challenge for the physician is to recognize the limitations of this remodeling process and work within the boundaries of this potential.

Specific Anatomic Structures

Bone

Although a child's bone is historically lamellar in pattern, there remains enough flexibility in the skeleton to permit what has been called "biological plasticity," a phenomenon not nearly as extensive in adult bone. Essentially, this allows a bone to "bend without breaking" and is responsible for some of the unique types of fractures seen in the pediatric age groups, specifically buckle and greenstick fractures (Figs. 7.1 and 7.2).

In addition, the mechanical properties of a child's bone vary from those of the adult. Such characteristics as modulus of elasticity, ultimate tensile strength, and yield point all reflect the increased elasticity and plasticity unique in this age group. However, the overall "strength" tends to be less than that of the adult in certain modes of loading, such as tension and shear.

D. B. Kraft · J. N. Delahay · R. S. Murray (✉)
Department of Orthopaedic Surgery, MedStar
Georgetown Univeristy Hospital, Washington, DC,
USA
e-mail: Ryan.S.Murray@gunet.georgetown.edu

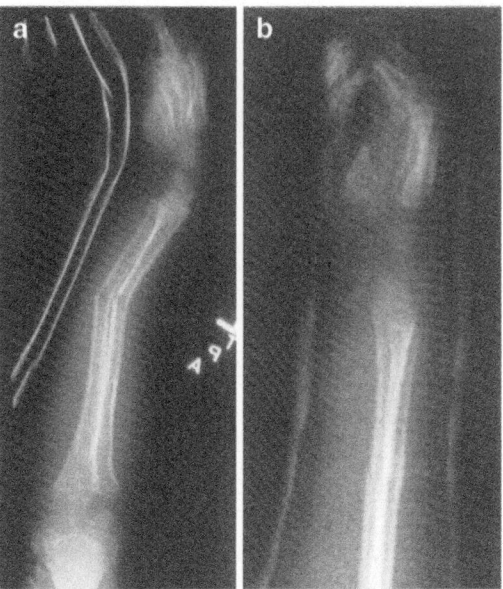

Fig. 7.1 (**a**) Lateral radiograph of a greenstick forearm fracture of both bones. The dorsal cortex angles without completely fracturing (plastic deformation). (**b**) Lateral radiograph obtained after reduction. (From Tachdjian MO. Pediatric Orthopedics, 6th ed. Philadelphia, PA: Herring; 2022. Reprinted with permission)

Ligament

As a tissue, ligament is one of the most age-resistant tissues in the human body. The tensile strength in the child and the adult is virtually the same. Therefore, these structures remain constant in the musculoskeletal system. While the strength of bone, cartilage, and muscle tends to change, the ligamentous structures remain unchanged with growth and development.

Periosteum

The outer covering of the bone is a dense fibrous layer, which in the child is significantly thicker than that of the adult. The periosteum of the child has an outer fibrous layer and an inner cambial or osteogenic layer. Hence, the child's periosteum confers both mechanical strength and biologic activity. The effect of these biologic differences is far reaching when one discusses fractures in children. Due to this thickened periosteum, fractures do not tend to displace to the degree seen in

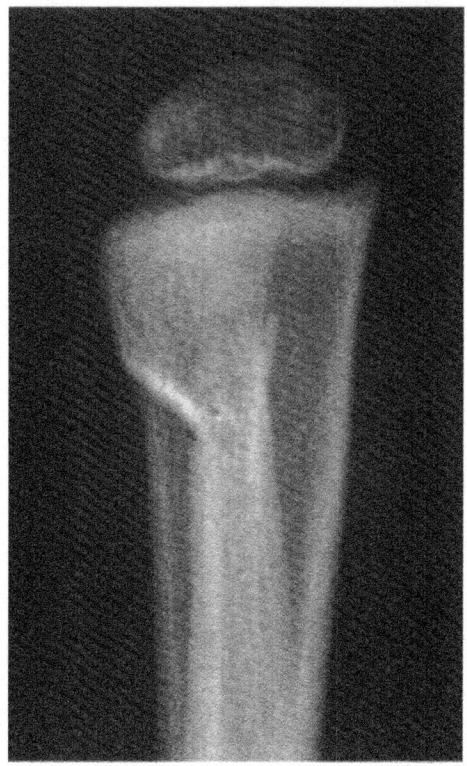

Fig. 7.2 Lateral radiograph of the distal radius showing a buckle fracture of the dorsal cortex. The volar cortex is uninvolved, and the dorsal cortex is not completely fractured. (From Tachdjian MO. Pediatric Orthopedics, 6th ed. Philadelphia, PA: Herring; 2022. Reprinted with permission)

adults, and the intact periosteum can be used as an aid in fracture reduction and maintenance. In addition, fractures will heal significantly faster than similar injuries in adults due to all the cellular precursors that are already present.

The osteogenic layer supplies active osteoblasts, ready to make bone for the fracture callus. There are some injuries where the periosteum can be torn or entrapped in the fracture site, creating a block to reduction or source of future growth disturbance.

Cartilage

The skeleton is developed embryologically within a cartilage model. At birth, large portions of any given bone remain largely cartilaginous. Cartilage is not seen on standard radiographs.

The cartilage anlage is very labile and dramatically affected by external influences such as mechanical loading. It is important to realize that, in examining an X-ray, one should not be lulled into a false sense of security if all appears well; what you do not see (i.e., the cartilage) is more important than what you do! Aberrant cartilaginous growth will drastically affect the ultimate shape of bones and, more importantly, joints. The best example is the proximal femur where most of the upper end is cartilaginous. Adverse influences due to eccentric loading seen in developmental dysplasia of the hip can have far-reaching effects when applied to the immature cartilage of the neonatal hip.

The Growth Plate

Far and away, the most unique characteristic of the immature skeleton—indeed, what is the defining component of the immature skeleton—is the growth plate, or the "physis" (Fig. 7.3). The physis is a cartilaginous plate interposed between the epiphysis (the secondary ossification center) and the metaphysis. It is essential for long-bone growth to occur. The downside is that this ana-tomic structure creates a point of mechanical weakness. The physis historically has four zones, each with its own physiologic role:

- Resting zone: The top layer of flattened cells is germinal and metabolically stores materials for later use, since they will ultimately "move their way" down the plate toward the metaphysis. The chondrocytes in this zone also are synthetic, as they fabricate the matrix in which they lie.
- Proliferating zone: The cells in this region are actively replicating and extending the plate. Their appearance has been described as a "stack of plates." In this region, the cells use the materials that they have previously stored for their "trip to the metaphysis."
- Hypertrophic zone: Having extended the plate in the former zone, the cells now swell and switch over to a catabolic state. They prepare the matrix for calcification and ultimately for conversion to bone. Due to large swollen cells and the disorganized matrix, this zone has been cited as being the weakest mechanically; hence, it is here that failure tends to occur. Most, however, would agree that fracture propagation can be seen throughout all zones in the case of trauma.

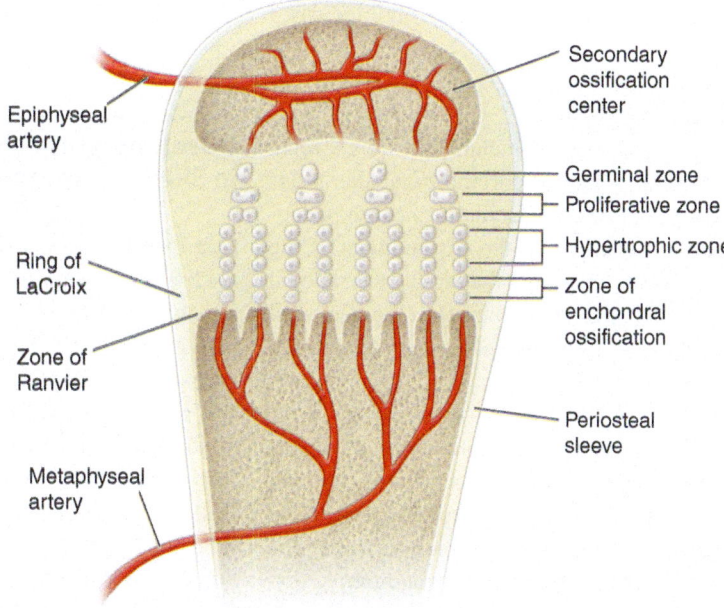

Fig. 7.3 Anatomy of a physis. Most injuries occur just above the area of provisional calcification within the hypertrophic zone. Subsequently the germinal layer frequently remains intact and attached to the epiphysis. (From Tachdjian MO. Pediatric Orthopedics, 6th ed. Philadelphia, PA: Herring; 2022. Reprinted with permission)

Secondary ossification center

Epiphyseal artery

Germinal zone
Proliferative zone
Hypertrophic zone
Zone of enchondral ossification

Ring of LaCroix

Zone of Ranvier

Periosteal sleeve

Metaphyseal artery

- Calcified zone: Metabolically, the matrix has been readied for the deposition of calcium salts, and the task of forming the osteoid is left for this lowest region of the plate. In the adjacent metaphysis, small vascular twigs can be seen arborizing toward the basal layers of the plate.

Peripheral Structures of the Plate

Two histologic regions have been identified with specific functional roles in skeletal development.

- Zone of Ranvier: Around the circumference of the plate is an identifiable clustering of cells that are responsible for latitudinal growth of the plate.
- Perichondral ring of La Croix: As the periosteum is continuous around the margins of the plate, this fibrous structure is apparent. Its function is to provide mechanical support against translational movement.

Factors Affecting the Skeletal Growth

Numerous factors, both intrinsic and extrinsic, affect the way in which the skeleton develops. Some examples are noteworthy and indicated below.

- Genetic
  - Inborn errors of metabolism (e.g., renal rickets) as well as chromosomal alterations (e.g., Down's syndrome) can cause phenotypic variations in the development of the skeleton. Abnormal histology, aberrational growth, and variational development will affect the ultimate shape and behavior of the skeleton.
- Nutrition
  - Vitamins and proteins are required for normal skeletal development and without appropriate levels, abnormalities will be seen. Rickets, for example, will alter the shape of the metaphysis, in addition to disrupting normal physical development.

- Endocrine
  - Hormonal influences play a significant trophic or permissive role in the development of the skeleton. Shortages or excesses, therefore, will disrupt the way in which the skeleton matures. Thyroid hormone is a good example whereby disrupted epiphyseal development is a hallmark of cretinism.
- Environmental
  - Mechanical effects as well as environmental toxins and drugs can adversely affect the development of the skeleton. Fetal alcohol syndrome and the use of illicit narcotics by the mother are just two examples of the growing compendium of skeletal aberrations due to externally applied toxins.
- Coexistent Disease
  - Neuromuscular diseases of children, such as cerebral palsy, polio, and muscular dystrophy, provide good examples of the secondary effects seen in the skeleton due to extrinsic disease. In these examples, the final common pathway in the pathophysiology of the deformities is muscle imbalance; hence, eccentric mechanical loading and aberrational mechanical loading of the immature skeleton produce changes such as joint dislocations and deformities (e.g., scoliosis).

Developmental Variations in Skeletal Growth

One of the most common reasons that children are brought to a physician is to evaluate the position of their lower extremities, particularly the way in which they stand and walk. Intoeing and toeing-out, as well as knock knees and bowlegs, are a major preoccupation of parents—and a major source of orthopedic referrals. The simple fact is that most of these children—well over 90%—are normal children who are simply reflecting variational growth and development. Dr. Mercer Rang, a preeminent pediatric orthopedist, has tried to emphasize this important fact by referring to these conditions as "non-disease." Rang further suggested that the appropriate management for "non-disease" is "non-treatment." It is important to recognize the difference between doing nothing and "non-treatment." As the physician seeing the child, one must recognize the variational patterns and differentiate them from pathologic states. Once that has been accomplished, the physician may embark on a program of aggressive "non-treatment" which might include such things as the following:

- Careful examination of the normal child
- Reassurance of parents and grandparents
- Supply educational information to strengthen one's diagnosis and approach
- Offer the option of yearly follow-up "to be sure that the non-disease is getting better"

Torsional Variations

The skeletal variations in the newborn reflect the intrauterine position and environment. This "molding" usually, but not always, results in an internally rotated position of the lower extremities and the ultimate manifestation of this rotation is intoeing when the child begins to walk. The two most typical variations leading to intoeing are internal tibial torsion and femoral anteversion.

Axial rotation of the tibias can best be identified by examining the child supine with hips and knees flexed and evaluating the transmalleolar axis at the ankle for its relation to the knee axis. Normally, it should lie 10–30° externally rotated from that of the knee. Neonates typically have an internally rotated axis which causes intoeing with the initiation of walking and spontaneously corrects after about 1 year of walking. Tibial external rotation can occasionally be seen but is far less common. Neither requires any specific treatment other than those recommended for "non-treatment."

The plane of the femoral head and neck in the normal adult lies 15° externally rotated from that of the transcondylar plane of the distal femur. In the newborn, this relationship is more extreme: the head/neck plane is about 45° external to that

of the transcondylar plate, and it corrects spontaneously at a rate of about 2° per year (Fig. 7.4). Persistence of this infantile pattern beyond the age of walking will cause intoeing as the leg internally rotates at the hip so that the femoral head sits properly in the acetabulum. The rate of correction varies widely, and "non-treatment" is usually all that is required.

Most believe that external femoral torsion represents the persistence of an infantile external rotational contracture of the soft tissues posterior to the hip; despite its etiology, spontaneous correction of this variation can similarly be anticipated.

When examining the child for femoral rotational patterns, it is best accomplished with the child prone, hips extended, and knees flexed 90°. Internal and external rotation of the hips can then be easily estimated using the leg as an angle guide (Fig. 7.5).

Knock knees (genu valgum) and bowlegs (genu varum) are another common source of physician referrals. Recognition of the normal allows relatively easy determination of pathologic states.

Newborns demonstrate 4–10° of genu varus, which tends to spontaneously correct by 18–24 months of age. Thus, a child who presents with bowlegs would be diagnosed as "physiologic genu varum." After 18–24 months of age, a child develops knock knees, which increases until about age 4 or 5 and then begins to improve. By age 7 or 8, most children have assumed more of an adult pattern: 5–7° of valgus in males and 7–9° of valgus in females.

Differential Diagnosis

Recognizing that the vast majority of children with angular patterns are normal and require "non-treatment," it is important to realize that angular deformities can be a manifestation of pathologic states.

Physiologic angular deformity is virtually always symmetric; the finding of asymmetry should, therefore, suggest a pathologic state and trigger an appropriate workup (Table 7.1).

Fig. 7.4 Degree of normal femoral torsion in relation to age. The curve represents the mean; the vertical lines represent the standard deviation. (From Tachdjian MO. Pediatric Orthopedics, 6th ed. Philadelphia, PA: Herring; 2022. Reprinted with permission)

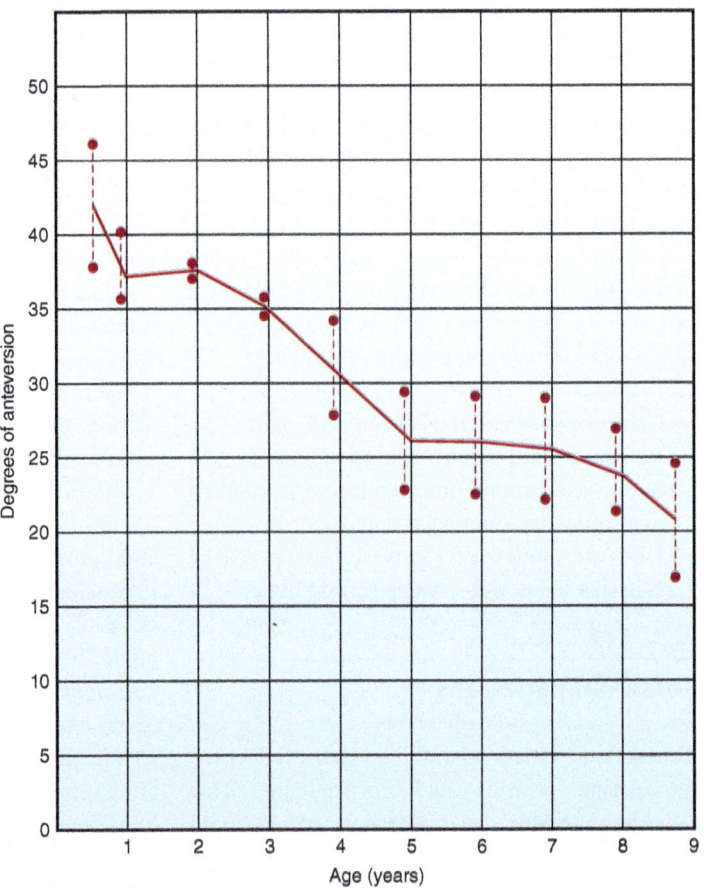

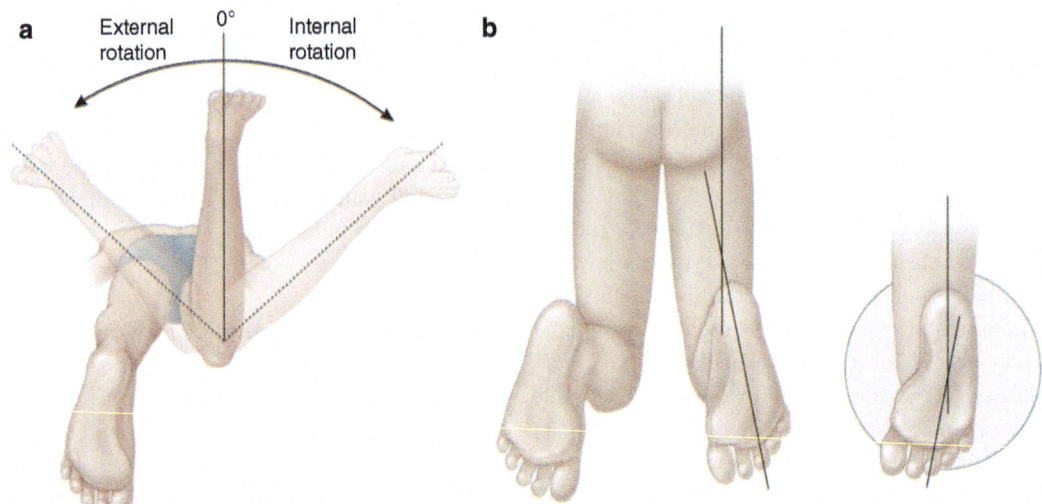

Fig. 7.5 Torsional profile examination with the patient prone. The examiner can expediently assess the thigh–foot axis to estimate tibial torsion and examine the shape of the lateral border of the foot to assess the presence of metatarsus adductus (**a**) and to determine the amount of internal and external rotation of the hip as an indication of the amount of femoral anteversion (**b**). (From Tachdjian MO. Pediatric Orthopedics, 6th ed. Philadelphia, PA: Herring; 2022. Reprinted with permission)

Table 7.1 Differential for genu valgum and genu varum

Knock knees (genu valgum)	Bowlegs (genu varum)
Physiologic	Physiologic
Renal rickets	Blount's disease
Skeletal dysplasias	Rickets (nutritional)
Physeal injury	Skeletal dysplasias (e.g., achondroplasia)
Trauma	Physeal injury
	Trauma

General Affectations of the Pediatric Skeleton

There are many diseases that have skeletal manifestations. This makes it impossible in one short chapter to fully discuss the vast array of pathologic states that have an impact on the musculoskeletal system. Rather, by being introduced to several specific examples in each disease category, one can appreciate some of the general ways in which the skeleton will react to various insults. This chapter will now focus on some of the vascular, infectious, arthritic, metabolic, and neurodevelopmental diseases that produce skeletal manifestations. An entire chapter of this book is devoted to a discussion of tumor and one to injury; therefore, these will only be mentioned insofar as their effects are unique to the growing skeleton.

Infection

Osteomyelitis

The pediatric skeleton is a prime location for bone and joint infections. In part, this is due to the many bacterial infections that small children seem to have—hence providing organisms capable of hematogenous spread from skin, ear, and nasopharynx. In addition, the unique metaphyseal blood supply in the child establishes the battlefield for the host–organism interaction. Since the physis creates a barrier to the vessels, they must double back on themselves, forming end-loop capillaries and creating an area of stasis in the bony metaphysis (Fig. 7.6). This area of stasis "catches" bacteria as they are showered hematogenously from distant sites. Once entrenched, the bacteria establish a focus of infection, and the classic case of osteomyelitis develops. It is important to recognize that the changes are not simply the result of the damage the bacteria do to the bone but also the reparative changes initiated by the bone in an effort to localize the infection.

The result of this activity is a mixture of bony destruction by the organisms and new bone formed to wall off the infection and shore up the areas of damage. The dead and dying bony fragments are referred to as "sequestra," and the new viable bone being formed is called "involucrum."

Clinical Features

One should inquire about a history of trauma, as well as infections elsewhere, that may have provided a source for the organism. Occasionally, no such history will be available, and the child presents with pain in a limb and fever. The combination of these two findings—pain in an extremity and fever—should be presumed to be infectious until proven otherwise. In children under 1 year of age, the findings may be more nonspecific and poorly localized—e.g., irritability, changes in feeding habits, and few signs of sepsis. Pseudoparalysis (failure to use the limb) may be the only localized finding. Localized physical findings such as swelling, heat, localized tenderness, erythema, and signs of systemic sepsis are frequently seen in the older child.

Diagnosis

Standard laboratory studies will usually show an elevated white blood cell (WBC) count, sedimentation rate (ESR), and C-reactive protein (CRP). The ESR and CRP are both acute phase reactants; however, the latter responds more rapidly to the presence of infection and, therefore, tends to be a more sensitive measure of skeletal involvement. X-rays initially may be negative, since it takes at least 10 days for the pathology to become demon-

Fig. 7.6 Metaphyseal circulation of the long bones in children. The nutrient artery terminates in end arterioles, which make a hairpin turn adjacent to the physis and feed into larger venous sinusoids. The resultant turbulent circulation enables bacteria to enter the extravascular space. (From Tachdjian MO. Pediatric Orthopedics, 6th ed. Philadelphia, PA: Herring; 2022. Reprinted with permission)

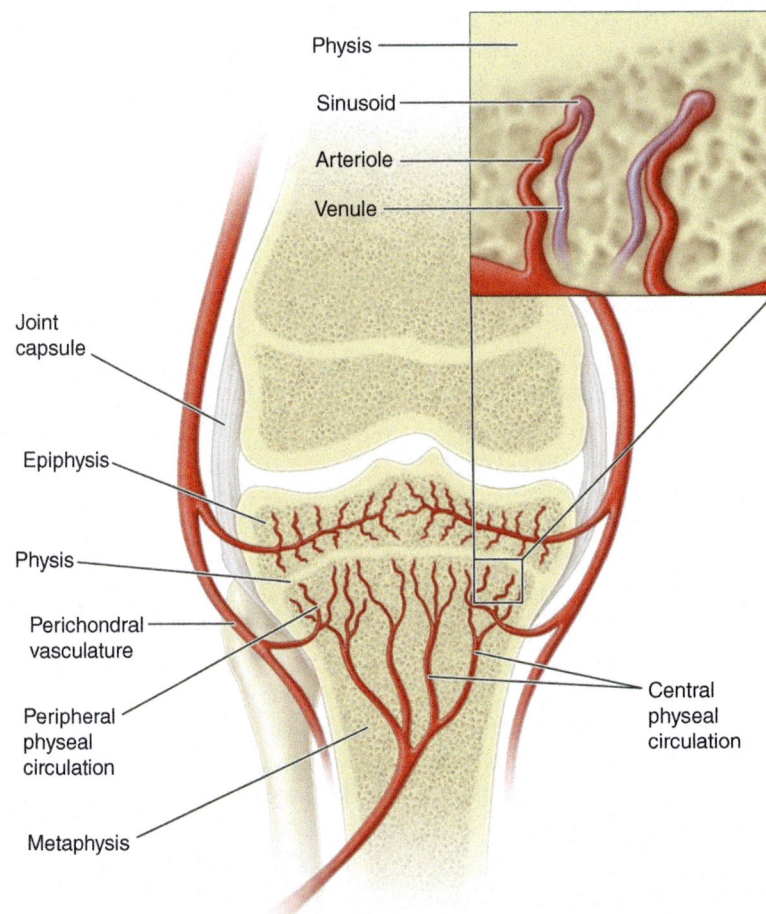

strable radiographically, they should nevertheless always be acquired. Bone resorption and new periosteal bone formation are the characteristic changes. However, neither of these may be seen initially. An MRI with contrast is helpful in the evaluation of these children.

Appropriate cultures are essential. Blood cultures are positive in up to 50% of cases of acute hematogenous osteomyelitis. The organisms vary slightly with age, but either *Staphylococcus aureus* or *Streptococcus species* should be anticipated. In neonates, one needs to consider the possibility of gram-negative organisms. Management may involve empiric intravenous antibiotics that covers the most likely organism, typically based on the local community acquired *S. aureus* sensitivities, and dosing is typically two to three times the standard to ensure peak bactericidal titer. The

duration of intravenous medication varies based on the severity of the illness and laboratory value response, such as CRP. If empiric treatment fails, the next step is either bone aspiration with a large bore needle or surgical irrigation and debridement with intraoperative culture.

In contrast to acute osteomyelitis, subacute osteomyelitis often lacks signs of systemic infection with normal labs and negative cultures.

Treatment

Diagnosis is critical prior to initiating antimicrobial treatment. All too often broad-spectrum antibiotics are given before a bacteriologic diagnosis is made. The result is a "partially treated osteomyelitis." These children present a challenging problem since the classical physical findings tend to be dampened or eradicated completely. The problem, however, is that the organisms are frequently not killed—they only await antibiotic withdrawal before initiating a new wave of bony destruction. The principles of management have been established for many years and are best summarized as follows: (1) complete bacteriologic diagnosis, (2) appropriate antibiotic selection, (3) antibiotic delivery by the appropriate route and for the appropriate duration, (4) immobilization to decrease the risk of pathologic fracture, and (5) surgical drainage of any abscesses. For many years, the tradition of intravenous (IV) antibiotic delivery has been accepted as essential. Although some would argue that the oral route is adequate, the IV route is still considered by most to be the standard mode of

delivery despite the inconvenience caused to child, family, and physician. The traditional duration of 6 weeks has been altered in some protocols to 3 weeks intravenous and 3 weeks oral, based on clinical response and the isolated organism. The indication for surgical drainage is the presence of loculated pus or infection resistant to antibiotics.

Typically, purulent loculations will be seen within the metaphysis and/or under the periosteum (Fig. 7.7). These subperiosteal abscesses typically follow breakthrough of the thin cortical bone in the metaphyseal region. As these subperiosteal collections strip the periosteum from the underlying cortex, the cortex is devascularized and segments become avascular. In severe cases of acute hematogenous osteomyelitis, it is not uncommon to see sequestration of the entire bony diaphysis.

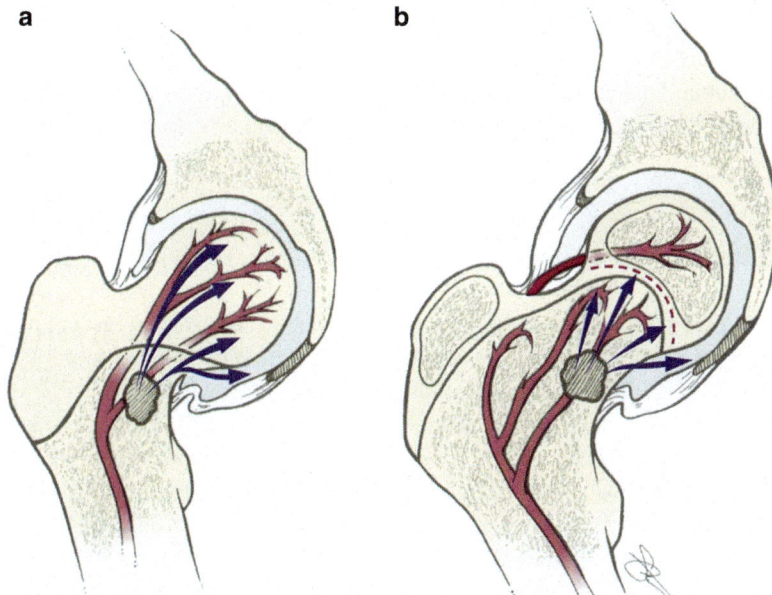

a   b

Fig. 7.7 Vascular anatomy of the proximal femur. (**a**) In the neonate, the entire epiphysis shares a blood supply with the metaphysis. Thus, infection in the metaphysis can spread into the epiphysis and can produce devastating osteonecrosis of the proximal femur. (**b**) After development of the secondary ossification center, the epiphysis and metaphysis have separate blood supplies. Thus, in the older child, the physis prevents the spread of infection into the epiphysis. However, the metaphysis remains intraarticular, and infection may decompress into the joint and produce septic arthritis. (From Tachdjian MO. Pediatric Orthopedics, 6th ed. Philadelphia, PA: Herring; 2022. Reprinted with permission)

Septic Arthritis

Infection of a child's joint typically results from one of the three pathologic mechanisms:

1. Hematogenous spread: Just as in osteomyelitis, organisms can localize in the joint finding the highly vascular synovium a favorable location for replication.
2. Breakthrough from a metaphyseal osteomyelitis: This occurs in specific joints where a portion of the metaphysis is intraarticular. Anatomically, the synovial reflection extends beyond the physis and includes a portion of metaphyseal cortical bone. The transverse Volkmann's canals provide a conduit for pus in the metaphysis to access the joint. In doing so, a secondary septic arthritis results. This phenomenon of breakthrough is most typical in the hip but can also occur in the elbow, where the radial head is intraarticular, the shoulder, and the ankle, where the fibular physis is intraarticular.
3. Penetrating trauma: This results in joint sepsis when organisms are directly injected into the joint.

Clinical Features

Joint swelling and redness are the typical physical findings that one would expect. Systemic signs of sepsis are also usually readily apparent. In contradistinction to acute hematogenous osteomyelitis, children affected with septic arthritis tend to be more toxic, exhibiting high fevers, listlessness, and poor feeding. In addition, these children will resist any attempt to move the involved joint.

Diagnosis

A workup like that for osteomyelitis should be carried out and at the risk of appearing repetitious, one cannot seriously consider this diagnosis in the differential without having made an attempt to retrieve organisms from the joint. It is important to be sure that the joint is, indeed, being aspirated and this frequently will require fluoroscopic control, especially if the joint in question is the hip. The pediatric hip is often difficult to enter under the best of circumstances and radiographic control using an arthrogram or ultrasound is recommended.

The most common organism retrieved in the child is *S. aureus*. As is the case with osteomyelitis, neonates should be suspected of having unusual organisms, including gram negatives. In the adolescent patient, one must never forget the common cause of septic arthritis: *Neisseria gonorrhoeae*.

Treatment

Septic arthritis, unlike acute hematogenous osteomyelitis, is a surgical emergency. It is imperative that the pus be removed from the joint as soon as possible. The articular cartilage is extremely vulnerable and easily damaged by enzymes—both those produced by the microorganisms and those produced by the white cells. It is, therefore, NOT enough to simply kill the organisms in the joint. The joint must be rid of all WBCs, bacterial byproducts, and enzymes. In most young children, this requires an arthrotomy. Occasionally, in the older child, arthroscopy is an appropriate technique for cleaning out a more accessible joint, such as the knee.

Repeated needle aspirations are rarely effective in cleaning the inflamed joint. In addition, repetitive aspiration in the child is yet another example of "man's inhumanity to man." Antibiotic management is similar to that for osteomyelitis regarding the choice of antibiotic and the route of delivery. The duration of administration, however, is frequently shortened. The prognosis for septic arthritis in a child depends on early diagnosis, aggressive drainage, and appropriate antibiotic management. Delay in diagnosis or delay in adequate surgical drainage can have disastrous long-term effects on the joint, typically producing irreversible changes (Fig. 7.8).

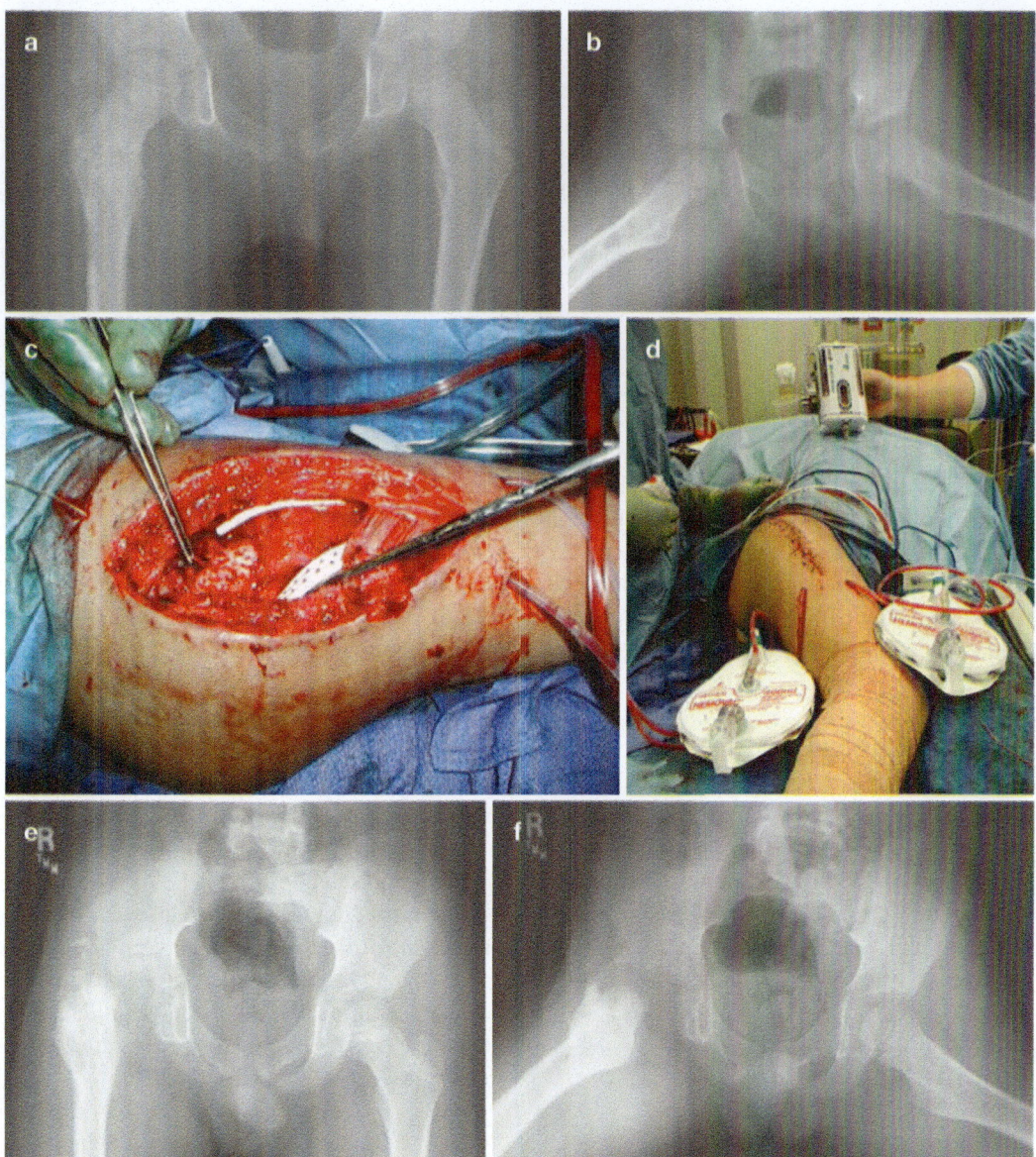

Fig. 7.8 This 11-year-old boy with a 2-week delay in presentation developed septic arthritis of the right hip and osteomyelitis of the proximal femur. Plain radiographs (**a** and **b**) after nine surgical procedures for irrigation and débridement (**c** and **d**) demonstrate involucrum associated with the proximal femur and a cortical window used for débridement. Radiographs taken 6 months later (**e** and **f**) demonstrate autolytic destruction of the femoral head and loss of the proximal femur. (From Tachdjian MO. Pediatric Orthopedics, 6th ed. Philadelphia, PA: Herring; 2022. Reprinted with permission)

Complications of Bone and Joint Infections

Long-term sequelae can result from bacterial damage to these relatively vulnerable tissues. In addition to the bone and articular cartilage, the child has a physis, which is likewise exposed to the insult.

Septic Joint Destruction

Loss of articular cartilage and arthrofibrosis ultimately result in joint contracture, deformity, and occasionally bony ankylosis (fusion). Salvage of the irreparably damaged articulations is difficult at best and frequently impossible.

Physeal Damage

Injury to the growth plate can have long-term effects, especially when it occurs in a very young child with significant growth remaining. Complete arrest and subsequent limb-length inequality or partial physeal arrest and the resultant angular deformity are the two standard patterns of postinjury deformity.

Pathologic Fracture

Although infected bone will frequently look denser (i.e., sclerotic) on X-ray, it should not be assumed that it is mechanically stronger. The dense bone is disorganized, its lamellar pattern disrupted, and, therefore, it is mechanically weaker. Pathologic fracture can occur even in the immobilized limb, although the risk is decreased.

Chronic Infection

Despite aggressive treatment, some infections are not completely eradicated, and a "stalemate" is established between the host and the organism. Occasionally, at times of physiologic stress, the infection will reactivate and cause additional damage.

Arthritis in Childhood

Juvenile Rheumatoid Disease

The polyarticular form of the juvenile idiopathic arthritis (JIA), as the name implies, takes its toll on the joints but is not associated with systemic findings. The hands and wrists are frequently involved, over 5 joints are affected, and is typically symmetric. Polyarticular JIA has a 60% remission rate.

Pauciarticular JIA is the most common and benign form of the disease. Typically, it is a monoarticular arthritis, with the knee, elbow, and ankle most commonly involved. Frequently, children suffering from the pauciarticular form of the disease present with an isolated chronically swollen joint. This finding should trigger a diagnostic workup. **Diagnostic blood studies are usually negative (rheumatoid factor is positive in only 15% of cases).** X-rays usually only show juxta-articular osteopenia, and frequently, a synovial biopsy may be needed. The histology of the synovium is like that of the adult disease—namely, hyperplasia and villous hypertrophy of the synovium. It is imperative to recognize that JIA is the leading cause of blindness in children due to the destructive iridocyclitis that can accompany the joint disease. All children with JIA should be under the care of an ophthalmologist since eye involvement does NOT parallel the degree of joint involvement; those with minimal joint disease can have the most severe eye changes.

Still's disease is acute onset JIA and the most common connective tissue disease in children. Children have systemic symptoms—fever, rash, hepatosplenomegaly—and develop polyarticular arthritis. This is the most virulent and destructive form of the disease and leaves multiple destroyed joints in its wake (Fig. 7.9). It typically occurs in ages 5–10 years and has no gender predilection.

Treatment should be directed toward control of the synovitis with medications, physical therapy to maintain joint motion, psychologic support for chronically impaired children, and ultimately arthroplasties or fusions for those joints most severely involved.

Hemophilia

Children with bleeding dyscrasias frequently have repeated hemarthroses. Initially, the blood in the joint simply distends the capsular structures and causes a mild synovitis. With repeated bleeds, the synovium becomes hyperplastic and ultimately pannus formation is seen. At this point, the joint changes appear very similar to those seen in rheumatoid disease—e.g., osteopenia, enzymatic cartilage degradation, bony erosions, and lysis.

Fig. 7.9 Radiographic changes of juvenile idiopathic arthritis of the wrist. Carpal destruction and volar subluxation are common findings. (From Tachdjian MO. Pediatric Orthopedics, 6th ed. Philadelphia, PA: Herring; 2022. Reprinted with permission)

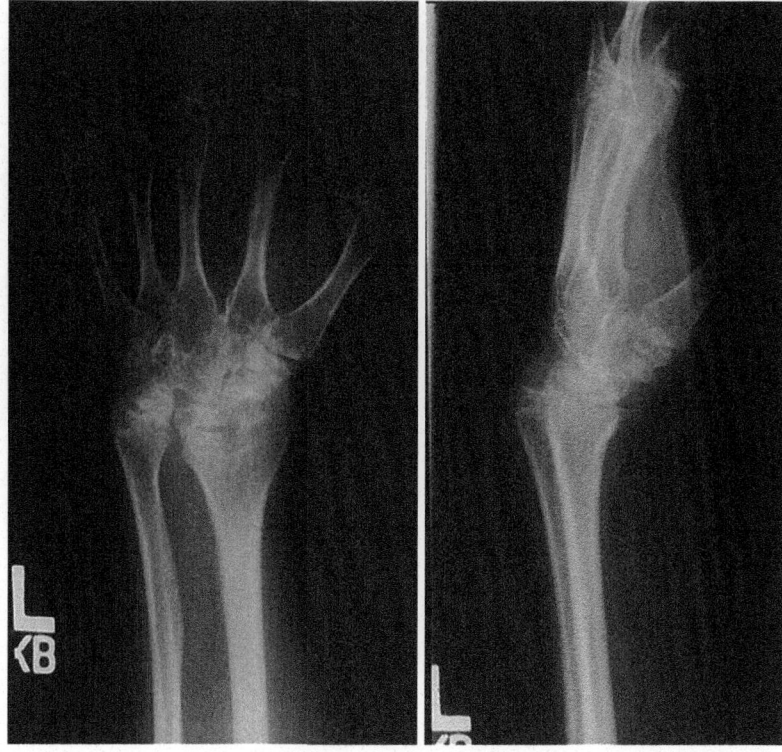

Lyme Disease

In the endemic regions of the Northeast and Middle Atlantic states, the child who presents with a swollen knee needs to be considered as a potential victim of Lyme disease. This infectious arthritis is due to a specific spirochete, *Borrelia burgdorferi*. The organism is transmitted to the human host by the bite of a deer tick. These ticks are significantly smaller than the common wood tick, and they are barely visible with the naked eye. Unfortunately, a history of a bite is rare and usually the diagnosis is reached by a high index of suspicion in a susceptible host. The combination of endemic region, erythematous annular skin lesions, and monoarticular arthritis should lead the physician to order a Lyme titer. Treatment is generally successful if begun early. Occasionally, despite adequate treatment, the arthritis can progress to chronic joint destruction mandating further care. Treatment is usually oral antibiotics.

Metabolic Disease

The classic metabolic disease to affect the pediatric skeleton is rickets (Fig. 7.10). The etiologies of rickets are multiple (Table 7.2), but the important pathophysiologic step is a relative paucity of vitamin D. Vitamin D is essential for normal progression of physeal bone development, and without it, provisional calcification will not occur in the deepest layer of the growth plate. As a result, physeal disorganization can be anticipated with subsequent physeal widening, trumpeting of the metaphysis, and aberrant enchondral bone growth. The clinically apparent changes of knobby joints, beading of the costochondral joints, and genu varum are all phenotypic reflections of the underlying histologic disruption of bone formation. Depending on the etiology of the rickets, the histologic pattern will vary slightly, but the overall skeletal changes remain relatively constant.

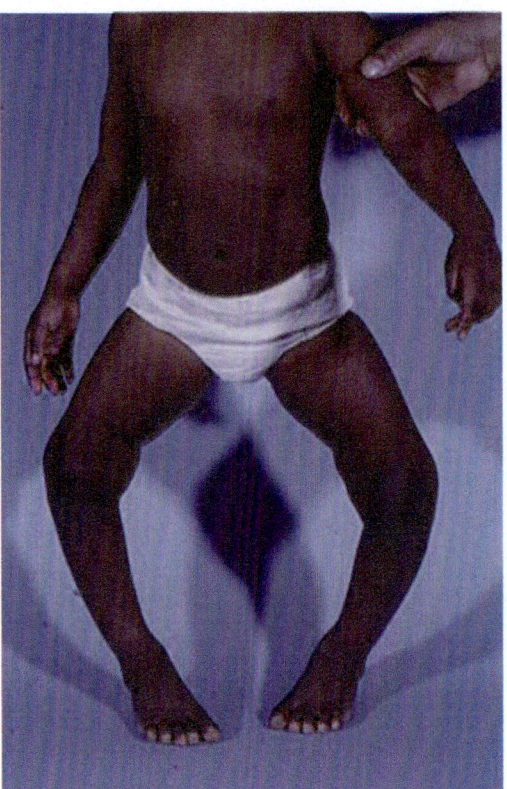

Fig. 7.10 A child with severe bowlegs, termed genu varus. (From Tachdjian MO. Pediatric Orthopedics, 6th ed. Philadelphia, PA: Herring; 2022. Reprinted with permission)

Table 7.2 Etiologies of rickets

1. Vitamin D dietary deficiency
2. Malabsorption states
3. Renal rickets
   (a) Tubular defects (congenital)
   (b) Glomerular disease (acquired)
4. Miscellaneous
   (a) Neurofibromatosis
   (b) Phenytoin-associated

Hematologic Disease

Sickle Cell Disease

The red cell deformation that occurs in sickle cell patients due to the abnormal hemoglobin is responsible for the skeletal changes. The abnormally shaped cells cause stasis and sludging in small arterioles and capillaries, resulting in disrupted flow and bony necrosis. The bony infarcts seen in sickle cell disease can occur anywhere in the bone but are more typical in the metaphysis.

These children are also predisposed to osteomyelitis due to the already sludged vessels in the metaphysis, predisposing the bone to bacterial trapping. Even though Staphylococcus is the most common organism retrieved, this patient population is also susceptible to infection with Salmonella. This organism gains access to the circulatory system through small infarcts in the intestinal wall and then enters the bone hematogenously. The treatment for the infarcts is appropriate hematologic care—hydration, analgesics, etc. Antibiotic selection for osteomyelitis should take into consideration the incidence of salmonella.

Leukemia

This is the most common malignancy of childhood, and the skeleton is not spared its ravages. The bones by X-ray will show nondescript lytic changes most characteristically seen in the metaphyseal region and referred to as "metaphyseal banding." The areas of osteopenia parallel and adjacent to the physis; although suggestive of leukemia, they are *not* pathognomonic of it.

Usually, the diagnosis has been made well before skeletal complications develop; however, occasionally a child will present for the evaluation of "growing pains" only to have a workup reveal this disease. Ordinarily "growing pains" occur in children 2–7 years of age, affect primarily the legs, are symmetric (although not simultaneous), occur in early evening or just after going to bed, and are NOT associated with any systemic complaints. Any variation from the usual pattern should suggest a basic workup to include X-rays and a complete blood count with further diagnosis made with bone marrow biopsy. Patients with leukemia usually present before 4 years of age with recurrent infections, bleeding, fatigue, and lymphadenopathy.

Congenital and Neurodevelopmental

This is the largest and most nondescript "wastebasket" of pathologic states, many of which have severe impact on the pediatric skeleton. Included here are congenital birth defects of no known etiology, such as proximal femoral focal deficiency, as well as genetic diseases transmitted in classic Mendelian fashion (e.g., hemophilia) or due to chromosomal defects (e.g., Down's syndrome). In addition, the neuromuscular diseases frequently have an immense impact on the skeleton, as aberrant and eccentric muscular forces are created. Unfortunately, it is difficult to find many common themes that make an appreciation of the skeletal impact easier to understand.

Osteogenesis Imperfecta

This disease is transmitted in a classic autosomal dominant pattern with only rare exception. The basic defect is one of abnormal collagen synthesis due to impotent osteoblasts. For this reason, it has been grouped with other "sick" cell syndromes. Certainly, the osteoblasts are normal in number but incapable of normal synthetic activity. The collagenous product of their incompetence is poorly formed and poorly cross-linked, making it weak.

The subsequent bone that is made is similarly architecturally thin and mechanically weak (Fig. 7.11). The severity of the disease is as expected—a function of the dose of abnormal genetic material. Some of the severe homozygotes are stillborn due to intracranial bleeds occurring in the perinatal period. As with most genetic diseases, penetrance varies such that some children have multiple fractures and severe shortening and others less involved have only the occasional fracture.

Typically, the bones are osteopenic with thinned cortices and decreased diameter. Multiple fractures with resulting deformities are expected. These fractures respond to appropriate treatment, and healing is only slightly prolonged. Occasionally, it is necessary to correct long-bone deformities operatively by performing multiple osteotomies in a single bone and lining the resultant fragments up on an intramedullary rod that is capable of lengthening with subsequent growth (Fassier-Duval growing rod, Fig. 7.12).

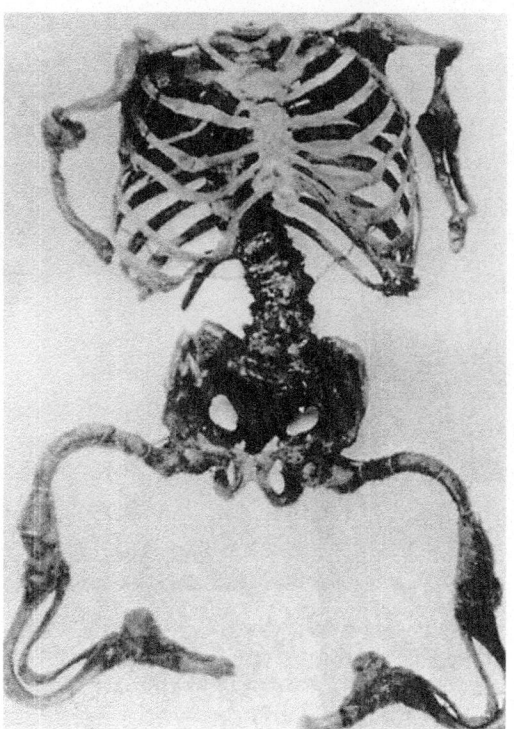

Fig. 7.11 The skeleton in severe osteogenesis imperfecta. (From Tachdjian MO. Pediatric Orthopedics, 6th ed. Philadelphia, PA: Herring; 2022. Reprinted with permission)

Scoliosis can also complicate this disease, and its management can be very challenging, especially if surgical management is required to correct the deformity. It is very difficult to use spinal instrumentation in the face of this osteopenic, softened bone.

Almost all patients with osteogenesis imperfecta are seen by geneticists and primary care clinics who guide the administration of bisphosphonates. Bisphosphonates inhibit osteoclasts which increase the cortical diameter and cancellous bone density to effectively reduce fracture incidence, pain, and improve ambulation in this population.

Down Syndrome

First described in England by Langdon Down in the 1800s, this syndrome has been shown to result from a trisomy of the number 21 chromosome. It

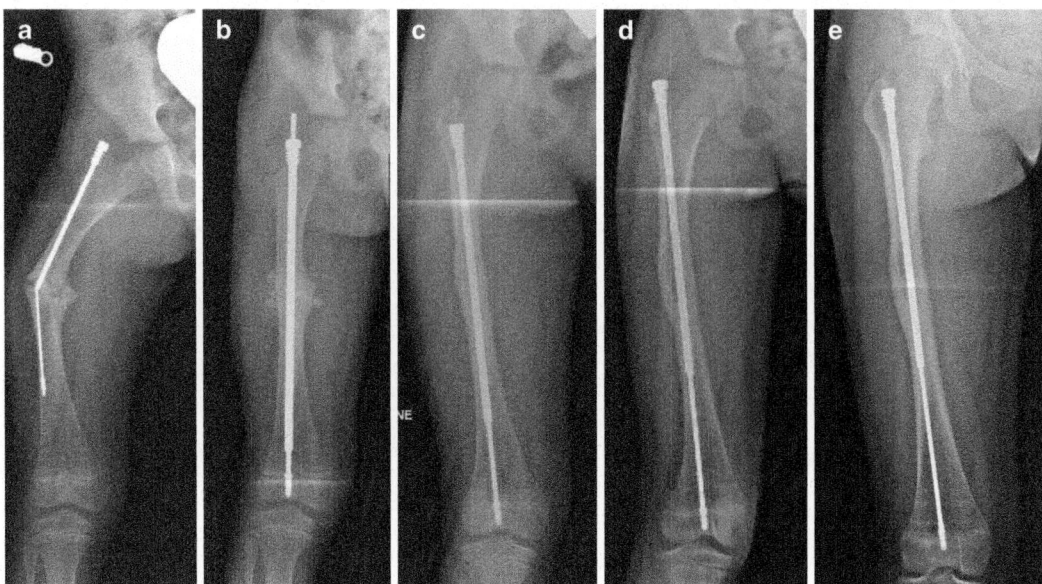

Fig. 7.12 A 6-year-old girl with osteogenesis imperfecta treated with a Fassier-Duval (FD) rod. (**a**) Patient had acute bending of the male component after a fall. The FD rod was placed 4 years earlier. Radiograph also shows loss of anchoring of the distal threaded portion of the male component from the distal femoral epiphysis and proximal migration. (**b**) Radiograph after revision of the FD rod with a larger diameter rod and a longer distal threaded portion on the male component. (**c**) At age 8, distal migra- tion of the threaded head of the female component distal to the greater trochanter was noted. (**d**) Revision of the female component and repositioning of the threaded head to the tip of the greater trochanter and bone grafting is shown. (**e**) Follow-up radiograph at age 12 shows tele- scoping of the rod. (From Tachdjian MO. Pediatric Orthopedics, 6th ed. Philadelphia, PA: Herring; 2022. Reprinted with permission)

is the most common chromosomal abnormality and it occurs in approximately 1 in 500 live births. Because of its frequency, it is the prototype for the other chromosomal abnormalities and the ortho- pedic manifestations tend to be somewhat com- mon to all.

The many musculoskeletal problems experi- enced by children with Down syndrome are largely related to the hypotonia, joint hypermo- bility, and ligamentous laxity that typify the group. The ligamentous laxity results from an inordinate number of elastic fibers relative to the number of collagen fibers in ligament and joint capsule. The joint changes typical of this disease and other chromosomal diseases can be traced directly to this ligamentous laxity. Specific mani- festations include the following:

- C1–C2 instability: Due to laxity of the trans- verse ligament of the odontoid process, anterior translation of C1 on C2 occurs, frequently at alarming degrees. Routine lateral cervical spine radiographs in flexion and extension should be regularly obtained in these children to evaluate them for this problem. This is particularly important in the pre-participation evaluation for competition in sporting activities.

- Hip subluxation and dislocation can occur insidiously over time, again resulting from the capsular laxity about the joint.

- Patellar subluxation is the cause of the typical gait seen in the older child with Down syn- drome. These children often walk with a stiff- legged gait in an effort to preclude patellar subluxation.

- Hypermobile flatfeet and bunions are com- mon, and management is primarily directed at controlling the deformity, if possible, and minimizing the pain, which is rarely a signifi- cant problem. Despite fixed deformities, it is frequently surprising how well these children compensate.

- Scoliosis is common and managed similarly to those with idiopathic scoliosis.
- SCFEs are also common and more likely to be unstable and high grade at presentation with higher rates of osteonecrosis.

Skeletal Dysplasias

There are several hundred recognized skeletal dysplasias, each with its own unique clinical characteristics and specific skeletal abnormalities (Fig. 7.13). It is impossible to recall all of the features, which define a given dysplastic condition, especially in light of the fact that each is quite rare. At best, generalizations can be employed to assist in the diagnosis of a specific patient and thereby guide the appropriate workup and referral to an individual skilled in definitive diagnosis. The anticipated orthopedic problems, treatment, and prognosis will hinge on the diagnosis.

When presented with an individual displaying dysplastic findings, especially short stature, chromosomal evaluation and standard X-rays are good starting points once appropriate history (especially family history) and a careful physical examination have been carried out. The X-rays should include a lateral of the cervical and thoracolumbar spine, an anteroposterior view of the pelvis, and anteroposterior views of the wrists and the knees. These views will allow one to evaluate epiphyseal, physeal, metaphyseal, and diaphyseal growth and their aberrations.

Most of the dysplasias tend to affect a specific region of the bone; by assessing each region, clues regarding the specific type of dysplasia can narrow the differential. For example, spondyloepiphyseal dysplasia affects primarily epiphyseal growth as the name implies. One should expect to see deformities of the epiphyseal nuclei and disordered apophyseal growth. Conversely, achondroplasia is a defect in physeal growth and will, therefore, produce significant shortening; in fact, it is the most common cause of pathologic short stature.

Most of the skeletal dysplasias are genetically transmitted, and a careful family history will define the pattern. Many, however, are spontaneous mutations or without a defined etiology. It is important to keep in mind that by definition a skeletal dysplasia is a GENERALIZED affectation of the skeleton with all bones showing some changes. Obviously, the end of the bone growing more rapidly will demonstrate the defect to a greater degree; thus, the knee and wrist films are more likely to show changes than the hip or elbow films.

Achondroplasia

As an example of how a dysplasia affects the skeleton, one should consider the most common, achondroplasia. Transmitted as an autosomal dominant mutation in FGFR3 in most cases, it is usually apparent at birth. The infant will be rhizomelically shortened; that is to say, the proximal segment of the limbs is relatively shorter than the middle or distal segments. In addition, the child is disproportionately built since the limbs are preferentially involved and, therefore, very short relative to the spine and trunk. These children follow the growth curve but several standard deviations below normal, achieving a mature height between 3 and 4 ft. As with all of the true dysplasias, intelligence is not impaired and life expectancy is near normal.

Clinical Features

The child's head shows flattening of the nasal bridge and prominent frontal bones (Fig. 7.14). Both findings are due to the disparity between the normal intramembranous calvarial growth and the retarded enchondral growth of the basilar portions of the skull. The extremities are short, with each of the bones being short in length, but relatively normal in girth since periosteal bone formation remains relatively unaffected. The spine and pelvis also show some decrease in height but of greater significance is the decrease in the interpedicular distance which effectively creates spinal stenosis. This, coupled with a hyperlordotic

Hyperplasias   **Hypoplasias**

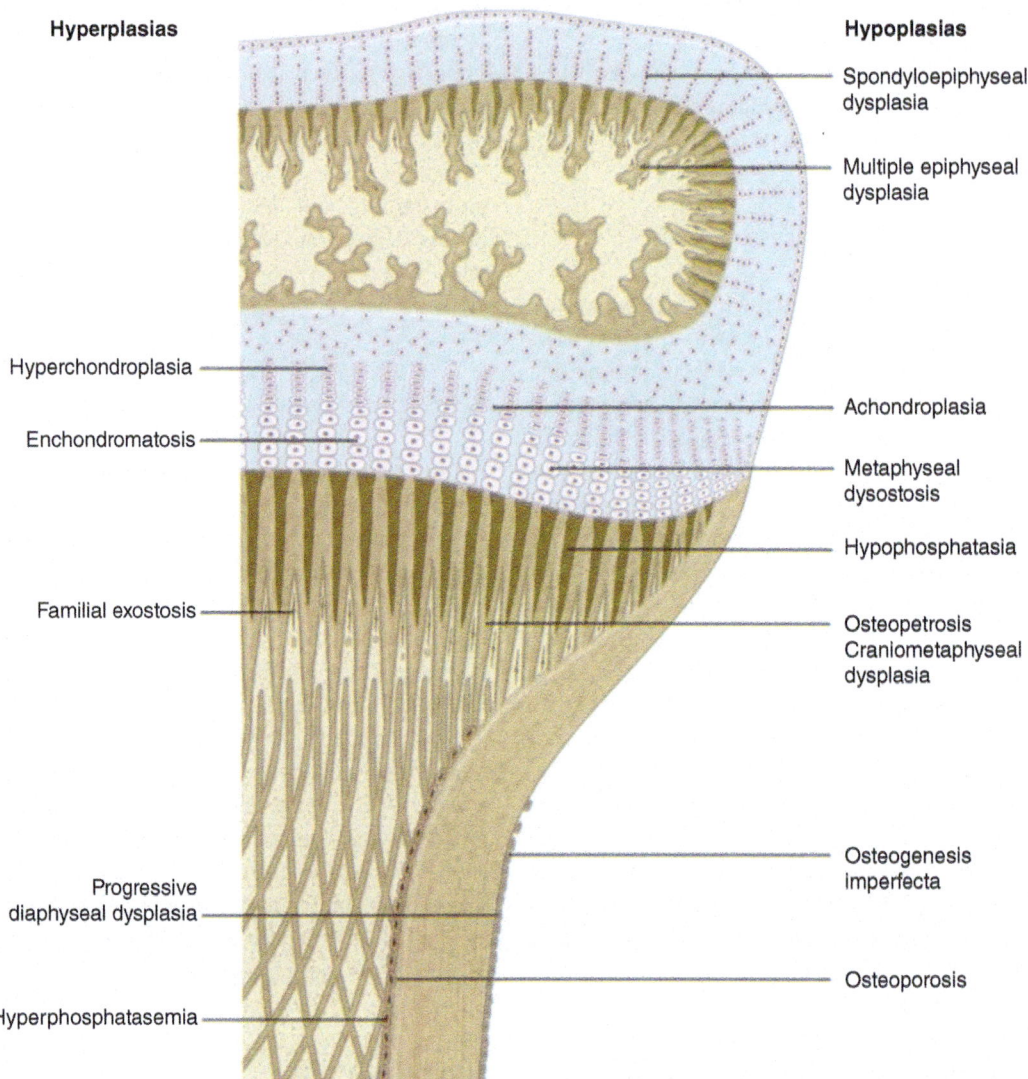

Fig. 7.13 Dynamic classification of bone dysplasias. (From Tachdjian MO. Pediatric Orthopedics, 6th ed. Philadelphia, PA: Herring; 2022. Reprinted with permission)

lumbar spine, leads to the development of symptoms at an early age. A major problem of the older adolescent is obesity, which complicates many of the other abnormalities. As adults, problems with multiple tendonitises and bursitises are commonplace.

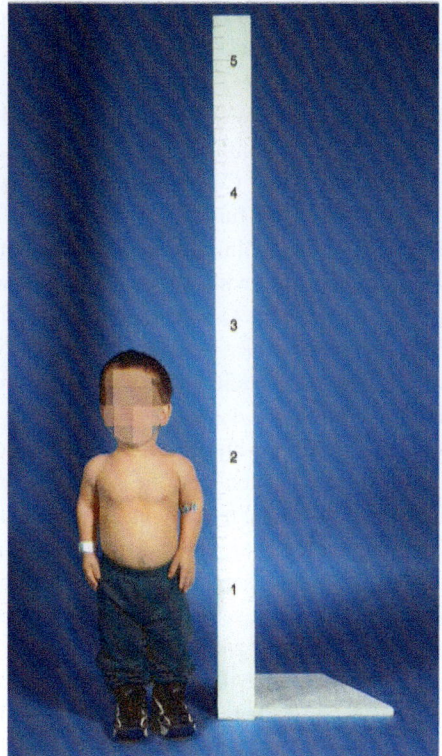

Fig. 7.14 A 6-year-old child with achondroplasia. Note that his fingers reach to the level of his hips. (From Tachdjian MO. Pediatric Orthopedics, 6th ed. Philadelphia, PA: Herring; 2022. Reprinted with permission)

Neuromuscular Disease

Unlike the skeletal dysplasias which are intrinsic abnormalities of the skeleton, neuromuscular disorders are extrinsic but drastically alter the normal skeleton due to the muscle imbalances they create.

Common themes can be seen that emphasize the fact that the problem is disparity in the agonist–antagonist relationship. Major joints tend to dislocate, with the hip being a prime example. The flexor pattern tends to become dominant, causing the femoral head to dislocate posteriorly. Scoliosis should be expected as asymmetry of spinal muscle action alters normal balance. If the neurologic defect is asymmetric, as in polio, then the growth plates in one leg will experience a different muscle pull than those of the other and a leg-length discrepancy can be anticipated.

Cerebral Palsy (CP)

CP is a **static** neurologic disease of children due to an insult to the immature brain during the perinatal period. The defect is, therefore, central, damaging the normal inhibitory influences on the peripheral gamma efferent system. Without central dampening, the peripheral reflex arc functions autonomously, and the result is increased tone or spasticity.

Cerebral palsy can be classified physiologically or geographically.

Physiologic Classification
- Spastic: Hypertonia, hyperflexia, and contractures are seen. This is the most common form of the syndrome.
- Athetoid: This is far less common today than it was in years past. Rh incompatibility and erythroblastosis fetalis were a common etiology of this form.
- Rigid.
- Ballismic.
- Mixed.

Geographic Classification
- Hemiplegia: The most common form, affecting one side of the body (upper and lower extremity), frequently associated with seizures.
- Diplegia: Both lower extremities predominate the pattern, the person is usually still ambulatory.
- Quadriplegia: The most severe cases involve children, with total body involvement, many of whom exhibit cognitive deficits and few of whom will ever walk.

Cerebral palsy is really a syndrome rather than a disease, and no two children are the same. This makes comparison of procedures and other treatments extremely difficult. The muscles all tend to be spastic; however, the muscle imbalance is created between spastic and more spastic muscles. Contractures, joint dislocations, limb deformities, and scoliosis should all be anticipated.

Polio

With the introduction of the Salk vaccine in 1954, this disease has become rare in the United States; however, it is certainly not eradicated and may be seen particularly in areas with high immigration rates. The polio virus has unique predilection for the anterior horn cells of the cord and the bulbar portion of the brain. In most cases, the involvement is spotty, and the degree of paralysis is variable. The victim is left with a mix of normal muscle, weak muscle, and absent muscle, creating a broad spectrum of muscle imbalance in an asymmetric distribution. It is important to remember that the sensory fibers are NOT affected, which gives these children a clear and distinct benefit over the children with spina bifida.

Spina Bifida

Despite the improvement in antenatal testing, many children with myelodysplasia are born in the United States each year (Fig. 7.15). Due to open cord defects at a certain level, these children have congenital paraplegia, lacking motor and sensory modalities below the level of the defect. The higher their level of defect, the poorer their

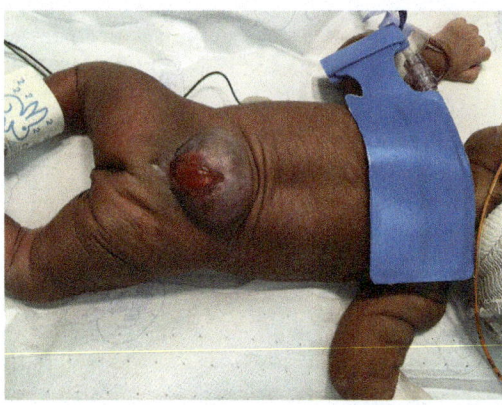

Fig. 7.15 Clinical appearance of untreated myelomeningocele sac. Note the large protrusion of the meninges, without protective skin. Breakdown of the sac usually occurs, followed by further neurologic injury, meningitis, and potentially encephalitis. (From Tachdjian MO. Pediatric Orthopedics, 6th ed. Philadelphia, PA: Herring; 2022. Reprinted with permission)

function, and hence, the prognosis. For example, a child with a T12 level (the spinal roots that are the last to function are T12) has no motor power and no sensation below the waist. These children will be wheelchair-confined and have bowel and bladder compromise. Conversely, children with an S1 level (the last functioning spinal level is S1) will have only minimal motor involvement and will usually walk without braces. Their major problems are the bowel and bladder malfunction.

The absence of sensation below the level of the lesion creates many additional problems for these children. Not unlike a diabetic patient with severe neuropathy, children with spina bifida are prone to foot ulceration, infection, and the development of neuropathic joints. One recently identified problem in this group is latex allergy. Perhaps due to repeated catheterization with latex rubber catheters, these patients can become severely sensitized to all latex contact, to the point of anaphylaxis. Specific protocols are now used at the time of surgical procedures to avoid contact with any latex products, including gloves, catheters, and IV tubing.

Lastly, it is important to realize that these children, as well as many of those with cerebral palsy, are multiply handicapped. They can have learning difficulties, perceptual problems, hearing and visual impairments, and emotional issues—all of which require a coordinated effort by multiple specialists to provide optimal care.

Regional Orthopedic Problems

The Pediatric Hip

Most of the showcase pediatric orthopedic maladies affect the hip. Several unique anatomic features predispose this joint to long-term problems following septic, vascular, developmental, and traumatic insults.

In the newborn, the upper end of the femur is entirely cartilaginous, representing the secondary ossification centers of both the greater trochanter and the femoral head (capital femoral epiphysis) as a composite chondroepiphysis. The two bony ossification centers will develop within this one cartilage mass and grow differentially to their ultimate adult size and shape. Implicit in this fact is that the growth of one is dependent on the growth of the other. Normally, the bony centrum of the capital femoral epiphysis should be radiographically visible by 3–6 months of age.

The growth of this epiphysis is dependent primarily on the blood supply of the upper end of the femur. Up until 1 year of age, there is communication between the metaphyseal and epiphyseal circulations that protects the capital femoral epiphysis from isolation in the event of an insult to the epiphyseal side.

Unfortunately, as the physis thickens and matures by 18 months of age, it becomes an impenetrable barrier between the two circulations, leaving the epiphysis of the head totally dependent on the epiphyseal vessels for its viability. Less than 10% of the femoral head is supplied by the branch of the obturator artery through the ligamentum teres. The epiphyseal vessels are supplied by the medial and lateral circumflex branches of the femoral artery (Fig. 7.16). This vascular isolation of the upper end of the femur is largely responsible for the disastrous complications of developmental dislocation of the hip (DDH), Perthes' disease, and slipped capital femoral epiphysis (SCFE).

The acetabulum develops from two cartilage segments. The first is the triradiate cartilage, a bilaminar physis that forms at the junction of the ilium, ischium, and pubis. Integrity of this growth plate is essential for acetabular height to be normal. The depth of the acetabulum is a function of the cartilaginous labrum that circumferentially surrounds the developing acetabulum. The acetabulum and proximal femur are forming simultaneously throughout development, and aberrations of one will affect the normal development of the other.

Developmental Dysplasia of the Hip (DDH)

The previous nomenclature "congenital dislocation" was changed to "developmental dislocation" in recognition of the fact that most of these hips are located at birth and go on to dislocate in the postnatal period. The incidence of this condition is about 1 per 1000 live births and is more common in females. Although it is fair to say that the etiology is unknown, it is important to recognize that there are both genetic and environmental factors; hence, it is considered a multifactorial trait. DDH is a true dysplasia (i.e., aberrant growth), and NOT simply a femoral head that is not located in the acetabulum. It is important to stress this fact to the parents to assist them in understanding the pathology. DDH encompasses a spectrum of pathology ranging from acetabular dysplasia to a subluxatable hip to dislocatable hip to dislocated hip (Fig. 7.17).

Early diagnosis is the key to optimal treatment and the best prognosis. First, consider the risk factors:

- First-born
- Female
- Intrauterine breech positioning
- Positive family history
- Oligohydramnios
- Macrosomia

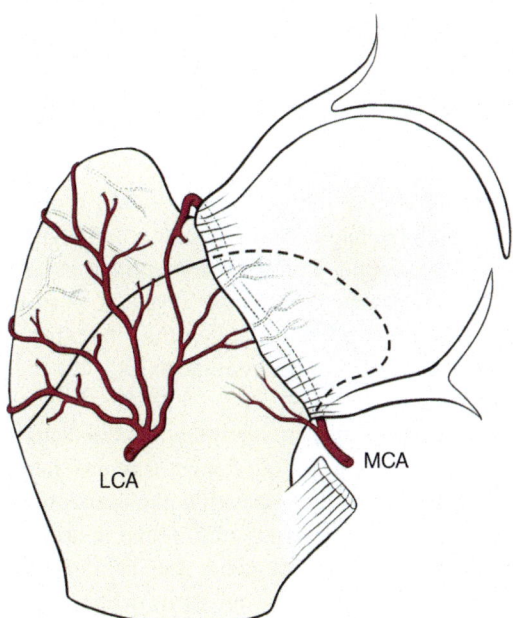

Fig. 7.16 Blood supply to the femoral head from the medial circumflex artery (*MCA*) and lateral circumflex artery (*LCA*), branches of the profunda femoris artery at the level of the tendinous portion of the iliopsoas muscle. (From Tachdjian MO. Pediatric Orthopedics, 6th ed. Philadelphia, PA: Herring; 2022. Reprinted with permission)

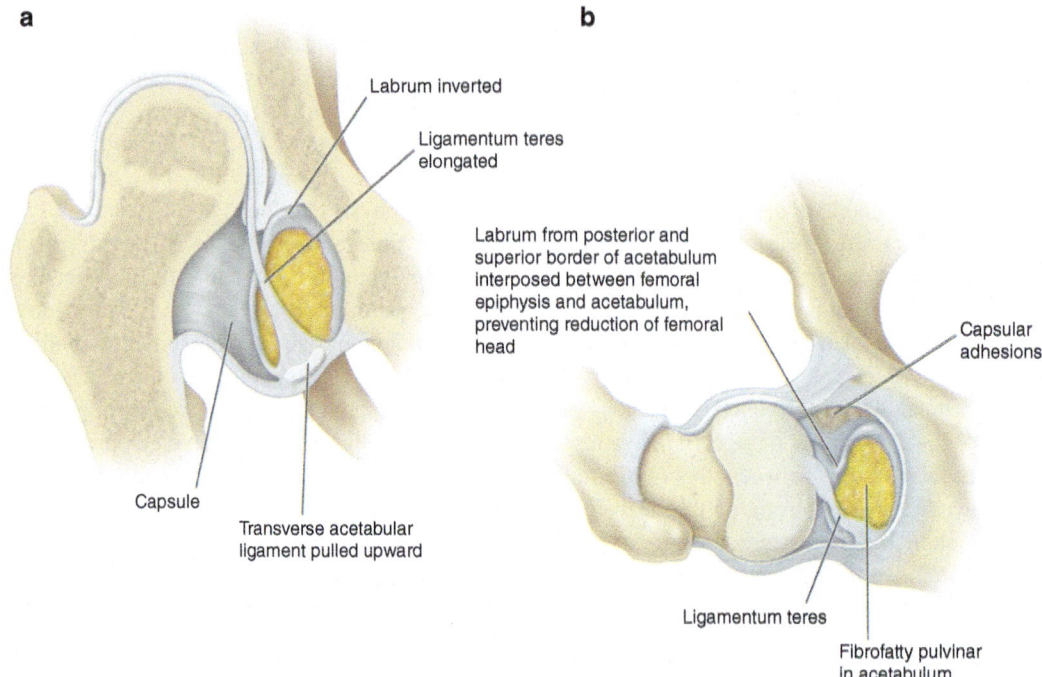

a

Labrum inverted

Ligamentum teres
elongated

Labrum from posterior and
superior border of acetabulum
interposed between femoral
epiphysis and acetabulum,
preventing reduction of femoral
head

Capsule

Transverse acetabular
ligament pulled upward

b

Capsular
adhesions

Ligamentum teres

Fibrofatty pulvinar
in acetabulum

Fig. 7.17 Pathology of the dislocated hip that is irreducible as a result of intraarticular obstacles. (**a**) The hip is dislocated. (**b**) The hip cannot be reduced on flexion, abduction, or lateral rotation. Obstacles to reduction are inverted limbus, ligamentum teres, and fibrofatty pulvinar in the acetabulum. The transverse acetabular ligament is pulled upward with the ligamentum teres. (From Tachdjian MO. Pediatric Orthopedics, 6th ed. Philadelphia, PA: Herring; 2022. Reprinted with permission)

With these in mind, a careful physical examination of the hips is the logical next step. In the newborn, one should attempt to demonstrate laxity and instability. The Barlow test is performed with the infant supine and the hips flexed (Fig. 7.18). As the hips are brought from the abducted to adducted position, a positive test is noted as the femoral head subluxates posteriorly over the posterior rim of the acetabulum. This would indicate instability. The Barlow is a provocative test: the hip is located, and the maneuver dislocates it. Conversely, the Ortolani test is a reduction maneuver; the hip is dislocated, and the test reduces it (Fig. 7.19). This is accomplished by abducting the adducted hip and noting a palpable (but rarely audible) "clunk" as the femoral head reduces over the posterior acetabular rim.

As the child gets older (by 3 months), the dislocated hip tends to become fixed in that position, and the classic signs of instability disappear in favor of those indicating a fixed dislocation deformity. Limited abduction is the most important finding to note. Examining the child on a firm surface, subtle differences in the degrees of hip abduction may herald a dislocated hip on the restricted side. Similarly, viewing knee height with the child supine and the hips and knees flexed may reveal a positive Galeazzi sign-one knee higher than the other—again indicating a dislocation on the low side (Fig. 7.20).

Imaging studies are important in both diagnosis and treatment. Before 3 months of age, much of the proximal femur is cartilaginous and therefore not visible on X-ray, ultrasound is used up until this time. Ultrasound has been helpful in the diagnosis of DDH, as well as in defining relatively subtle degrees of acetabular dysplasia (Fig. 7.21). The value of ultrasound after the child is 3 months old decreases, and standard X-rays assume a more central role. After 3 months, many classic measurements are made

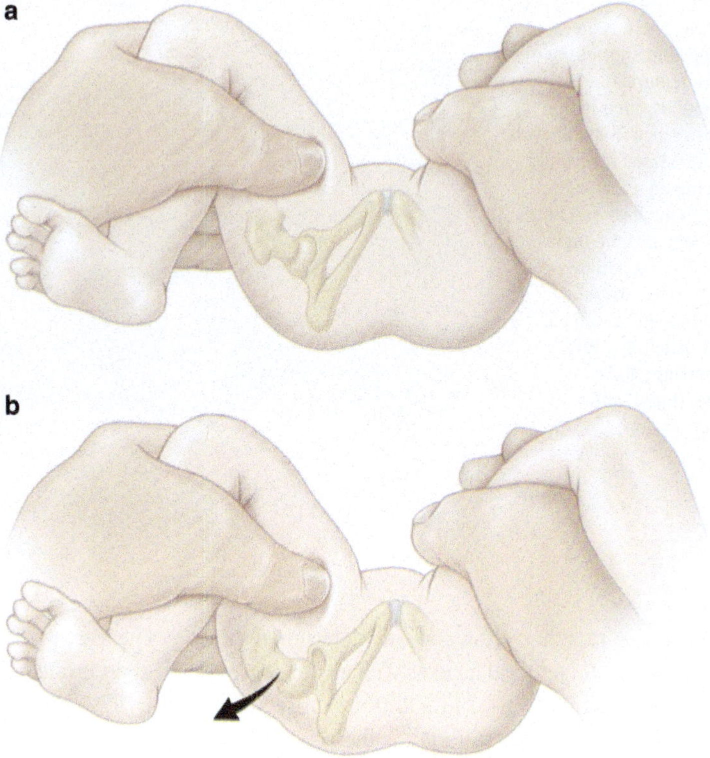

Fig. 7.18 The Barlow test for developmental dislocation of the hip in a neonate. (**a**) With the infant supine, the examiner holds both of the child's knees, gently *adducts* one hip, and pushes posteriorly. (**b**) When the examination is positive, the examiner will feel the femoral head make a small jump (*arrow*) out of the acetabulum (Barlow sign). When the pressure is released, the head is felt to slip back into place. (From Tachdjian MO. Pediatric Orthopedics, 6th ed. Philadelphia, PA: Herring; 2022. Reprinted with permission)

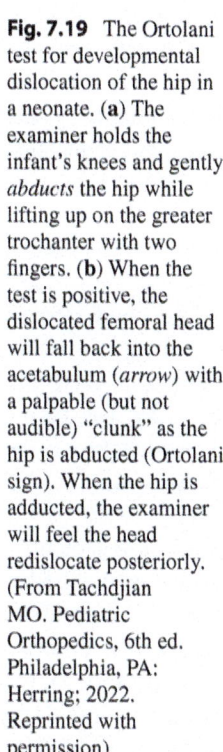

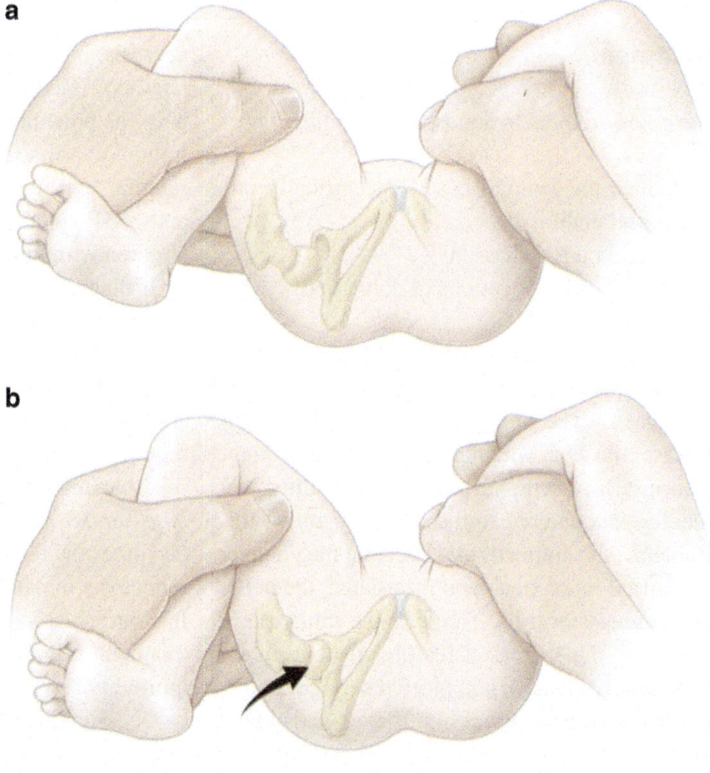

Fig. 7.19 The Ortolani test for developmental dislocation of the hip in a neonate. (**a**) The examiner holds the infant's knees and gently *abducts* the hip while lifting up on the greater trochanter with two fingers. (**b**) When the test is positive, the dislocated femoral head will fall back into the acetabulum (*arrow*) with a palpable (but not audible) "clunk" as the hip is abducted (Ortolani sign). When the hip is adducted, the examiner will feel the head redislocate posteriorly. (From Tachdjian MO. Pediatric Orthopedics, 6th ed. Philadelphia, PA: Herring; 2022. Reprinted with permission)

Fig. 7.20 The Galeazzi sign. There is an apparent shortening of the femur as demonstrated by the difference in knee levels as assessed for a child lying on a firm table with the hips and knees flexed at right angles. (From Tachdjian MO. Pediatric Orthopedics, 6th ed. Philadelphia, PA: Herring; 2022. Reprinted with permission)

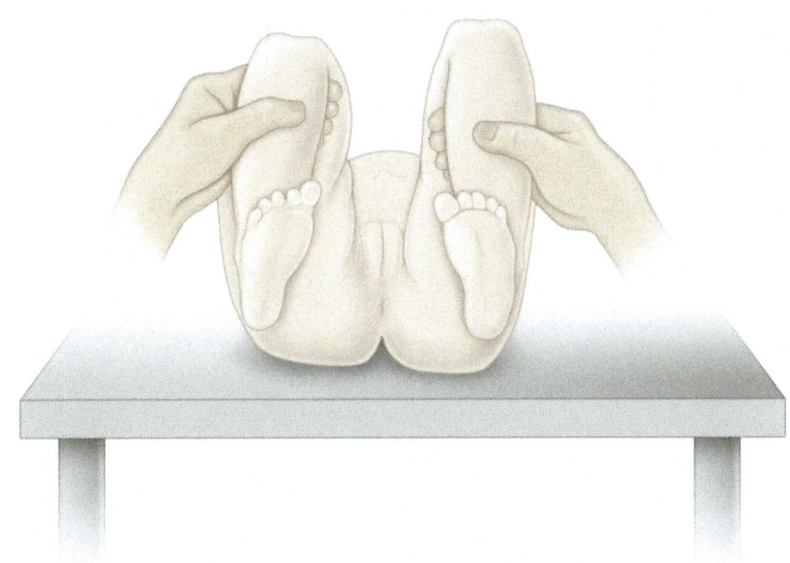

on this X-ray that allow one to determine the location of the femoral head as well as the degree of acetabular dysplasia. In addition, subsequent X-rays are important to monitor the progress of treatment.

Treatment

The goals of DDH treatment are the following:

- Reduce the femoral head concentrically into the acetabulum.
- Maintain this reduction.
- Avoid the complications of doing both.

The pitfalls in accomplishing these apparently simple goals qualify more as "land mines." The adage, "The first physician to treat DDH is the last physician with the opportunity to achieve a normal hip," emphasizes the difficulties frequently encountered in the management of this problem. Also implied is the fact that the younger the child is when treatment is initiated, the better the prognosis will be. The later the initiation of treatment, the increased likelihood of need for increasingly invasive and morbid surgical procedures to create a normal hip, if even possible at later ages.

The use of a Pavlik harness as initial treatment in the infant is the international standard (Fig. 7.22). For the child under 3 months of age with a frank dislocation or with persistent, appropriate application and use of a Pavlik harness will assure a normal hip in about 80% of cases. The device, however, is not foolproof, with avascular necrosis, inferior dislocation, erosion of the acetabulum (Pavlik disease), and femoral nerve palsy as potential complications, not to mention failure to achieve a reduction. One should be familiar with the appropriate use of this device and NOT randomly apply it as a panacea to all children with hip clicks.

If diagnosis is delayed and the child presents after 6 months for treatment, more aggressive modalities are generally required to achieve a reduction. Closed reduction under anesthesia, adductor tenotomy, or open reduction may be required, followed by immobilization in a spica cast to maintain the reduction.

After 18 months of age, pelvic osteotomies and proximal femoral osteotomies are required to reduce the hip and to reconform the acetabulum. It is rarely possible to produce a normal hip when treatment is initiated after the age of walking, but morbidity and time to future need for arthroplasty can be significantly improved with these treatments.

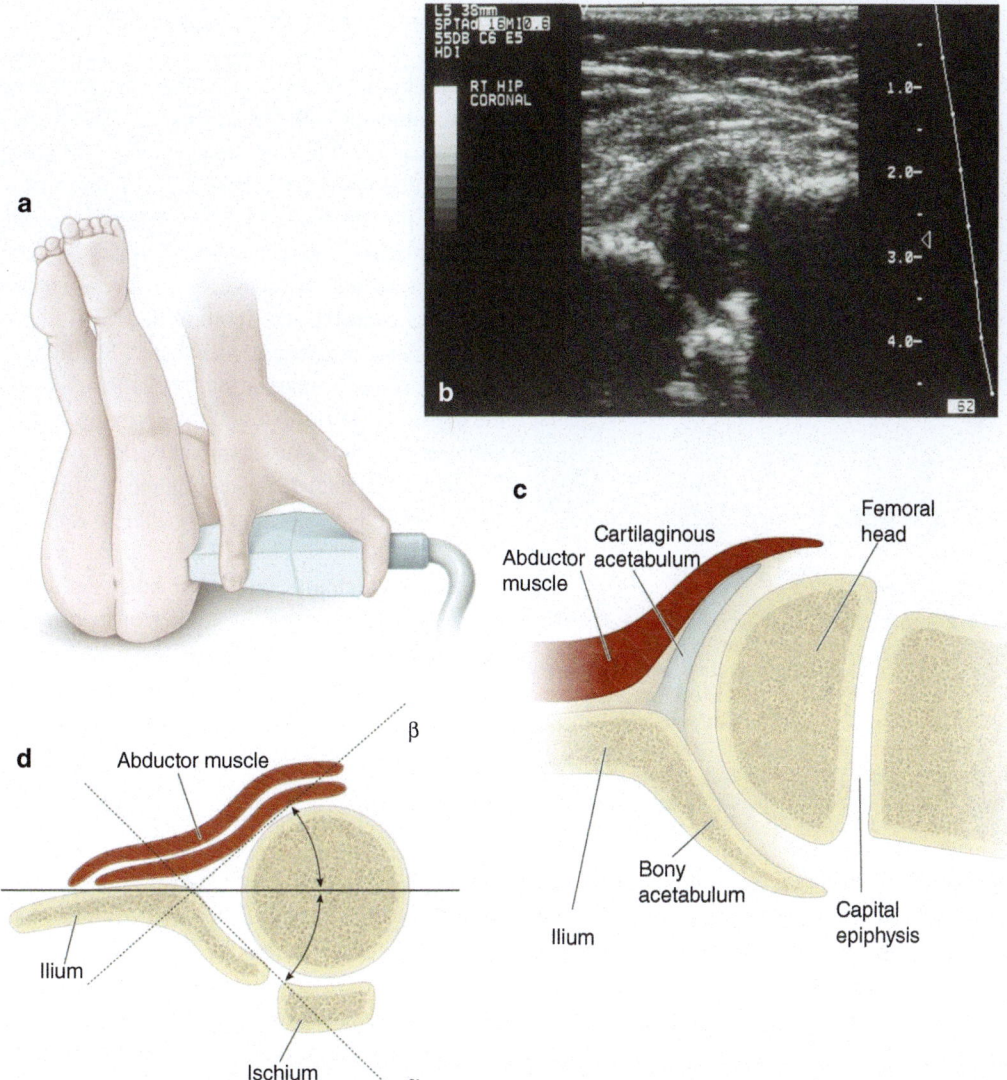

Fig. 7.21 Ultrasonographic evaluation of the infant hip. (**a**) The sonogram should be obtained with the child in the lateral decubitus position. (**b**) Ultrasonographic scan showing hip structures in a child. (**c**) Highlights of the anatomic structures shown on the sonogram. (**d**) Measurement of alpha (α) and beta (β) angles on ultraso-nography scans to establish Graf class. The alpha angle is the angle between the baseline and the roof of the bony acetabulum. The beta angle is the angle between the base-line and the cartilaginous acetabular roof. (From Tachdjian MO. Pediatric Orthopedics, 6th ed. Philadelphia, PA: Herring; 2022. Reprinted with permission)

The prognosis for DDH is very good when the diagnosis is made early, and treatment initiated in infancy. With delay in diagnosis and, therefore, in treatment, the prognosis worsens. The most dreaded complication, avascular necrosis, can occur at many points in the treatment algorithm despite the advances in treatment.

Perthes' Disease

Idiopathic avascular necrosis of the femoral head in the child was originally described in 1909 by multiple authors: Legg in Boston, Calvé in France, and Perthes in Germany. Unfortunately, all authors interpreted that the observed changes were due to nontuberculous sepsis. Slowly, it has

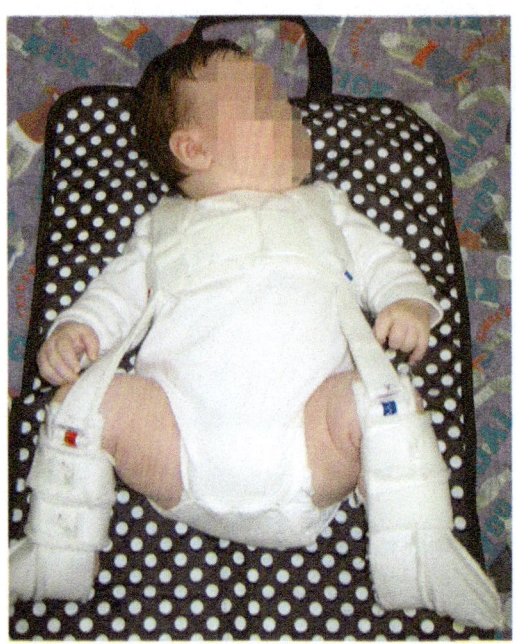

Fig. 7.22 The Pavlik harness. The transverse chest strap should be placed just below the nipple line. The hips should be flexed to 120°, and the posterior straps should not produce forced abduction. (From Tachdjian MO. Pediatric Orthopedics, 6th ed. Philadelphia, PA: Herring; 2022. Reprinted with permission)

been recognized that this femoral head ischemia is of unknown etiology, with genetic and environmental factors playing various roles. The changes cannot be produced by a single period of avascularity, but multiple episodes may cause the characteristic pathologic changes. The exact trigger for this vascular disruption has remained elusive.

The affected children are typically Caucasian males from a lower socioeconomic status, geographically in cities and further from the equator, aged 4–9 years, and slightly delayed in skeletal growth. Generally, the child presents with a limp, absence of any systemic symptoms, and pain that varies with activity levels. Clinically, the child will usually have restricted hip motion, especially rotational, and some adductor muscle spasm. Local findings of tenderness and erythema are not seen. Since standard laboratory studies are usually normal, imaging studies are paramount in the diagnosis and treatment of the disease.

Pathologically, the disease progresses through four stages, and these are reflected by the X-rays

and magnetic resonance imaging (MRI) scans. Initially, the stage of synovitis, which lasts 2–3 weeks, produces an irritable hip syndrome easily confused with toxic synovitis. The X-rays are negative at this time. Subsequently, the stage of avascularity onsets, lasting 2–3 months, during which time the femoral head necrosis occurs. Fragmentation changes of the capital femoral epiphysis herald this stage. Once the avascular event has occurred, the femoral head will revascularize and the process will "heal," resulting in the stage of revascularization. The critical issue is the degree of deformation of the normally spherical femoral head before complete healing occurs. Eccentric mechanical loads applied to the softened, diseased head frequently alter its sphericity. The healing phase lasts approximately 2 years, at which time only the residual deformity remains as the permanent marker of the disease (Fig. 7.23).

The treatment principles for this disease are really no more advanced than they were 30 years ago. Nevertheless, certain facts seem generally accepted. The prognosis hinges on two basic features. First is the patient's age at onset of the disease. Children under age 5 will do well left untreated, which is the current recommendation. Those over age 8 do poorly, despite treatment. The other factor is the extent of head involvement. Obviously, the head that is completely necrotic is more likely to sustain permanent deformation than a head only partially involved. For children of intermediate age, 5–8 years, the principle of "containment" continues to be accepted. Conceptually, the thought is to place the softened femoral head concentrically into the acetabulum, which will in turn act as a mold or template as the head revascularizes. This can be accomplished in the smaller child by using an abduction orthosis and in the larger child by using either a femoral or acetabular osteotomy to improve congruity prior to deformation. The treatment for the older child with an already deformed hip is highly controversial. In general, the prognosis is good for the younger children, whereas many of those diagnosed after age 9 require total hip replacement in early adulthood.

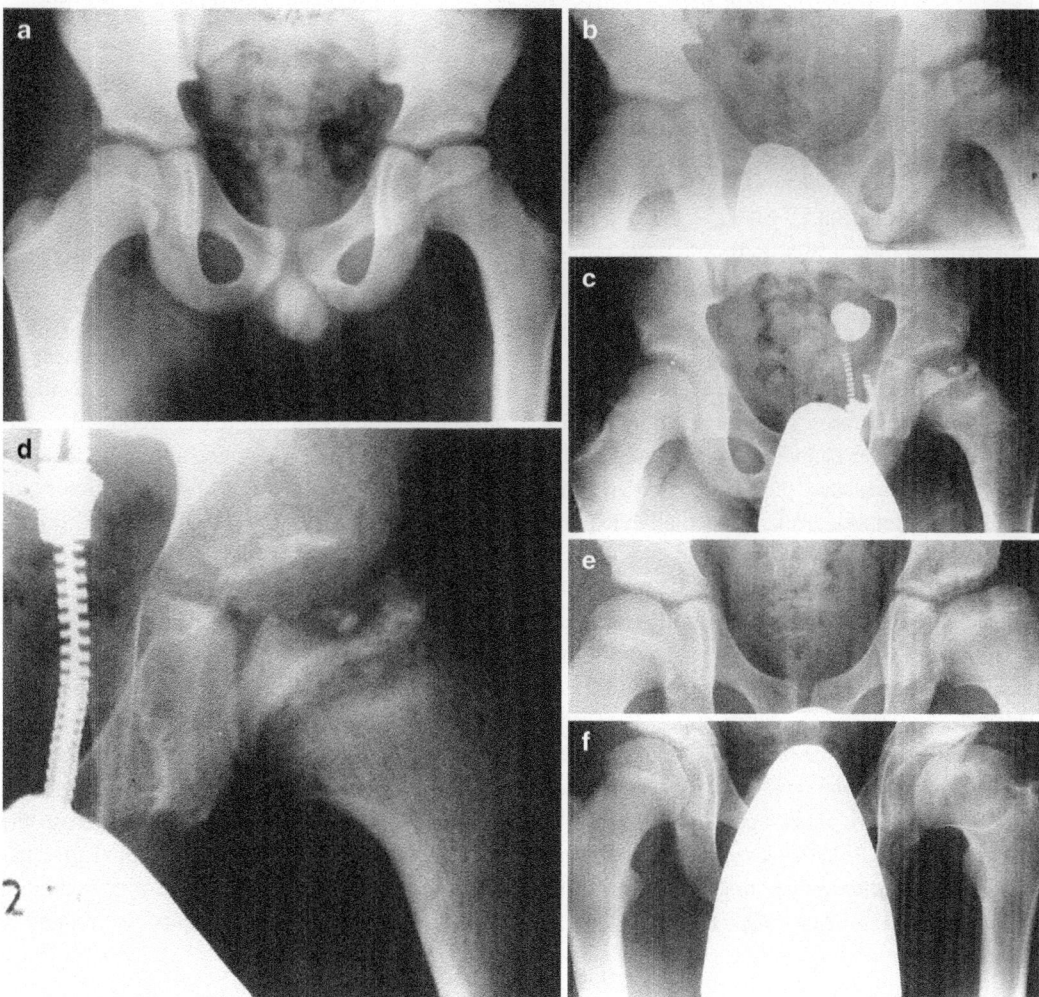

Fig. 7.23 Radiographic evolution of Legg-Calvé-Perthes disease, with onset in a boy at 10 years 11 months of age. Despite the late age of onset, the femoral head remodels well as the patient approaches skeletal maturity. (**a**) Anteroposterior (AP) radiograph obtained at onset of the disorder shows increased density in the femoral head and apparent widening of the joint space (Waldenström's initial stage). (**b**) AP radiograph obtained 9 months after onset shows the head entering the fragmentation stage. The central fragment remains dense and has collapsed relative to the lateral portion (lateral pillar) of the femoral head. The lateral pillar is lucent but has not collapsed, and the hip is classified as group B in the lateral pillar classification system. The joint space has widened further. (**c**) AP radiograph obtained 17 months after onset shows early reossification of the femoral head (the healing stage). (**d**) A closer view of the femoral head at 22 months after onset of disease. There is still widening of the joint space, and the acetabulum has a bicompartmental appearance. (**e**) AP radiograph obtained 4 years after onset. The femoral head is healed and in the residual state. There is still widening of the joint space and incongruity of the head with the acetabulum. (**f**) AP radiograph obtained 6 years after onset shows improved roundness of the femoral head and better joint congruity. (From Tachdjian MO. Pediatric Orthopedics, 6th ed. Philadelphia, PA: Herring; 2022. Reprinted with permission)

Slipped Capital Femoral Epiphysis (SCFE)

Hip pain in the adolescent should always raise suspicion of this entity. In fact, many of these patients present with pain along the medial side of the thigh radiating to the knee. This referred pain in the obturator distribution is quite typical. These children also share a common body habitus: they tend to be quite obese, with delayed secondary sexual characteristics.

Many of these children have been limping for several months before they present for evaluation. Pathologically, the capital femoral epiphysis has "slipped" or translated posteriorly and medially relative to the femoral neck. It is actually the femoral neck that is moving anteriorly and laterally relative to the head which remains located in the acetabulum. This displacement ultimately results in an irritated hip which is manifested by a limp, pain, and external rotational deformity of the leg. This deformity is usually readily apparent on physical examination: as the hip is flexed, the leg obligately externally rotates. Diagnosis is made with X-rays of the pelvis including an AP and frog-leg lateral of the hip. If one traces a line up the femoral neck, and line should does not intersect with the epiphysis, SCFE may be diagnosed (Fig. 7.24).

There have been multiple suggestions as to the etiology of the slipped capital femoral epiphysis. Many authors feel that these children are hormonally predisposed and with the superimposed stress of obesity, the perichondral ring is no longer able to "girdle" the physis; hence, the slip occurs. Typically, the slip is said to occur through the hypertrophic zone of the physis, but the displacement may actually transcend the entire physis. Children have chronic slips if they had symptoms for over 3 weeks. Acute SCFE was often considered the result of an acute injury and therefore, frequently considered by some authors to be a fracture through the physis. When the child had a history of limping and then a superimposed acute injury, the resultant slip is referred to as an acute on chronic slip.

Slips are also classified into stable and unstable groups defined by the ability of the child to walk with crutches. Children with unstable slips are unable to ambulate even with assistive devices.

Treatment involves an "in situ" pinning with a centrally placed compression screw across the physis. A reduction may be attempted in acute slips due to the mobility of the recent injured segment; however, any attempt to reduce a

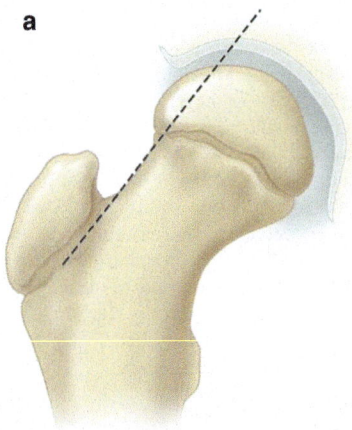
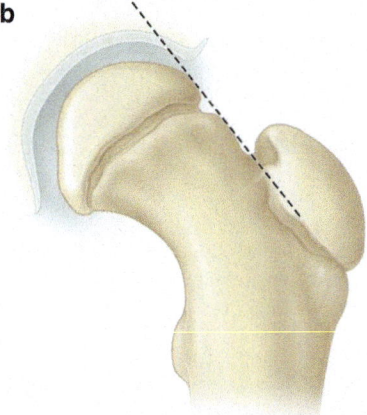
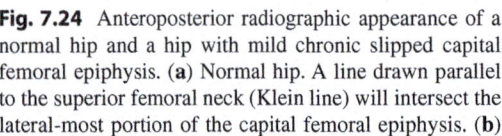

Fig. 7.24 Anteroposterior radiographic appearance of a normal hip and a hip with mild chronic slipped capital femoral epiphysis. (**a**) Normal hip. A line drawn parallel to the superior femoral neck (Klein line) will intersect the lateral-most portion of the capital femoral epiphysis. (**b**) Hip with mild chronic slip. Klein line does not intersect the capital epiphysis (Trethowan sign). Lateral radiographs will confirm the diagnosis. (From Tachdjian MO. Pediatric Orthopedics, 6th ed. Philadelphia, PA: Herring; 2022. Reprinted with permission)

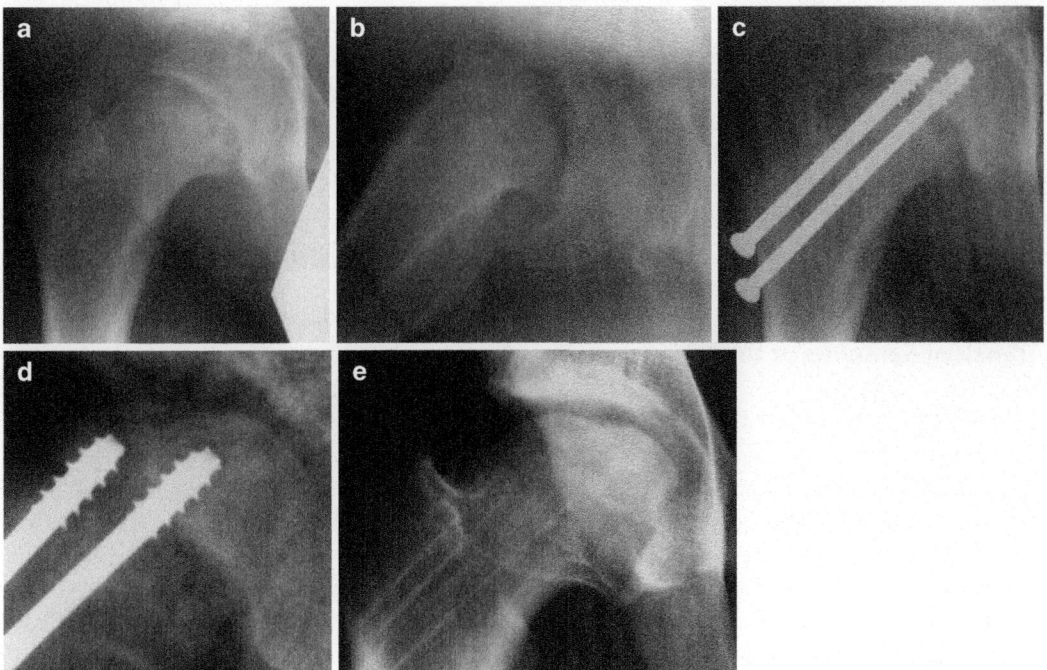

Fig. 7.25 Unstable slipped capital femoral epiphysis (SCFE) with resolving segmental avascular necrosis (AVN). (**a**) Initial radiograph of a patient who presented with a mild, stable SCFE. Admission was delayed for the mutual convenience of the family and surgeon. (**b**) The patient fell in the bathroom the day after the diagnosis was made, developing an unstable slip with further deformity. (**c**) The slip was treated immediately by closed reduction and percutaneous in situ pinning. (**d**) On follow-up, segmental AVN of the capital epiphysis and mild collapse were noted. The patient was asymptomatic. (**e**) At 2-year follow-up, the capital epiphysis appeared to have recovered. The patient remained asymptomatic. This case illustrates the importance of urgent fixation of slips when the diagnosis is made. Both the surgeon and patient were fortunate that a higher price was not paid for their mutual convenience, because resolution of AVN without segmental collapse is an uncommon outcome of this complication. (From Tachdjian MO. Pediatric Orthopedics, 6th ed. Philadelphia, PA: Herring; 2022. Reprinted with permission)

chronic slip may result in high rates of physeal or vascular damage resulting in avascular necrosis (Fig. 7.25).

Slips are graded based on the degree of displacement and, should severe slipping have occurred, resulting in excessive deformity, most authors would recommend that this deformity be corrected as a second stage once the physis has fused; however, some recommend one attempt at reduction prior to pinning.

The complications of the disease and its treatment can be devastating. Avascular necrosis is primarily a complication of the treatment rather than the disease itself. Aggressive reduction maneuvers and femoral neck osteotomies have both been implicated in the etiology of avascular necrosis. There is literature to suggest, however, that avascular necrosis may be a complication of high-grade slips.

The other concern is chondrolysis. This phenomenon can occur as a result of the disease itself or secondary to treatment in cases of screw penetration into the joint. It appears to be a particular concern in African-Americans, leading some to suggest an immunologic link. If affected, one observes degradation of the articular cartilage with resultant joint space narrowing and severe hip stiffness.

It should be recognized that this condition primarily affects adolescents. Therefore, when it is diagnosed in a younger child, one should consider specific endocrine abnormalities or metabolic diseases such as hypothyroidism, hyperparathyroidism, or chronic renal failure. In cases of particularly young children (calculated by the modified Oxford score) or those with these metabolic disorders, it may prudent to prophylactically fix the contralateral hip. There is a 10–30% risk of contralateral slip in all patients with unilateral SCFE.

With early and adequate treatment, specifically pinning "in situ," excellent long-term results can be anticipated.

Transient Synovitis of the Hip

By far and away, the MOST COMMON cause of limp and hip pain in a child is the "irritable hip syndrome," also called "transient" or "toxic synovitis." Frequently, these children will have a history of an upper respiratory infection (URI) or ear infection in the recent past, leading many to believe that this condition is a postinfectious inflammation of the hip.

Clinically, such children are not sick; they remain active, eat well, and are afebrile. Their lab studies, including X-rays, are usually normal. On exam, the hip is irritable, with additional findings of an antalgic limp, decreased range of motion, and pain with log rolling of the leg.

The treatment is supportive and includes nonsteroidal anti-inflammatory drugs (NSAIDs) and activity reduction, the latter being key. The process is self-limited, with the limp disappearing in 5–7 days. If it persists longer, one should suspect that the child has remained too active.

The Pediatric Knee

Unlike the hip, the affectations that one sees about the knee in a child are, for the most part, all benign and generally respond to simple treatment measures.

Osgood–Schlatter's Disease

Traction apophysitis of the tibial tuberosity is one of the more common causes of knee pain, especially of the preadolescent age group. It is more commonly seen in males and is associated with patella alta. Although the name implies inflammation, there is little present. Essentially, this disorder of enchondral ossification results from a powerful muscle group pulling on an open growth plate producing an overload strain, resulting in irritation of the local tissues.

These children have local swelling and tenderness over the tibial tuberosity without other findings. The key to successful treatment is activity restriction, followed by activity modification until the growth plate closes. It is important for the children to accept responsibility for their knee care: decreasing activity, using ice after activity, and occasionally using a lightweight knee sleeve primarily for psychological support. It is equally important to reassure the parents that, no matter how much pain their child has, he or she is not damaging the knee in any permanent way. Within 1–2 years, nearly all children have complete resolution of their symptoms.

Osteochondritis Dissecans (OCD)

OCD is an avascular necrosis of a portion of the subchondral bone that is acquired, reversible, and idiopathic. Classically, it affects the lateral aspect of the medial femoral condyle, adjacent to the intercondylar notch. However, it can occur on any of the condylar surfaces and is also commonly seen in the elbow at the capitellum. It is a disorder of the subchondral bone which affects the overlying cartilage surface to varying degrees.

Clinically, the child presents with vague knee pain, which is poorly localized. Occasionally, an effusion will be present. The diagnosis is usually made radiographically, especially if an intercondylar notch view is obtained (Fig. 7.26). Generally, short-term activity restriction, ice, and NSAIDs are adequate to relieve acute symptoms and are much more successful in younger patients with widely open physes. An MRI is often obtained to further characterize the lesion and determine its stability. Unstable lesions (those that are loose, hinged, or with fluid surrounding the lesion) may benefit from drilling or additional fixation. Should a loose fragment be identified, it can be removed or fixed into place as well.

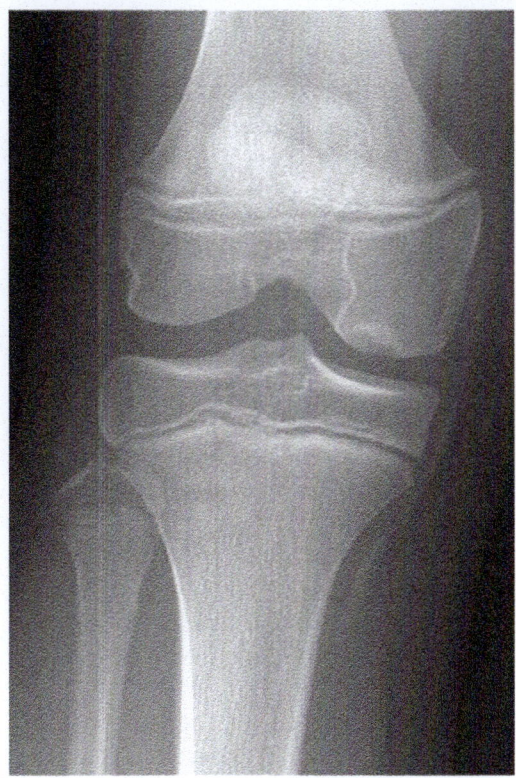

Fig. 7.26 Typical radiographic appearance of osteochondritis dissecans of the right knee medial femoral condyle. A region of subchondral bone is demarcated by radiodense convex margin. (From Tachdjian MO. Pediatric Orthopedics, 6th ed. Philadelphia, PA: Herring; 2022. Reprinted with permission)

The Discoid Meniscus

The menisci develop embryologically from a cartilaginous plate referred to as the interzone. The cartilage plates normally thin out to become shaped like the letter "C" on the medial side and the letter "O" on the lateral side of the knee. Should this hollowing out NOT occur on the lateral side, a thick cartilage plate persists as a discoid meniscus. This structure can cause the child to have knee pain and occasional effusion beginning around age 3–5 years; however, some may be asymptomatic until adolescence or even diagnosed incidentally at older ages. On exam, most dramatic is a prominent audible and palpable "clunk" or snap seen when the knee is flexed and extended with some rotation applied. This results from a hypermobile meniscus that is lacking the

normal peripheral capsular attachments. The discoid meniscus is not only abnormal in overall shape but in the collagenous composition as well. It is thicker with less vascularity, decreased quantity and more disorganized collagen, and frequent intrameniscal mucoid degeneration all of which predispose this tissue to tearing. If symptoms warrant, arthroscopic removal of the central portion of the discoid meniscus is required, contouring it to the normal shape. Discoid menisci may be associated with a lateral femoral condyle OCD lesion as well, and intraoperatively, it has been noted that around one quarter are associated with various cartilage lesions.

Popliteal Cysts

A localized mass in the popliteal space can occur in small children. Typically, this is a cyst containing gelatinous fluid. As with any mass, these cysts are a source of great concern to the parents, who can benefit a great deal from reassurance as to the correct diagnosis. These can be seen at a young age, frequently just after the child begins to walk.

Typically, the cyst presents between the tendon of the semitendinosus and the medial head of the gastrocnemius; thus, it lies medial in the popliteal space. An X-ray should be negative, and an ultrasound will confirm a cystic structure. A more extensive workup should be considered if the mass is atypical—that is, on lateral side, painful, or enlarging. Because most of these cysts will disappear in time, surgical excision should be reserved for the ones that cause symptoms. It is important to note that in children these are rarely associated with intraarticular pathology, whereas in the adult that association is the norm.

The Pediatric Foot

Foot deformities in children are common and a frequent cause for orthopedic referrals. There are as many developmental variations in foot configuration as there are children who have feet. It seems that no two pairs of feet are exactly alike.

The challenge then for the physician is to determine which of these feet are pathologic. Although a number of guidelines have been suggested, none is as helpful as the axiom "Feel the foot." The pathologically deformed foot cannot be positioned normally by manual manipulation; hence, it is rigid. Conversely, if the abnormally positioned foot can be reduced to a normal configuration with only modest manual pressure, the foot should be considered flexible and the result of excessive intrauterine molding. It is generally true that most flexible "deformities" are considered "non-disease" and as such require no specific treatment. However, rigid deformities usually present a definite therapeutic challenge.

Flatfoot or Pes Planovalgus

As the name implies, the longitudinal arch is low to nonexistent. Officially, the foot is pronated, and the heel is typically in valgus or everted. Flatfeet can be flexible or rigid, and the difference is critical. Besides feeling the foot, the other technique that is helpful in differentiating the two is simply to examine the child sitting, standing, and standing on the toes. The rigid flatfoot will remain flat in all three positions, whereas the flexible foot is only flat when standing. When seated (not weight-bearing) and when toe-standing, the arch reconstitutes itself and the foot appears to normalize. This is no longer considered an abnormality and is currently viewed as a normal variant. Three pain syndromes do occasionally occur which generally respond to simple therapeutic measures:

- Arch pain: The child with flatfoot will occasionally develop a strain pattern in the arch. This is easily treated with simple, inexpensive, commercially available supports.
- Calf pain: Typically, this is caused by tight heel cords and can be treated simply with stretching exercises and arch supports.
- Accessory navicular syndrome: A modest percentage of children, approximately 14%, will have a separate ossicle in the posterior tibial tendon adjacent to the tarsal navicular that is

rarely symptomatic. The prominence of this bone may cause symptoms, which generally respond to padding or occasionally excision of the accessory navicular.

Rigid Flatfoot

The pronated foot that does not correct on toe-standing should be studied for the presence of a tarsal coalition. These bony, cartilaginous, or fibrous bridges, usually talonavicular or calcaneonavicular coalitions, are genetically determined and usually can be diagnosed by appropriate X-rays and advanced imaging modalities. Pain occurs from this rigid deformity around ages 8–13 years (ages of ossification) from reduced subtalar motion and hindfoot valgus. Treatment is based on location and severity of symptoms, ranging from nonoperative to coalition resection to fusion.

Another cause of a rigid flatfoot when seen in a newborn is congenital vertical talus. This results in abnormal positioning of the talus, with the navicular dorsally dislocated onto the talar neck. As a result, the foot is beyond flat—the arch is convex (rather than concave) and frequently referred to as a "rocker bottom deformity." This uncommon pathologic foot requires initial treatment with casting to stretch the tissues followed by surgical correction.

Congenital Clubfoot

Similar to DDH, this deformity is multifactorial in origin. Environmental factors applied to a genetically predisposed individual result in this pathologic deformity. As with DDH, it is important to make it clear to the parents that this is NOT a postural deformity. Rather, there is an anatomic abnormality of the talus. Due to the abnormal medial and plantar deviation of the talar neck, there are a number of secondary deformities. The tarsal navicular is dislocated dorsally onto the talar neck; soft tissue contractures develop, and the resultant configuration is characteristic. The forefoot is adducted, the hindfoot is in varus (inverted), and the entire foot is in equinus. The deformity can be remembered with the pneumonic "CAVE"—cavus, adductus, varus, and equinus.

A clubfoot, as is the case with most pathologic feet, is rigid on clinical exam (Fig. 7.27). X-rays can be used to confirm the diagnosis but are not needed. Since clubfeet are frequently seen in association with other abnormalities, every effort should be made to evaluate the whole child. Syndromes often associated with clubfeet include myelodysplasia, arthrogryposis, and diastrophic dwarfism. Clubfoot treatment in syndromic children is usually exceedingly difficult and surgery is almost always required eventually.

In the case of the "standard" congenital clubfoot, occurring in an otherwise normal child, the recommended initial treatment is stretching and serial casting. The Ponseti method is the standard of treatment. Using this method of manipulation in conjunction with serial casting, many authors are reporting successful initial correction by closed treatment in 95% of cases but with recurrence approaching 50%. Should closed treatment fail or should recurrent deformity be observed, surgical correction is the usual next step. Most authors recommend surgical correction between 6 and 9 months of age if closed treatment has been unsuccessful. Risk of recurrence can be decreased with compliance with post-casting brace wear.

The overall success of various treatment protocols is largely dependent on the initial severity of the deformity. In addition, the need for late procedures to correct residual deformity will similarly be a function of initial severity as well as the success of initial correction techniques. In general, if correction is complete and achieved prior to the age of walking, an excellent prognosis can be anticipated, with the Ponseti method achieving favorable long-term outcomes in 85% of cases. It is, however, important to point out to the family that congenital clubfoot involves not only the foot but the soft tissues of the leg itself. Therefore, an overall decrease in the girth of the calf should be expected and leg-length discrepancy may occur.

Metatarsus Adductus

Metatarsus adductus is the most common problem seen in a child's foot in infancy. Many cases are simply the result of excessive uterine cramming and, therefore, are best considered "nondisease." The supple postural deformities are

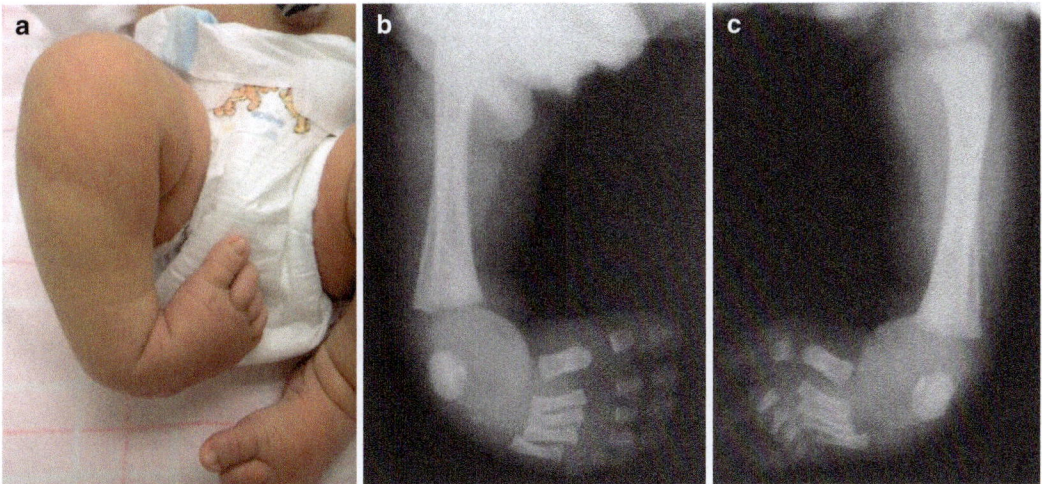

Fig. 7.27 Talipes equinovarus in a newborn. (**a**) Clinical appearance of an untreated clubfoot. (**b** and **c**) Initial radiographic appearance of bilateral untreated clubfeet.

(From Tachdjian MO. Pediatric Orthopedics, 6th ed. Philadelphia, PA: Herring; 2022. Reprinted with permission)

essentially normal variants and will correct without specific treatment. The clinical problem, however, is that some of these feet are, in fact, pathologic rather than postural and, therefore, do need appropriate care.

Typically, metatarsus adductus presents with medial deviation of the forefoot in relation to the hindfoot with variable supination (Fig. 7.28). When viewed from the plantar surface, the foot with metatarsus adductus has a typical "kidney bean" appearance. Again, on examination it is critical to "feel the foot." By doing so, these feet can be grouped into three clinical types. First, type I (mild): foot is supple and easily corrects with digital stroking of the lateral side of the foot. Type II (moderate): gentle, manual pressure is required on the medial forefoot for correction. Type III (severe): moderate force is required for correction; even so, some cases may not be correctable.

The mild and moderate deformities frequently correct spontaneously and do not require aggressive treatment. Simple shoeing or occasionally serial casts are used in these children to gain initial improvement. The severe feet and some of the tighter moderate feet clearly deserve serial casting at the very least. Certainly, in some cases, when serial casting fails, surgical intervention may be required.

For the majority of cases, the prognosis is excellent. Even those children with mild persistent deformity have virtually no functional or cosmetic problems with their feet. Unfortunately, persistent severe metatarsus adductus can cause problems such as shoe fitting, pain, and cosmetic deformity. Late reconstruction of these feet usually requires osteotomies through the midfoot.

The Pediatric Upper Extremity and Neck

In general, the vast majority of upper extremity problems in children that require orthopedic evaluation are traumatic in origin. Fractures of the elbow and forearm are common and treatable. Nontraumatic conditions of the upper extremity are far less common and are primarily congenital in nature.

Sprengel's Deformity

Congenital elevation of the scapula is generally due to persistence of a fibrous cartilaginous or bony bar that persists between the spine and the superior medial border of the scapula. This omovertebral bar prevents the scapula from migrating inferiorly from its embryonic position adjacent to the cervical spine to the normal adult position. Sprengel's is associated with cervical and renal anomalies that must be evaluated.

Sprengel's deformity usually presents as asymmetry of the neck or shoulder and physical examination is generally adequate for diagnosis. Since most children have no significant functional defi-

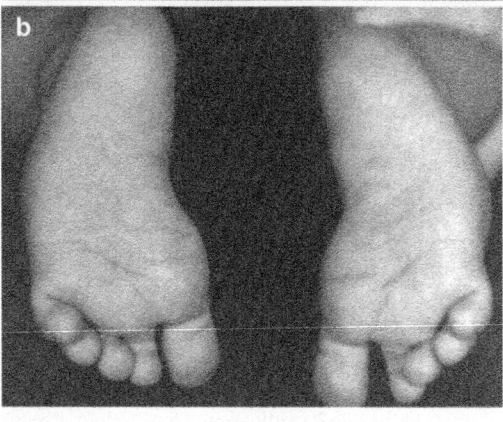

Fig. 7.28 Bilateral mild metatarsus adductus. (**a**) Dorsal view showing medial deviation of all the metatarsals. (**b**) Plantar view showing the "bean-shaped" foot. This type of foot is easily corrected with serial casting. (From Tachdjian MO. Pediatric Orthopedics, 6th ed. Philadelphia, PA: Herring; 2022. Reprinted with permission)

cits, surgical treatment is usually not recommended. Cosmesis is an occasional complaint and can be managed by simple excision of the upper portion of the scapula. If a functional deficit such as restricted range of motion does exist, several operative procedures have been developed to reduce the scapula to its normal position.

Congenital Muscular Torticollis

Although not truly an upper extremity problem, children with this condition present with a wry neck and asymmetry. Physical examination is usually adequate to make the diagnosis and differentiate it from some of the other causes of asymmetry in this region: Klippel–Feil anomaly, congenital scoliosis, and Sprengel's deformity. Essentially, the problem is a contracture within the sternocleidomastoid muscle. The exact etiology of this contracture has been the subject of some controversy. Intrauterine hemorrhage within the muscle, local compartment syndrome, and fibrotic bands have all been proposed. Despite the etiology, the net result is a newborn presenting with a torticollis and facial asymmetry. Typically, the head is tilted TO the side of the lesion and the face and chin are turned AWAY from the side of the lesion.

The deformity usually responds to simple physical therapy, stretching by the parents, and positioning the crib to encourage the infant to look TO the side of the lesion, thereby stretching the tight sternocleidomastoid. Occasionally, nonsurgical treatment is not adequate, and operative release is required. This should be done before the child is 18 months to 2 years of age, most importantly, to level the eyes. Worthy of note is the coincidence of this condition and developmental hip dysplasia. Since 20% of these children have abnormal hips, careful screening in this group is strongly recommended.

Radial Anomalies

The most common long-bone deficiencies in the upper extremity involve the radius. Partial or complete absence of this bone, with or without adjacent hand deficiencies, can be seen as an isolated finding or in association with several syndromes. Fanconi anemia and VACTERL syndromes should be considered when the radial dysplasia is bilateral. Further workup will usually reveal the renal defect or the thrombocytopenia, which are life-threatening. The hand tends to deviate to the radial side and is referred to as "radial clubhand." Early treatment is nonoperative and based on stretching and bracing. Later surgical reconstruction of the extremity to improve wrist function is appropriate.

Congenital Trigger Thumb

Perhaps it is best not to use the term "congenital" since the defect is rarely noticed at birth or, for that matter, in the first 6 months. It is usually appreciated when the child begins using the hand for grasping. At this point, the flexed interphalangeal joint is noticed by the parents. Initially, stretching will straighten the digit, but as the tendinous nodule of the flexor pollicis longus enlarges, it will no longer slide under the flexor pulley. The thumb is then "stuck" in flexion. Some will respond to simple stretching, but most require surgical tenolysis after 12 months of age. The vast majority of those treated in this way have an excellent result and no recurrence.

Pediatric Trauma

The basic principles of injury to the immature skeleton have been discussed in part elsewhere. The unique features of pediatric fractures are primarily due to the biologic differences between child and adult, specifically, the presence of an open growth plate, the periosteum, the ability of pediatric bone to plastically deform, and the ability to remodel this deformity.

The physis is a point of mechanical weakness. Many loading modes are capable of causing failure through the physis. These fractures were classified many years ago by Salter and Harris. Their classification was based on the direction that the fracture line took through the physis and adjacent osseous structures. Purportedly, this classification correlates with prognosis—the higher the number of fracture type, the poorer the prognosis. Although true within certain limits, this is not always the case. For example, a Salter II fracture of the distal radius is a common, benign injury, whereas a Salter II fracture of the distal femur is frequently complicated by a partial physeal arrest in more than 50% of cases (Fig. 7.29). Fractures of the physis heal rapidly in 3–4 weeks, but parents should be warned about potential growth plate arrest and subsequent limb-length discrepancy or angular deformity. Physeal fractures that cross the plate and/or enter the joint may require operative restoration of normal anatomy to minimize the risk of this complication.

The periosteum, as previously noted, is thicker, more vascular, and more osteogenic than that of an adult. The mechanical benefits provided by the periosteum tend to minimize fracture displacement, act as an aid in reduction, and assist in maintenance of reduction. Biologically, the active osteogenic potential allows fractures to heal in half the time required for a similar bone in the adult.

The biologic plasticity of pediatric bone is responsible for the typical fracture patterns seen in the pediatric diaphysis. The incomplete fractures—greenstick and buckle—represent the ability of these bones to bend, but not break all the way through. In general, this phenomenon is not seen in the adult bone due to the progressive stiffening of cortical bone that occurs with aging. Occasionally, this feature presents a therapeutic dilemma. In the forearm, a plastically deformed ulna will act as a spring to re-deform the already fractured radius. The solution is to complete the fracture of the ulna by osteoclasis. This will allow one to align the forearm acceptably and prevent re-deformation.

Finally, the extensive remodeling ability of pediatric bone has corrected many seemingly unacceptable reductions without the need for multiple closed reductions (Fig. 7.30). There are limits to the amount of correction that can be anticipated. One should not be overly secure, expecting "Mother Nature" to correct all malposition. In general, angular deformity will remodel to variable degrees. Greater correction can be expected if the deformity is in the plane of motion of the joint. Similarly, the closer the fracture to the joint, the more complete will be the correction. Translational deformity (i.e., displacement) at all levels tends to completely remodel.

Rotational malalignment does NOT remodel; therefore, it is important to correct rotatory deformity to within acceptable parameters, which vary by location. Complications of pediatric fractures are uncommon with adequate treatment; however, when they do occur, management may be problematic. The reason for this is the growth remaining in the skeleton. Any injury compromising the growth mechanics of a long bone will only compound itself over time as the deformity appears to worsen. Periarticular fractures and physeal fractures tend to present more problems in this regard than do those in the diaphysis.

The treatment principles, then, are directed toward fracture reduction and maintenance

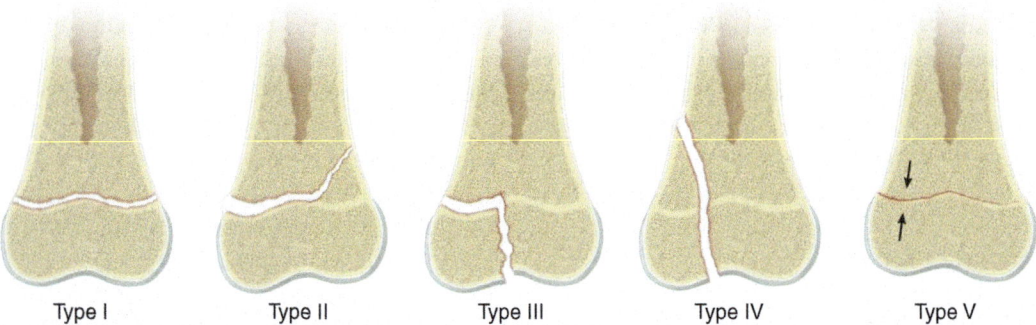

Fig. 7.29 Salter-Harris classification of physeal fractures. (From Tachdjian MO. Pediatric Orthopedics, 6th ed. Philadelphia, PA: Herring; 2022. Reprinted with permission)

Fig. 7.30 (**a**) Antero-posterior (AP) radiograph of a proximal humerus fracture in an 8-year-old boy. The fracture has healed with significant angulation. (**b**) AP radiograph obtained 1 year after injury demonstrates extensive remodeling of the proximal humerus. (From Tachdjian MO. Pediatric Orthopedics, 6th ed. Philadelphia, PA: Herring; 2022. Reprinted with permission)

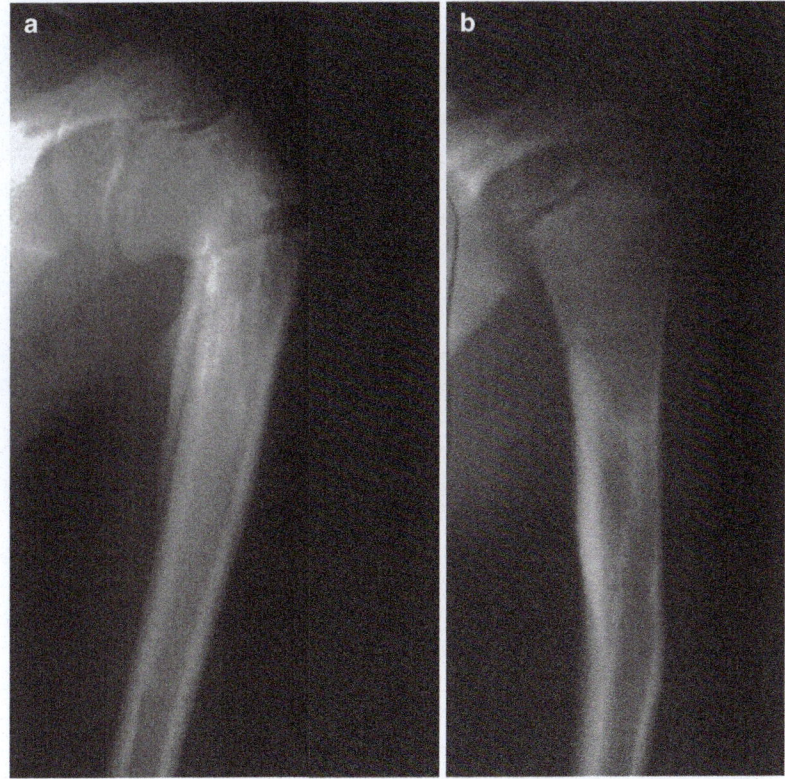

while avoiding complications—goals similar to those in the adult. Operative treatment of certain physeal injuries is common, and there is now current interest in operative treatment of more diaphyseal fractures, especially of the femur, in an effort to decrease length of hospital stay and improve early mobilization. Regardless of the reduction approach, the need for immobilization is undisputed. Children by definition are non-compliant; premature removal of immobilizing devices usually has disastrous results. One need not be concerned about joint stiffness or a cast-induced atrophy in children. It is far more important to continue the immobilization until the fracture is healed. Physical therapy following cast removal is rarely needed since the activity level of a normal child, unhampered by a cast, is more than adequate to mobilize the extremity. It is especially important NOT to subject the child with an elbow injury to a well-meaning but overaggressive physical therapist. This will only aggravate the joint stiffness and delay resolution.

In summary, children's fractures necessitate management similar to the adult: reduction, maintenance, and avoidance of complications. However, due to generally permissive biologic mechanisms, the tolerances in treatment are much greater. Successful results require adequate recognition of the unique qualities of the pediatric skeleton and the special problems that may follow trauma to it.

Non-accidental Trauma

No discussion of pediatric skeletal trauma would be complete without mention of non-accidental trauma. Child abuse is the second most common cause of death in children, and 50% of fractures in children prior to walking age are due to this non-accidental trauma. The sociologic implications are extensive for the patient, the family, and the physician. Child abuse rarely occurs as an isolated event, and the result of returning the child to the home may be disastrous. It then becomes important to recognize the signs and symptoms of "non-accidental" trauma. Failure to recognize or suspect this syndrome will likely result in continued abuse.

The diagnosis is usually based on finding a constellation of manifestations, rarely is it based on an isolated fracture. Rather, several fractures in multiple stages of healing, a fracture that does not correlate with the reported history, notable skin changes such as ecchymosis outside that expected for the fracture, and metaphyseal fractures more reliably indicate abuse. Other red flags to watch out for include delay in seeking care, no history of injury or inconsistent story regarding the injury, scapula fractures, sternal fractures, posteromedial rib fractures, transphyseal distal humerus fracture, and spinous process fractures. Non-accidental trauma typically presents with findings in multiple areas, including the following:

- General neglect: Beware the child who fails to make eye contact with parents or physician. The child who is dirty and uncared for and who exhibits evidence of psychological and nutritional neglect should raise one's suspicions.
- Skin and soft tissue injury: "Imprinting" of the skin due to blows with specific objects, such as belt buckles, coat hangers, and ropes, should be searched out. Evidence of cigarette and radiator burns can commonly be found. Eye-ground hemorrhages and forehead hematomas indicate "shaken baby syndrome."
- Craniocerebral injury: Subdural or epidural hematomas with or without non-parietal skull fractures are highly suggestive of abuse.
- Rib fractures: Multiple fractures especially in a line typically indicate a kicking injury.
- Metaphyseal-epiphyseal fractures: "Bucket-handle" and "teardrop" fractures of the metaphyseal region generally suggest shaking the child while holding the limb.
- Diaphyseal fractures: Spiral fractures of the distal humerus and fractures of the femoral shaft in a nonambulatory child are the most typical of abuse.

This tragic problem is becoming more commonly diagnosed in recent years, primarily due to heightened societal awareness of the problem.

Physicians need to be vigilant and knowledgeable of the hallmarks of child abuse; only then they can meet their legal reporting requirements, thereby saving a child from return to an abusive environment. If non-accidental trauma is suspected, a skeletal survey should be obtained. Early involvement of social work and pediatricians is important. Physicians are mandatory reporters and legally obligated to report suspected abuse or neglect.

Evaluation of a Limp

The limping child is a relatively common problem, and yet one that is difficult to evaluate. Multiple etiologies, the child's difficulty in localizing pain, and a vague history make it essential that the physician has a systematic approach to this problem. Rather than order multiple unpleasant and expensive diagnostic studies, it is usually more valuable to carefully observe and examine the child, especially in a sequential fashion.

Generically, a limp is any uneven or laborious gait or, for that matter, any alteration in normal gait sequence. Normal gait classically occurs in two phases for each extremity: stance and swing. The stance phase is initiated at heel strike for a given limb and terminated with toe-off of that extremity. Stance accounts for 60% normally, leaving 40% of the cycle for swing when the foot is off the ground. Three classic aberrations of the gait cycle have been described in children:

- Antalgic limp: Pain is the etiology of this gait aberration. Due to pain in the limb with ground contact, the stance phase is shortened, and the patient unloads the extremity more quickly. Many etiologies will cause an antalgic limp, such as a fracture in the foot or toxic synovitis of the hip.
- Trendelenburg limp (gluteus medius lurch): Frequently referred to as an abductor lurch, this pattern is due to the incompetence of the abductor lever arm to stabilize the pelvis. If one remembers that a moment is created by a force acting over a distance, it can be appreciated that altering either factor will cause a Trendelenburg limp:

– Force alteration: Muscle weakness, as seen in polio
– Distance alteration: Shortened lever arm, as seen in DDH or malunited femoral neck fracture
• Short leg limp: Leg-length discrepancy will be manifested as an apparent limp with the pelvis dropping on the short side. A careful history should investigate a past traumatic event, systemic symptoms, and the effect on activity. Physical findings such as fever, focal findings of swelling, limitation of motion, and muscle spasm should be sought. Age itself may be a clue to the etiology since each group seems particularly prone to certain ailments.
    – 1–3 years old: Trauma, infection, DDH, new shoes
    – 5–9 years old: Transient synovitis, Perthes' disease, JRA, Lyme disease
    – Over 12 years: SCFE

Extending the diagnostic workup, one should first consider standard X-rays, especially of the hips. An MRI is the second-line study if the source of the pain or abnormality is apparent. Unfortunately, it is not possible to specifically outline the studies to be routinely obtained. Reaching the correct diagnosis is all too often the result of coinciding historical data, physical findings, laboratory data, and a "gut" sense. Several diagnostic algorithms have been proposed that emphasize the basic factors in evaluating pediatric limp:

• Is there a history of trauma?
• Are there systemic symptoms?
• Are there focal findings?

By answering these questions, a workup can be fashioned that should ultimately reveal the etiology.

Conclusions

Children are different. They are not small adults. Biologically and mechanically their musculoskeletal systems predispose them to patterns of injury and disease unique to their age group. By understanding these differences, one can anticipate some of the patterns, thereby permitting appropriate treatment and minimizing complications.

The seven categories of disease—vascular, infections, tumor, arthritis, metabolic, injury, and neurodevelopmental—all produce changes in the skeleton that reflect the unique feature of childhood: growth. Simple insults can be made worse over time due to aberrational growth and conversely potentially disastrous insults can be palliated by the innate remodeling potential of the pediatric skeleton.

Pediatric Spine

Scoliosis

Scoliosis refers to abnormal coronal curvature of the spine. The human spine is normally straight when viewed from behind, but, because of the potential implications of unnecessarily labeling a child as "having" scoliosis, minor deviations from normal (less than 10°) may be considered within normal limits. Scoliosis has been discussed in the medical and orthopedic literature since antiquity and is widely believed by the lay population and medical professionals to be a debilitating or disabling condition, resistant to treatment, and with a grave prognosis.

Advances in both operative and nonoperative treatment, as well as a better understanding of the natural history of scoliosis, have removed much of the stigma from this condition. A variety of conditions may cause or be associated with scoliosis. The most common type of scoliosis is referred to as idiopathic, meaning that the cause of the disorder is unknown. Hereditary factors have been implicated, and research is ongoing as to other possible causes of idiopathic scoliosis. While it is likely that the development of idiopathic scoliosis is multifactorial, genetic, hormonal, biochemical, biomechanical, and neuromuscular abnormalities continue to be investigated. Idiopathic scoliosis can be broken down by age at diagnosis: curvature of the spine diagnosed up to age 3 years is defined as infantile idiopathic scoliosis, a diagnosis between the ages of 4 and 10 is juvenile idiopathic scoliosis, and curves diagnosed after the age of 10, or the onset of adolescence, is referred to as adolescent idiopathic scoliosis. Most cases of idiopathic scoliosis are identified during the adolescent growth spurt and are therefore considered adolescent curves.

Numerous other conditions either cause or are associated with scoliosis and must be considered when evaluating an individual for scoliosis. Congenital abnormalities of the vertebrae, resulting in congenital scoliosis or congenital kyphosis, represent some of the more common etiologies of spinal deformity. Neuromuscular disorders such as polio, cerebral palsy, muscular dystrophy, spinal muscular atrophy, or myelomeningocele are frequently associated with spinal deformity. Other conditions, such as neurofibromatosis or Marfan syndrome, may result in spinal deformity and scoliosis is also seen secondary to intraspinal anomalies such as syringomyelia (cystic degeneration of the central aspect of the spinal canal) or a tethered spinal cord. There is also a known association between non-adolescent scoliosis and certain congenital conditions, such as congenital heart disease.

While 1.5–3% of the population are believed to have curves over 10°, only 0.2–0.3% of the normal population have curves over 30°, a magnitude where treatment is typically instituted. The natural history of idiopathic scoliosis has been well established. Most curves are identified in early adolescence. Progression is variable and is more likely in younger patients, in skeletally immature patients (in particular, premenarchal girls), and in larger curves. Finally, while mild curves are as common in boys as in girls, progressive curves and curves requiring treatment are far more common in girls.

The implication of scoliosis in adulthood entails consideration of curve progression, pain, disability, and mortality. It has been established that an idiopathic curve of greater than 50° is at significant risk for progression even in adulthood. While curve progression is a possibility, the presence of scoliosis does not necessarily place the patient at risk for back pain. Some patients with scoliosis appear to have pain related to the curve, but it has been demonstrated that patients with idiopathic scoliosis are not at any increased risk, when compared to the general population, for the development of disabling low back symptoms. Similarly, pulmonary dysfunction and significant functional disability are rare occurrences. The mortality rate of individuals with idiopathic scoliosis does not differ from that of the general population. Finally, scoliosis does not have an adverse impact on a woman's ability to bear children nor is the curve more likely to progress during pregnancy than at other times.

Management

The management of a child with documented or suspected scoliosis begins with a thorough evaluation. Most cases are picked up during school screening or by the patient's primary care physician. The Adam's forward bend test is the key to checking a child for possible scoliosis. Asymmetry of the spine and trunk is identified by asking the child to bend forward at the waist with the knees straight and the hands hanging toward the floor. The observer is seated behind the patient (Fig. 7.31). Asymmetry of the ribs from right to left is considered a positive test and merits further evaluation by an orthopedist. Other possible signs of scoliosis include pelvic or shoulder asymmetry or asymmetry of the waist creases.

Evaluation for scoliosis should be a routine part of a pediatrician's well-child physical examination and is very sensitive for picking up most cases of scoliosis.

In evaluating the patient with possible scoliosis, important historical points include a family history of spinal deformity, any abnormality or delay in reaching developmental milestones, and associated neurologic symptoms involving the lower extremities or urogenital system, including gait abnormalities, paresthesias, and recent onset of enuresis. Physical examination includes the above evaluation as well as a thorough inspection of the skin, looking for café au lait spots, palpation of the spine, looking for an occult spina bifida, examination of the lower extremities, and looking for calf or foot atrophy or asymmetry. Neurologic examination should also be carried

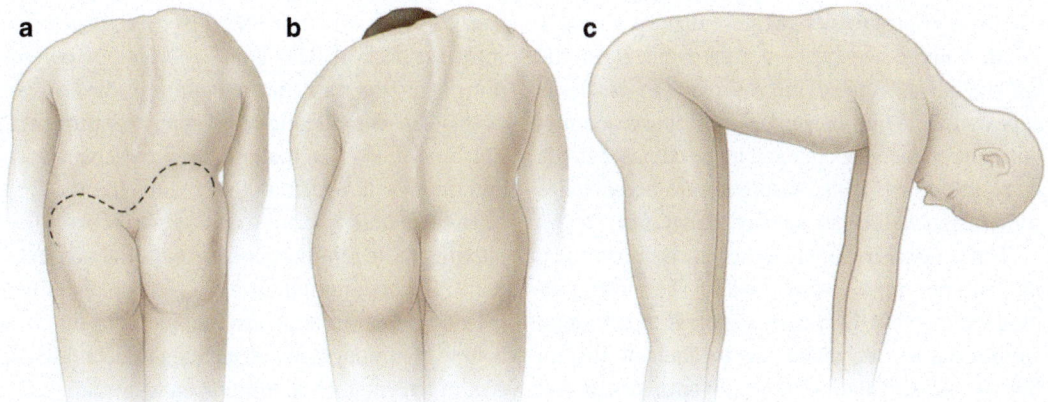

Fig. 7.31 Assessing spinal deformity. (**a**) A patient with limb-length inequality exhibits prominence of the entire length of the long side of the trunk during forward bending because of pelvic obliquity. *Dotted line*, Iliac wings. (**b**) A patient with true scoliosis has truncal prominence localized to the convexity of the curve(s)—in this exam-

ple, a right thoracic deformity. (**c**) When viewed from the side, a patient with a kyphotic deformity has an increased or sharply localized kyphosis when in the forward-bending position. (From Tachdjian MO. Pediatric Orthopedics, 6th ed. Philadelphia, PA: Herring; 2022. Reprinted with permission)

out, including assessment of deep tendon reflexes, superficial skin reflexes, and testing for Babinski's sign. Any sign or symptom suggestive of central nervous system abnormality merits a more detailed workup, possibly including imaging of the brain stem, spinal cord, or cauda equina.

Radiographic evaluation is carried out on any patient suspected of having scoliosis. The size of the curve is measured by the Cobb angle, which is the angle between the most tilted vertebrae on the top and bottom of the curve. A standing posteroanterior view (PA) of the full spine, including the pelvis, will demonstrate the presence or absence of significant deformity. The pelvis is inspected for evidence of skeletal maturity, manifested by closure of the iliac apophysis. In some cases, obtaining a hand film for bone age may be helpful. Because there is a known association between scoliosis and spondylolisthesis (see below), a lateral X-ray of the spine should be obtained, including visualization down to the sacrum.

Treatment options available for the growing child with scoliosis include observation, bracing, and surgery. Previous attempts at curve control utilizing physical therapy, chiropractic, exercises, or electrical stimulation have proven ineffectual and are not recommended. Observation, with repeat radiographs every 4–6 months, is appro-

priate in the child with scoliosis less than 25–30°. Curves that have been documented to progress beyond 25° or curves measuring beyond 30° at first presentation, in a child with significant growth remaining, are treated with a brace.

Current braces are underarm orthoses, such as the Boston or Wilmington brace, are fitted to the patient and relatively subtle to wear for significant periods of time. The recommendation is to wear the brace 18 h a day, with notable loss of efficacy if worn less than 13 h. Notably, boys tend to be less compliant with bracing than girls. These braces have proven effective at controlling most thoracic and thoracolumbar idiopathic curves, avoiding the need for surgery in approximately 80% of cases, and have become the current standard for the management of curves of moderate magnitude in skeletally immature patients. Unfortunately, successful bracing means preventing any further progression of the scoliosis but does not result in improvement of the curve.

When a curve exceeds 40° or 45°, it becomes increasingly difficult to control with an external orthosis. Because of this, as well as the increasing risk of progression into adulthood with curves greater than 50°, surgery is generally recommended for curves that progress into the range of 50°. The goals of the surgical treatment of scoliosis include the arrest of progression, achievement of a solidly fused, balanced spine, and improvement in the curve with associated improvement in cosmetic appearance. While upward of 50% curve correction can routinely be obtained in the adolescent, the more important goals of surgery are achieving a solid fusion well balanced over the sacrum.

The surgical treatment of scoliosis constitutes, first and foremost, a spine fusion. The most common approach to this fusion is posterior, although certain curves are amenable to anterior fusion. Spinal instrumentation has evolved over the last quarter of a century and newer implants, utilizing multiple points of fixation along the spine, are more easily contoured to help the surgeon restore physiologic alignment in three planes, as there is a significant rotational component to the deformity (Fig. 7.32).

In the adolescent with idiopathic scoliosis, curve correction using modern techniques aver-

ages 50–70%. About 95–98% of patients go on to solid fusion with less than 10% loss of correction. Infection and thromboembolic disease are occasional complications of spinal instrumentation and fusion, although they are seen more commonly in adults than in adolescents. The most feared complication of surgery for scoliosis, paraplegia, is rare particularly with the advancement of neuromonitoring. Neurophysiologic monitoring of intraoperative spinal cord function is now commonplace and appears to decrease the risk of irreversible neurologic catastrophe.

Congenital Scoliosis

Individuals with congenital abnormalities of the spine represent an unusual but well-defined subset of patients with spinal deformity. Failure of formation (hemivertebrae), failure of segmenta-

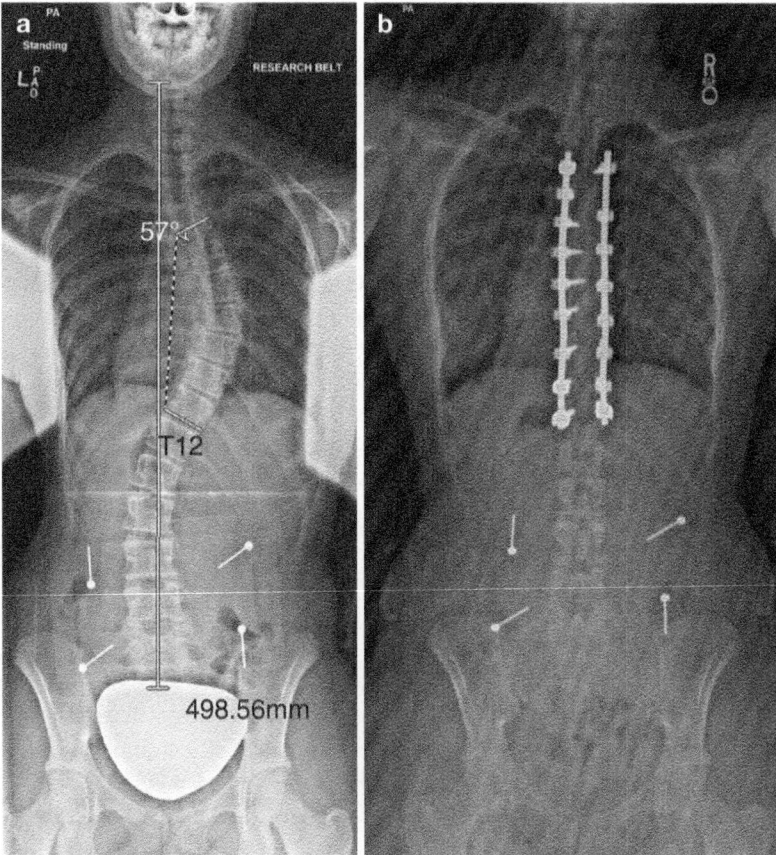

Fig. 7.32 Lowest instrumented vertebra fusion selection for a 1A curve. (**a**) The preoperative standing anteroposterior film demonstrates a 57° right thoracic curve with a compensatory lumbar curve A modifier center sacral vertical line (CSVL, between the pedicles) and CSVL last touching T12. (**b**) The 2-year radiographs following a posterior spinal fusion and instrumentation from T4 to T12 with nice coronal plane correction and overall excellent balance. (From Tachdjian MO. Pediatric Orthopedics, 6th ed. Philadelphia, PA: Herring; 2022. Reprinted with permission)

tion (bars), and mixed deformities are seen. The prognosis varies depending upon the type of anomaly present, but the patient with congenital scoliosis, in particular with a failure of segmentation, is certainly at higher risk for progression than the patient with an idiopathic curve. There is a known association between congenital spine deformity and congenital anomalies of the urogenital system and all patients with congenital scoliosis or kyphosis should be referred for imaging of the genitourinary (GU) system. Congenital heart disease is also more common in this population.

In addition to the increased risk of progression, which approaches 100% in curves involving a unilateral unsegmented bar, congenital curves are resistant to bracing. While progressive congenital scoliosis in a growing child is still routinely treated with an orthosis to prolong time to surgery, the orthopedic surgeon, the pediatrician, and the patient and family need to be aware that there is a high risk for further progression necessitating surgical intervention. Congenital deformities can, on occasion, result in quite severe curves in very young children, but postponing surgery in this setting only results in a more difficult reconstructive problem at a later date.

Neuromuscular Deformity

Neuromuscular causes of scoliosis include polio, cerebral palsy, muscular dystrophy, posttraumatic paraplegia, and myelomeningocele. At one time, polio was the most common cause of scoliosis in this country. Neuromuscular curves have a characteristic long, C-shaped appearance. Extension of the curve into the pelvis, with pelvic obliquity on sitting or standing, is common and complicates both surgical and nonsurgical treatment. The risk of scoliosis varies among these conditions but may be as high as 60–70%. All neuromuscular curves have a propensity, once progression ensues, for rapid collapse of the spine into a severe curve. Because of the respiratory difficulty associated with many of these conditions, it is imperative to screen patients carefully for scoliosis, to monitor them closely for

progression, and to institute early and aggressive treatment when indicated.

Brace treatment with a well-molded, total contact thoracolumbosacral orthosis (TLSO) is instituted for curves measuring beyond 30° in the growing patient. Progression despite adequate bracing, resulting in progressive loss of function, is believed in most cases to be an indication for surgery in this patient population. In these patients, surgical treatment is fraught with a high rate of complications, including instrumentation failure secondary to osteoporosis, increased rates of infection, and postoperative respiratory failure.

Kyphosis

Kyphosis refers to forward curvature, or rounding, of the spine in the sagittal plane. Kyphosis is normal in the mid and upper thoracic spine, with a normal range of thoracic kyphosis from 20° to 45° in children and adolescents. Excessive kyphosis, as measured on a standard lateral radiograph exceeding 45–50°, has several possible etiologies.

The child or adolescent presenting with hyperkyphosis of the thoracic spine is frequently accompanied by a parent giving a long history of "poor posture." While postural kyphosis is not uncommon, other causes of the deformity should be considered. The most prominent among these is juvenile kyphosis, known as "Scheuermann's disease." Although the etiology of Scheuermann's kyphosis remains unknown, several theories have been proposed, including avascular necrosis of the anterior cartilaginous ring apophysis of the vertebral body, the presence of Schmorl's node (herniation of intravertebral disc material through the endplate), relative osteoporosis leading to anterior compression fractures, altered biomechanics leading to anterior growth arrest, endocrine or nutritional abnormalities, and metabolic bone disease.

Scheuermann's kyphosis is the most common form of nonpostural kyphosis. The criteria for diagnosis in the thoracic spine include excessive thoracic kyphosis with associated radiographic abnormalities including vertebral wedging of greater than 5° at three consecutive vertebrae, endplate irregularity, and the presence of Schmorl's nodes. The reported prevalence of this disorder varies among authors but is approximately 1%. Although the postural abnormality may be identified earlier, radiographic changes are usually not seen until 11–12 years of age.

Most cases of thoracic hyperkyphosis represent primarily cosmetic abnormalities. Mild postural kyphosis will frequently resolve spontaneously or following a thoracic extension exercise program. Most patients with Scheuermann's kyphosis lead normal lives, with no functional limitations and an incidence of disabling back pain that is not increased over the normal population. There is some evidence, however, that adults with kyphosis in excess of 65–70° may have an increased incidence of thoracic back pain and mild to moderate functional limitations. Neurologic complications secondary to Scheuermann's disease are rare but have been reported. There is no evidence that cardiopulmonary dysfunction is a complication of this condition.

Congenital kyphosis is a rare condition that must be ruled out, due to the possibility of severe progression and subsequent neurologic abnormality (Fig. 7.33). As in congenital scoliosis, congenital kyphosis can result from failure of formation or failure of segmentation. In contrast to congenital scoliosis, however, congenital kyphosis secondary to failure of formation (congenital hemivertebrae) is the more malignant type, with an exceedingly high rate of progression. Congenital kyphosis in association with a hemivertebrae has the highest rate of neurologic impairment of any of the spinal deformities. Tuberculosis should also be considered in the child or adolescent with excessive kyphosis, particularly if there is a history of travel outside the United States or a positive family history.

Management of the patient with hyperkyphosis begins with a thorough physical examination. Differentiation between Scheuermann's disease and postural kyphosis is facilitated by viewing the patient, in the forward flexed position, from the side. Patients with postural kyphosis have a smooth, round curve which reverses on voluntary extension. The typical deformity in Scheuermann's kyphosis involves a sharp, angular gibbus that does not correct on extension of the spine. A minimal scoliosis of the spine may also be noticed on forward bending. A thorough neurologic examination is mandatory to rule out spastic paraparesis, which would suggest other possible diagnoses including congenital kyphosis, intraspinal anomaly, or thoracic disc herniation. Standing PA and lateral

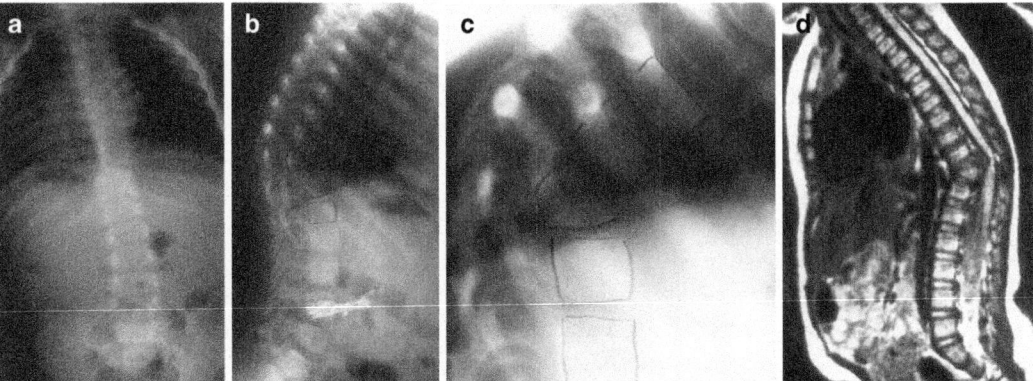

Fig. 7.33 (**a–c**) Chest radiographs obtained in a 14-month-old girl to evaluate an upper respiratory tract infection showed an abnormality at T11. On further radiographic evaluation, the abnormality was determined to be kyphosis caused by failure of vertebral body formation. A 51° kyphosis was measured. (**d**) Magnetic resonance imaging demonstrated abrupt angulation of the spinal cord at this level. The child was neurologically normal. (From Tachdjian MO. Pediatric Orthopedics, 6th ed. Philadelphia, PA: Herring; 2022. Reprinted with permission)

radiographs of the entire spine are obtained. It is important to check for the presence of spondylolisthesis, which is increased in patients with Scheuermann's disease.

Observation, frequently accompanied by a program of thoracic extension exercises, is utilized in patients with postural kyphosis or without evidence of progression in cases of Scheuermann's disease. Bracing is indicated for patients with curves 60–80° with a Jewett type brace with a high chest pad. Unlike scoliosis, Scheuermann's kyphosis can respond with curve correction, typically about 10°, following successful brace treatment. Spine fusion is reserved for patients with curves over 80° which are not likely to respond to bracing and create a significant functional or cosmetic deformity. The fusion extends from just above to just below the area of kyphosis, typically over 10–12 vertebral levels.

Spondylolisthesis

"Spondylolisthesis" refers to the forward slippage of one vertebrae on that below it. Spondylolisthesis is most common in the lower lumbar spine, particularly at L5–S1, and is a common cause of back pain in children and adolescents. Degenerative spondylolisthesis occurs in middle-age and older adults because of degenerative changes in the discs and facet joints allowing subluxation and is most common at L4–L5. In pediatric patients, the most common type of spondylolisthesis is isthmic spondylolisthesis, caused by a defect in the pars interarticularis at L5, resulting in slippage of L5 anteriorly over S1. The pars defect, referred to as spondylolysis, is believed to be a stress or fatigue fracture. It is present in 6–7% of adolescent athletes and responsible for almost 50% of back pain in this population. Spondylolisthesis is more common in males, Caucasian patients, and athletes who participate in sports demanding hyperextension, such as gymnasts or football lineman.

In children and adolescents, spondylolysis or spondylolisthesis may present as back pain, frequently associated with hamstring spasm. Other less common causes of back pain in the pediatric population include disc space infection, benign tumors such as osteoid osteoma, lumbar disc herniation, or urologic and gastric pathology. Because back pain is such a ubiquitous complaint, the relationship between a patient's complaint of back or leg pain and the presence of spondylolisthesis is often difficult to determine. While acute pars fractures are occasionally seen, there is usually no history of trauma. The patient typically presents with low back pain, which radiates into the buttock and, on occasion, down the leg. Physical examination may demonstrate tenderness in the area of the L5–S1 facet joint and often painful extension can be elicited. The most telltale sign in the adolescent is hamstring spasm, which can be quite severe. In patients with a high-grade slip, flattening of the buttocks and a transverse abdominal crease may be seen. Neurologic findings are rare, although in more advanced cases L5 nerve root findings may be present.

Plain radiographs should be obtained in the standing position. Most pars defects are visible on the lateral radiograph. If the diagnosis is uncertain, fine-cut CT scanning may be used to diagnose occult defects in the pars interarticularis and MRI imaging is useful to identify nerve root compression in the L5–S1 foramen in patients with neurologic symptoms. The treatment of patients with spondylolysis or spondylolisthesis depends on the degree of slippage as well as the patient's symptoms, as this is frequently diagnosed incidentally, and patients are asymptomatic. The Meyerding classification accounts for the percent slip from 0 to 100% and has been broken down as grades I (0–25%), II (25–50%), III (50–75%), and IV (75–100%) or V (>100%, or spondyloptosis) (Fig. 7.34).

In patients who are asymptomatic regardless of slip grade, full activity, sometimes with a 3-month contact sport hiatus, is allowed with radiographic follow-up to evaluate for slip progression, which is quite rare. Patients with symptomatic low-grade spondylolisthesis are treated with physical therapy including hamstring stretching for 6 months, most improve with this alone. Bracing may be considered for patients with an acute pars reaction spondylolysis or those

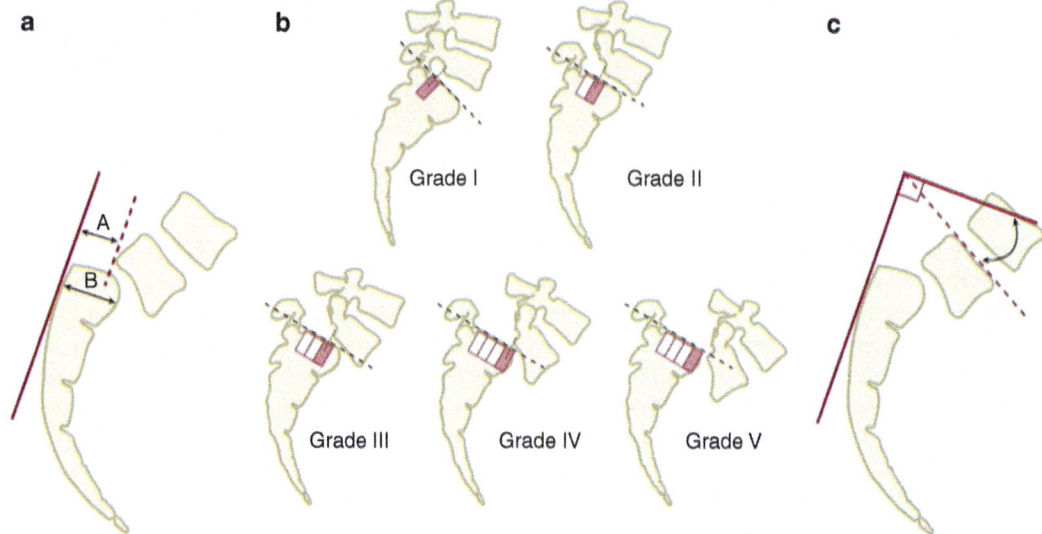

Fig. 7.34 (**a**) Percentage of forward slippage, A/B, described by Taillard. (**b**) Meyerding grades I–V. The degree of spondylolisthesis is determined by dividing the sacral body into four segments. Grade V is complete spondyloptosis. (**c**) The slip angle is measured from the superior border of L5 and a line is drawn perpendicular to the posterior edge of the sacrum. (From Tachdjian MO. Pediatric Orthopedics, 6th ed. Philadelphia, PA: Herring; 2022. Reprinted with permission)

that have not responded to physical therapy. Operative treatment is recommended for skeletally immature patients who fail to respond to conservative measures, with either pars repair or fusion with or without reduction of the listhesis. The results of surgery are usually quite rewarding, particularly in the pediatric population. Complications of surgery include failure of fusion, progressive slippage, persistent or recurrent pain, and neurologic injury.

Conclusions

The pediatric spine is susceptible to unique pathology compared to the adult, and while many conditions are appropriately treated with reassurance and nonoperative conservative therapies, surgical intervention is sometimes warranted, particularly in cases of neurologic compromise or deformity progression. It is important to be aware of the most common disease processes and their most common populations, so as to direct patients toward the appropriate care.

Further Reading

Hosseinzadeh P, Milbrandt T. The normal and fractured physis: an anatomic and physiologic overview. J Pediatr Orthop B. 2016;25(4):385–92. https://doi.org/10.1097/BPB.0000000000000245. PMID: 26523532.

Erkilinc M, Gilmore A, Weber M, Mistovich RJ. Current concepts in pediatric septic arthritis. J Am Acad Orthop Surg. 2021;29(5):196–206. https://doi.org/10.5435/JAAOS-D-20-00835. PMID: 33273402.

Ravelli A, Martini A. Juvenile idiopathic arthritis. Lancet. 2007;369(9563):767–78. https://doi.org/10.1016/S0140-6736(07)60363-8. PMID: 17336654.

Tortolani PJ, McCarthy EF, Sponseller PD. Bone mineral density deficiency in children. J Am Acad Orthop Surg. 2002;10(1):57–66. https://doi.org/10.5435/00124635-200201000-00008. PMID: 11809051.

Shirley ED, Ain MC. Achondroplasia: manifestations and treatment. J Am Acad Orthop Surg. 2009;17(4):231–41. https://doi.org/10.5435/00124635-200904000-00004. PMID: 19307672.

Shrader MW, Wimberly L, Thompson R. Hip surveillance in children with cerebral palsy. J Am Acad Orthop Surg. 2019;27(20):760–8. https://doi.org/10.5435/JAAOS-D-18-00184. PMID: 30998565.

McCarthy JJ, D'Andrea LP, Betz RR, Clements DH. Scoliosis in the child with cerebral palsy. J Am Acad Orthop Surg. 2006;14(6):367–75. https://doi.org/10.5435/00124635-200606000-00006. PMID: 16757676.

Lomita C, Ezaki M, Oishi S. Upper extremity surgery in children with cerebral palsy. J Am Acad Orthop Surg. 2010;18(3):160–8. https://doi.org/10.5435/00124635-201003000-00005. PMID: 20190106.

Tai TH, Wong CC. Legg-Calvé-Perthes disease. N Engl J Med. 2022;386(23):e62. https://doi.org/10.1056/NEJMicm2118649. PMID: 35675179.

Zhang S, Doudoulakis KJ, Khurwal A, Sarraf KM. Developmental dysplasia of the hip. Br J Hosp Med (Lond). 2020;81(7):1–8. https://doi.org/10.12968/hmed.2020.0223. Epub 2020 Jul 6. PMID: 32730146.

Sucato DJ. Approach to the hip for SCFE: the North American perspective. J Pediatr Orthop. 2018;38(Suppl 1):S5–12. https://doi.org/10.1097/BPO.0000000000001183. PMID: 29877938.

Niu EL, Lee RJ, Joughin E, Finlayson CJ, Heyworth BE. Discoid meniscus. Clin Sports Med. 2022;41(4):729–47. https://doi.org/10.1016/j.csm.2022.05.009. PMID: 36210168.

Hopwood S, Khan F, Kemp J, Rehm A, Ashby E. Clubfoot: an overview and the latest UK guidelines. Br J Hosp Med (Lond). 2023;84(1):1–7. https://doi.org/10.12968/hmed.2022.0380. Epub 2023 Jan 16. PMID: 36708340.

Kuznia AL, Hernandez AK, Lee LU. Adolescent idiopathic scoliosis: common questions and answers. Am Fam Physician. 2020;101(1):19–23. PMID: 31894928.

Sports Medicine of the Hip and Knee

8

William F. Postma and Nicholas Apseloff

Introduction

Sports medicine is a multidisciplinary field involving the medical and surgical care of athletes and active individuals, both on and off the field. The goal of sports medicine as an orthopedic subspecialty is the diagnosis and treatment of both acute and chronic athletic injuries, returning athletes to their pre-injury activity level and preventing further injury. Outside of orthopedics, other fields such as internal medicine and family medicine are often involved in the medical management of athletes.

Over the past several decades, advances in arthroscopy have provided sports medicine specialists with improved tools for treating intra-articular injuries, leading to improved outcomes with a less invasive approach compared with traditional open surgery. As a surgical subspecialty, orthopedics sports medicine focuses primarily on soft tissue injuries of the musculoskeletal system including injuries to ligaments (e.g., anterior cruciate ligament [ACL] in the knee, ulnar collateral ligament [UCL] in the elbow), tendons (e.g., Achilles tendon, patellar tendon), fibrocartilaginous structures (e.g., meniscus in the knee, labrum in the hip and shoulder), and articular cartilage.

The purpose of this chapter is to focus on the biologic tissues involved in sports injuries, followed by an overview of the basic principles of the evaluation and management of these injuries.

Musculoskeletal Tissues

Articular Cartilage

Articular cartilage injury is often associated with trauma to a joint. When diffuse and occurring over a period time, this process can result in osteoarthritis; however, there is an additional subset of these injuries that are more focal and result from a direct injury, often referred to as osteochondral injuries. Functional restoration of focal injury to articular cartilage remains one of the most challenging of orthopedic problems within the sports medicine field.

Articular cartilage composition and thickness varies from joint to joint and is directly age dependent. The patellofemoral joint in the knee has the thickest articular cartilage in the body, likely to support the high forces placed across

W. F. Postma (✉)
Department of Orthopedic Surgery, MedStar
Georgetown University Hospital,
Washington, DC, USA
e-mail: William.F.Postma@gunet.georgetown.edu

N. Apseloff (✉)
MedStar Georgetown Orthopedic Institute,
Georgetown University School of Medicine,
Washington, DC, USA

Department of Orthopedics, University of Pittsburgh,
Pittsburgh, PA, USA

this joint (Fig. 8.1). The tissue typically is composed of 75–80% water and dense extracellular matrix consisting of 50–75% of type II collagen and 15–30% of proteoglycan macromolecules. A remarkable characteristic of articular cartilage is its relative acellularity, as chondrocytes occupy less than 10% of this tissue. Chondrocytes maintain the extracellular matrix of articular cartilage and aid in cellular homeostasis. The collagen provides tensile strength to articular cartilage, while the proteoglycans and extracellular matrix provide its more important compressive role.

Structurally, articular cartilage is highly organized into four zones of depth from the articular surface to the underlying subchondral bone. Zone 1, the *superficial layer*, makes up approximately 10% of cartilage, determines its load-bearing ability, and serves as a gliding surface. Within this layer, chondrocytes arranged with collagen fibers are parallel to the joint surface to provide high tensile strength and stiffness and provide a low coefficient of friction for smooth gliding between joint surfaces. Zone 2, the *transitional layer,* is composed of chondrocytes and randomly oriented collagen fibers. This layer has a higher

concentration of proteoglycans and lower concentration of collagen as compared to Zone 1. Zone 3, the *deep layer*, is composed of collagen fibers and clusters of chondrocytes oriented perpendicular to the underlying subchondral plate, providing compressive strength. Zone 4, the *calcified layer*, is a relatively acellular layer which acts to join the deep zone of uncalcified cartilage to the subchondral bone. The clearly defined boundary between the uncalcified and calcified cartilage layers is termed the tidemark.

Articular cartilage is an avascular as well as aneural tissue. As an avascular tissue, it exchanges gases, nutrients, and waste products through diffusion from the synovial fluid. Nutrient transplant is thought to be assisted by movement of fluid in and out of cartilage in response to cyclic loading of joints. This poor blood supply of articular cartilage is responsible for the poor healing response seen after acute injury or chronic wear of the articular surface.

Injuries to articular cartilage are best described by the Outerbridge classification system. This system characterizes the injury to articular cartilage based on its qualitative appearance at the time of surgery: grade I, softening with swelling; grade II, fragmentation and fissuring; grade III, fragmentation and fissuring down to subchondral bone; and grade IV, exposed subchondral bone. Grade I/II lesions are thought to involve superficial injury and are best left untreated, while grade III/IV lesions represent full thickness cartilaginous injuries and are best treated surgically.

Tendons

Tendons are strong, relatively inextensible tissues that attach muscle to bone, allowing the muscle to exert an action resulting in movement. They are composed of densely packed collagen bundles within a proteoglycan matrix. Fibroblasts are the predominant cell type within tendon and are arranged in parallel orientation between the bundles of collagen fibers. The tendon fibroblasts act to produce both collagen and proteoglycan within the tendon unit. Collagen is the major constituent of tendon. Type I collagen comprises

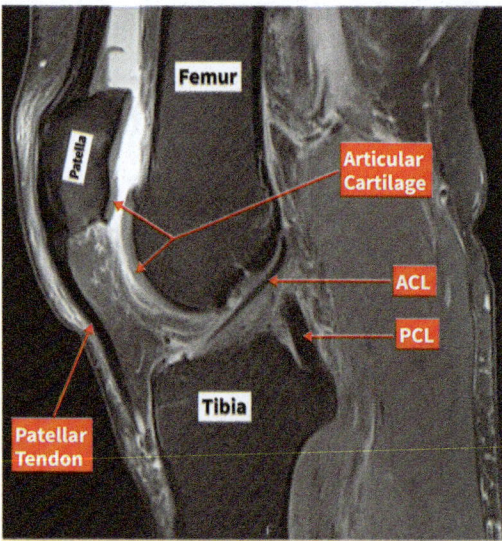

Fig. 8.1 Labeled sagittal MRI of a knee. The articular cartilage on the patella and trochlea of the femur (patellofemoral joint) are labeled with arrows. The patella does have relative loss of cartilage of about 50% in this patient. Also labeled in this image are the cruciate ligaments of the knee (ACL/PCL) and the patellar tendon

86% of a healthy tendon's dry weight, while type III is found in lesser amounts. It is the high concentration of collagen in combination with its parallel orientation that gives tendons their high tensile strength. Collagen chains are linked together to form fibrils that, in turn, are bound together by a proteoglycan matrix to form a fascicle, the primary unit in tendon structure. Fascicles, in turn, are bound by the endotenon, a layer of elastin-containing loose connective tissue that supports the blood, lymphatic, and neural supply to the tendon unit. It is the endotenon that is contiguous with both the muscle fibers and periosteum at the musculotendinous and tenoosseous junctions, respectively.

Acute tendon injuries may be direct, occurring as a result of laceration or contusion, or indirect, occurring secondary to tensile overload. Tensile overload is a common injury within the field of sports medicine (i.e., patellar tendon, quadriceps tendon Achilles tendon ruptures) (Fig. 8.2). Acute traumatic tendon ruptures typically occur due to a forceful eccentric contracture of the muscle. During an eccentric contracture, the muscle attempts to contract while it is lengthening. In the majority of these cases, avulsions at the insertion of the tendon and musculotendinous junction ruptures are far more common than midsubstance ruptures of tendon because most tendons can withstand tensile forces greater than can be exerted by their muscular or bony attachments.

Chronic tendon overload injuries occur at the sites of high exposure to repetitive tensile overload (e.g., Achilles tendonitis from running, patellar tendonitis in jumping sports, lateral epicondylitis of the elbow in tennis). Whether or not inflammation has a role in the early stages of these overuse injuries is unclear. However, in cases that are not responsive to short periods of rest with persistence of symptoms, similar findings can be seen histologically, reflecting a more degenerative process. Disruption of collagen fibrils, hyaline degeneration, and proliferation of vasculature are classic in these entities and termed angioplastic fibroplasia and result in tendinosis or breakdown of the corresponding tendinous unit. At this stage this is not an inflammatory process, as no acute or chronic inflammatory infiltrates are demonstrable on these histologic specimens. Tendinosis is also observed in cases of spontaneous tendon rupture and may be clinically silent until rupture occurs. An example is an Achilles tendon rupture seen in middle-aged athletes participating in strenuous sports.

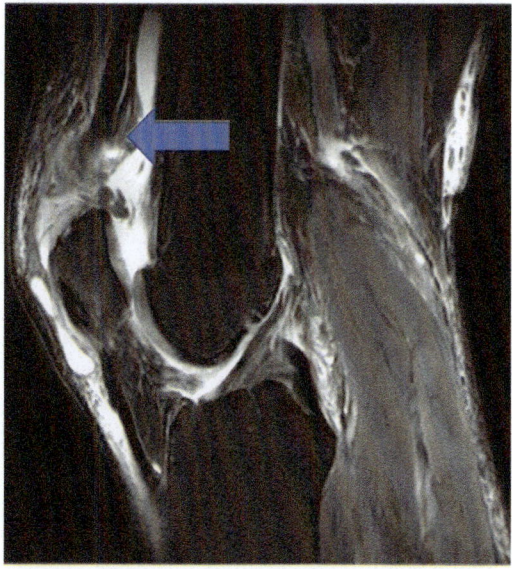

Fig. 8.2 Sagittal MRI of the knee demonstrating an acute quadriceps tendon rupture. The thick dark band of the quadriceps (blue arrow) on a T2 MRI should normally attach to the superior pole of the patella. In this image, there is a disruption of the tendon insertion indicative of a complete rupture

Ligaments

Ligaments are bands of connective tissue that serve to connect two bones. Like tendons, these are very organized hierarchical structures composed primarily of collagen with high tensile strengths. Type I collagen makes up approximately 70% of the dry weight of ligaments. Small amounts of elastin are combined with fibroblasts in a complex extracellular matrix. This collagen matrix comprises a series of fibers forming a subfascicular unit. Multiple subfascicular units are then bound together to form a fasciculus. These fasciculi can in turn be oriented in a simple longitudinal fashion such as the medial collateral ligament (MCL) of the knee or can spiral to form a more helical structure such as the anterior and posterior cruciate ligaments (ACL and PCL) of the knee (Fig. 8.3).

At their attachments to bone, the transition from ligament to bone occurs gradually in a series of distinct phases. These phases range from ligament to fibrocartilage, from fibrocartilage to mineralized fibrocartilage, and from mineralized fibrocartilage to bone. The size of each zone varies from ligament to ligament and is related to its structural properties. Collagen fibers, known as Sharpey's fibers, run in continuity throughout this zone of transition and have an important role in securing the ligament to bone. While somewhat similar to tendons in their microscopic organization and composition, ligaments and tendons are structurally and biochemically different. Ligaments contain a lower percentage of collagen and a higher percentage of extracellular matrix. There is also a more random alignment of collagen fibers within ligaments compared to tendons.

Unlike injuries to tendons that can be both acute and chronic processes, ligamentous injuries occur as a result of acute trauma and represent a macrotraumatic process. When a stress is applied

to a ligament, an injury or sprain occurs, whose severity (grades I–III) depends on the amount of stress applied. A grade I sprain represents the least traumatic episode where some ligamentous fibers are torn on a microscopic level, while the overall structural integrity is maintained. An example of this is a common ankle sprain where traditionally the anterior talofibular ligament (ATFL) is injured. In a grade II sprain, some fibers are macroscopically torn in combination with microscopic damage, resulting in a stretching of the ligament. While the biomechanical properties of the ligament are compromised in this scenario, some structural integrity of the ligament remains. An example of this injury is an injury to the medial collateral ligament (MCL) of the knee. When examining a patient with a grade II injury of the MCL, the knee demonstrates increased laxity to a valgus load but an endpoint is still felt, signifying some remaining structural integrity. In a grade III sprain or "tear/rupture," the ligament completely fails with no structural integrity remaining. After rupture of the anterior cruciate ligament, there is an increase in anterior translation of the tibia relative to the femur with a force directed from posterior to anterior on the tibia. This represents a complete structural failure of the ligament.

Intra-articular (inside of a joint) and extra-articular (outside of a joint) ligaments differ in their response to acute trauma (Fig. 8.4). This is influenced by a difference in the local vascular supply of these entities, the presence of synovial fluid within joints, the degree of ligamentous injury, and whether or not a significant gap forms between the two ends of ligamentous rupture. Typically, extra-articular ligaments have a high potential for healing and gradually heal with predominantly type I collagen within a 6- to 12-week time frame. Maturation of this ligament scar can sometimes take up to 1 year, despite histologic evidence of healing as early as 6 weeks. Contrastingly, intra-articular ligaments such as the anterior cruciate ligament have a poor healing potential due to the intra-articular milieu. In cases of complete disruption of this structure, dissociation of the midsubstance "mop ends" results in significant gap formation with inhibition of the

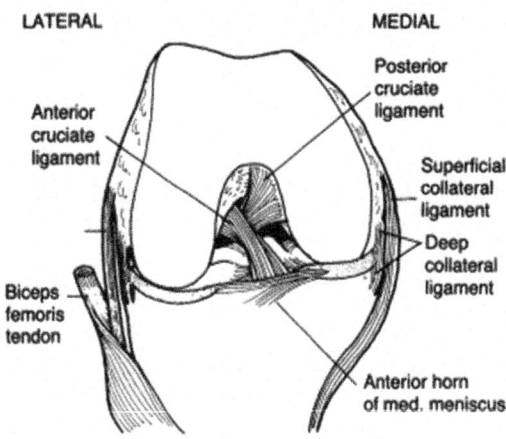

Fig. 8.3 Ligamentous anatomy of the knee. The two cruciate ligaments (anterior cruciate ligament [ACL] and posterior cruciate ligament [PCL]) are intra-articular structures that resist translational and rotational forces in the knee. (Printed with permission from Springer Publishing from: Brown, C.H., Steiner, M.E. (1994). Anterior Cruciate Ligament Injuries. In: Siliski, JM. (eds) Traumatic Disorders of the Knee. Springer, New York, NY)

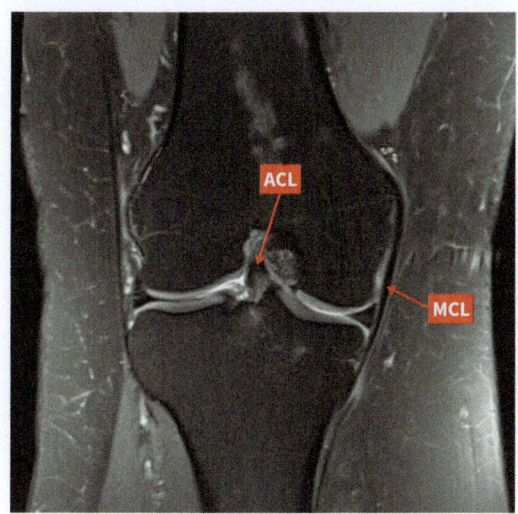

Fig. 8.4 Coronal MRI of the knee demonstrating the anterior cruciate ligament (ACL) and medial collateral ligament (MCL). The ACL is inside of the knee joint (intra-articular), while the MCL is outside of the joint (extra-articular). This difference in location contributes to the different healing capacities of the two structures. MCL injuries have a higher propensity to heal without surgery due to their extra-articular location with richer blood supply. The ACL is an intra-articular structure with a less robust blood supply and is bathed in synovial fluid, leading to a diminished healing capacity after injury

healing process. These differences result in varied treatment approaches as extra-articular ligamentous injuries (e.g., MCL) are frequently treated conservatively, while intra-articular injuries (e.g., ACL) are typically treated surgically secondary to a poor healing response.

Muscle

Injuries of skeletal muscle and the musculotendinous junction commonly lead to prolonged clinical disability. Muscle strains alone account for up to 50% of injuries in particular sports.

Active force generation within the muscle depends on its contractile apparatus. The contractile apparatus is composed of actin and myosin myofilaments that are arranged into functional units called sarcomeres. Muscle contraction consists of an energy-dependent process of cross-bridge unlinking and advancement of the myofilaments within the sarcomere. Either aerobic or anaerobic processes provide cellular energy for this process. Muscle fibers may be characterized by their capacity for aerobic respiration. Oxidative (red) fibers are characterized by slower sustained contractions (slow-twitch) under aerobic conditions, while glycolytic (white) fibers contract rapidly (fast-twitch) under anaerobic conditions. Fiber-type composition varies significantly between muscular groups and among different individuals. The force of muscle contraction is directly related to its cross-sectional area, which is reflective of its number of parallel contractile elements.

Muscular injury can result from tensile failure (e.g., during eccentric contracture of a muscle), direct injury (e.g., contusions, lacerations), or indirect mechanisms such as vascular or neurologic injury as seen in cases of acute or chronic (exercise-induced) compartment syndrome.

Muscular strains or tears involve either partial or complete disruption of the muscle–tendon unit. Clinical and experimental observations suggest that most muscular strain injuries occur at the musculotendinous junction. Common examples involve hamstring and adductor strains surrounding the hip. This usually occurs with passive stretch or with lengthening during muscular contraction (eccentric contraction). Complete injuries are often associated with muscle retraction, hematoma formation, and local inflammation, while lesser degree strains involve more microscopic failure. Functional recovery is dependent on the coordinated specific repair of the contractile elements with their surrounding connective tissues and neurovascular structures. This process can take up to 6 months in some cases. While individual muscular fibers may contract normally after repair and regeneration post-injury, whole muscle contractile function rarely returns to normal after gross skeletal muscular injury.

Less common are muscular contusions that are a result of direct trauma. In these cases, skeletal muscle damage results from non-penetrating, high-energy force directed to the muscular group. These forces can result in the temporary or permanent loss of vascular and neurologic function secondary to direct trauma imparted to the musculature. These injuries are often characterized by a large associated hematoma. Ultimate recovery is often related to the magnitude of original injury. A relatively infrequent complication of muscle contusions is myositis ossificans. In this condition, normal mesenchymal cells involved in the healing process differentiate into osteoblasts, resulting in the formation of bone within the healing muscle. This abnormal ectopic bone often results in a palpable prominence in the injured area with associated pain at times.

Meniscus

The knee contains two menisci: the medial meniscus and lateral meniscus (Fig. 8.5). The menisci are semilunar fibrocartilaginous structures sitting atop the medial and lateral tibial plateaus (Fig. 8.6). The menisci are composed primarily of type I collagen oriented circumferentially. It is this circumferential collagen orientation that gives this tissue its unique force loading characteristics and function within the knee. As the femoral condyle contacts the tibial plateau during knee joint loading (e.g., during ambulation), some of this force gets dispersed through these parallel collagen fibers of the menisci in a mechanism termed "hoop stress." The compressive force at the knee joint is effectively converted to a tensile force within the fibrocartilaginous menisci, thus distributing the load to the meniscus and offloading the force seen at the articular cartilage. This results in not only shock absorption but more even force distribution throughout the tibial plateau and articular cartilage. Without a functional meniscus, the articular cartilage of the femoral condyle and tibial plateau experiences significantly greater forces and "point loading" rather than force distribution which accelerates the development of osteoarthritis of the knee (Fig. 8.7).

Meniscal injuries are best categorized by the location and morphology of the tear, as these dictate treatment and prognosis of healing. Like articular cartilage, the menisci have poor vascularity. The medial and lateral menisci receive their blood supply from branches of the medial and lateral middle geniculate arteries, respec-

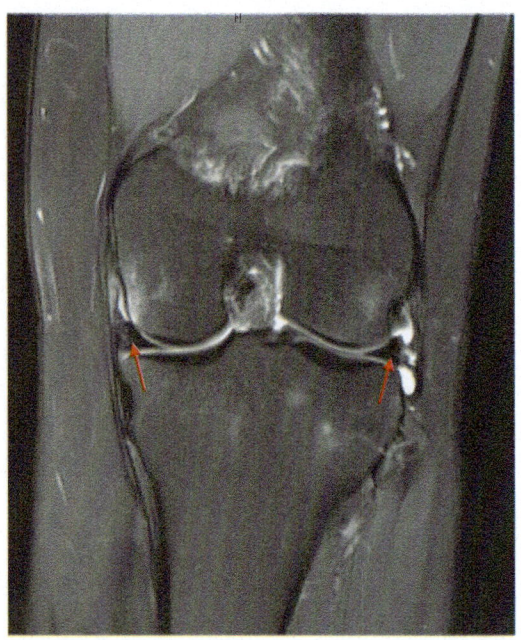

Fig. 8.5 Coronal MRI of the knee demonstrating medial and lateral menisci (arrows) atop the medial and lateral tibial plateaus. In cross-section, the menisci appear triangular in shape

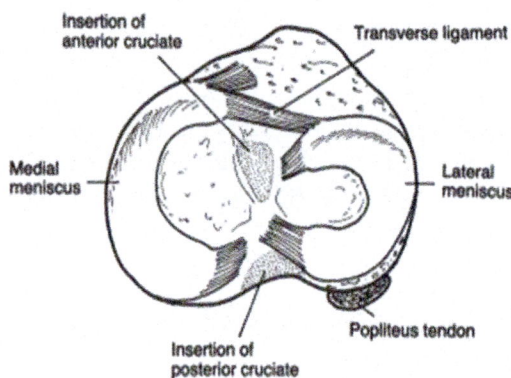

Fig. 8.6 Depiction of the medial and lateral menisci atop the tibial plateau, viewed from above. Shaded areas in the center of the image demonstrate the footprints of the anterior cruciate ligament (ACL) and posterior cruciate ligament (PCL). (Printed with permission from Springer Publishing from Brown, C.H., Steiner, M.E. (1994). Anterior Cruciate Ligament Injuries. In: Siliski, JM. (eds) Traumatic Disorders of the Knee. Springer, New York, NY)

tively. The menisci have been classically described as having three zones of vascularity (Fig. 8.8). The peripheral third of the meniscus (red-red zone) is vascularized and has the poten-

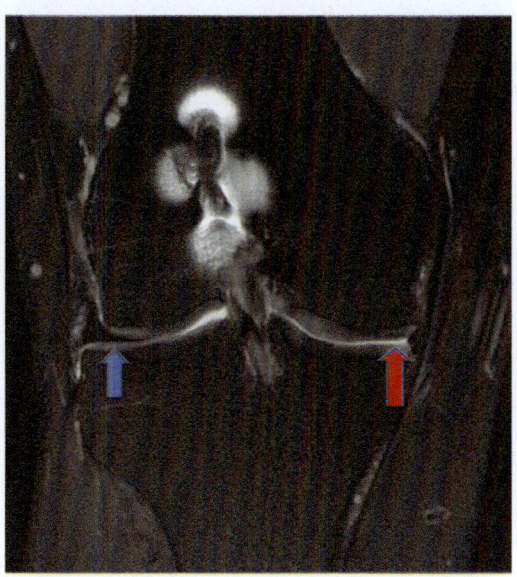

Fig. 8.7 Coronal MRI of the knee demonstrating medial meniscus deficiency after an ACL reconstruction. On the left-hand side of the image, the triangle-shaped lateral meniscus (blue arrow) is present. On the right-hand side of the image, the medial meniscus is missing a significant portion (red arrow) due to a combination of chronic meniscal degeneration and prior surgery (partial meniscectomy)

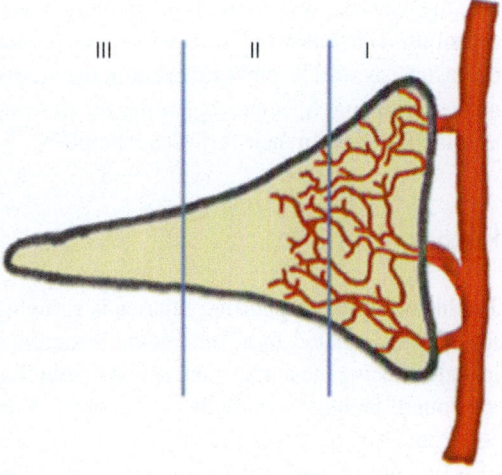

Fig. 8.8 Depiction of the vascular zones of the meniscus. The right-hand side of the image demonstrates the periphery of the meniscus with the highest vascularity and best propensity to heal after injury (zone I or the red–red zone). The central segment has an intermediate vascular supply and intermediate propensity to heal after injury (zone II or the red–white zone). The left-hand side of the image demonstrates the central portion of the meniscus with the least vascularity and lowest propensity to heal after injury (zone III or the white–white zone). (Published with permission from Springer Publishing from Balke, M., Almqvist, K.F., Vansintjan, P., Verdonk, R., Verdonk, P., Hoeher, J. (2016). Traumatic Lesions in a Stable Knee: Masterly Neglect—Meniscectomy—Repair. In: Hulet, C., Pereira, H., Peretti, G., Denti, M. (eds) Surgery of the Meniscus. Springer, Berlin, Heidelberg)

tial to heal after being torn. The middle third of the meniscus (red-white zone) is partially vascularized and has intermediate healing potential. The central third of the meniscus (white-white zone) is avascular and has poor healing potential. In general, tears in the white-white zone are debrided, while tears in the red-red zone are repaired. It is important to preserve as much functional meniscus tissue as possible when debriding meniscal tears, as complete meniscectomy will lead to accelerated osteoarthritis.

Evaluation of Common Sports Medicine Injuries

The principles involved in the initial evaluation of the injured athlete focus on history and a focused physical examination. Oftentimes injuries to the athlete are seen in real time which helps better understand the mechanism of injury and narrows the differential diagnosis For example, a football player who gets tackled from the side and sustains a valgus blow to the knee would likely have an MCL injury, whereas a player who is cutting or pivoting and feels a pop in their knee without contacting another player would be more likely to have an ACL tear. The on-field sports medicine physician also has a "golden window" of time to evaluate the injury before the effects of swelling, pain, and muscle spasm complicate the physical exam. Additionally, significantly displaced fractures or joint dislocations may be more easily reduced in this immediate post-injury setting while still on the field. The sports medicine physician is frequently asked about the safety of a player returning to play after specific injuries. The return-to-play decision is based on a variety of factors including the type and severity of injury, as well as the nature of the sport and the player's position in that sport. Knowledge of the common injuries, as well as the sporting activities themselves, is important in making these decisions. The following sections will focus on the history as well as physical exam in the sports medicine setting. Specifics regarding the injuries are elaborated on in their respective chapters.

History

The history in many sporting injuries is straightforward and related to acute trauma. Examples include twisting the ankle when coming down for a rebound, feeling the shoulder "pop out" when being tackled, or hearing a "pop" within one's knee on cutting cross-field. Important in this history is the mechanism of injury, as this often relates very closely with the structure injured. With the history alone, the diagnosis can be made or at least narrowed to a few potential diagnoses. Thus, the history is just as important and oftentimes more important than the physical examination. In contrast to acute traumatic sporting injuries, overuse injuries typically have no specific identifiable mechanism of injury. Examples can include plantar fasciitis, shin splints, and patellar tendinitis. For these insidious conditions, it is important to obtain the specifics of recent activity, including changes in activity level or type of activities (number of miles run per week), changes in shoe wear or other equipment, or changes to the surface utilized (track to road, flat surface to hills, etc.). Other pertinent details include whether this problem has occurred before, and if so, how it happened, what type of treatment was rendered, and what the outcome was. Previous problems may alert the clinician to a different treatment problem to prevent recurrence of the injury. Examples include the management of "first time" as opposed to recurrent shoulder dislocations.

Symptoms that occur with activity and improve with rest are typical of overuse injuries. Pain that awakens a patient from sleep usually indicates more serious injury or an underlying systemic disorder. Are there any specific activities that might cause symptoms? In the athlete with intermittent knee symptoms, pain in the anterior aspect of the knee that is worse with stair climbing or with prolonged sitting suggests problems related to the patellofemoral joint. Symptoms that occur predictably with cutting and pivoting activities, accompanied by swelling and instability, suggest an internal derangement of the knee such as a meniscus injury or tear of the anterior cruciate ligament.

Physical Examination

The specific examination depends on the nature of the symptoms and the region affected. Each anatomic region and orthopedic condition has pertinent special tests. All physical examinations, however, should begin with inspection and observation of the extremity. After acute injury, one should compare the injured limb in question to its opposite side. Inspection for skin changes such as ecchymoses, abrasions, and associated swelling should be performed. Determining range of motion of the joint in question, both actively and passively, is imperative. First, have the athlete move the joint in question and observe for associated pain or asymmetry as compared to the opposite side. Examples include a patient who presents with shoulder pain of insidious onset whose active and passive range of motion is asymmetric and limited on the affected side, suggesting an adhesive capsulitis as a diagnosis. This is compared to a rotator cuff injury where passive range of motion would be full despite a limited active range of motion. Other examples include the inability to actively extend the knee after an acute injury, despite nearly full passive range of motion. This suggests an injury (rupture) of the extensor mechanism that can be seen in patellar tendon or quadriceps tendon ruptures, as well as some patella fractures.

Strength assessment is an important component to the exam of any joint-related injury. During strength assessment, weakness may be due to direct injury to a musculotendinous unit responsible for joint function. However, pain, guarding, or reflex inhibition of muscular contraction can also be responsible for perceived weakness on examination. The ability of the sports medicine professional to examine the athlete in the acute setting shortly after the injury (before pain and swelling set in) is especially helpful in obtaining an accurate assessment of strength. Although relatively uncommon, injuries to nerve and vascular structures can and do occur and should be ruled out as a precipitating cause of injury especially in the acute setting. Their examination is an essential component of a complete physical exam.

On initial examination, one should always keep an open mind for referred symptoms. In addition to examining the joint in question, one should also focus particularly on the adjacent joints, as well as the spine, for a contributing role in the symptoms. Examples include a slipped capital femoral epiphysis (SCFE) of the hip in an adolescent with knee pain or a cervical disc herniation as a cause for shoulder discomfort.

Applying special examination techniques specific to the area in question and suspected diagnosis completes the physical examination. These techniques can be found in their respective chapters according to the area in question. Examples of special tests include impingement signs in case of shoulder pain or apprehension in the case of shoulder instability as the arm is placed in a position of abduction and external rotation.

Special Tests

Every joint has special tests associated with them to aid in specific injuries. These are very important to diagnosis confirmation and are included to a certain extent in the specific chapters and sections focused on those specific diagnoses.

X-Rays

Plain radiographs, or X-rays, are a useful tool in the initial work-up of acute traumatic injuries that occur in sports. X-rays are useful at identifying fractures of bones or dislocations of joints. While soft tissue injuries may not demonstrate any positive findings on an X-ray, it is still important to rule out fracture or dislocation as causes of pain or swelling after an acute injury. When X-rays remain negative but there is a high suspicion for injury to an important structural or

functional soft tissue (e.g., anterior cruciate ligament, rotator cuff), then further advanced imaging can be obtained such as magnetic resonance imaging (MRI), computed tomography (CT), or ultrasound. Specifically obtained radiographic stress views can be useful in assessing joint integrity. Common examples include stress views taken for grade III injuries of the acromioclavicular (AC) joint or stress views of lateral malleolus ankle fractures to assess for injury to the syndesmosis.

Magnetic Resonance Imaging

Magnetic resonance imaging (MRI) is a useful diagnostic imaging tool within sports medicine. MRI provides for a high-resolution assessment of soft tissues that cannot be visualized on X-ray or CT. While X-ray and CT are the gold-standard for evaluation of acute fractures, MRI is more sensitive at identifying stress fractures. Endurance athletes such as long-distance runners who report chronic bone or joint pain with activity may have negative X-rays but ultimately end up having an occult stress fracture that is only seen on MRI. Common locations for stress fractures in athletes include the tibia, navicular, calcaneus, metatarsals, and femoral neck. The addition of intra-articular contrast (MRI arthrogram) is especially helpful in the shoulder and hip to aid in the diagnosis of labral tears. MRI should be used judiciously as it is expensive compared to plain radiographs, and it is common to identify incidental age-related changes that often do not need intervention. It is critical to first start with history and physical exam before proceeding with MRI to further assess a suspected diagnosis.

Arthroscopy

Most commonly applied to the knee, shoulder, ankle, elbow, and hip, arthroscopy is the goldstandard tool for definitive diagnosis and treatment of intra-articular injuries. Arthroscopy involves the use of an "arthroscope," which is a minimally invasive tool comprised of a thin tube with a video camera and light source which is inserted into a joint through a small incision. The joint is then insufflated with fluid to expand the

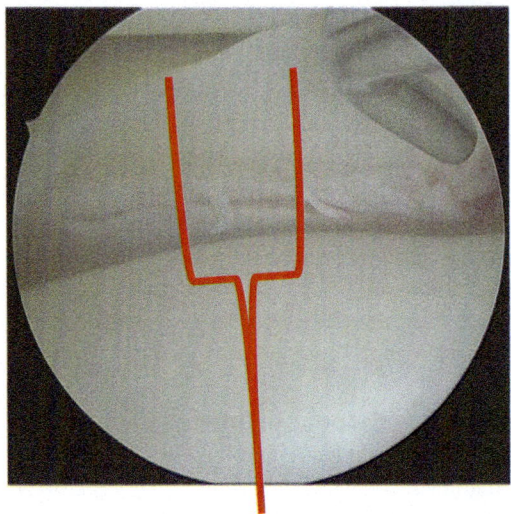

Fig. 8.9 Intraoperative picture taken during a knee arthroscopy demonstrating a meniscal tear (outlined by red bar). In this image, the broad white surface along the bottom is the articular cartilage of the tibial plateau. Above this lies the meniscus, which is flipped up with a metal probe (right) to demonstrate an undersurface longitudinal meniscal tear

joint and allow for improved visualization and insertion of tools (Fig. 8.9). Its utility in diagnosis alone is not often utilized but can be especially helpful in situations where all other diagnostic testing has not been successful in establishing a diagnosis. The overwhelming use of arthroscopy in the field of sports medicine, however, is for the treatment of joint injuries once a diagnosis is reached (e.g., arthroscopically assisted ACL reconstruction).

Treatment of Sports Injuries

Treatment of sports injuries follows an algorithmic approach. The goals of treatment are to initially reduce pain, inflammation, swelling, and stiffness, followed by increasing strength and function to allow expeditious return to normal function and athletic activity. Treatment varies based on whether it is an acute traumatic injury versus a chronic overuse injury. For acute traumatic injuries, treatment can be divided into three distinct but overlapping phases: immediate, early, and late.

Acute Traumatic Injuries

Immediate
Immediate treatment begins at the time of injury. For acute traumatic injuries, it is often helpful to provide some sort of immobilization to the injured extremity to reduce pain and provide stabilization pending further imaging, if necessary. An example of this would be placing a knee immobilizer on a football player who gets tackled and feels a pop followed by immediate knee pain. The mnemonic "RICE" (rest, ice, compression, elevation) is helpful in this immediate and early period to minimize local soft tissue edema and pain. If the sports medicine physician is present at a sporting event when an injury occurs, then an immediate physical examination can be performed to aid in forming a differential diagnosis and guide further management.

Early
Early treatment involves establishing a definitive diagnosis and minimizing the sequelae of trauma, including joint stiffness and muscle atrophy. Additional testing is often required at this stage to help formulate both the diagnosis and the definitive treatment plan. An accurate diagnosis at this stage is critical, as important time-sensitive decisions need to be made (e.g., surgical versus nonsurgical management, early range of motion versus more prolonged immobilization, return-to-play timing). Nonsteroidal anti-inflammatory drugs (NSAIDs) are a useful tool to manage pain and inflammation during this period.

Late
The majority of sports injuries are successfully treated without surgery. Physical therapy is often necessary to allow patients to regain their pre-injury strength and range of motion. This rehabilitation and recovery period can take weeks to months depending on the injury. Specific indications for operative management vary depending on the specific injury pattern, as well as the athlete's goals and expectations both on and off the athletic field. Surgical intervention may involve traditional open techniques, arthroscopic techniques, or a combination of both.

Chronic Overuse Injuries

In the treatment of chronic overuse injuries, rest is frequently employed in the form of activity modification. In general, any activity that exacerbates symptoms should be avoided. The injured tissues must be allowed to rest in order to heal and resolve the inflammatory process causing the symptoms. Often for the athlete, this involves temporary restriction from their sport.

During the period of activity modification, a variety of techniques can be helpful to further relieve pain and inflammation in order to restore normal function. This can begin with the use of nonsteroidal anti-inflammatory drugs (NSAIDs) for symptom relief but not treating the underlying problem in most cases. Various modalities such as ice, heat, electrical stimulation, ultrasound, and massage can all be helpful in decreasing pain and swelling.

Although activity modification is the mainstay of treatment, a prolonged period of inactivity can result in muscular atrophy, joint stiffness, and overall de-conditioning. Definitive treatment for these injuries often involves a dedicated physical therapy program aimed at restoring the athlete's strength and endurance required for a return to sport. Focus on the athlete's biomechanics is also an essential component in treating overuse injuries to prevent recurrence. Attention to the specifics of the supporting structures is often helpful in this regard. Alignment problems are often identified in this phase of treatment for lower extremity injuries. Fabrication of a shoe lift orthotic for a previously unrecognized limb length discrepancy or a medial longitudinal arch support for over-pronation can lead to a more successful return to activity. Sometimes video analysis of the activity is helpful to identify, correct, and prevent improper biomechanics.

Occasionally, overuse injuries do not respond to non-operative measures and surgical correction is required. Conditions that are occasionally associated with failure of conservative treatment include lateral epicondylitis ("tennis elbow"), shoulder impingement, and patellar/Achilles tendonitis. Conservative treatment is trialed for prolonged periods—often 6 months to 1 year—before resorting to surgical intervention. Rarely, stress fractures in high-risk areas (e.g., femoral neck) or those which fail to respond to adequate immobilization will require surgical intervention.

Common Pathologies Treated by Sports Medicine Specialists

Hip: Femoroacetabular Impingement (FAI)

The hip is a ball-and-socket synovial joint where the ball (femoral head) articulates with the cup (acetabulum). In individuals with normal anatomy, the femoral head is spherical and the acetabulum is hemispherical. In a disease process known as femoroacetabular impingement (FAI), commonly referred to as "hip impingement," the femoral head and/or acetabulum has a shape that does not match each other, resulting in structural impingement.

Bony overgrowth at the femoral head–neck junction is referred to as a "cam lesion," resulting in cam impingement. Cam lesions are most commonly located at the anterosuperior aspect of the femoral head–neck junction and are more commonly seen in males. With hip flexion, adduction, and internal rotation (the so-called FADIR maneuver), the cam lesion impinges on the acetabular labrum, causing pain, labral tearing, and in severe cases leads to articular cartilage delamination. With repeated injury to the articular cartilage over time, severe FAI can lead to osteoarthritis of the hip.

Bony overgrowth of the acetabular rim is referred to as a "pincer lesion" resulting in pincer impingement. This so-called acetabular overcoverage can be focal or global. Pincer lesions are most commonly located over the anterior or anterosuperior acetabular rim. When the hip is brought into FADIR, the pincer lesion on the acetabulum impinges on the femoral neck. Mixed lesions refer to the presence of both cam and pincer morphologies.

Patients typically present with insidious anterior or anterolateral hip pain although acute injuries can occur. Pain occurs with activity, especially flexion activities such as squats and lunges although sitting pain is commonplace as the problem progresses as that position often brings the impinging surfaces together, thus compressing or stressing the labrum and underlying tear. The workhorse of the special test is the FADIR test maneuver for that reason as well.

Initial evaluation of FAI includes radiographs of the involved hip and pelvis (Fig. 8.10). Specific radiographs for FAI include an AP view of the pelvis, frog-leg lateral view (hip abducted 45°), Dunn lateral view (hip flexed 90° and abducted 20°), modified Dunn lateral view (hip flexed 45° and abducted 20°), cross-table lateral view, and false profile view (pelvis rotated 60° toward the side being imaged). The Dunn and frog-leg lateral views are helpful in detecting femoral head–neck asphericity (cam lesions), while the cross-table lateral and false profile views are helpful for evaluating acetabular over-coverage (pincer lesions). The classic finding on an AP pelvis view of a severe cam lesion is called a "pistol grip deformity." Magnetic resonance imaging (MRI) of the hip may be obtained to evaluate the labrum and articular cartilage (Fig. 8.11).

The initial treatment for patients with FAI is conservative, starting with activity modification and physical therapy. For patients who fail conservative treatment, the first-line surgical treatment is hip arthroscopy with specific procedures performed to address the patient's specific pathology. Through an arthroscopic approach, cam and pincer lesions can be resected, and the labrum can be repaired, debrided, or reconstructed with allograft. Hip arthroscopy has made it possible to treat FAI through a minimally invasive approach. Prior to hip arthroscopy, the treatment involved open surgical hip dislocation (which is still required in some severe cases). For patients with end-stage osteoarthritis as a result of FAI, the treatment is total hip arthroplasty.

Knee: Anterior Cruciate Ligament (ACL) Injury

The ACL is an intra-articular ligament in the knee that spans from the medial wall of the lateral femoral condyle to the middle of the intercondylar area of the tibial plateau. The ACL prevents anterior translation and rotation of the tibia relative the femur. There are two distinct bundles of the ACL. The anteromedial (AM) bundle is tight in knee flexion and primarily resists anterior translation of the tibia relative to the femur. In contrast, the posterolateral (PL)

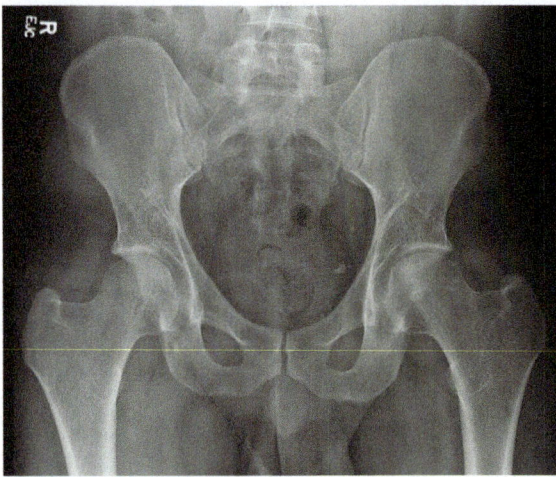 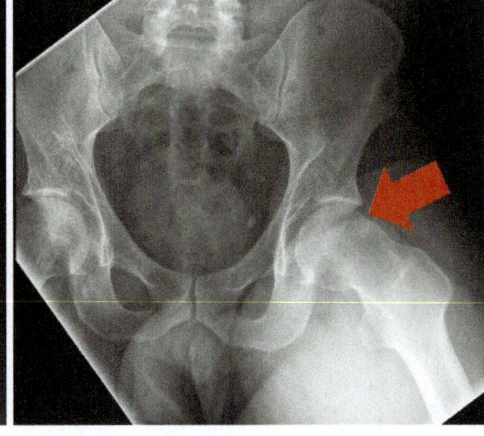

Fig. 8.10 *Left*: AP pelvis X-ray. *Right*: Modified Dunn lateral X-ray of the left hip. The left hip in the images above demonstrates a cam lesion. The cam lesion (red arrow) is more evident on the modified Dunn lateral view, as this hip positioning places the lesion located along the anterosuperior femoral head–neck junction perpendicular to the X-ray beam

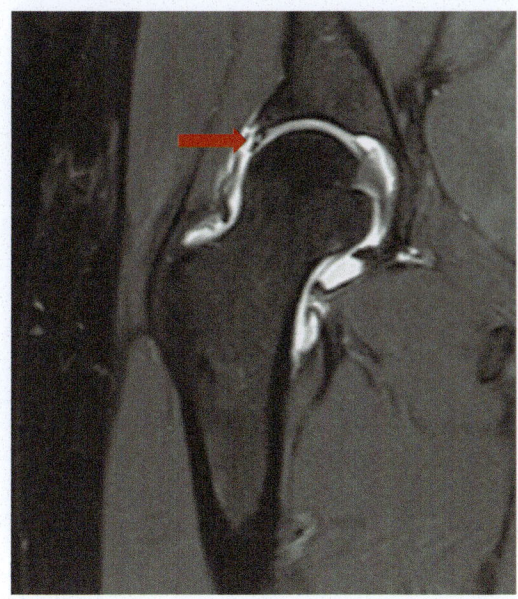

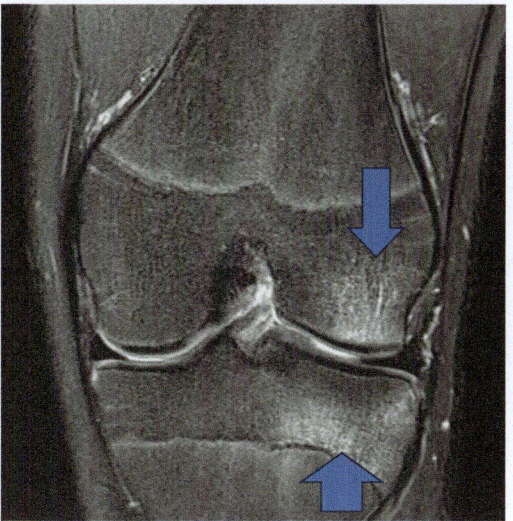

Fig. 8.11 Coronal MRI arthrogram demonstrating hip labral tearing (red arrow) in the setting of femoroacetabular impingement

Fig. 8.12 Coronal MRI of the knee demonstrating the bone bruise pattern (white areas in the bone denoted by the arrows) seen after anterior cruciate ligament (ACL) injury. On T2 MRI, there is hyperintensity (indicative of a bone bruise) along the lateral femoral condyle and posterior aspect of the lateral tibial plateau

bundle is tight in knee extension and primarily resists rotation of the tibia relative to the femur.

ACL tears most commonly occur due to a non-contact pivoting injury (e.g., when an athlete plants their foot and twists to change direction). The ACL receives blood supply from branches of the middle geniculate artery. When the ACL is torn, this blood supply is disrupted leading to hemarthrosis or blood inside of the knee joint. Intra-articular ligament injuries (e.g., ACL and PCL) lead to hemarthrosis due to their presence inside of the joint, whereas extra-articular injuries (e.g., MCL, LCL) bleed outside of the knee joint capsule and do not form hemarthrosis.

On physical examination, the most sensitive test to detect an ACL tear is the Lachman test, while the most specific test is the pivot shift test. The Lachman test is performed by positioning the patient supine with the involved knee flexed to 20–30°. The examiner stabilizes the femur, grasps the tibia, and attempts to translate the tibia anteriorly relative to the femur. A positive Lachman test is indicated by increased anterior tibial translation compared to the contralateral uninjured side. A positive Lachman test can be graded according to severity with grade 1 being 3–5 mm anterior translation of the tibia, grade 2 being 5–10 mm translation, and grade 3 being >10 mm translation.

The pivot shift test is performed with the patient supine and the examiner initially holding the involved extremity with the knee in extension. A valgus force and axial load are applied to the knee along with slight internal rotation of the tibia, leaving the tibia in an internally subluxated position in the setting of ACL injury. The knee is then slowly brought into flexion. A positive pivot shift is denoted by a palpable clunk or shift in the knee which occurs around 30–40° flexion, corresponding to the subluxated lateral tibial plateau reducing onto the lateral femoral condyle. This reduction and shift occur at roughly 30–40° knee flexion. The mechanism behind this shift is not fully understood but may be partially due to the iliotibial (IT) band transitioning from a knee extensor to a knee flexor as the knee goes from a fully extended to flexed position.

On MRI of knees with a torn ACL, there is a classic bone bruise pattern involving the midportion of the lateral femoral condyle and the posterior aspect of the lateral tibial plateau (Fig. 8.12). These bone bruises occur secondary to the lateral femoral condyle impacting the lateral tibial pla-

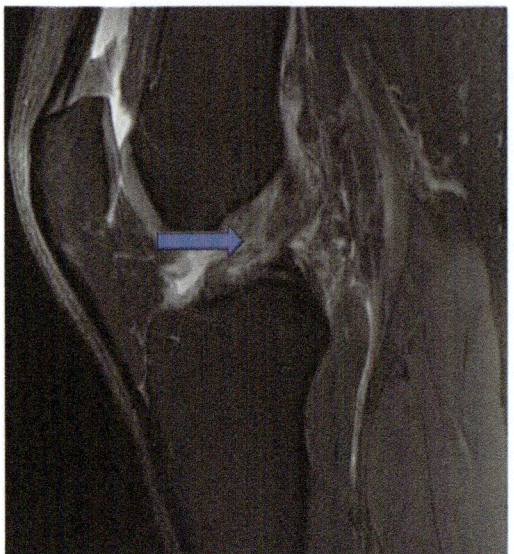

Fig. 8.13 Sagittal MRI of the knee demonstrating anterior cruciate ligament (ACL) tear

teau during the pivot shift subluxation that occurs at the time of ACL injury. MRI also serves to confirm the diagnosis of an ACL tear and identify concomitant injuries around the knee (e.g., meniscal tears, collateral ligament tears) (Fig. 8.13).

The gold-standard surgical treatment for ACL tears is an ACL reconstruction with tendon graft. The most common autograft sources are patellar tendon (with bone plugs from the patella and tibia, also known as a "bone–patellar tendon–bone" graft), hamstring tendon (semitendinosus/gracilis), and quadriceps tendon. Alternatively, a variety of different allograft (cadaver) options are available. The surgery is performed with arthroscopic assistance, and the graft is passed through tunnels drilled through the anatomic footprints of the native ACL on the proximal tibia and lateral femoral condyle. Postoperatively, patients undergo functional physical rehabilitation with an emphasis on progressive range of motion, strengthening, and agility with the goal of returning to full sport roughly 9–12 months after surgery.

Shoulder

Sports medicine surgeons treat a variety of shoulder pathology, including glenohumeral instability (shoulder subluxations and dislocations), labral tears, and rotator cuff tears. For more detailed information, see Chap. 9.

Summary and Conclusion

Sports medicine has evolved to encompass care of not only those participating in sports but of all active individuals. As patients continue to remain active into their older age, the sports medicine physician's role has expanded to include everyone from children on youth soccer teams to octogenarian pickleball players. The field of sports medicine has significantly advanced over the past several decades with continual innovation in arthroscopic surgery techniques and rehabilitation protocols. As our knowledge of the basic science of musculoskeletal tissues advances, so do our techniques for treating them when injured. Patients are now able to return to sports and activities after injury quicker and safer than before.

Further Reading

1. Miller MD, Thompson SR. DeLee, Drez, & Miller's orthopaedic sports medicine: principles and practice. 5th ed. Philadelphia, PA: Elsevier; 2019.
2. Madden CC, Putukian M, McCarty EC, Young CC, editors. Netter's sports medicine. 3rd ed. Philadelphia, PA: Elsevier; 2022.
3. Azar F. Orthopaedic knowledge update (OKU): sports medicine 6. Rosemont, IL: American Academy of Orthopaedic Surgeons; 2020.
4. Miller MD. Operative techniques in sports medicine surgery. 3rd ed. Philadelphia, PA: Wolters Kluwer; 2021.

The Shoulder

Evan Michaelson and Brent Wiesel

Functional Anatomy

The shoulder girdle includes three bones (scapula, clavicle, and proximal humerus) (Fig. 9.1), three joints (glenohumeral, acromioclavicular, and sternoclavicular), an additional articulation (scapulothoracic), and some 17 musculotendinous units. These individual elements function in a synchronous and interdependent manner in order to maximize the power and range of motion of the shoulder girdle. The clavicle is the sole bony link between the upper extremity and the axial skeleton.

The Glenohumeral Joint

The glenohumeral (GH) joint is the articulation of the proximal humeral epiphysis (ball) with the glenoid fossa (socket) of the scapula. This joint contributes to the majority of motion in the shoulder girdle. As only 20–30% of the humeral head is in contact with the glenoid fossa at any point in the shoulder's arc of motion and the radius of curvature of the glenoid is greater than that of the humeral head, there is little inherent bony stability of the GH joint. The joint has often been compared to a golf ball sitting on a tee turned on its side. As a result, the soft tissues surrounding the joint are responsible for maintaining joint stability and congruity while still permitting the tremendous range of motion required of the GH joint. These soft tissue stabilizers include the joint capsule, glenohumeral ligaments, glenoid labrum, long head of the biceps tendon, and the rotator cuff musculature. The burden placed upon these soft tissues leads to the majority of degenerative and traumatic conditions affecting the shoulder girdle.

The Glenohumeral Ligaments

The capsule of the shoulder is a specialized structure that contains distinct thickenings referred to as ligaments (Fig. 9.2). The glenohumeral ligaments are named for their origin from the glenoid rim. This ligamentous complex includes the superior glenohumeral ligament (SGHL), the middle glenohumeral ligament (MGHL), and the inferior glenohumeral ligament. These ligaments function as static stabilizers of the glenohumeral joint. The SGHL is the primary restraint to inferior translation and external rotation with the arm in adduction. The MGHL is the primary stabilizer to anterior translation with the arm in 45° of

E. Michaelson · B. Wiesel (✉)
Georgetown University School of Medicine, Washington, DC, USA

MedStar Orthopedic Institue, MedStar Georgetown University Hospital, Washington, DC, USA
e-mail: Brent.B.Wiesel@gunet.georgetown.edu

W. F. Postma et al. (eds.), *Essentials of Orthopedic Surgery*,
https://doi.org/10.1007/978-3-031-66215-7_9

Fig. 9.1 Anterior view of the shoulder demonstrates the skeletal anatomy and two of the four articulations, the glenohumeral and acromioclavicular joints

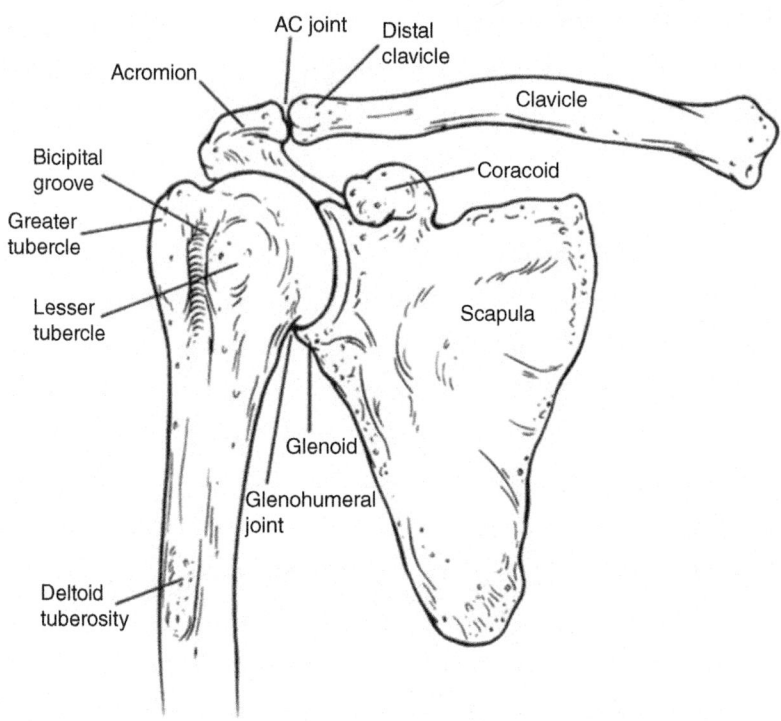

abduction. The inferior glenohumeral ligament complex includes an anterior band (AIGHL), posterior band (PIGHL), and an intervening sling or pouch. The inferior glenohumeral ligament complex becomes taut when the arm is abducted to 90°. In this position, the anterior band resists anterior translation with external rotation, and the posterior band resists posterior translation with internal rotation forces. The sling supports the humeral head.

The Labrum

The labrum is a fibrous structure of variable anatomy that attaches to the rim of the glenoid cartilage through a fibrocartilaginous zone, increasing the depth of the glenoid concavity by 50%. The labrum functions to increase the surface contact area with the humeral head; to act as a static stabilizer through a buttress effect; and to serve as an attachment site for the shoulder capsule, glenohumeral ligaments, and long head of the biceps tendon. The labrum has a variable cross-sectional anatomy, with the superior aspect of the labrum

more triangular shaped and well defined and the inferior aspect of the labrum more rounded and less distinct. Common anatomic variations include a sublabral hole (foramen) or an absent labrum in the anterior-superior quadrant of the glenoid. The combination of a cord-like MGHL and absent anterosuperior labrum has been termed a Buford complex. It is important that the surgeon recognize variations in labral anatomy as inappropriate repair of a sublabral foramen or Buford complex will lead to significant postoperative stiffness.

The Rotator Interval

The rotator interval is the triangular region between the superior aspect of the subscapularis tendon and the anterior aspect of the supraspinatus tendon whose base is the coracoid. The rotator interval includes a number of fibrous structures including the coracohumeral ligament (CHL), the SGHL, and the transverse humeral ligament. The coracohumeral ligament is the most significant structure in the

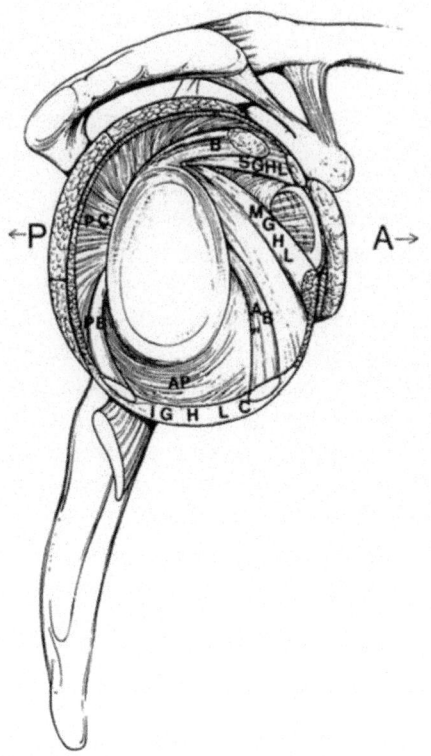

Fig. 9.2 In this cutaway view of the shoulder joint, the humeral head has been removed, allowing visualization of the interior of the normal glenohumeral anatomy. Notice the discrete ligaments that constitute the anterior shoulder capsule, namely the superior (*SGHL*), middle (*MGHL*), and anterior inferior glenohumeral ligaments. In this illustration, the most important anterior restraining structure, the inferior glenohumeral ligament complex (*IGHLC*) is shown to be further subdivided into having anterior (*AB*) and posterior (*PB*) bands and an axillary pouch (*AP*). (From Rockwood CA Jr., Matsen FA III eds. *The Shoulder*. Vol 1. Philadelphia, PA: Saunders; 1990. Reprinted with permission)

rotator interval and is extra-articular. It originates from the lateral base of the coracoid, fanning out to envelope the supraspinatus tendon inserting on the greater tuberosity and the subscapularis tendon inserting on the lesser tuberosity. The CHL is a primary restraint to inferior translation and external rotation in the adducted arm. The transverse humeral ligament forms the apex of the rotator interval and contributes to the superior soft tissue sling that stabilizes the long head of the biceps tendon as it passes through the interval to enter (or exit) the glenohumeral joint.

The Long Head of the Biceps Tendon

The long head of the biceps tendon (LHBT) remains somewhat enigmatic with respect to its function in the shoulder girdle but is nonetheless a potential source of pain and disability. The long head of the biceps enters/exits the glenohumeral joint at the rotator interval by way of the bicipital groove and is an intra-articular structure. The LHBT originates from the superior glenoid tubercle and blends with the fibers of the superior labrum. This intimate relationship of the LHBT with the superior labrum is a significant source of morbidity in the throwing athlete.

Although there is conflicting data, the long head of the biceps is thought to be a humeral head depressor and may contribute to glenohumeral instability. Potentially more relevant is the theory of the "peel-back" mechanism of SLAP (superior labrum anterior posterior) tears. This theory suggests that the LHBT and superior labrum can be torn from the superior glenoid in the late cocking position of a baseball pitch as the LHBT becomes taut and "peels back" the superior labrum off the glenoid rim. Whether or not this theory is correct, SLAP tears can be a significant problem in the throwing athlete. Tendinitis of the LHBT is also a common source of morbidity in the shoulder and is often a component of the impingement syndrome.

The Rotator Cuff

The rotator cuff consists of four muscle-tendon units including the subscapularis, supraspinatus, infraspinatus, and teres minor. These muscles originate on the scapula and insert onto the tuberosities of the proximal humerus. The subscapularis originates on the anterior surface of the scapula and inserts onto the lesser tuberosity. The remaining rotator cuff muscles originate from the posterior surface of the scapula and insert along the greater tuberosity. The roles of the rotator cuff are to keep the humeral head centered in the glenoid fossa throughout the range of shoulder motion and to contribute to the rotation and elevation of the extremity. As such, the rotator cuff is the primary dynamic stabilizer of the glenohumeral joint. Traumatic and overuse injuries to the rotator cuff are the most common problems in the shoulder girdle.

The Subacromial Space

The subacromial space is a potential space beneath the acromion and above the rotator cuff. The subacromial bursa outlines the subacromial space and provides frictionless gliding of the rotator cuff beneath the acromion and coracoacromial arch. Bony osteophytes on the undersurface of the anterior acromion have been postulated to narrow the subacromial space, irritate the subacromial bursa, and contribute to rotator cuff tears.

The Acromioclavicular Joint

The acromioclavicular (AC) joint is a true diarthrodial joint containing a fibrocartilaginous disc. The AC joint helps link the appendicular skeleton with the axial skeleton through the clavicle. Because there is little intrinsic bony stability to the AC joint, a number of ligaments and other soft tissues serve to stabilize this articulation (Fig. 9.3). The superior AC ligament is the most important horizontal stabilizer. The coracoclavicular (CC) ligaments, consisting of the conoid ligament (medial) and the trapezoid ligament (lateral), provide the primary restraint to vertical displacement of the clavicle. A significant amount of rotation occurs in the clavicle throughout the arc of elevation of the upper extremity. Approximately 10% of this rotation occurs at the acromioclavicular joint.

Fig. 9.3 In this anterior view, note the acromioclavicular joint surrounded by the capsule (acromioclavicular ligament), in addition to the supporting coracoclavicular ligaments, the conoid and trapezoid. (From Rockwood CA Jr., Matsen FA III eds. *The Shoulder.* Vol 1. Philadelphia, PA: Saunders; 1990. Reprinted with permission)

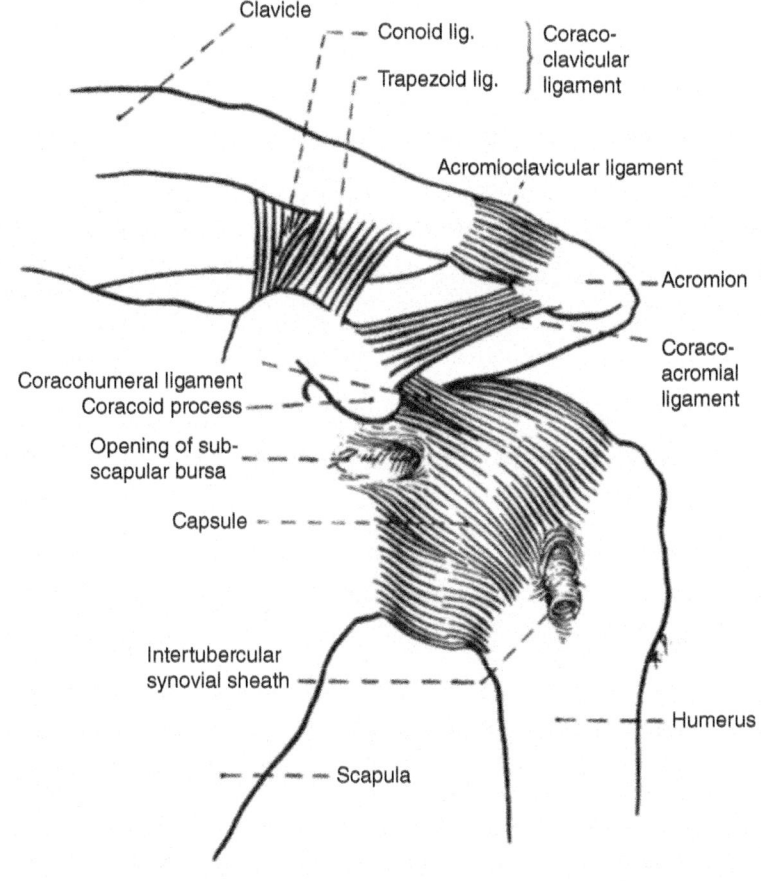

The Sternoclavicular Joint

The sternoclavicular (SC) joint is the only bony connection the upper appendicular skeleton has to the axial skeleton and has the least bony stability of any major joint. The majority of clavicular rotation occurs at the sternoclavicular joint, but less than 50% of the bulbous, medial clavicle is in contact with the shallow, sternal articular fossa. Thus, the soft tissues provide stability to the sternoclavicular joint. The ligamentous anatomy of the SC joint includes the intra-articular disk ligament, the costoclavicular ligament, the interclavicular ligament, and the capsular ligament. Of these, the posterior sternoclavicular joint capsule has been shown to be the most important structure for preventing both anterior and posterior displacement of the medial clavicle.

The Scapulothoracic Articulation

The scapulothoracic articulation includes the scapula, posterior thorax, and interposed bursae which provide frictionless motion between the scapula and posterior thorax. The scapulothoracic articulation provides a significant percentage of motion to the shoulder girdle. Specifically, the glenohumeral joint and scapulothoracic articulation function in a synchronous fashion to provide full forward elevation of the upper extremity in a 2:1 ratio. The scapular stabilizer muscles include the trapezius, levator scapulae, rhomboids, latissimus dorsi, and serratus anterior. Dysfunction of scapulothoracic motion, seen clinically as scapular winging, may be a result of nerve injury or muscle dysfunction. Damage to the spinal accessory nerve results in trapezius dysfunction and lateral scapular winging. Long thoracic nerve injury leads to serratus anterior dysfunction and medial scapular winging. Pain and loss of motion in the glenohumeral joint can lead to overuse and fatigue of the scapular stabilizer muscles resulting in pseudo winging of the scapula.

The Brachial Plexus

The brachial plexus is comprised of the ventral rami of cervical roots C5, C6, C7, C8, and ventral thoracic root T1. With the exception of the spinal accessory nerve (XI) which innervates the trapezius, all of the muscles contributing to the function of the shoulder girdle and upper extremity are innervated by nerves originating from the brachial plexus. The brachial plexus includes five nerve roots, three trunks (superior, middle, and inferior), six divisions (three anterior, three posterior), three cords (lateral, medial, and posterior), and six terminal branches (musculocutaneous, ulnar, medial cord branch to median nerve, lateral cord branch to median nerve, axillary, and radial). With the exception of the divisions, nerves originate from each level of the brachial plexus to innervate muscles of the shoulder girdle. Brachial plexus injuries are relatively common with traumatic shoulder girdle injuries such as proximal humerus fractures, glenohumeral dislocations, and fracture/dislocations.

Clinical Examination of the Shoulder Girdle

The history of present illness is critical in the evaluation of shoulder girdle pathology and should be used to develop a reasonable differential diagnosis based on the patient's story, age, and the epidemiology of shoulder pathology. For example, a high school athlete with activity-related shoulder pain is more likely to have instability or labral pathology than a rotator cuff tear. Conversely, a 65-year-old who has shoulder pain with activities of daily living is more likely to have rotator cuff disease than a labral tear or instability. The physical examination is used to narrow the differential diagnosis and make the definitive diagnosis. Most of the time, an accurate diagnosis can be made using only the history and physical examination. Indiscriminate use of imaging studies and additional testing is not recommended. Prior to ordering additional studies, the examiner must have a clear understanding of how the study will contribute to the evaluation and treatment of the patient.

History

Patients with shoulder pathology most often complain of pain, stiffness, instability, and weakness. When pain is the chief complaint, the examiner must characterize the pain, with particular attention to location. Pain from the glenohumeral joint and its surrounding soft tissues typically is localized to the anterosuperior aspect of the shoulder. Localization of the pain to the deltoid insertion in the arm is common in rotator cuff or subacromial pathology. Pain emanating from the neck or to the posterior scapular region is frequently due to cervical spine disease. Pain and crepitation in the periscapular region, however, may be related to scapulothoracic bursitis.

The timing and frequency of shoulder pain must also be given careful consideration. Activity-related pain can provide valuable clues as to the underlying diagnosis. Pain with overhead activities of daily living is common in rotator cuff pathology. Pain with sporting activities such as swimming, throwing, or serving is often related to the labrum or glenohumeral instability. In overhead athletes it is important to determine the phase of the throwing motion during which the pain occurs. Night pain is often reported with shoulder girdle pathology, especially in the setting of rotator cuff tears. Patients will often report the inability to sleep on the affected side. Rest pain is uncommon but may occur with severe arthropathy or radicular pain from the cervical spine. If rest pain is the predominant complaint, the examiner should consider infection or malignancy as a possible source of pain.

The relationship of pain to injury is important to establish. Pain that begins with a traumatic event such as a fall on an outstretched hand, direct blow to the shoulder, or shoulder dislocation may represent significant damage to the rotator cuff, ligaments, or bony structures. Pain that begins days or weeks after a seemingly innocuous event such as shoveling snow, trimming hedges, or painting may represent tendonitis or early capsulitis. Pain that begins more insidiously

or over time is more likely to be related to degenerative lesions of the shoulder girdle such as rotator cuff tears or osteoarthritis.

Complaints of shoulder instability are relatively common. The patient may describe the shoulder "slipping out of place" or "getting stuck" in extreme positions. It is important to establish whether a frank shoulder dislocation was ever documented. True traumatic shoulder dislocations are the result of significant trauma and require a manipulative reduction. Unfortunately, subsequent dislocations may occur with less trauma. Patients who have shoulders which "slip out of place" and "slide back in" on their own are more likely to have multidirectional instability as opposed to traumatic instability.

Weakness or loss of shoulder function is also a frequent complaint. In the absence of pain, a neurologic origin of the deteriorating function should be considered. Insidious onset of pain with deteriorating function may represent a degenerative condition of the shoulder or adhesive capsulitis.

A careful review of systems is important to document as there are a number of disease processes remote from the shoulder girdle that can result in shoulder pain. Cervical spine pathology, cardiac disease, gallbladder disease, and lung disease (pancoast tumor) can present with shoulder pain. A history of cancer is also important to document as metastatic cancer can present with shoulder pain and lesions in the shoulder girdle.

Functional Assessment

In addition to establishing the history of present illness, it is imperative to establish the functional status of the patient. Important patient factors to note include the handedness (right, left, or ambidextrous) of the patient, the vocation of the patient, extracurricular/sporting activities enjoyed by the patient, assistive devices used for ambulation, and, most importantly, the expectations of the patient regarding their shoulder problem. Understanding the patient's functional demands and expectations allows the clinician to prescribe appropriate treatment regimens and to provide reasonable expectations for functional recovery.

Inspection

The physical examination begins with inspection of the shoulder girdle. The region must be adequately exposed for the examination. The inspection begins with assessment of symmetry between the involved and uninvolved shoulder girdles. Gross deformities such as distal clavicle prominence in an AC separation, prior surgical incisions, skin discoloration, or open wounds are readily appreciated. A more subtle finding is muscle atrophy which may be the result of disuse or injury. Patients with longstanding rotator cuff tears will often have atrophy of the supra- and infraspinatus fossae resulting in prominence of the spine of the scapula. Traumatic injuries can produce subtle deformities. In the setting of an anterior dislocation, the anterior aspect of the shoulder may appear "full" and the posterior aspect may lose its normal contour making the posterior acromion appear more prominent. Inspection should continue through the entire exam as some deformities such as scapular winging may only be revealed during provocative testing.

Palpation

The primary importance of palpation is to localize the source of pain. Palpation of bony prominences and superficial joints yields the most information. In the absence of trauma, palpation includes the SC joint, AC joint, the greater and lesser tuberosities, and the bicipital groove. Tenderness on palpation at any of these sites can be a valuable clue in making a diagnosis. When the presenting complaint is neck or periscapular pain, palpation of the posterior elements of the cervical spine and bony elements of the scapula is warranted. In the setting of trauma, palpation of all bony structures and areas of deformity is critical to localize the zone of injury.

Range of Motion

The evaluation of range of motion is straightforward. The examiner directs the motions and observes for symmetry. The standard motions include forward elevation, external rotation, internal rotation, and abduction. Forward elevation occurs in the plane of the scapula and is a combination of scapulothoracic and glenohumeral motion. When testing range of motion, scapulothoracic motion and other compensating mechanisms must be observed and controlled for accurate measurements. Loss of glenohumeral motion can lead to scapulothoracic substitution and scapular winging. External rotation is evaluated with the arms at the side to prevent scapulothoracic contribution to rotation. Internal rotation is evaluated by having the patient place his or her hands as high as possible along the midline of the back. Internal rotation is graded by the approximate vertebral level the patient is able to reach. Assessment of abduction, including internal and external rotation in abduction, is critical for unmasking subtle losses of motion. Throwing athletes often lose some internal rotation in abduction while gaining external rotation in abduction in their throwing arm. There is no net loss of motion, only a resetting of the range of motion relative to the non-throwing shoulder.

When loss of active motion is identified, the examiner must assess the passive range of motion. If there is loss of active and passive motion, there is likely a soft tissue contracture or a physical block to motion (dislocation, loose body, or osteophyte). In the absence of trauma, loss of both active and passive motion usually represents adhesive capsulitis (frozen shoulder) or glenohumeral arthritis. If there is loss of active motion with preserved passive motion, the examiner must consider tendon (rotator cuff) rupture or, potentially, nerve damage. When examining the rotator cuff muscles, the examiner must appreciate lag signs.

A lag sign can be documented when the patient has a loss of active motion with preservation of passive motion. The examiner positions the shoulder at the end range of full passive motion and instructs the patient to maintain the position. If the patient is unable to maintain the position and the extremity falls away, the patient is considered to have a positive lag sign. The horn blower's sign is the lag sign for the abducted, externally rotated position and is suggestive of a massive rotator cuff tear involving the posterior cuff.

Strength Assessment

The relative strength of muscle groups can be assessed during the physical examination. In order to assess strength, the examiner manually resists the patient's active motion in a defined plane such as abduction, adduction, and internal or external rotation. Asymmetric weakness on the involved side can provide additional diagnostic information. Weakness or paralysis of the scapular stabilizer muscles can be assessed by having the patient perform pushups against a wall. Scapular winging can be elicited using this technique.

Neurologic Examination

In the absence of trauma or brachial plexopathies, most neurologic lesions about the shoulder involve a peripheral nerve. Common peripheral neuropathies in the shoulder girdle include the suprascapular, spinal accessory, and long thoracic nerves. Although these conditions can be painful, many patients report dysfunction or cosmetic deformity as the presenting complaint. These lesions are appreciated during the inspection, range of motion and strength testing of the shoulder girdle. Suprascapular neuropathy can occur at the level of the suprascapular notch or proximal and involve both the supra- and infraspinatus tendons resulting in prominence of the scapular spine and weakness of forward elevation and external rotation. Suprascapular nerve lesions at the level of the spinoglenoid notch involve only the infraspinatus muscle resulting in atrophy of the infraspinatus fossa and weakness of external rotation. Compression in this area is often the result of a paralabral cyst associated with a labral tear and is common in overhead athletes. Spinal accessory nerve injury is often iatrogenic from a posterior cervical node biopsy or a radical neck dissection for malignancy. Injury to the spinal accessory nerve (cranial nerve XI) results in trapezius dysfunction and lateral scapular winging. Long thoracic nerve injury is thought to be secondary to traction or contusion and affects the serratus anterior muscle resulting in medial scapular winging. Medial or lateral refers to the direction toward which the inferior border of the scapula is directed. Nerve lesions in the shoulder girdle should be further evaluated with electromyography (EMG) and nerve conduction testing. The majority of these nerve lesions (except iatrogenic laceration) recover without surgical intervention.

Special Tests and Signs

There are many special tests or maneuvers that have been described to evaluate individual structures or reveal specific pathology. Physical examination of the shoulder can be challenging, as exam findings may overlap multiple diagnoses, patients may have multiple coexisting pathologies, and shoulder disorders may have variable presentations. The examiner should elect to perform specific maneuvers and evaluate the results of these tests in the context of the patient demographics, history, and complaints. A few of these tests and signs are reviewed below.

Rotator Cuff

The most commonly used tests attempt to recreate the pain that occurs with rotator cuff impingement under the coracoacromial (CA) arch by rotating the greater tuberosity under the acromion. The painful arc sign occurs when the patient experiences pain while elevating the upper extremity from 70° to 120°. The Neer impingement sign is positive when shoulder pain is reproduced as the upper extremity is passively elevated in the scapular plane with the scapula stabilized (Fig. 9.4). Unrestricted passive range of motion is required specifically for a positive Neer impingement sign. Hawkins's impingement sign is tested by passively internally rotating the humerus when the arm is at 90° of forward flexion with the elbow flexed. A positive test is defined as shoulder pain with this maneuver. The drop arm test is performed by placing the upper extremity at shoulder level (90°) in the scapular plane with the thumb pointing downward. The test is considered positive when the patient is unable to maintain the extremity in this position and is indicative of superior rotator cuff pathology.

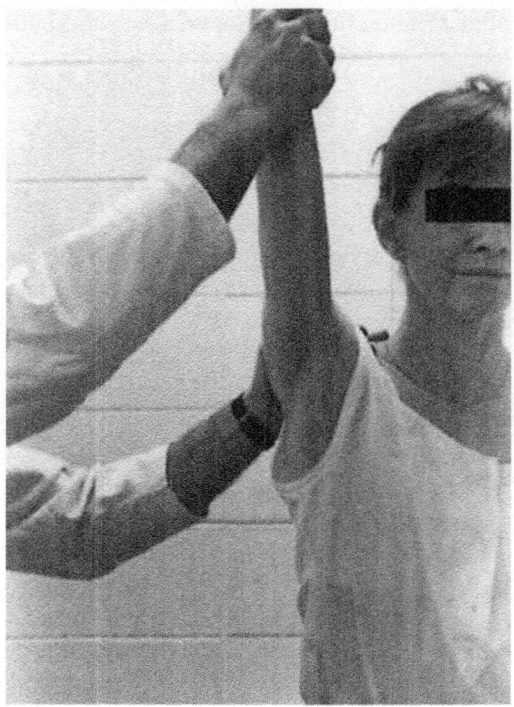

Fig. 9.4 Impingement of the rotator cuff is demonstrated by passively elevating the shoulder against the fixed scapula. Pain suggests the possibility of mechanical compression of the rotator cuff against the anterior inferior acromion, a process known as impingement. (From DeLee JC, Drez D Jr. *Orthopaedic Sports Medicine: Principles and Practice.* Vol 1. Philadelphia, PA: Saunders; 1994. Reprinted with permission)

Multiple tests have been described to evaluate the subscapularis. The lift-off test is performed by having the patient place his or her hands behind the back with the arm internally rotated and the elbow flexed. The patient is then asked to lift the hands off the back without extending the elbows. If the patient is unable to perform the lift-off, the test is considered positive and indicative of subscapularis insufficiency. For patients who are unable to reach behind their back, the belly press test can be used to evaluate the subscapularis. The belly press test is performed by having the patient place his or her hands on the abdomen and, while pressing the hands to the abdomen, bringing the elbows anterior to the coronal plane of the body. Inability to perform the belly press maneuver is a positive test. The bear-hug test is performed by having the patient place the pathologic arm in 90° of forward flexion with the hand resting on the contralateral AC joint. The examiner then attempts to lift the hand off the contralateral shoulder by applying an external rotation force to the forearm. Inability of the patient to actively maintain hand position on the contralateral shoulder is positive and indicative of subscapularis pathology.

Biceps Tendon (Long Head and Superior Labrum)

Speed's test is used to evaluate the long head of the biceps tendon. The test is performed by having the patient maintain forward elevation of the upper extremity at shoulder height against resistance with the elbow extended and the forearm supinated. The test is considered positive when pain is produced in the area of the bicipital groove with the maneuver. Yergason's test is performed by having the patient actively supinate the forearm against resistance with the arm at the side and the elbow in 90° of flexion. A positive finding for biceps pathology is seen with pain localized to the bicipital groove.

The active-compression test, or O'Brien's test, is used to evaluate the superior labral-biceps tendon complex. The test is performed in two steps. The upper extremity is brought to shoulder height in forward flexion with the forearm fully pronated (thumb down) and adducted approximately 15°. The patient resists the examiner's downward pressure from this position. If this maneuver elicits pain in the shoulder, the test is repeated with the forearm supinated. If the pain is reduced or absent with the second maneuver, the test is considered positive. A positive test indicates that the biceps tendon-superior labral complex is torn or detached from the superior glenoid. The examiner should be aware that pain localized to the top of the shoulder during active-compression testing is likely related to the AC joint rather than the superior labrum. Cross-body adduction testing, positive with pain when the shoulder is flexed to 90° and the arm passively adducted across the body, is indicative of AC joint pathology and can be used to differentiate AC joint pain from labral pathology in the setting of an uncertain active-compression finding.

Shoulder Instability

A number of tests have been described to evaluate shoulder instability. All of the following tests can be performed with the patient supine on the examining table. The apprehension test is performed with the shoulder abducted to 90° and externally rotated to 90° in the coronal plane of the body. From this position, the examiner continues to externally rotate the shoulder. If the patient experiences apprehension (fear of the shoulder dislocating), the test is considered positive. If the patient has a positive apprehension test, the examiner can reduce the subluxated humeral head by applying a posterior directed force against the proximal humerus, thereby reducing the humeral head. If the apprehension is relieved, the relocation test is positive. The examiner can then release the proximal humerus. If apprehension recurs with release of the posterior directed force, the release test is positive. The posterior apprehension test employs a similar concept, but with the arm in a position at risk for posterior instability. The shoulder and elbow are flexed 90° with the arm in adduction and internal rotation. The examiner stabilizes the scapula with one hand while applying a posteriorly directed axial load through the elbow. Posterior apprehension is positive when pain or apprehension is elicited.

The load-and-shift test is used to assess the direction and degree of shoulder laxity. The examiner uses one hand to apply a longitudinal load to the humerus directed toward the glenohumeral joint. This hand is located at the elbow with the elbow flexed. The other hand is used to apply a perpendicular force to the proximal humeral shaft in an attempt to shift (subluxate or dislocate) the humeral head relative to the glenoid. The test is performed while maintaining the upper extremity in the coronal plane of the body. The degree of abduction/rotation and the direction of the applied force can be varied to evaluate the various glenohumeral ligaments. The test is graded by the examiner who determines through tactile sense whether the humeral head translates to the glenoid rim (1+); over the glenoid rim but spontaneously reduces (2+); or over the rim requiring manual reduction (3+). This test is often more useful in the anesthetized patient due to guarding in the awake patient.

Imaging Studies and Other Diagnostic Tests

The use of routine imaging studies and tests to evaluate the shoulder girdle for diagnostic purposes is not recommended. At the conclusion of the history and physical examination, the examiner should have a reasonable diagnosis. Additional tests or studies are used to answer specific questions. If the clinical diagnosis is frozen shoulder but the examiner is concerned that the patient has glenohumeral arthritis, it is reasonable to order radiographs to rule out osteoarthritis since the natural history and treatment of osteoarthritis and adhesive capsulitis are dissimilar. If the clinical diagnosis is rotator cuff impingement or tendonitis, there is no reason to obtain further studies initially as they will not change the recommended course of treatment.

Radiographs

The standard shoulder series includes an anteroposterior (AP) X-ray in the plane of the scapula; a Y-outlet view; and an axillary view. This series of X-rays is mandatory in the evaluation of shoulder girdle trauma. Unfortunately, the axillary view is often not obtained, yet it is the most sensitive for documenting shoulder dislocations. The Velpeau view may replace the axillary view if the patient is not able to participate in the axillary view due to pain or range of motion restrictions. AP views with the humerus internally and externally rotated may be used to critically evaluate greater tuberosity fractures or calcific tendinitis. The scapula is approximately 30° oblique to the coronal plane of the body; therefore, in order to obtain a true AP view of the glenohumeral joint, the X-ray beam must be obliquely oriented to the coronal plane of the body (Fig. 9.5). The AP view is useful for evaluating the clavicle, AC joint, glenohumeral joint space, glenoid, scapular body, proximal humeral shaft, surgical neck, and greater tuberosity. The Y-outlet view is useful for evaluating the scapular spine, scapular body, cor-

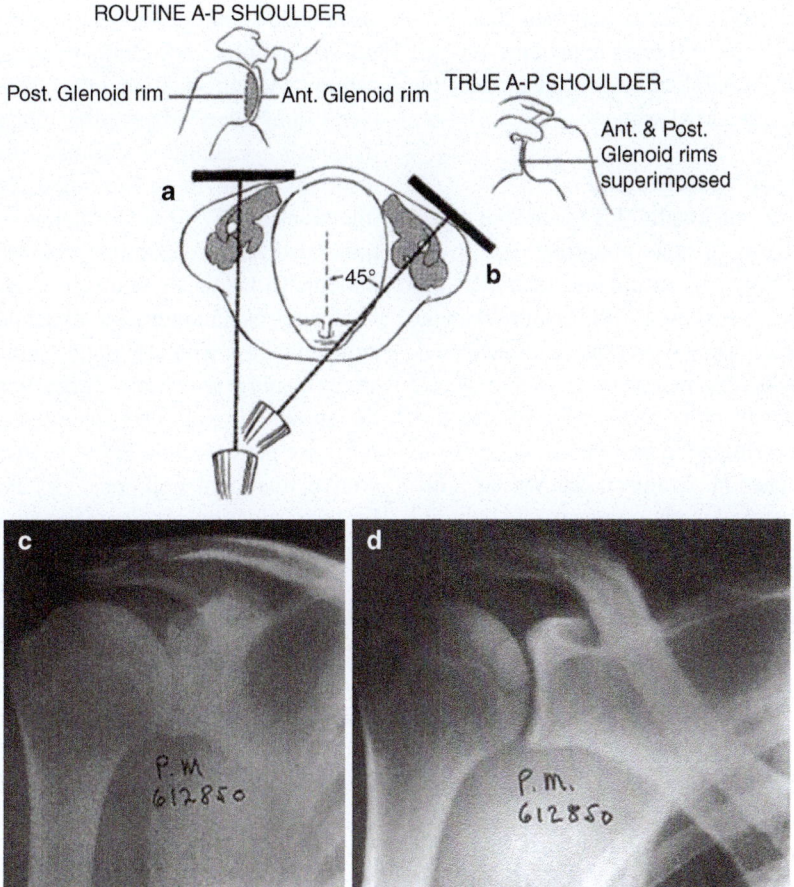

Fig. 9.5 These illustrations and X-rays demonstrated the importance of obtaining a "true" anteroposterior (AP) perspective of the glenohumeral joint. In X-ray (**a**), note that the AP view is actually one of the thoraxes, yielding an X-ray which shows overlap of the glenohumeral joint. When the beam is angled, however, as in (**b**), a "true" AP view of the glenohumeral joint is obtained. Note the differences in appearance in these views in (**c**) (AP view of the thorax) and (**d**) (true AP view of the glenohumeral joint). (From Rockwood CA Jr., Matsen FA III eds. *The Shoulder*. Vol 1. Philadelphia, PA: Saunders; 1990. Reprinted with permission)

acoid, shape of the acromion, and spur formation in the CA ligament. The axillary view is critical in evaluating glenohumeral joint congruence. Anterior or posterior dislocations are best seen on the axillary view.

Magnetic Resonance Imaging

The magnetic resonance imaging (MRI) scan is commonly employed to evaluate the soft tissues of the shoulder girdle and is considered the gold standard for evaluating the rotator cuff tendons. Subacromial fluid, tendon inflammation, and rotator cuff tears are all visible with MR imaging. MRI scans can be performed with an arthrogram (intra-articular contrast dye) to better delineate intra-articular structures such as labral tears and articular-sided partial rotator cuff tears. Standard MRI views of the shoulder include coronal oblique, sagittal oblique, and axial cuts. The coronal and sagittal views are termed oblique because they are obtained in the plane of the scapula which is oblique to the coronal and sagittal planes of the body. Although the MRI scan is a powerful tool in the evaluation of shoulder problems, it is a very sensitive test. Positive findings, therefore, may correlate poorly with a patient's clinical presentation. For example, MRI scans obtained on patients with normal, pain-free shoulders have documented a greater than 50% incidence of rotator cuff tears in patients over the age of 60. It is therefore important to treat the patient and not the MRI scan.

Computerized Tomography

Computerized tomography (CT) scans are useful in the evaluation of bone abnormalities. In the setting of complex or comminuted shoulder girdle fractures, CT scanning with or without image reconstruction is a powerful tool for clinical decision making and/or preoperative planning. CT scans are useful in the evaluation of shoulder instability, providing the best characterization of humeral impaction fractures, known as Hill-Sachs lesions, and both posterior and anterior glenoid bone loss. CT scans are also valuable in assessing bone deficiencies such as glenoid wear and are commonly obtained prior to shoulder arthroplasty in any patients with significant glenoid deformity.

Electrodiagnostic Testing

Electromyography (EMG) and nerve conduction velocity (NCV) testing are commonly used to evaluate neurologic lesions of the shoulder girdle. EMG testing involves placing small needle electrodes into the muscles to record resting potentials and firing patterns. NCV testing is used to document the speed with which an impulse is conducted along a peripheral nerve. Abnormalities such as a conduction block may indicate severe nerve injury. Electrodiagnostic testing is useful in documenting both the presence and recovery of peripheral nerve lesions as well as identifying the anatomic origin of nerve compression.

Evaluation and Treatment of Common Shoulder Problems

The majority of common shoulder girdle problems result from degenerative changes, overuse, or traumatic injury. Atraumatic shoulder pain is common and includes rotator cuff disease, arthropathy, adhesive capsulitis, calcific tendinitis, and multidirectional instability. Most

atraumatic shoulder pain is initially treated with activity modification, anti-inflammatory medication, and physical therapy. Treatment regimens may vary depending on the specific diagnosis. Calcific tendinitis, for example, responds well to subacromial corticosteroid injections. The physical therapy prescription may also vary depending on the diagnosis. Patients with adhesive capsulitis require stretching exercises, in contrast to patients with rotator cuff tendonitis who are treated with rotator cuff strengthening exercises. Surgical treatment in the atraumatic population is generally reserved for those patients who fail to respond to nonoperative treatment regimens. A basic algorithm for the evaluation of atraumatic shoulder pain is provided in Fig. 9.6.

Traumatic injuries to the shoulder girdle are common and include both soft tissue and bony injury. Treatment is individualized based on the age of the patient, functional status of the patient, and the severity of the injury. Depending on the injury, nonoperative or operative treatment may be appropriate. Common traumatic injuries to the shoulder girdle include shoulder dislocations, AC joint injuries, clavicle fractures, and proximal humerus fractures and are reviewed in the skeletal trauma chapter. Contrary to popular belief, traumatic rotator cuff tears are relatively uncommon although they should always be considered in the setting of weakness following a traumatic injury to the shoulder.

Rotator Cuff Disease

Degenerative and overuse injuries of the rotator cuff (RC) are common sources of shoulder pain and disability. Anterosuperior shoulder pain emanating from the rotator cuff under the coracoacromial arch has historically been called impingement syndrome, encompassing a spectrum of pathology in the subacromial region including subacromial bursitis, RC tendinopathy, partial-thickness RC tears, and full-thickness RC tears. Abnormalities in scapulothoracic movement, also known as scapular dyskinesia, may contribute to symptoms of impingement. Partial

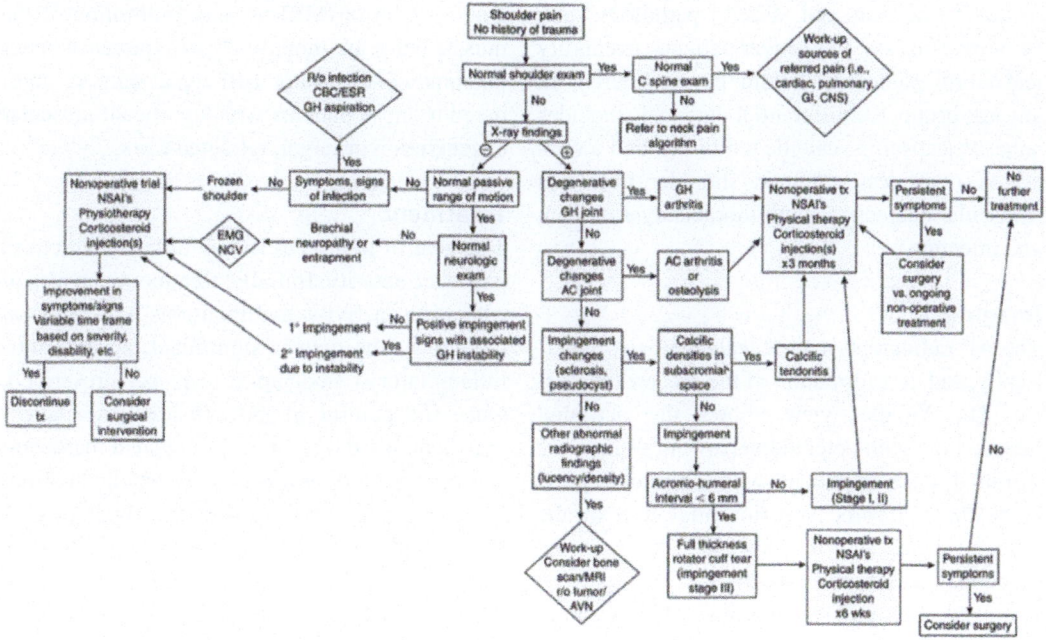

Fig. 9.6 Algorithmic approach to the diagnosis and treatment of atraumatic shoulder pain

and full-thickness tears of the rotator cuff become more prevalent with increasing age. It is unusual for patients under the age of 40 years to present with rotator cuff tears in the absence of significant trauma. Conversely, older patients may present with massive rotator cuff tears after an innocuous event. There are two main theories which attempt to explain such degenerative cuff tears. The external impingement model suggests an extrinsic cause of rotator cuff tears such as abrasion of the anterosuperior cuff under the acromion and coracoacromial arch. The intrinsic model suggests that a relatively poor blood supply to the critical zone of the rotator cuff in combination with high stresses across the cuff leads to RC tears. The true pathophysiology likely results from a combination of these models.

History

The chief complaint is usually anterosuperior shoulder pain which often radiates to the lateral deltoid region. The pain is typically worse with overhead activities, arm movements away from the body, and at night. The patient may recall a minor traumatic event, or the pain may have started insidiously.

Examination

Inspection of the shoulder girdle usually reveals symmetry, but patients with degenerative cuff tears may present with atrophy of the supra- or infraspinatus fossae. The patient typically has discrete tenderness at the cuff insertion on the greater tuberosity. The active range of motion is generally normal; however, some patients with large RC tears may exhibit loss of active motion with preservation of passive motion. In this setting, the clinician may be able to document lag signs. Strength testing may reveal weakness of the supraspinatus or infraspinatus tendons. Special tests include the Neer and Hawkins's impingement signs. If the patient has concomitant biceps tendon pathology, there may be tenderness at the bicipital groove and Speed's test may be positive. Tenderness over the AC joint may indicate that the AC joint is contributing to the painful condition. A cross-body adduction test recreating pain at the AC joint is considered confirmatory.

Differential Diagnosis

The differential diagnosis varies with the age of the patient. In older patients, the differential diagnosis includes arthritis, cervical spine pathology, metastatic disease, and visceral pathology such as cardiac disease. In younger patients, instability and labral pathology should be considered. In any age group, the differential diagnosis includes adhesive capsulitis, calcific tendinitis, and a variety of other less common shoulder problems (avascular necrosis, scapulothoracic dysfunction, and infection).

Imaging

The AP radiograph may reveal sclerosis, hypertrophy, and cyst formation of the greater tuberosity. The Y-outlet view shows the acromial morphology with potential narrowing of the subacromial space. In patients with longstanding RC tears, there may be superior migration of the humeral head and the distance between the humerus and acromion on the AP view may be narrowed. The axillary view illustrates the joint space and may reveal an os acromiale. An MRI scan is useful for a number of reasons. Confirmation of rotator cuff disease (and exclusion of other etiologies) is reassuring, but not necessary. The MRI scan is extremely useful for assessing the RC tendons and muscle bellies (Fig. 9.7). The presence, size, and chronicity of a RC tear directly impacts patient care (surgical options), recovery, and, ultimately, prognosis. Patients with smaller tears and less muscle degen-

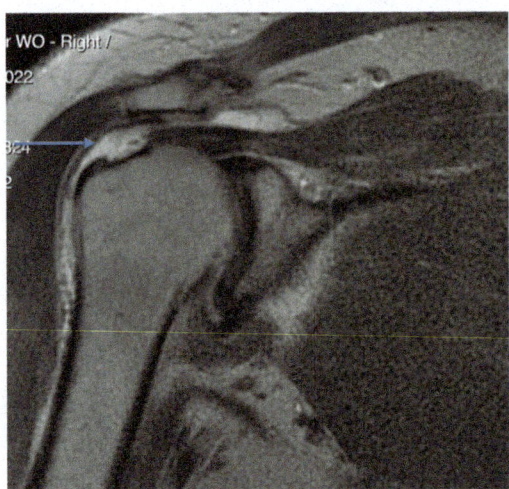

Fig. 9.7 A tear of the supraspinatus tendon with fluid in the gap is appreciated in this coronal oblique magnetic resonance imaging (MRI) scan of the glenohumeral joint

eration, seen on MRI as fatty infiltration of the muscle belly, are more likely to experience better outcomes after rotator cuff repair surgery compared to those patients with significant muscular degeneration or larger, retracted tears.

Treatment

The goal of treatment is to return the patient to pain-free activity. Initially, treatment consists of education, activity modifications and physical therapy. If the pain is significant, an oral anti-inflammatory medication can be prescribed. Once the painful period subsides, the patient may benefit from a course of physical therapy to strengthen the rotator cuff and scapular stabilizers, stretch any stiff regions, and improve posture. A subacromial corticosteroid injection can be considered in a patient who fails to respond to the initial treatment over 1–2 months or patients with so much initial pain that they cannot participate in physical therapy. Patients who fail to respond to nonoperative management over 3–6 months may benefit from surgical treatment. Most surgeons will obtain an MRI scan to assess the degree of rotator cuff pathology or tear prior to surgical treatment. For patients who present with rotator cuff symptoms and weakness after an initial traumatic event, MRI may be warranted to assess for rotator cuff tearing and to determine if surgical intervention is indicated.

In the absence of a rotator cuff tear, surgeons may recommend arthroscopic subacromial decompression. This involves removing the inflamed subacromial bursa, releasing the coracoacromial ligament, and shaving the undersurface of the acromion (acromioplasty) to create more room in the subacromial space for the rotator cuff. Subacromial decompression is rarely needed as an isolated procedure since the vast majority of patients without a full-thickness rotator cuff tear will improve with the nonoperative management strategies described above.

Patients who have reparable RC tears are treated with primary repair, and most surgeons will perform an acromioplasty, especially if there is a downsloping acromion or large bone spur, although several studies suggest this may be unnecessary. RC repairs can be done with open, mini-open, and arthroscopic techniques (Fig. 9.8). Arthroscopic rotator cuff repair has become the standard of care as it allows for better visualization of the tear pattern and a more anatomic repair. Results of arthroscopic repair are now equivalent or superior to open repair in recent studies.

Care should be taken to preserve the CA ligament in patients with large tears and multiple tendon tears to prevent superior migration of the humeral head if the repair fails. There are a variety of options for patients with irreparable tears, including arthroscopic debridement, partial tendon repair, superior capsular reconstruction, and tendon transfers. Rotator cuff arthropathy is the end-stage of irreparable rotator cuff disease, and will be discussed, along with treatment options, in the next section. If biceps tendon pathology is found at the time of surgery, either tenodesis or tenotomy can be performed. Patients who are noted to have AC joint arthropathy and pain prior to surgery may benefit from a distal clavicle resection, which can also be done arthroscopically. Recovery

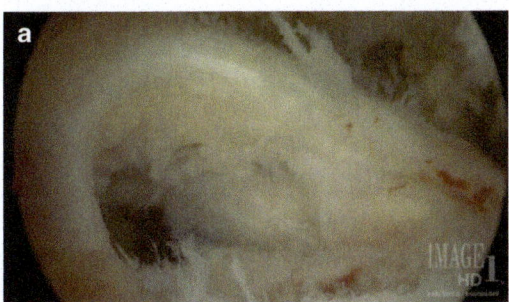
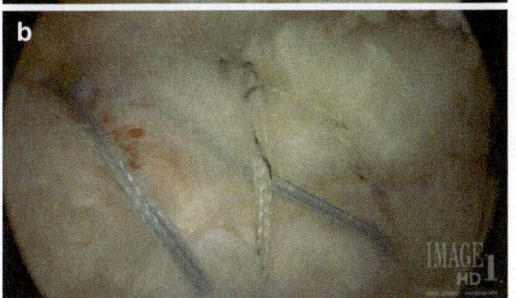

Fig. 9.8 (**a**) Arthroscopic photography of a right shoulder with a full-thickness tear of the supraspinatus tendon. (**b**) Arthroscopic photography following arthroscopic repair of the tear with suture anchors

from RC surgery can take anywhere from 4 to 6 months. The goal of early (4–10 weeks) post-operative physical therapy is recovery of passive shoulder motion. Restoration of strength and function is the goal of subsequent postoperative therapy. Failure of the patient to adhere to postoperative physical therapy can result in a poor outcome. New work is underway to explore biological augmentation to rotator cuff repair in order to improve healing rates, especially in degenerative and irreparable tears.

Rotator Cuff Arthropathy

Rotator cuff arthropathy (RCA) is the end-stage outcome of rotator cuff disease often resulting in significant shoulder pain and dysfunction. The primary roles of the rotator cuff are to stabilize the humeral head in the glenoid fossa throughout shoulder motion and to create a force couple with the deltoid to enable effective overhead shoulder motion. When chronic rotator cuff injury with degeneration is present, a variety of clinical and radiographic findings can be seen. The spectrum of dysfunction ranges with the severity of the condition and the physical demands on the individual patient. Although less active patients are sometimes able to compensate for their dysfunction with scapulothoracic mobility or the contralateral arm, many patients present with complaints of pain with motion, significant weakness, or pseudoparalysis. There is characteristic anterior-superior escape of the humerus, as the shoulder loses the inferior and medial directed stabilizing force of the rotator cuff.

History
Patients will often complain of chronic pain and weakness with shoulder elevation and movements away from the body. In patients without associated arthritis, pain will often be limited at rest. Night pain is common and patients often report being unable to sleep on the affected side.

Examination
Inspection may demonstrate disuse atrophy of the shoulder girdle. Passive range of motion will

be intact prior to the development of arthritis, with significantly limited active range of motion, especially in forward elevation. As arthritis progresses, passive range of motion will become progressively restricted. There will be significant weakness in rotator cuff testing, and lag signs can be seen most commonly in forward flexion, external rotation at the side, and Hornblower's sign in abduction and external rotation. A thorough motor and neurovascular exam should be performed including strength testing of all three heads of the deltoid.

Differential Diagnosis

The spectrum of rotator cuff disease including tendonitis and rotator cuff tear will have a similar presentation. Adhesive capsulitis may cause a similar degree of dysfunction, but with limited passive motion and lacking radiographic pathology. It is important to differentiate RCA from osteoarthritis (where the rotator cuff is typically intact), as this distinction may influence surgical decision-making.

Imaging

A standard shoulder X-ray series combined with physical examination is usually sufficient for diagnosis. The AP radiograph may show superior translation of the humerus, calcification of the CA ligament, and acetabularization of the CA arch with femoralization of the humeral head. The Scapular-Y view will show loss of the subacromial space, and the axillary view may show anterior escape of the humeral head. As RCA progresses, all views may demonstrate arthritic progression (Fig. 9.9). Glenoid wear should be evaluated on the AP and axillary radiographs, as superior glenoid wear frequently occurs. If there is severe glenoid deformity, a CT scan can be obtained for surgical planning purposes. Once superior migration of the humeral head is seen on the AP radiograph, MRI of the shoulder is not needed to make the diagnosis of RCA. If an MRI is obtained, it will demonstrate significant rotator cuff pathology often involving massive tears of 2 or more tendons with retraction of the tendon edges past the joint line and atrophy of the rotator cuff muscle bellies.

Treatment

Initial treatment is nonoperative combined with activity modification. Physical therapy includes strengthening the deltoid and remaining rotator cuff muscles to improve function. Oral anti-inflammatories and intra-articular steroid injections may provide pain relief. Nonoperative treatment measures generally provide mild and temporary symptomatic improvement. When nonoperative intervention and activity modification fail to provide adequate relief, operative intervention is indicated.

The primary surgical option for patients with RCA is reverse total shoulder arthroplasty (RTSA). In RTSA, the ball-and-socket anatomy of the shoulder is reversed (Fig. 9.10). The rounded implant, known as the glenosphere, is placed on the glenoid, and the socket is implanted on the humeral side of the shoulder. Reversing the anatomy of the shoulder creates a few significant advantages in the setting of RCA. The shoulder joint becomes more constrained, recreating stability lost with rotator cuff dysfunction and enabling elevation of the shoulder by the deltoid without superior translation of the humeral head. The center of shoulder rotation is moved inferiorly and medially, thereby partially substituting for the inferior, medial, and compressive force of the rotator cuff that enables effective force coupling with the deltoid in the native shoulder. An increased deltoid moment arm and higher deltoid muscle tension increases the stability of the shoulder and efficacy of the deltoid to elevate the arm without the assistance of the rotator cuff musculature. Overall, RTSA is a highly effective procedure that provides durable relief for patients with significant pain and functional limitations.

Osteoarthritis

Degenerative arthritis, or osteoarthritis (OA), occurs in the glenohumeral joint but is less common than in the hip or knee joints. Osteoarthritis of the glenohumeral joint has the same pathophysiology as in other joints with progressive articular cartilage destruction.

Fig. 9.9 AP, scapular-Y, and axillary radiographic views of a shoulder with rotator cuff arthropathy. Characteristic superior and anterior escape can be seen as well as greater tuberosity hypertrophy and coracoacromial calcification

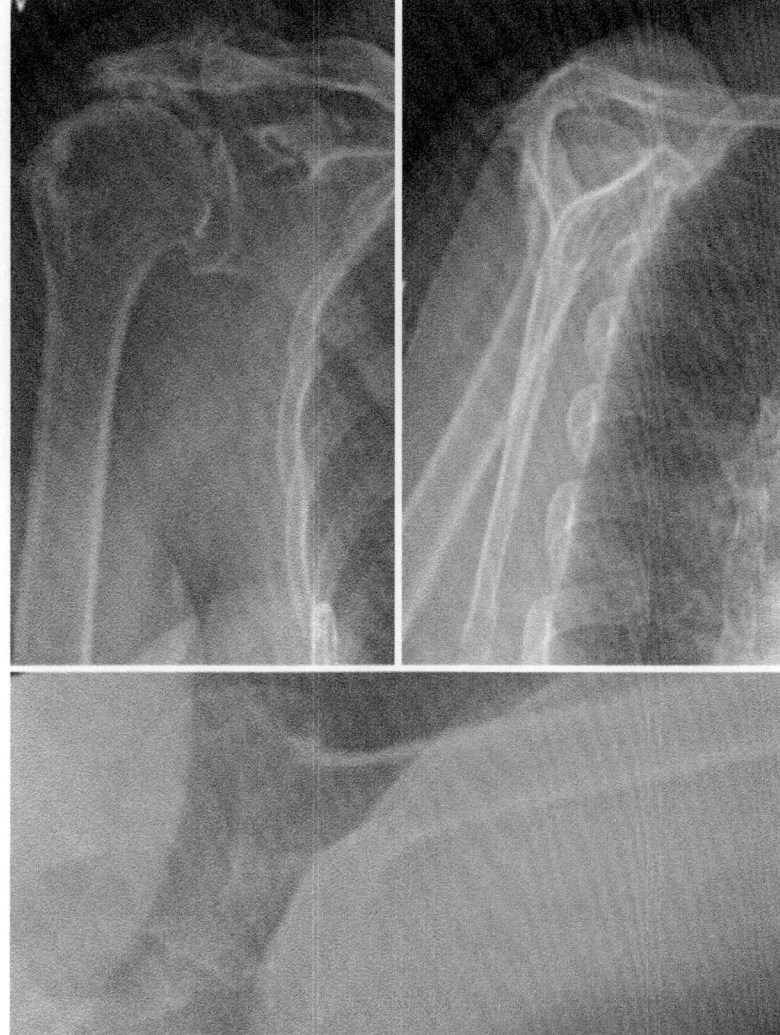

History

Patients with early osteoarthritis may have a clinical syndrome that is virtually indistinguishable from impingement syndrome. In patients with advanced osteoarthritis, pain is more likely to be chronic, occur at rest, and be resistant to standard analgesics and anti-inflammatory medications. In addition, loss of shoulder motion is a common complaint. Patients may have trouble sleeping, often not able to sleep on the affected shoulder.

Examination

Patients with early osteoarthritis may examine similarly to those with impingement syndrome. In more advanced OA, generalized disuse atrophy of the shoulder girdle may be noticeable and there is often significant crepitus of the glenohumeral joint. In general, there is a progressive loss of active motion in all planes, but loss of external rotation with the arm at the side is often the most dramatic. Passive motion is similarly decreased and there is often a significant amount of pain associated with passive stretching of the joint capsule near the end ranges of motion. It is important to look for scars indicative of prior surgeries to the shoulder. A thorough strength and neurovascular exam should also be performed, paying specific attention to axillary nerve function, along with deltoid and rotator cuff strength.

Fig. 9.10 AP, scapular-Y, and axillary views of a patient with rotator cuff arthropathy after reverse total shoulder arthroplasty

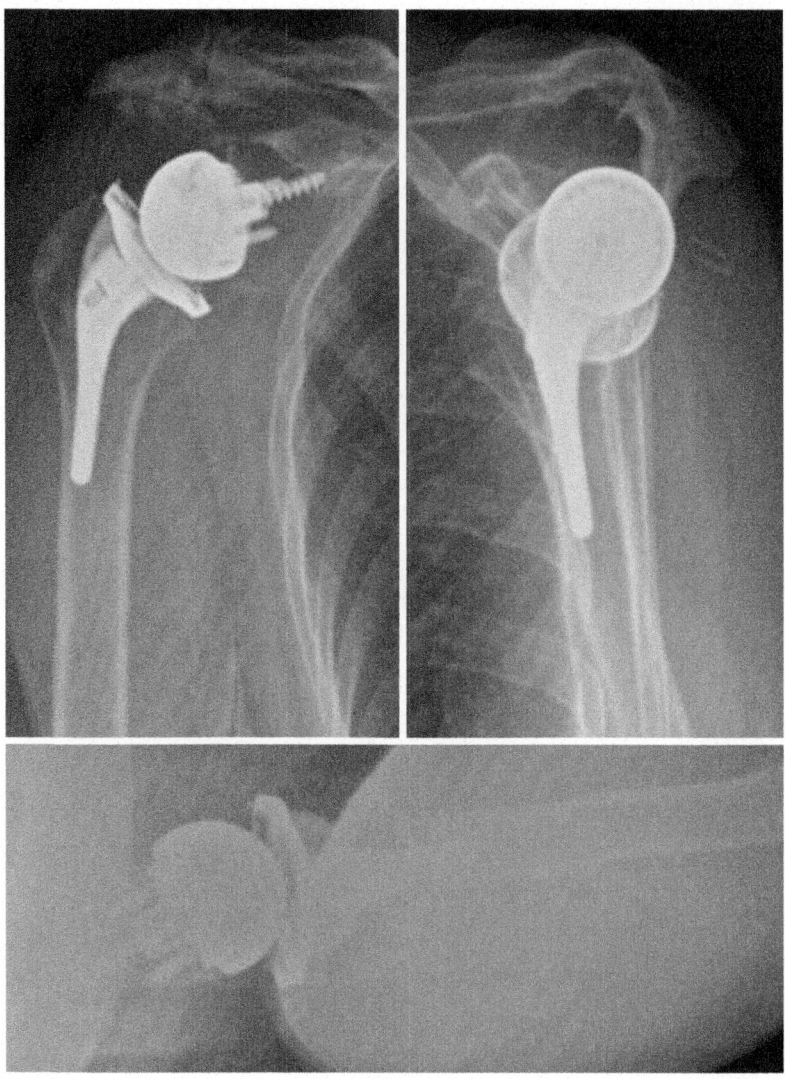

Differential Diagnosis

Adhesive capsulitis can have a similar presentation to and is distinguished from glenohumeral arthritis via radiography. Inflammatory arthropathy and septic arthritis can have similar presentations, with medical history, onset, and signs of infection differentiating these conditions. The examiner must have a high index of suspicion for locked posterior shoulder dislocations in older patients who are poor historians as a result of dementia or stroke.

Imaging

A standard shoulder series is recommended. Joint space narrowing, subchondral sclerosis, osteophytes, and subchondral cyst formation are classic findings in osteoarthritis and are best seen on the AP and axillary view (Fig. 9.11). In the glenohumeral joint, inferior humeral osteophytes predominate. Often, eccentric posterior glenoid wear is present. MRI scans are generally not used in the evaluation of OA. A CT scan to assess the glenoid for eccentric wear or bone loss is common during preoperative evaluation for shoulder arthroplasty. In patients with greater deformity, many surgeons will utilize 3-D surgical planning software prior to shoulder replacement surgery to create preoperative shoulder templates from CT scans.

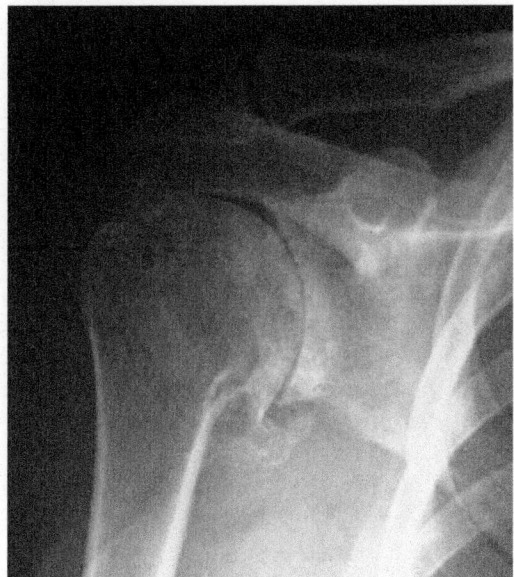

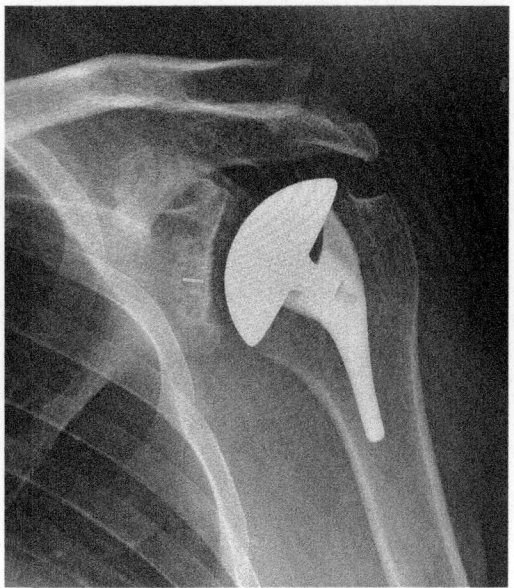

Fig. 9.11 All of the classic findings of osteoarthritis are present in this true AP X-ray of the glenohumeral joint, including joint space narrowing, subchondral sclerosis, osteophyte formation, and subchondral cyst formation

Fig. 9.12 A total shoulder arthroplasty is demonstrated in this true AP X-ray of the glenohumeral joint. This metallic humeral component is placed via press-fit into the proximal humerus but may also be cemented. The pegged polyethylene glenoid component is cemented into the glenoid and is represented by the reproduction of the joint space. The central peg of the polyethylene glenoid component is identified by the horizontal radiopaque marker

Treatment

Initial treatment for OA includes education, rest, activity modification, and anti-inflammatory medications. Physical therapy for stretching and maintenance of motion is an important component of nonoperative treatment. Intra-articular corticosteroid injections often delay the need for surgical intervention but provide inconsistent and incomplete pain relief in this setting. When nonoperative management is no longer able to control the patient's pain, surgical management is a reasonable option. In select younger patients with concentric wear, some joint space preservation, and reasonable motion, improved symptoms may be obtained from arthroscopic debridement. The goal of debridement is pain relief and postponement of prosthetic joint arthroplasty. This intervention may include a combination of loose body removal, osteophyte debridement, chondroplasty, capsular releases, subacromial decompression, biceps tenodesis, and axillary neurolysis.

In the setting of painful, end-stage OA, prosthetic joint replacement with either an anatomic total shoulder arthroplasty (aTSA) (Fig. 9.12) or RTSA is recommended, depending on the amount of bony deformity and status of the rotator cuff. For aTSA, a plastic glenoid component is cemented onto the patient's glenoid in addition to replacement of the humeral head. aTSA introduces the risk of glenoid-sided prosthetic loosening and wear which may require revision surgery and, similar to a native shoulder, requires a well-functioning rotator cuff for good shoulder function. Similar to the reverse shoulder arthroplasty, surgery is performed via the deltopectoral interval. The subscapularis muscle must be detached in order to access the joint. The muscle is repaired following placement of the implant, but the repair must be protected during the early phase (first 6 weeks) of postoperative rehabilitation, as the survival of the anatomic arthroplasty is dependent on the healing of the subscapularis. In many situations, especially in older patients who may have degeneration of the rotator cuff or patients with significant boney deformity, RTSA is now being used to treat patients with glenohumeral arthritis.

Miscellaneous Arthropathy

A variety of other disease processes can lead to glenohumeral joint destruction. Inflammatory arthropathy, such as rheumatoid arthritis, can lead to joint destruction as a result of synovial disease. While the clinical presentation may be similar to osteoarthritis with pain and loss of motion, there are some important differences. In particular, rheumatoid arthritis can result in rotator cuff deficiency and incompetence. In these patients, anatomic total shoulder arthroplasty is contraindicated since glenoid loosening in the setting of rotator cuff deficiency is a common problem. If arthroplasty is required in the setting of significant destruction of the rotator cuff, then reverse total shoulder arthroplasty is the procedure of choice. Progressive bony destruction of the humeral head and glenoid can result from rheumatoid arthritis, making prosthetic arthroplasty difficult. Avascular necrosis can occur as a result of trauma, corticosteroid use, alcoholism, and other less common etiologies. Avascular necrosis of the humeral head can lead to pain and loss of motion in the glenohumeral joint. Hemiarthroplasty is an option for young patients with humeral head collapse and chronic pain. Total shoulder arthroplasty is indicated when secondary destruction of the glenoid is present. Charcot or neuropathic arthropathy is typically a painless condition that results in severe joint destruction. Charcot arthropathy in the glenohumeral joint is commonly related to a cervical spine syrinx and an MRI of the cervical spine should be obtained in any patient presenting with possible Charcot arthropathy. There are no reliable surgical options for Charcot arthropathy.

Adhesive Capsulitis

Adhesive capsulitis, or frozen shoulder, is a painful condition in which the synovial lining of the glenohumeral joint is inflamed. Adhesive capsulitis is a clinical diagnosis in which examination reveals an equal loss of active and passive motion. Primary adhesive capsulitis is idiopathic meaning that no trigger can be identified. It occurs in middle-aged persons and is associated with dia-

betes and thyroid dysfunction. Secondary adhesive capsulitis implies that a trigger or cause of the disease process can be identified. Trauma, surgery, and concomitant shoulder girdle pathology may result in secondary adhesive capsulitis.

History
The patient reports an insidious onset of shoulder pain and progressive decreased range of motion. Pain often occurs during rotational movements such as reaching behind the back, putting on a coat, or fastening a bra. Often the patient may recall a minor event that precipitated the condition. Pain at night is common. It is important to obtain a past medical and surgical history to identify possible risk factors. Insulin-dependent diabetes is a strong risk factor for adhesive capsulitis. Symptoms may depend on the stage of the disease: the initial inflammatory phase will manifest as pain throughout the range of motion, whereas during the frozen phase patients will report significant motion restrictions and pain at the end range of motion.

Examination
In the absence of prior trauma or surgery to the shoulder girdle, the inspection and palpation portions of the exam are usually unremarkable. Active motion can be extremely limited in all planes of motion, and the passive motion is similarly restricted. The patient often experiences pain at the end range of motion (active or passive). Rotator cuff strength is intact within the confines of the limited motion.

Differential Diagnosis
Early adhesive capsulitis can mimic rotator cuff pathology. Subtle losses of internal and external rotation in abduction may be the only clues to differentiate between the two diagnoses. Unrecognized trauma (locked posterior shoulder dislocations) and glenohumeral joint arthropathy can mimic adhesive capsulitis, but these entities can be easily excluded with standard radiographs.

Imaging
A standard shoulder series is useful in excluding other diagnoses; however, there are no radiographic findings for adhesive capsulitis. MRI may demonstrate general inflammation and cap-

sular thickening but is not routinely ordered unless there is concern for concomitant pathology such as rotator cuff tear, and further studies are generally not indicated unless additional pathology is suspected.

Treatment

Once the diagnosis is made, education of the patient is paramount. In general, the treatment of adhesive capsulitis is twofold: treatment of the synovial inflammation and restoration of motion. Anti-inflammatory medications can be used, but a corticosteroid injection into the glenohumeral joint space is more efficient and effective for treating the synovial inflammation. Patients should be educated that the goal of inflammation control is to relieve pain, so they are able to participate fully in stretching and physical therapy. The patient must start a stretching program to regain motion in all planes. Initially, supervised physical therapy is helpful, but the patient must independently perform a battery of home stretching exercises daily. A gradual restoration of motion is the anticipated course although this can often take 12–18 months. In patients who fail to show any response to nonoperative treatment after 3–6 months, surgery may be a reasonable option. Historically, patients with diabetes have a higher failure rate of nonoperative treatment compared to patients without risk factors. Additionally, patients with secondary adhesive capsulitis from trauma or prior shoulder surgery often fail to respond fully to nonoperative treatment. Manipulation of the shoulder under anesthesia was once the preferred treatment and continues to be a reasonable option. However, proximal humerus fractures can occur with manipulations under anesthesia, and osteoporosis is a risk factor for this complication. Arthroscopic capsular release is a more invasive, yet more anatomic, procedure. The surgery involves releasing the shoulder capsule under direct vision with a combination of biters and electrofrequency devices. The axillary nerve is at particular risk during release of the inferior capsule. Aggressive physical therapy with active-assisted and active range of motion is mandatory to maintain the postoperative range of motion and should be started on the day of surgery. Shoulder strengthening and resistance therapy is instituted only after restoration of full, active shoulder motion.

Calcific Tendinitis

Calcific tendinitis of the rotator cuff is a painful condition of the shoulder girdle and is a common clinical problem (Fig. 9.13). The etiology of calcific tendinitis is a matter of debate. The pathogenesis of calcifying tendinitis includes various stages of tendon degeneration, calcium deposition, and calcium resorption. In the formative phase of calcium deposition, there may be little or no pain. Typically, the resorptive phase is more painful and clinically relevant, related to the inflammatory process of calcium resorption.

History

In the resorptive phase, the patient may present with an acute onset of severe shoulder pain that may mimic a septic shoulder joint. In the formative phase, the patient may present with more chronic symptoms that mimic impingement syndrome.

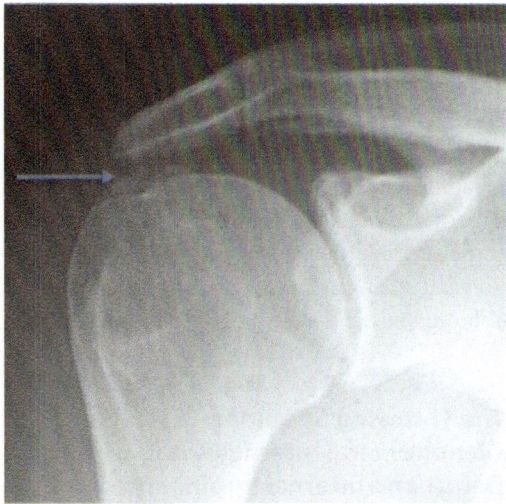

Fig. 9.13 A calcium deposit is present in the supraspinatus tendon immediately medial to its attachment site on the greater tuberosity in this true AP X-ray of the glenohumeral joint

Examination

Acute bursitis in the resorptive phase may lead to fullness of the anterosuperior shoulder, but otherwise the inspection is typically unremarkable. Typically, there is tenderness at the rotator cuff insertion corresponding to the calcium deposition. There may be a loss of active motion secondary to pain, but passive motion and rotator cuff strength testing, although painful, is generally intact. Impingement signs are often positive.

Differential Diagnosis

The differential diagnosis includes rotator cuff disease and adhesive capsulitis. Referred pain from cardiac origin or other visceral organs and radicular pain from the cervical spine should be considered. Septic arthritis may need to be ruled out in the acute, severely painful phase.

Imaging

The appearance of calcific tendinitis on radiographs varies depending on the phase of the disease. In the formative phase, the calcium deposit is usually well circumscribed and easily identified. In the resorptive phase, the deposit may appear fluffy and less well defined. In addition to the standard shoulder series, internal and external rotational AP views can be helpful for identifying more subtle deposits. Additional studies are not usually indicated.

Treatment

Treatment generally involves pain management. Noninvasive treatment options include anti-inflammatory medications and extra-corporeal shock wave therapy. More invasive options include corticosteroid injections and lavage therapy. Surgical treatment is a last resort and involves arthroscopic debridement of the calcium deposit.

The Throwing Shoulder: Glenohumeral Internal Rotation Deficit and Internal Impingement

Glenohumeral internal rotation deficit (GIRD) results from a physiologic adaptation in the osseous structure and capsular balance to repetitive overhead throwing activities. A thickened, contracted posterior capsule is a hallmark of GIRD, leading to an anterior humeral shift and the characteristic loss of shoulder internal rotation compared to the contralateral side. GIRD is a risk factor for the development of symptomatic pathology, especially internal impingement. Internal impingement is abnormal contact between the greater tuberosity or rotator cuff and the posterior glenoid or superior labrum in the abducted and externally rotated shoulder position. This impingement can be symptomatic, and it may lead to other attritional pathology including partial-thickness articular-sided rotator cuff tears, posterior labral tears, or SLAP tears (Fig. 9.14).

History

Symptomatic patients with GIRD will localize pain posteriorly and deep in the shoulder, worst in the late cocking phase of the throwing motion. Throwing athletes may also complain of decreased velocity and loss of throwing control. Patients will often have no pain at rest. Onset of symptoms is generally insidious, without an inciting event.

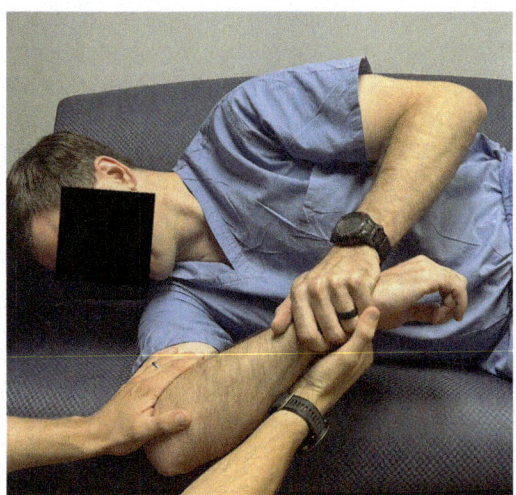

Fig. 9.14 Patient participating in sleeper stretch, moving hand down towards the table to create shoulder internal rotation and stretch the posterior shoulder capsule

Examination

The hallmark of GIRD is decreased shoulder internal rotation in the throwing side compared to the contralateral shoulder. As mentioned earlier, the throwing side almost always has an increase in external rotation and a decrease in internal rotation when compared to the opposite side; however, the total arc of motion should remain the same. In GIRD, the total arc of rotation is reduced due to the pathologic loss of internal rotation. Cross-body adduction may also be limited. Shoulder rotation should be measured with the arm in 90° of abduction. Pain may be elicited with forced shoulder abduction and external rotation. Scapular mechanics should be carefully visualized to identify any winging or dyskinesia. The Jerk and posterior load-and-shift tests are useful for identifying any posterior labral pathology.

Differential Diagnosis

Labral pathology and rotator cuff impingement should be considered. Patients with increased range of motion should be evaluated for multidirectional instability. Physeal injuries should be ruled out in younger throwing athletes.

Imaging

A standard shoulder X-ray series should be used to evaluate for physeal injury in adolescent throwers, often seen as widening of the physis. A Bennett lesion, or posteroinferior extra-articular ossification, may be seen on the axillary radiograph. The axillary may also reveal glenoid retroversion. An MRI or MRA is useful to evaluate for advanced labral pathology, and specifically an MRI with the arm in the abduction external rotation (ABER) position may be useful to evaluate for internal impingement.

Treatment

Most patients will be successfully treated nonoperatively with a focus on physical therapy. Strengthening the lower extremities, core, scapular stabilizers, and rotator cuff is crucial to improve the transfer of energy for throwing and to take stress off the shoulder. Surgical intervention is generally reserved for patients with more advanced pathology.

Superior Labrum and Biceps Tendon Pathology

The long head of the biceps tendon is intimately associated with the superior labrum, as it inserts into the superior labrum and supraglenoid tubercle. Conditions associated with this complex can range from biceps tendinitis to acute or chronic SLAP tear. Injuries generally occur in athletes with repetitive overhead activities such as throwers, volleyball players, and swimmers. Alternatively, acute SLAP tears may occur after single traumatic events that involve traction or compression to the shoulder. Classification of SLAP tears is based on the amount of labral or biceps tendon involvement and the displacement of the injured structure.

History

Patients may complain of pain associated with loss of throwing velocity and stamina. The pain is localized deep in the shoulder joint and may radiate along the proximal biceps tendon. The patient may notice painful shoulder crepitus with throwing and shoulder rotation. The onset and degree of pain will depend on the nature of the injury, but even patients sustaining traumatic SLAP tears may present with chronic symptoms associated with activity.

Examination

Pain may be elicited with palpation of the long head of the biceps tendon. In overhead throwers, the range of motion testing often shows increased external rotation and decreased internal rotation as seen in GIRD. Special tests include Speed's and Yergason's tests, which are commonly positive for weakness or pain in the setting of biceps tendinitis. The O'Brien's active-compression test is sensitive for SLAP tears. Strength testing is generally intact.

Differential Diagnosis

Chronic SLAP tears should be distinguished from GIRD and internal impingement, with one theory suggesting that these are different points in the same pathology spectrum. Rotator cuff tendonitis should be considered in the setting of overuse injury. The differential diagnosis in the setting of a traumatic event includes fracture, dislocation, and rotator cuff injury.

Imaging

A standard shoulder series will rule out fracture about the shoulder girdle. An MRI in acute injuries or MRA in chronic complaints will demonstrate the presence and morphology of a SLAP tear. Discontinuity of and fluid under the superior labrum, tearing of the long head of the biceps tendon, and displacement of the superior labrum or biceps tendon inferiorly are signs of SLAP tear. MRI is also useful to rule out associated diagnoses including Bankart or rotator cuff injuries. MRI will show fluid in the bicipital groove in the setting of biceps tendinitis. MRI should be evaluated with consideration of the history and physical exam, as SLAP tears have been commonly identified on MRI in patients over the age of 30 with asymptomatic shoulders. SLAP tears found on MRI are often not the source of symptoms, and the imaging studies should always be correlated with the complaints of the patient.

Treatment

Initial treatment is nonoperative in the form of rest, anti-inflammatory medications, and physical therapy. Physical therapy will specifically involve strengthening of the rotator cuff and scapular stabilizing musculature, along with posterior capsular stretching. Any motion or core deficits should be addressed. In overhead athletes with attritional pathology, nonoperative management and physical therapy should be trialed for at least 3 months prior to surgical intervention. Surgical treatment is indicated if there is a failure of nonoperative measures, and the type of surgical intervention depends on the patient demographics and type of tear. Surgery is generally arthroscopic, with options including SLAP debridement, repair of the labrum and biceps anchor for any unstable lesions, or biceps tenodesis in patients older than 30–40 years. Any other instability lesions can be addressed at the time of arthroscopy. The surgeon should be cautious when repairing the superior labrum of overhead athletes, as many of these patients will demon-

strate posterosuperior labral instability on arthroscopy related to the physiologic adaptation of the "peel-back" phenomenon. Overhead athletes should be educated that a SLAP repair will likely limit their external rotation capacity after recovery and return to sport, especially at high levels, is unpredictable.

Multidirectional Instability

Shoulder instability is a complex problem with a spectrum of pathology ranging from atraumatic multidirectional shoulder instability to traumatic, unidirectional shoulder dislocations. Multidirectional instability (MDI) generally refers to shoulder pain and disability caused by excessive laxity of the static shoulder stabilizers (capsule and glenohumeral ligaments).

History

In the overhead athlete (pitchers, swimmers, and volleyball players), MDI can present with activity-related pain, scapular winging, and occasionally neurologic symptoms down the arm. Other patients may present with shoulder subluxations and dislocations that may easily reduce on their own but are a significant source of disability and distress to the patient. Patients with generalized laxity or collagen disorders such as Ehlers-Danlos Syndrome may present with multidirectional instability. In these patients, symptoms often develop bilaterally.

Examination

Scapular winging may be noticeable on inspection during range of motion and strength testing. The active and passive ranges of motion are often excessive compared to the average shoulder. Additionally, the patient may exhibit generalized ligamentous laxity at other joints, as measured with the Beighton score. The sulcus sign (hollowing of the subacromial region with downward traction on the arm) may be noticeable and indicative of shoulder laxity. Provocative shoulder testing such as the apprehension or posterior apprehension tests may produce pain rather than apprehension. Other patients may have true apprehension. Load-and-shift testing often reveals subluxation or dislocation in multiple directions.

Differential Diagnosis

The differential diagnosis includes rotator cuff disease, labral pathology, and peripheral nerve injury in the setting of scapular winging.

Imaging

The standard radiographs are typically unremarkable although bony abnormalities such as glenoid hypoplasia can be identified. An MRI arthrogram often does not demonstrate specific structural injuries but can be useful to exclude labral injury (Bankart lesion) and document a patulous capsule.

Treatment

The mainstay of treatment for MDI is rehabilitation. Physical therapy is focused on strengthening the dynamic stabilizers of the shoulder girdle, including the rotator cuff and scapular stabilizers. More specialized therapy can be prescribed for athletes and is based on their specific sport and needs. Patients who fail rehabilitation may be candidates for surgical treatment. In most cases, rehabilitation should be continued for at least 6–12 months. Surgical treatment involves decreasing the volume of the shoulder joint by surgically altering the capsule (capsulorrhaphy). Surgery may be performed by arthroscopic or open methods. Arthroscopic methods tend to preserve motion better and may be preferable in athletes who would not tolerate minor losses of motion. Open surgical treatments historically have had lower rates of recurrent instability. Criticisms of open procedures such as the inferior capsular shift include loss of motion and potential subscapularis deficiency.

Summary

The shoulder is a complex structure that provides tremendous versatility and power to the upper extremity. The majority of painful shoulder girdle conditions are readily diagnosed with a thorough history and physical examination. Successful treatment of shoulder girdle problems is often accomplished by following a relatively simple algorithm of rest, activity modification, nonsteroidal anti-inflammatory drug therapy, and physical therapy. More invasive treatment options, such as arthroscopic and open surgery, are highly effective in appropriately selected patients.

Further Reading

Nicholson G, editor. Orthopaedic knowledge update: shoulder and elbow. 5th ed. Rosemont, IL: American Academy of Orthopaedic Surgeons; 2020.

Iannotti JP, Williams GR Jr, Miniaci A, Zuckerman JD. Disorders of the shoulder: diagnosis & management. 3rd ed. Philadelphia, PA: Lippincott Williams & Wilkins; 2013.

The Spine

10

Joseph L. Ferguson and Douglass C. Johnson

Introduction

In this chapter, we will separate pathology into the cervical and lumbar regions. In the cervical region, the spinal cord is present, and conditions such as myelopathy and cord compression can occur. These occur less frequently in the lumbar spine due to the spinal cord ending at approximately L1–L2 in adults and becoming the cauda equina, a collection of nerve roots traveling distally to their respective foramina. Additionally, the lumbar spine experiences all of the forces of the trunk and torso and is responsible for transmitting these forces to the lower extremities. As a result of these forces, disc herniations, degenerative disc disease, and spondylolisthesis are more common in the lumbar spine. The thoracic spine, due to the morphology of the facet joints and rib articulations, is relatively immobile when compared to the cervical and lumbar regions. Conditions addressed in this chapter occur less frequently in the thoracic region, and as a result will not be discussed. It should be noted that this chapter focuses solely on degenerative issues related to the cervical and lumbar spine. Back

and neck pain in the setting of recent trauma requires much different evaluation and management, and as such will not be discussed here.

Cervical Spine

Disorders of the neck are ubiquitous. Significant problems can arise from various types of arthritis as well as trauma. In each instance, recovery or improvement is the usual outcome, but can sometimes be disastrous, even resulting in quadriplegia. Every physician should be familiar with the signs and symptoms of the various diagnostic entities that occur in the cervical spine and be able to identify the serious problems that require immediate attention, such as an unrecognized myelopathy.

History

The location of the pain is the major point to obtain from a patient's history. The majority of patients complain of localized symptoms in the neck, with and without referral of pain between the scapulae or shoulders. The pain is described as vague, diffuse, axial, non-dermatomal, and poorly localized. The pathogenesis of this type of complaint is attributed to structures innervated by the sinuvertebral nerve or the nerves innervating the paravertebral soft tissues and is generally a localized injury.

Illustrations by Anna Beaufort.

J. L. Ferguson · D. C. Johnson (✉)
Department of Orthopedics, MedStar Georgetown
University Hospital, Washington, DC, USA
e-mail: Joseph.Ferguson@gunet.georgetown.edu;
Douglass.C.Johnson@medstar.net

© The Author(s), under exclusive license to Springer Nature Switzerland AG 2024
W. F. Postma et al. (eds.), *Essentials of Orthopedic Surgery*,
https://doi.org/10.1007/978-3-031-66215-7_10

Another group of patients will complain of neck pain with the addition of arm involvement. This arm pain is secondary to nerve root irritation and is termed radicular pain. The degree of nerve root involvement can vary from a monoradiculopathy to multiple levels of involvement. It is described as a deep aching, burning, or shooting arm pain, often with associated paresthesias. The pathogenesis of radicular pain can derive from soft tissue (herniated disc), bone (spondylosis/osteophyte), or a combination of the two—typically referred to as a disc-osteophyte complex.

Finally, a third group of patients will complain of symptoms secondary to cervical myelopathy, which is compression of the spinal cord and usually secondary to degenerative changes, although can be acute secondary to a severe soft disc herniation. The clinical complaints vary considerably. The onset of symptoms usually begins after 50 years of age, and males are more often affected. Onset is usually insidious, although there is occasionally a history of trauma. The natural history is that of initial neurologic deterioration followed by a plateau period lasting several months. This is referred to as a "stepwise deterioration" in neurologic function. The resulting clinical picture is often one of an incomplete spinal lesion with a patchy distribution of deficits. Disability varies with the number of vertebrae involved and with the degree of changes at each level.

Common presenting symptoms of cervical myelopathy include numbness and paresthesias in the hands, clumsiness of the fingers, weakness (greatest in the lower extremities), and gait disturbances. Patients will often report difficulty buttoning shirts, loss of fine motor skills, and worsening handwriting. Abnormalities of micturition are seen in about one-third of cases and indicate more severe cord involvement. Symptoms of radiculopathy can coexist with myelopathy and confuse the clinical picture. Sensory disturbances may show a patchy distribution. Spinothalamic tract (pain and temperature) deficits may be seen in the upper extremities, the thorax, or the lumbar region and may be in a stocking or glove distribution. Posterior column deficits (vibration and proprioception) are more commonly seen in the feet than in the hands. Usually there is no gross sensory impairment, but a diminished sense of appreciation of light touch and pinprick. A characteristic broad-based, shuffling gait may be seen, signaling the onset of functionally significant deterioration.

It should be noted that compressive neurologic pathologies are not mutually exclusive. Indeed, some patients may present with both radicular and myelopathic symptoms, known as cervical myeloradiculopathy. These should be evaluated and treated as a combined pathology, taking care not to exclude either in the process.

Physical Examination

The physical examination should begin with observation of the cervical spine and upper torso unencumbered by clothing. The physical findings are of two different types. One set can be categorized as nonspecific and found in most patients with neck pain, but will not help to localize the type or level of the pathological process. A decreased range of motion is the most frequent nonspecific finding. It can be secondary to pain or, structurally, to distorted bony or soft tissue elements in the cervical spine. Pain will often lead to muscle guarding, or spasm, in an attempt to "brace" the neck and prevent further movement. Hyperextension and excessive lateral rotation, however, will usually cause pain—even in a normal individual.

Tenderness is another nonspecific finding that can be quite helpful. There are two types of tenderness that must be considered. One is diffuse, elicited by inflammation of the paravertebral muscles, and is found over a wide area of the posterolateral muscle masses. The second type of tenderness is more specific and may help localize the level of the pathology. It can be localized by palpation over each intervertebral foramen and spinous process.

The next goal of the physical exam is to isolate the level or levels in the cervical spine responsible for the symptomatology. The exam is also important to rule out other sources of pain, which include compression neuropathies, thoracic outlet syndrome, and chest or shoulder pathology.

The major focus of the exam is directed at finding a neurologic deficit (Table 10.1). A dermatomal or myotomal deficit, such as decreased strength, sensory deficit (often decreased sensation to light touch), or diminished deep tendon reflex is most likely an objective finding in a patient with a radiculopathy. Although less reproducible, manual tests and maneuvers that increase or decrease radicular symptoms may be helpful. In the Spurling's test, the patient's head is extended, tilted laterally, and slightly rotated toward the symptomatic side, and then compressed to elicit reproduction or aggravation of the radicular symptoms. The axial manual traction test is performed in the presence of radicular symptoms in the supine position. With 20–25 lb of axial traction, a positive test is the decrease or disappearance of radicular symptoms. All these tests are highly specific (low false-positive rate) for the diagnosis of root compression, but the sensitivity (false-negative rate) is less than 50%. L'hermitte's sign is a feeling of electric shock extending distally down the axial spine with flexion at the neck, which can indicate spinal cord compression. It is worth noting that a C5 nerve root palsy is the most common palsy in the cervical spine. This can be seen preoperatively but is more commonly seen post-operatively after cervical decompression. Patients present with acute weakness of the deltoid and biceps as well as radicular pain in the C5 distribution. Patients should be counseled that in most cases this will likely resolve spontaneously within 6 months. The exact etiology of the C5 palsy is not known, but one proposed theory is that decompression and posterior translation of the spinal cord results in traction on the C5 nerve root, resulting in a palsy.

Myelopathic physical findings should also be specifically checked. These patients can have a gait disturbance, so they should be observed walking. Patients with myelopathy will have a characteristic broad-based shuffling gait that is due to their loss of balance and proprioception. The extent of motor disability can vary from mild to severe. Pyramidal tract weakness and atrophy are more commonly seen in the lower extremities and are the most common abnormal signs. The usual clinical findings in the lower extremities are spasticity and weakness.

Weakness and wasting of the upper extremities and hands may also be due to combined spondylotic myelopathy and radiculopathy. In this situation, the patient usually complains of hand clumsiness. A diminished or absent upper extremity deep tendon reflex can indicate compressive radiculopathy superimposed on spondylotic myelopathy. Hoffman's test is a sensitive but not specific abnormal reflex exam that can indicate myelopathy. The test is performed by securing the middle phalanx of the long finger and flicking the distal phalanx into an extended position. Resulting involuntary contraction of the thumb and/or index finger IP joint is a positive test, indicative of upper motor neuron pathology. The inverted supinator test (inverted brachioradialis reflex) is another sensitive but nonspecific exam maneuver that can indicate upper motor neuron pathology. The test is performed by tapping the brachioradialis at the level of the radial styloid. Absence of contraction of the brachioradialis and an abnormal response of finger flexion indicates a positive test. The Romberg test should additionally be performed to assess for ataxia. In this exam, patients are asked to stand with their feet side by side while closing their eyes and attempt to maintain their balance.

Table 10.1 Features of the cervical neurologic exam

Disk level	Nerve root	Sensory	Motor	Reflex
C2–C3	C3	Pinna of ear, mastoid process	None	None
C3–C4	C4	Upper trapezius	None	None
C4–C5	C5	Deltoid, anterior arm	Deltoid, Biceps	Biceps
C5–C6	C6	Thumb and index finger	Biceps, elbow flexion, wrist extension	Biceps
C6–C7	C7	Index and middle finger	Triceps	Triceps
C7–T1	C8	Ring and small finger	Intrinsics	None

Inability to maintain balance and posture indicates issues with proprioception that can be caused by myelopathy. Gait patterns should also be assessed in patients with concern for myelopathy. Myelopathic patients will have difficulty performing a tandem toe-to-heel walk and may have the characteristic wide-based, slow, shuffling gait.

Sensory deficits in spinothalamic (pain and temperature) and posterior column (vibration and proprioception) function should be documented. Usually there is no gross impairment of sensation; rather, a patchy decrease in light touch and pin-prick is seen. Hyperreflexia, clonus, and positive Babinski's signs are seen in the lower extremities. Hoffman's sign and hyperreflexia may be observed in the upper extremities.

In addition to a complete cervical exam, a detailed lumbar exam may also be indicated in cases of myelopathy to determine the extent of involvement and detect any neurologic deficits. Oftentimes with cord compression, there are distinct lower extremity issues related to upper motor neuron compression (Fig. 10.1).

Diagnostic Studies

In evaluating any pathologic process, one will usually have a choice of several diagnostic tests. The cervical spine is no exception. This section will deal with the most common ones that are routinely used. In general, all of these tests play a confirmatory role. In other words, the core of the information derived from a thorough history and physical examination should be the basis for a diagnosis; the additional tests are obtained to confirm this clinical impression. Trouble develops when these tests are used for screening purposes since most of them are overly sensitive and relatively nonselective. Thus, the studies discussed should never be interpreted in isolation from the overall clinical picture.

Plain Radiographs

Radiographic evaluation of the cervical spine is helpful in assessing patients with neck pain and the routine study should include standing anteroposterior and lateral views. Flexion-extension X-rays are indicated in defining stability, whether in the setting of trauma or suspected spondylolisthesis (Fig. 10.2). The generally accepted radiographic signs of cervical disc disease are loss of height of the intervertebral disc space, osteophyte formation, secondary encroachment of the intervertebral foramina, and osteoarthritic changes in the apophyseal joints (Fig. 10.3).

It should be stressed that the identification of some pathology on plain cervical X-rays does not, per se, indicate the cause of the patient's symptoms. In several series, large numbers of asymptomatic patients have shown radiographic evidence of advanced degenerative disc disease. At approximately age 40, some degeneration (narrowing) can be expected, particularly at the C5–C6 and C6–C7 levels. This is considered to represent a normal aging process. By age 70, cervical spondylosis is almost ubiquitous, though usually asymptomatic. The difficult problem with regard to radiographic interpretation is not in the identification of these changes, but rather in determining how much significance should be attributed to them.

Radiographic abnormalities of alignment in the cervical spine may also be of clinical significance, but they need to be correlated with the whole clinical picture; listhesis or slipping forward or backward (retrolisthesis) of one vertebra upon the vertebra below it is such a finding.

If instability is suspected, functional X-rays may be taken. These view the spine from the side, with the head flexed (bent forward) or extended (arched back); the spine normally flexes equally at each spinal level. If one vertebral level is unstable, that particular vertebra moves more or less and disrupts the symmetry of motion. Again, this finding must be correlated with the whole clinical picture as its mere presence may be asymptomatic.

Magnetic Resonance Imaging

Magnetic resonance imaging (MRI) provides an image on film that is obtained by measuring the differences in proton density between the various tissues evaluated. With the use of the computer, multiplanar images are obtainable. It is a safe test since it uses neither ionizing radiation nor invasive contrast agents.

Fig. 10.1 Dermatomal distribution chart

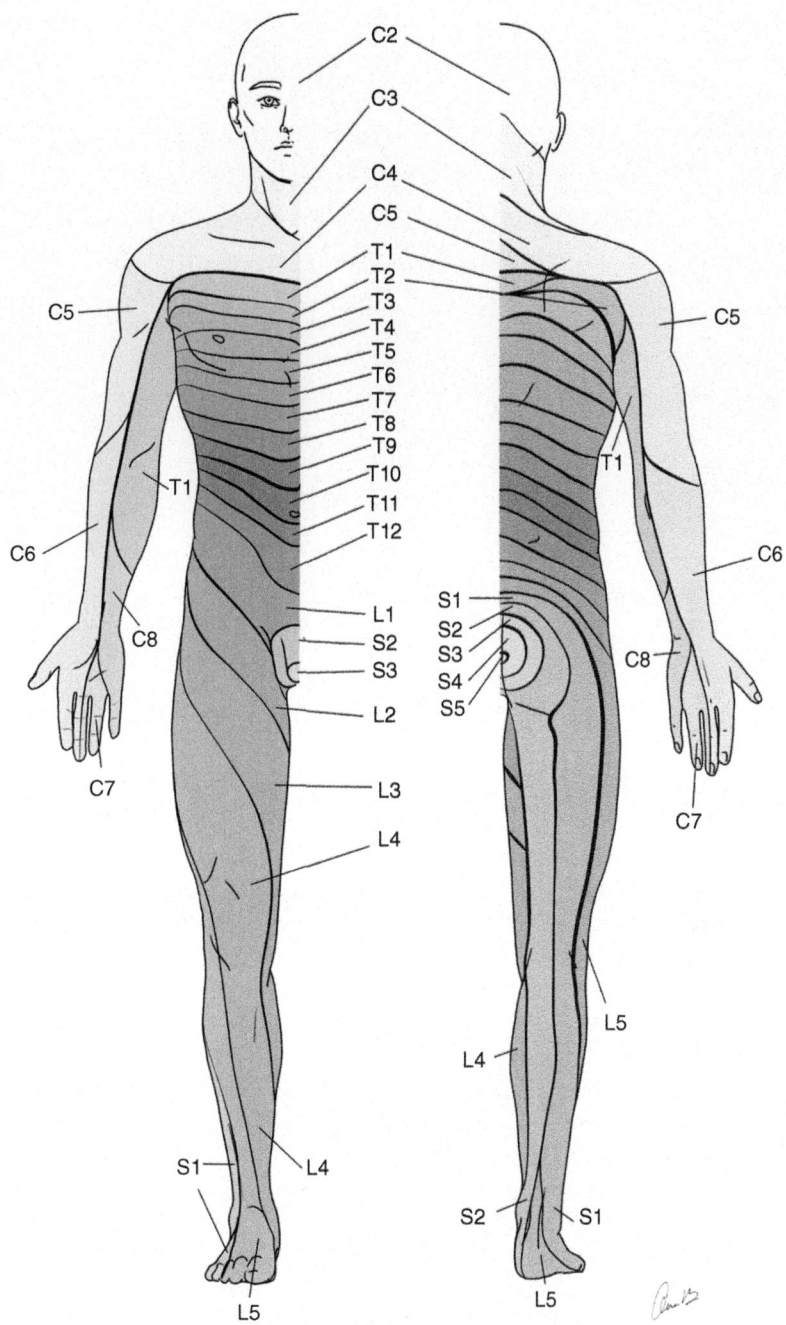

The technical advances in recent years have made MRI both more accessible, cost-effective, and useful. With the advent of 1.5 T and new 3.0 T coils with stronger magnetic fields, higher quality images are generated in less time. The distinction between soft tissues and bone and the relationship of both to the neural foramen are excellent (Fig. 10.4). MRI can also accurately detect rare conditions such as infection, tumor, or intrinsic abnormalities of the spinal cord. An excellent test, MRI can be combined with plain films to permit an accurate noninvasive evaluation of a cervical radiculopathy or myelopathy. It is currently the diagnostic study of choice in the cervical spine.

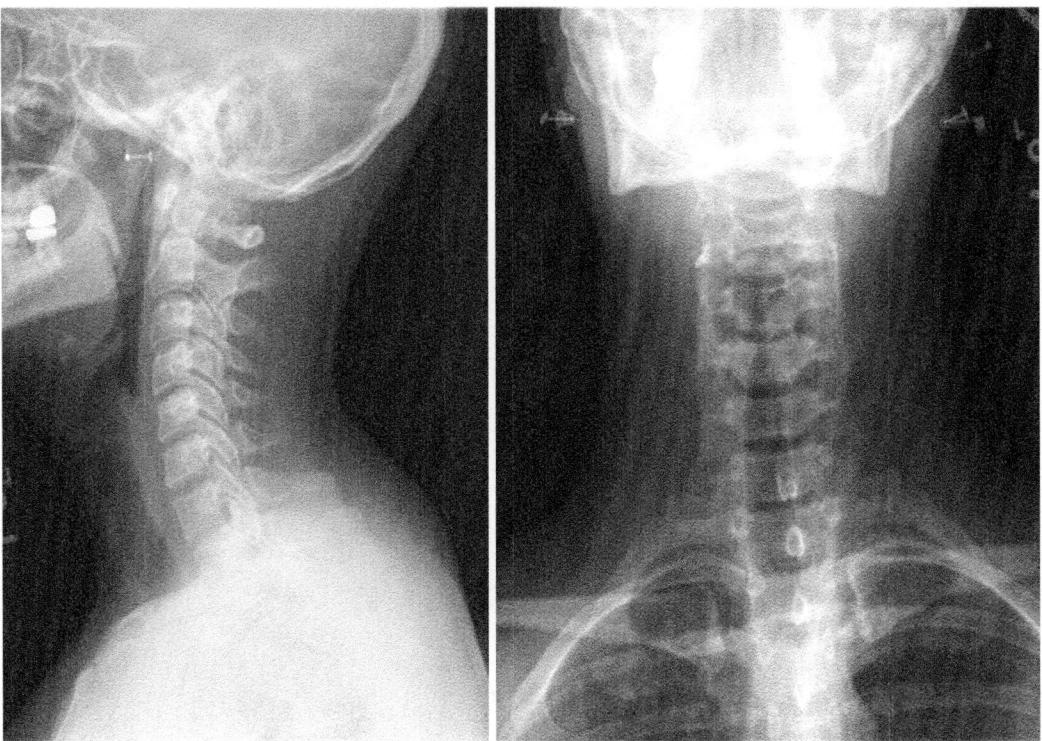

Fig. 10.2 Lateral and AP X-rays of a normal cervical spine

Review of MRI imaging should begin with axial and sagittal views of T2-weighted images compared side-by-side. These images alone can provide a comprehensive picture of bony structures, intervertebral discs, neural foramina, the thecal sac, and associated pathology. The MRI should be used as a confirmatory test to substantiate a clinical impression. It should not be used as a screening test since there are many false-positive as well as false-negative results. Thus, some normal people will have abnormal MRI findings, whereas some abnormal people will be found to have normal MRIs. The patient's symptoms and clinical exam MUST correlate to the MRI findings when formulating a diagnosis.

Myelography

A myelogram is performed by injecting a water-soluble dye into the spinal sac so that the outline of the sac itself, as well as each nerve root sleeve, can be evaluated. However, with recent advances and the relative accessibility of current MRI tech-

niques, myelograms are becoming less frequent in practice and are generally used when patients have contra-indications that preclude them from MRI such as pacemaker, spinal cord stimulator, or other indwelling metal artifacts.

Computerized Tomography

Computerized tomography (CT) permits one to create cross-sectional imaging of the cervical spine at any desired level. The advantages of CT include excellent differentiation of bone and soft tissue (disc or ligament) lesions, direct demonstration of spinal cord and spinal cord dimensions, assessment of foraminal encroachment. CT scans of the cervical spine are most commonly indicated for trauma and to rule out ossification of the posterior longitudinal ligament (OPLL).

Unfortunately, CT involves radiation exposure. It does, however, provide very good information and is especially useful for patients who, for a variety of reasons, cannot undergo MRI investigation.

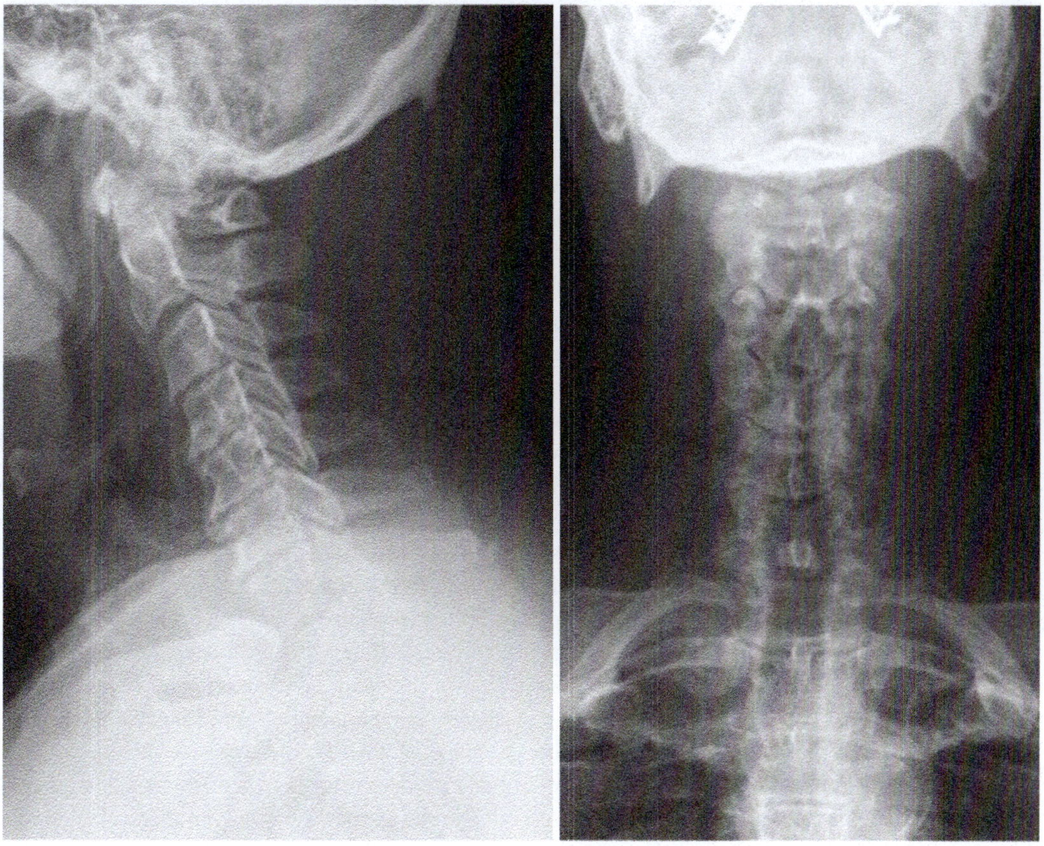

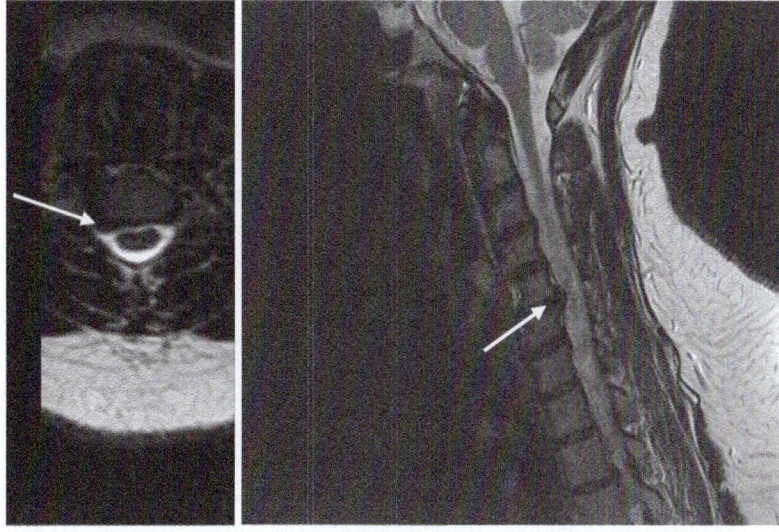

Fig. 10.3 Lateral and AP radiographs demonstrating degenerative changes in the cervical spine

Fig. 10.4 Axial and sagittal T-2 weighted images of the cervical spine demonstrating a disc-osteophyte complex at the C5–C6 level with foraminal stenosis and loss of cervical lordosis

Electromyography

Electromyography (EMG) is an electric test that confirms the interaction of nerve to muscle. The test is performed by placing needles into muscles to determine if there is an intact nerve supply to that muscle. The EMG is particularly useful in localizing a specific abnormal nerve root. It should be appreciated that it takes at least 21 days for an EMG to show up as abnormal. After 21 days of pressure on a nerve root, signs of denervation with fibrillation can be observed. Before 21 days, the EMG will be negative in spite of nerve root damage. It should be noted that there is no quantitative interpretation of this test. Thus, it cannot be said that the EMG is 25 or 75% normal.

EMG can also be useful in recognizing double-crush phenomenon in which asymptomatic compression of a nerve at one location such as the cervical spine can increase the susceptibility of a peripheral nerve to impairment at another more distal location [1].

The EMG is an electronic extension of the physical examination. Although it is 80–90% accurate in establishing cervical radiculopathy as the cause of pain, false-negative results do occur. If cervical radiculopathy affects only the sensory root, the EMG will be unable to demonstrate an abnormality. A false-negative examination can occur if the patient with acute symptoms is examined early (4–28 days from onset of symptoms). A negative study should be repeated in 2–3 weeks if symptoms persist. The accuracy of the EMG increases if both the paraspinal and extremity muscles innervated by the suspected root demonstrate abnormalities.

The EMG is not part of the routine evaluation of the cervical spine. It can help elucidate radiculopathy originating from the cervical or lumbar spine versus peripheral nerve compression originating more distally. It is indicated to confirm a clinical impression and localize pathology to a cervical nerve root or to rule out other sources of pathology, such as peripheral neuropathies or compressive neuropathies in the upper extremities.

Clinical Conditions

There are many conditions that may present as neck pain, with or without arm pain, in any particular individual. However, there are several that are quite common and will be presented in detail.

Myelopathy Versus Radiculopathy

Before progressing further, it is important to highlight the very important distinction between myelopathy and radiculopathy. Symptoms originate from the spinal cord and exiting nerve roots, respectively, but with different presentations and operative treatments.

Myelopathy is caused by compression of the spinal cord itself and affects upper motor neurons. It often presents with vague, non-dermatomal symptoms. Patients will note worsening clumsiness of the hands, worsening handwriting, generalized pain, and subtle loss of balance that many attribute to the aging process. It should be noted that myelopathy is often painless, which frequently delays the patient from seeking medical attention. The progression of myelopathy is in a stepwise fashion (Fig. 10.5). Patients will report an acute worsening that then stabilizes over time until the next insult to the cord which will again cause acute worsening of symptoms. Early operative intervention is important in myelopathy to relieve the compression on the spinal cord. However, it is important to educate patients that the surgery itself is not curative in nature. The goal is to halt progression of the stepwise decline, and often patients will not see significant improvement in their symptoms post-operatively.

Contrasted to myelopathy, which is compression of the spinal cord, radiculopathy is compression of the peripheral nerves as they exit the spine. This can initially present with neck pain in the acute setting, after a disc herniation for example, but will often also present with radicular pain with or without weakness in the extremity. When contrasted to myelopathy, the symptoms will be much more discrete and focal with pain generally in a dermatomal

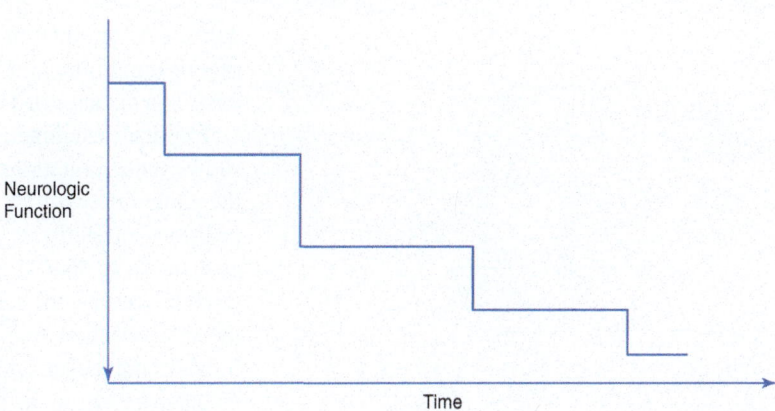

Fig. 10.5 The stepwise progression of myelopathy. Patients may be initially asymptomatic and then notice acute worsening of symptoms after an insult to the spinal cord. Symptoms will then stabilize until there is another insult to the cord resulting in further progression of symptoms

Neurologic Function

Time

distribution and focal weakness or hyperreflexia in the areas innervated by the affected nerve root. Nonoperative management is a mainstay in the treatment of radiculopathy, with a large number of patients experiencing resolution of symptoms with rest, NSAIDs, and physical therapy. However, the presence of progressive weakness is a sign of progressive damage to the affected nerve and should be considered for more urgent operative intervention.

Neck Sprain-Neck Ache

Neck sprain, while a misnomer, describes a clinical condition involving a nonradiating discomfort or pain about the neck area associated with a concomitant loss of neck motion (stiffness). While the clinical syndrome may present as a headache, most often the pain is located in the middle to lower part of the back of the neck. A history of injury is rarely obtained, but the pain may start after a night's rest or on simply turning the head. The source of the pain is most commonly believed to be the ligaments about the cervical spine and/or the surrounding muscles. The axial pain may also be produced by small annular tears without disc herniation or from the facet joints.

The pain associated with a neck sprain is most often a dull aching pain, which is exacerbated by neck motion. The pain is usually abated by rest or immobilization. The pain may be referred to other mesenchymal structures derived from a similar sclerotome during embryogenesis. Common referred pain patterns include the scapular area, the posterior shoulder, the occipital

area, or the anterior chest wall (cervical angina pectoris). Those referred pain patterns do not connote a true radicular pain pattern and are not usually mechanical in origin.

Physical examination of patients with neck ache usually reveals nothing more than a locally tender area or areas, usually just lateral to the spine. The intensity of the pain is variable and the loss of cervical motion correlates directly with the pain intensity. The presence of true spasm, defined as a continuous muscle contraction, is rare except in severe cases where the head may be tilted to one side (torticollis).

Since the radiograph in cervical sprain is usually normal, a plain X-ray is usually not warranted on the first visit. If the pain continues for more than 2 weeks or the patient develops other physical findings, then an X-ray should be taken to rule out other more serious causes of the neck pain such as neoplasia or instability. The prognosis for these individuals is excellent since the natural history is one of complete resolution of the symptoms over several weeks. The mainstay of therapy includes rest and gentle mobilization and exercises. Although medications such as anti-inflammatory agents or muscle relaxants may aid in the acute management of pain, they do not seem to alter the natural history of the disorder.

Acute Herniated Disc

A herniated disc is defined as the protrusion of the nucleus pulposus through the fibers of the annulus fibrosus (Fig. 10.6). Most acute disc her-

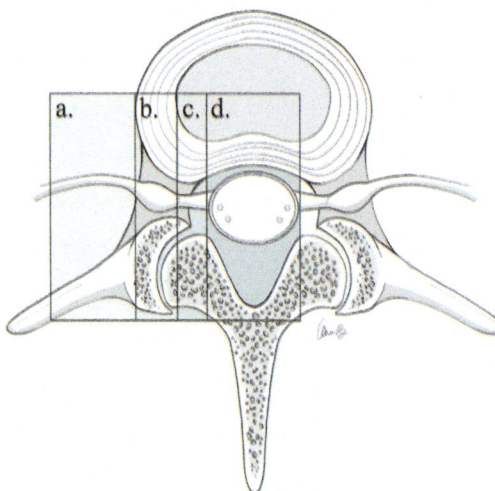

Fig. 10.6 Representative illustration of locations of disc herniation. (**a**) Far lateral (extra-foraminal), (**b**) foraminal, (**c**) lateral recess, and (**d**) central

niations occur posterolaterally and in patients around the fourth decade of life when the nucleus is still gelatinous. The most common areas of disc herniation are C5–C6 and C6–C7, whereas C7–T1, C3–C4, and C4–C5 are infrequent. Disc herniation of C2–C3 is very, very rare. Unlike the lumbar herniated disc, the cervical herniated disc may cause myelopathy in addition to radicular pain due to the presence of the spinal cord in the cervical region. Figure 10.7 demonstrates axial and sagittal MRI images of a central disc herniation at C5–C6 causing compression of the spinal cord.

The disc herniation usually affects the root numbered lowest for the given disc level; for example, a C3–C4 disc affects the C4 root, C4–C5 the fifth cervical root, C5–C6 the sixth cervical root, C6–C7 the seventh nerve root, and C7–T1 the eighth cervical root. Unlike the lumbar region, the disc herniation does not involve other roots, but more commonly presents some evidence of upper motor neuron findings secondary to spinal cord local pressure.

Not every herniated disc is symptomatic. The presence of symptoms depends on the spinal reserve capacity, the presence of inflammation, the size of the herniation, as well as the presence of concomitant disease such as osteophyte formation. Absolute stenosis in the cervical spine is

defined by an anterior–posterior canal diameter of <10 mm in the mid-sagittal axis. Relative stenosis is a distance of 10–12 mm.

Physical examination of the neck usually shows some limitation of motion and on occasion the patient may tilt the head in a "cocked robin" position (torticollis) toward the side of the herniated cervical disc. Extension of the spine will often exacerbate the pain since it further narrows the intervertebral foramina. Axial compression, Valsalva maneuver, and coughing may also exacerbate or re-create the pain pattern.

The presence of a positive neurologic finding is the most helpful aspect of the diagnostic workup, although the neurologic exam may remain normal despite a distinct radicular pattern. Even when a deficit exists, it may not be temporally related to the present symptoms but could be due to a prior attack at a different level. To be significant, the neurologic exam must show objective signs of reflex diminution, motor weakness, or atrophy. The presence of subjective sensory changes is often difficult to interpret and require a coherent and cooperative patient to be of clinical value. The presence of sensory changes alone is usually not enough to make a diagnosis firm, and peripheral nerve entrapments should be ruled out in this scenario.

Nerve root sensitivity can be elicited by any method which increases the tension of the nerve root. Radicular arm pain is often increased by the Valsalva maneuver or by directly compressing the head with the Spurling maneuver. While these signs are helpful when present, their absence alone does not rule out radicular pain.

The provisional diagnosis of a herniated disc is made by the history and physical examination. The plain X-ray is usually nondiagnostic, although occasionally disc space narrowing at the suspected interspace or foraminal narrowing on the oblique films will be seen. The value of the films is largely to exclude other causes of neck and arm pain. The MRI is a confirmatory examination and should not be used as a screening test since misinformation may ensue.

The treatment for most patients with a herniated disc is nonoperative since the majority of patients respond to conservative treatment over a

Fig. 10.7 T-2 weighted axial and sagittal MRI images demonstrating central herniation of the C5–C6 intervertebral disc resulting in stenosis and spinal cord compression

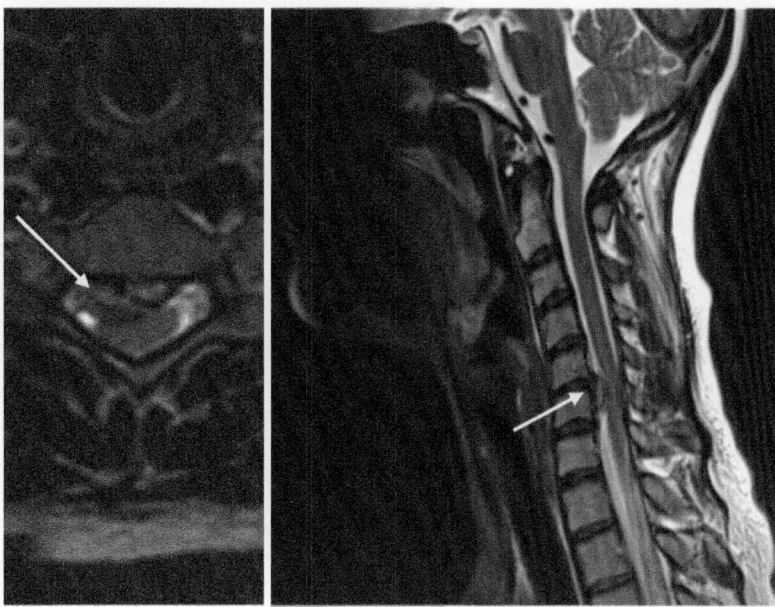

period of a few months. The efficacy of the non-operative approach depends heavily on the doctor–patient relationship. If a patient is well informed, insightful, and willing to follow instructions, the chances for successful nonoperative outcome are greatly improved.

The cornerstone to the management of a cervical herniated disc is rest and gentle mobilization, with physical therapy often offering significant help with safe progression. Most people will be able to return to work, or at least light duty, in a month.

Cervical Spondylosis

What was once commonly referred to as cervical degenerative disc disease is now more accurately named cervical spondylosis. Cervical spondylosis is a chronic process defined as the development of osteophytes and other stigmata of degenerative arthritis as a consequence of age-related disc disease, and can affect the intervertebral disc, the facet joints, and the uncovertebral "joints." Cervical spondylosis can be thought of similarly to arthritis in one of the major joints of the extremities. Radiographic features such as joint space narrowing, osteophyte formation, sclerosis, and cystic changes can be noted as the disease progresses over time. This process may produce a wide range of symptoms. However, it should be stressed that an individual may have significant spondylosis and be asymptomatic.

Cervical spondylosis is believed to be the direct result of age-related changes in the intervertebral disc. These changes include desiccation of the nucleus pulposus, loss of annular elasticity, and narrowing of the disc space with or without disc protrusion or rupture. In turn, secondary changes include overriding of facets, increased motion of the spinal segments, osteophyte formation, inflammation of synovial joints, and even microfractures. These macro- and microscopic changes can result in various clinical syndromes (spondylosis, ankylosis, central or foraminal spinal stenosis, radiculopathy, myelopathy, or spinal segmental instability).

The typical patient with symptomatic cervical spondylosis is over the age of 40 and complaining of neckache. Not infrequently, however, these patients will have very few neck pain symptoms and will present with *referred* pain patterns: occipital headaches; pain in the shoulder, suboccipital and interscapular areas and the anterior chest wall; or other vague symptoms suggestive of anatomic disturbances (e.g., blurring of vision, tinnitus). In patients with predominantly referred pain, a past history for neck pain is usually obtained.

Physical examination of the patient with cervical spondylosis is often associated with a dearth of objective findings. The patient will usually have some limitation of neck motion associated with midline tenderness. Not infrequently, palpation of the referred pain areas will also produce local tenderness and should not be confused with local disease. The neurologic examination is normal.

Anteroposterior (AP) and lateral radiographs of the cervical spine in cervical spondylosis show varying degrees of changes. These include disc space narrowing, osteophytosis, foraminal narrowing, degenerative changes of the facets, and instability (Fig. 10.3). As previously discussed, these findings do not necessarily correlate with symptoms. In large part, the radiograph serves to rule out other more serious causes of neck and referred pain such as tumors. Further diagnostic testing is usually not warranted.

Cervical spondylosis alone is treated by nonoperative measures. The mainstay of treatment for the acute pain superimposed on the chronic problem is rest and gentle mobilization/physical therapy. In addition, oral anti-inflammatory medications are the mainstay of pharmacologic management. Often these medications will need to be administered on a chronic basis or at least intermittently. Trigger-point injections with local anesthetics (lidocaine) and corticosteroids (prednisone or methylprednisolone) may be therapeutic as well as diagnostic. Further counseling with regard to sleeping position, automobile driving, and work is in order. Manipulation and traction are rarely needed and may, in fact, be deleterious to the patient. Chiropractic manipulation in the cervical spine is not recommended by the authors for this reason.

Cervical Spondylosis with Myelopathy

When the secondary bony changes of cervical spondylosis encroach on the spinal cord, a pathologic process called myelopathy develops. If this involves both the spinal cord and nerve roots, it is called myeloradiculopathy. Radiculopathy, regardless of its etiology, causes shoulder or arm pain, with or without objective neurologic (dermatomal/myotomal) changes.

Myelopathy is the most serious sequelae of cervical spondylosis and the most difficult to treat effectively. Less than 5% of patients with cervical spondylosis develop myelopathy and they are usually between 40 and 60 years of age. The changes of myelopathy are most often gradual and associated with posterior osteophyte formation (called spondylitic bone or hard disc) and spinal canal narrowing (spinal stenosis). Acute myelopathy is most often the result of a central soft disc herniation.

The characteristic stooped, wide-based, and somewhat jerky gait of the patient summarizes the chronic effects of cervical spondylosis with myelopathy. The spinal cord changes may develop from single- or multiple-level disease and as such may not present in a singular or standard manner. Subjectively patients may initially complain of sensory changes in the hands followed by difficulty with fine motor skills including handwriting and buttoning clothes. Lower extremity symptoms may predate the upper extremity symptoms and include sensory changes, loss of balance, and recurrent falls.

Objective physical exam findings include hyperreflexia, sensory deficits, weakness, spasticity, and clonus. Again it is important to obtain subjective symptoms from the patient in their history and then corroborate with objective physical exam findings.

Radiographs of the cervical spine in these patients will often reveal advanced degenerative disease, including spinal canal narrowing by prominent posterior osteophytosis, variable foraminal narrowing, disc space narrowing, facet joint arthrosis, and instability. Schmorl nodes can be seen on imaging which represent intravertebral disc herniation, often seen in degenerative disease and can contribute to the inflammatory response. Modic changes, seen on MRI range from low-grade Type I to high-grade Type III are an additional indicator of degenerative changes in both the cervical and lumbar spine. Signal intensity in the vertebral endplates represents bone marrow edema, inflammation, and eventually sclerosis. Congenital stenosis of the cervical canal is frequently seen, predisposing the patient to the development of myelopathy (Fig. 10.8). The MRI is quite striking and diagnostic. Effacement of the cerebrospinal fluid and flattening of the cord is indicative of stenosis. In addition, hyperintense signal can be seen within the cord on T2-weighted MRI images, termed myelomalacia. Though patients may remain asymptomatic despite presence of myelomalacia, this stenosis must be addressed with relative urgency as symptoms will invariably progress with time.

When myelopathy is diagnosed clinically and confirmed radiographically, the "conservative" treatment is surgical decompression. This is because the prognosis for compressive myelopathy is that the individual will experience a stepwise deterioration in neurologic function over time. There are situations where the patient may not be a good surgical candidate, and risks/benefits must be discussed with the patient and family. The goals of surgery in the myelopathic patient are to decompress the spinal canal to prevent further spinal cord compression and vascular compromise, and to prevent further neurologic decline. While some recovery may be possible, the goal of surgery is to halt the progression of neurologic decline. These indications may vary slightly from surgeon to surgeon because of the lack of absolute or definitive clinical data. Additionally, an in-depth conversation must be had with the patient to explain the goals of surgery, as full recovery of neurologic function is unlikely.

Rheumatoid Arthritis

Rheumatoid arthritis affects 2–3% of the population. Historically, about 60% of patients with rheumatoid arthritis exhibited signs and symptoms of cervical spine involvement, whereas up to 86% had radiographic evidence of cervical disease. However, with recent advancements in disease-modifying anti-rheumatic drugs (DMARDs), the prevalence of cervical disease in rheumatoid arthritis has decreased drastically.

Cervical spine involvement, secondary to the erosive, inflammatory changes of rheumatoid arthritis (synovitis), is divided into three categories: (1) atlantoaxial instability, (2) basilar invagination, and (3) subaxial instability. Atlantoaxial instability is the most common and most serious of the instability patterns affecting 20–34% of hospitalized patients. The evaluation of a patient

Fig. 10.8 Axial and sagittal T-2 weighted MRI demonstrating multi-level cervical stenosis with associated myelomalacia

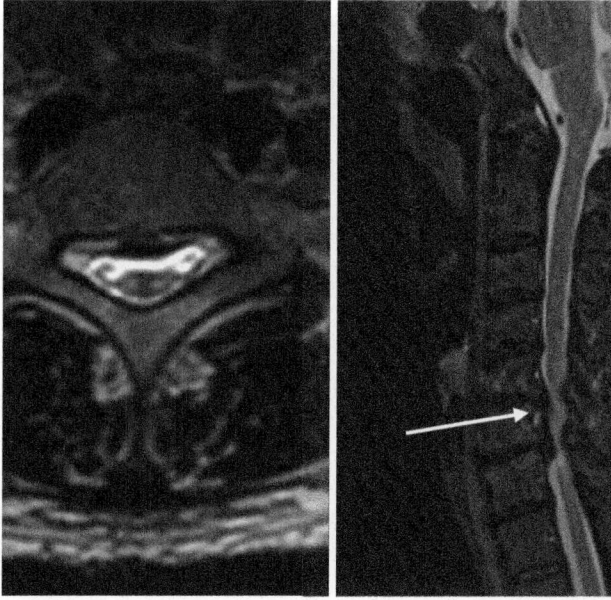

with rheumatoid arthritis is difficult due to the multiple system involvement. The physical examination should start with a careful neurologic evaluation to rule out upper motor neuron disease before moving to neck range of motion or other vigorous maneuvers that may harm the patient.

The evaluation of the patient with cervical rheumatoid arthritis begins with plain radiographs of the neck, which may reveal osteopenia, facet erosion, disc space narrowing, and subluxation of the lower cervical spine (stepladder appearance). To determine that atlantoaxial disease is present, dynamic flexion-extension views of the lateral upper cervical spine are required.

Basilar invagination is defined as upper migration of the odontoid projecting into the foramen magnum. The addition of a CT scan with and without contrast material in the upper cervical spine can provide valuable information as to the relationship of the bony elements to the spinal cord. Subaxial subluxations are identified by dynamic flexion-extension films.

The mainstay in nonoperative therapy is the cervical orthosis. Although this does not fully immobilize the atlantoaxial interval, it does produce symptomatic relief. Some authors have advocated intermittent home traction, but this must be used only with great caution under a physician's direction. Medications such as traditional NSAIDs have a definite role in the nonoperative management of rheumatoid disease. Secondary agents such as methotrexate, chloroquine, or oral steroids are best administered under the direction of a rheumatologist.

Cervical Hyperextension Injuries

Hyperextension injuries of the neck occur most often in motor vehicle collisions when a driver is struck from behind, causing sudden, forced extension of the cervical spine. This is also known as a "whiplash" injury.

Whiplash injuries can range from minor musculoskeletal strains to severe cord injury. Patients may be asymptomatic after the initial injury but will note worsening pain and stiffness over the next 12–24 h as swelling and inflammation increases. The anterior cervical muscles are often tender to the touch. The patient may have pain on mouth opening or chewing, hoarseness or difficulty swallowing, and will seek medical care.

A complete neurological examination is crucial. Any evidence of objective neurological deficit merits immediate diagnostic tests and advanced imaging to determine the cause. Although by definition hyperextension cervical injury causes damage only to the soft tissue structures of the neck, plain radiographs of the cervical spine should be obtained in all cases. Unsuspected fracture—dislocations of the cervical spine, facet fractures, odontoid fractures, or spinous process fractures—might be otherwise missed in the neurologically intact patient. Cervical spondylosis will be demonstrated on plain radiographs as well. Of course, if objective neurologic deficits are present, then further diagnostic aids are necessary, (e.g., head CT, spine CT, myelogram, MRI).

Since the majority of patients have no neurologic deficits, a reasonable medical routine is based on the premise of resting the involved injured soft tissues. A soft cervical collar helps significantly in relieving muscle spasm and preventing quick head turns. The collar should not be worn for more than 2 weeks, lest the recovering muscles start weakening from nonuse. Heat is helpful and should be applied by a heating pad, hot showers, or hot tub soaks. If neck pain is severe, a short period of bed rest may be necessary. Mild analgesics, nonsteroidal antiinflammatory drugs (NSAIDs), and muscle relaxants are all helpful and are generally indicated. Narcotic analgesics should be avoided if possible. Activity should be restricted as determined by the severity of the symptoms. Generally, driving should be avoided for the acute symptomatic period. After approximately 2 weeks of this regimen, significant improvement should be noted. If not, 2 more weeks of continued conservative care can be considered. If symptoms persist at 4 weeks post-injury, some further testing is necessary before emotional overlay is considered the cause. If headaches persist, a cranial MRI scan should be done. If normal at 4 weeks, the patient can be assured that no intracranial abnormality is present. If arm or shoulder pain persists, an MRI should be considered. If these tests are normal, the patient can be assured that no compression of neural structures is present.

Cervical Spine Algorithm

The task of the physician, when confronted with the cervical spine patient, is to integrate his or her complaints into an accurate diagnosis and to prescribe appropriate therapy. Achieving this goal depends on the accuracy of the physician's decision-making ability. Although specific information is not available for every aspect of neck pain, there is a large body of data to guide us in handling these patients. Using this knowledge, which has already been presented, an algorithm for neck pain has been designated.

An algorithm can be used as "a set of rules for solving a particular problem in a finite number of steps." It is, in effect, an organized pattern of decision-making and thought processes which can be found useful, in this instance, in approaching the universe of cervical spine patients. The algorithm can be followed in sequence (Fig. 10.9) and is also presented in table form (Table 10.2).

The primary objective for the physician is to return patients to their normal function as quickly as possible. In the course of achieving this goal, the physician must be concerned with other circumstances, which include making efficient and precise use of diagnostic studies, minimizing the use of unindicated surgery, and making therapy available at a reasonable cost to society. The algorithm follows well-delineated rules, established from the consensus of a broad segment of qualified spine surgeons. It allows the patient to receive the most helpful diagnostic and therapeutic measures at optimal times.

The algorithm begins with the universe of patients who are initially evaluated for neck pain, with or without arm pain. Patients with major trauma, including fractures, are not included. After an initial medical history and physical examination—and assuming that the patient's symptoms are originating from the cervical spine—the first major decision is to rule in or out the presence of a cervical myelopathy.

The character and severity of the myelopathy depends on the size, location, and duration of the lesion. Ventrolateral lesions encroach on the nerve roots and lateral aspects of the spinal cord, producing all the manifestations accompanying nerve root compression. The chief radicular signs are weakness, loss of tone, and volume of the muscles of the upper extremity, while the pressure on the spinal cord may produce pyramidal tract signs and spasticity in the lower extremities.

Midline lesions intrude on the central aspect of the anterior portion of the spinal cord. They produce no signs of nerve root compression. Both lower extremities are primarily involved, and the most common problem relates initially to gait disturbance. As the disease progresses, bowel and bladder control may be affected.

Once a diagnosis of cervical myelopathy is made, surgical intervention should be considered without delay. The best results are attained in patients with one or two motor units involved and with myelopathy of a relatively short duration. The longer pressure is applied to the neural elements, the poorer the results. A cervical MRI or CT-myelogram should be obtained in these patients to precisely define the neural compression and an adequate surgical decompression should be performed as soon as possible to achieve the best results.

After cervical myelopathy has been ruled out, the remaining patients, who constitute an overwhelming majority, should be started on a course of conservative management. At this stage of the patient's course, a specific diagnosis, whether it be a herniated disc or neck strain, is not important because the entire group is treated in the same fashion.

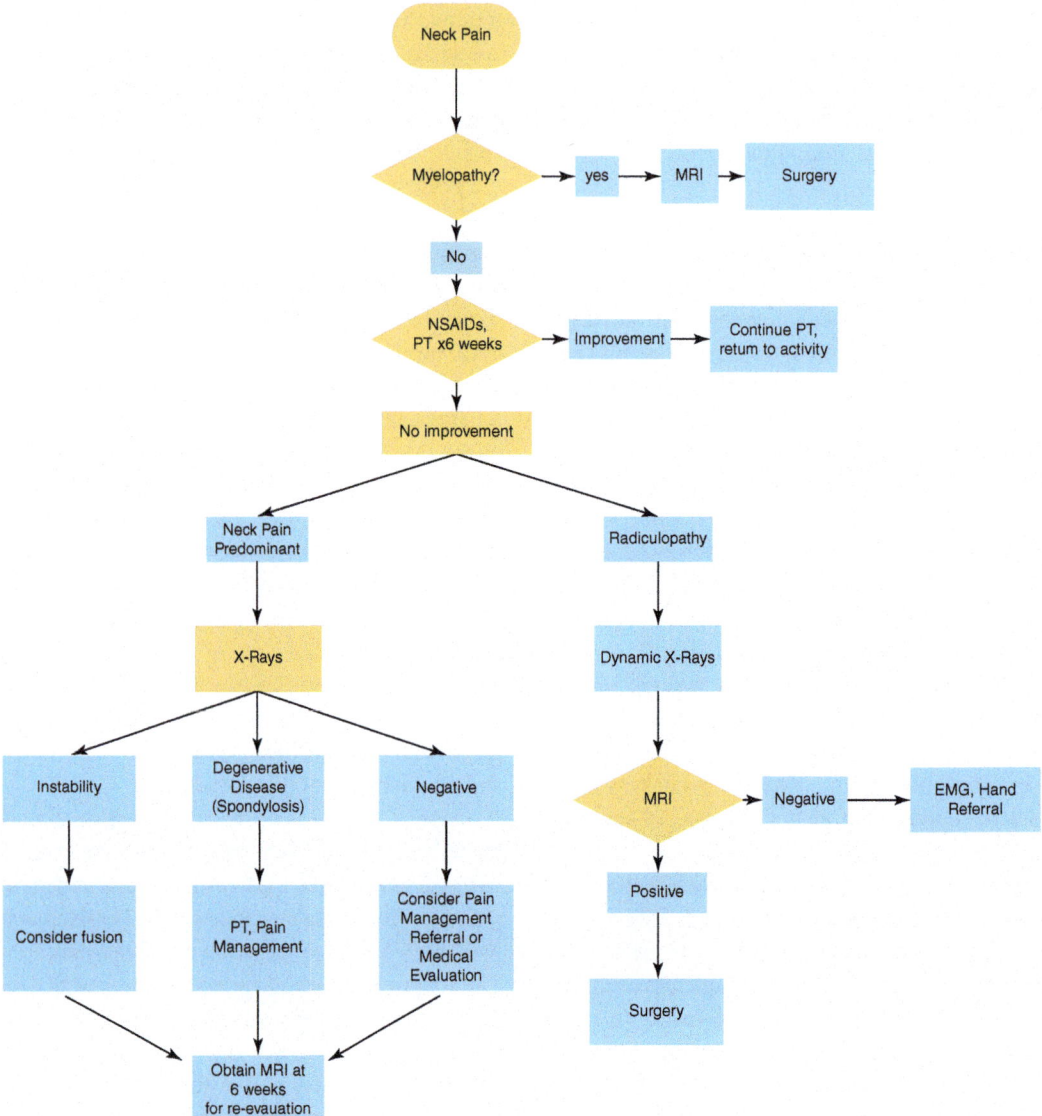

Fig. 10.9 Cervical spine algorithm

Table 10.2 Differential diagnosis of neck pain

	Pain	Compression test	Neurologic exam	Plain radiographs	Flex/Ext radiographs	CT scan	MRI	Inflammatory markers
Neck strain	Neck	–	–	–	–	–	–	–
Disc herniation	Arm	+	+	–	–	+	+	–
Instability	Neck	–	–	±	+	–	–	–
Degenerative disc	Neck	–	–	+	–	+	+	–
Myelopathy	Neck	–	–	+	–	+	+	–
Tumor	Neck	–	–	+	–	+	+	+
Spondy-loarthropathy	Neck	–	–	+	–	+	+	+

Conservative Treatment

The primary mode of therapy in both acute and chronic cervical spine disease is gentle mobilization. In the acute neck injuries, immobilization allows for healing of torn and attenuated soft tissues, whereas in chronic conditions, immobilization is aimed at reduction of inflammation in the supporting soft tissues and around the nerve roots of the cervical spine. This is best achieved by guided treatment in physical therapy and is often required by insurance before further imaging in our current healthcare climate.

The other mainstay of the initial treatment is drug therapy. It is directed at reducing inflammation, especially in the soft tissues. There are a variety of anti-inflammatory medications available; however, there is no one drug that has proven to be significantly better than all the others. The dosage must be adequate to achieve a therapeutic blood level. The efficacy of this treatment regimen is predicated on the patient's ability to understand the disease process and the role of each therapeutic modality. The vast majority of patients will respond to this approach in the first 10 days, but a certain percentage will not heal rapidly.

At this juncture, a local injection into the area of maximal tenderness should be considered. Localized tender areas in the paravertebral musculature and trapezii will be found in many individuals and are referred to as trigger points. Marked relief of symptoms is often achieved dramatically by infiltration of these trigger points with a combination of lidocaine (Xylocaine) and 1 mL of a steroid preparation. The object of the injection is to decrease the inflammation in a specific anatomic area. The more localized the trigger point, the more effective this form of therapy.

In the absence of neurologic deficit, the patient should be treated conservatively for up to 6 weeks. The majority of cervical spine patients will get better and should be encouraged to gradually increase their activities. The goal is a return to their normal lifestyles. An exercise program should be directed at strengthening the paravertebral musculature, not at increasing the range of motion.

The pathway along this top portion of the algorithm is reversible. Should regression occur, with exacerbation of symptoms, the physician can resort to more stringent conservative measures. The majority of patients with neck pain will respond to therapy and return to a normal life pattern within 2 months of the beginning of their problem. If the initial conservative treatment regimen fails, symptomatic patients are divided into two groups. The first is comprised of people who have neck pain as a predominant complaint, with or without interscapular radiation. The second group is made up of those who complain primarily of arm pain (brachialgia).

Neck Pain Predominant

After 6 weeks of conservative therapy with no symptomatic relief, plain X-rays with lateral flexion–extension films are carefully examined for abnormalities. One group of patients will have objective evidence of instability. In the lower cervical spine (C-3 through C-7), instability is identified by horizontal translation of one vertebra on another of more than 3.5 mm or of an angular difference of adjacent vertebrae of more than 11°. The majority of patients with instability will respond well to further nonoperative measures, including a thorough explanation of the problem and some type of bracing. In some cases, these measures will fail and a surgical fusion of the involved spinal segments will be necessary.

Another group of patients complaining mainly of neck pain will be found to have degenerative disease on their plain X-ray films. The radiographic signs include loss of height of the intervertebral disc space, osteophyte formation, secondary encroachment of the intervertebral foramina, and osteoarthritic changes in the apophyseal joint. The difficulty is not in identifying these abnormalities on the roentgenogram, but in determining their significance.

Degeneration in the cervical spine can be a normal part of the aging process. In a study of matched pairs of asymptomatic and symptomatic patients, it was concluded that large numbers of asymptomatic patients show roentgenographic evidence of advanced degenerative disease. The most significant radiographic finding relevant to symptomatology was found to be narrowing of the intervertebral disc space, particularly between C5–C6 and C6–C7. There was no difference between the two groups as far as changes at the apophyseal joints, intervertebral foramina, or posterior articular process.

These patients should be treated symptomatically with anti-inflammatory medication, support, and trigger-point injections as required. In the quiescent stages, they should be placed on isometric exercises. Finally, they should be reexamined periodically because some will develop significant pressure on the neurologic elements (myelopathy).

The majority of patients with neck pain will have normal X-rays. The diagnosis for this group is neck strain. At this point, with no objective findings, other pathology must be considered. These patients should undergo a bone scan and medical evaluation. The bone scan is an excellent tool, often identifying early spinal tumors or infections not seen on routine roentgenographic examinations. A thorough medical search may also reveal problems missed in the early stages of neck pain evaluation. If these diagnostic studies are positive, the patient is treated appropriately. If the above workup is negative, the patient should have a thorough psychosocial evaluation. This is predicated on the belief that a patient's disability is related not only to his or her pathologic anatomy, but also to the perception of pain and the stability in relationship to his or her sociologic environment. Drug habituation, alcoholism, depression, and other psychiatric problems are frequently seen in association with neck pain. If the evaluation reveals this type of pathology, proper measures should be instituted to overcome the disability.

Should the outcome of the psychosocial evaluation prove to be normal, the patient can be considered to have chronic neck pain. One must be aware that other outside factors such as compensation and/or litigation can influence a patient's perception of his or her subjective pain. Patients with chronic neck pain need encouragement, patience, and education from their physicians.

They need to be detoxified from narcotic drugs and placed on an exercise regimen. Many will respond to antidepressant drugs such as amitriptyline (Elavil). All of these patients need periodic reevaluation to avoid missing any new or underlying pathology.

Arm Pain Predominant (Radiculopathy)

Patients who have pain radiating into their arm may be experiencing their symptoms secondary to mechanical pressure and inflammation of the involved nerve roots. This mechanical pressure may arise from a ruptured disc or from bone secondary to degenerative changes. Other pathologic causes of arm pain should be carefully considered. Extrinsic pressure on the vascular structures or on the peripheral nerves is most likely imitators of brachialgia. Pathology in the chest and shoulder should also be ruled out.

A careful physical examination should be conducted. If there is any question about these findings, standing AP and lateral X-rays should be obtained. If patients fail 6 weeks of conservative management of their radicular symptoms, advanced imaging should be obtained to further evaluate the patient. MRI will often provide more information as to the source of pain and a reliable diagnosis. However, in the setting of an equivocal MRI, EMG can be obtained as a confirmatory tool or to evaluate peripheral sources of radiculopathy.

It has been repeatedly documented that unequivocal evidence of nerve root compression must be found for surgery to be effective. One must have a strong confirmation of mechanical root compression from the neurologic exam and a confirming study before proceeding with any surgery. The indications for surgery are the subjective complaint of arm pain and a neurologic deficit or positive EMG. An MRI must confirm the pathology. If the patient does not have these, there is inadequate clinical evidence to proceed with surgery. For patients who have met these criteria for cervical decompression, the results will usually be satisfactory: 95% can expect good or excellent outcomes.

Lumbar Spine

Low back pain occurs much more commonly than neck pain. The lifetime incidence of low back pain is estimated to be 65%. Every physician will be either personally affected (family/friends) or professionally challenged by this problem.

History

Upon initial evaluation of a new patient for lower back pain, it is important to obtain as much detail as possible regarding the nature of a patient's symptoms. Pain isolated to the lower back points toward musculoskeletal spasm or instability. Pain that begins in the low back and radiates in a dermatomal fashion down the legs points toward foraminal stenosis and disc herniation. Pain that is in the low back and associated with vague bilateral posterior thigh numbness points more so toward neurogenic claudication. Remember that the spinal cord ends at L1–2 in the adult, so cord compression and upper motor neuron pathologies are not possible with pathology below L2. However, compression of the conus medullaris is possible and should be considered at L1–2. A thorough history should be obtained to help elucidate the source of symptoms, and then supported with a detailed physical exam to assess sensory deficits or focal weakness.

A general medical review, especially in the older patient, is imperative. Metabolic, infectious, visceral, and malignant disorders may initially present to the physician as low back pain.

The location of the pain is one of the most important historical points. The majority of patients just have back pain with or without referral into the buttocks or posterior thigh. Referred pain is defined as pain in structures which have the same mesodermal origin. These patients have a localized injury and the referral of pain into the buttocks or thigh does not signify any compression on the neural elements. This type of pain is described as dull, deep, and/or diffuse.

Radiculopathy in the lumbar presents similarly to cervical radiculopathy, with pain that originates in the back, travels down the leg, often below the knee into the foot. It is described as sharp and radiating. It may be accompanied by numbness and tingling. Radiculopathy is caused by a mechanical compression of an inflamed nerve root where the pain travels along the anatomic course of the nerve. The compression can be secondary to either soft tissue (disc) or bone. The most common nerve roots affected are L5 and S1—levels that account for pain traveling below the knee. Finally, one should inquire about changes in bowel or bladder habits. Occasionally, a large midline disc herniation may compress several roots of the cauda equina (Fig. 10.10). This is termed cauda equina compression (CEC) syndrome. Urinary retention and incontinence of bowel or bladder are, along with severe pain and saddle paresthesia, the major symptoms.

Physical Examination

The physical examination is directed at finding the location of the pain. All patients with low back pain can have some nonspecific findings which vary in degree depending on the severity of the condition. These include a list to one side, tenderness to palpation and percussion and a decreased range of motion of the lumbar spine. The above findings can be present in both radiculopathy and referred pain patients. Their presence denotes that there is a problem but does not identify the etiology or level of the problem. The neurologic examination may yield objective evidence of nerve root compression if present (Table 10.3). A thorough neurologic evaluation of the lower extremities should be conducted on each patient, particularly to check the reflexes and motor findings. Sensory changes may or may not be present, but because of overlap in the dermatomes of spinal nerves, it is difficult to identify specific root involvement.

In patients with radiculopathies, there are several maneuvers that tighten the sciatic nerve and, in so doing, further compress an inflamed lumbar root against a herniated disc or bony spur. These maneuvers are generally termed tension signs or a

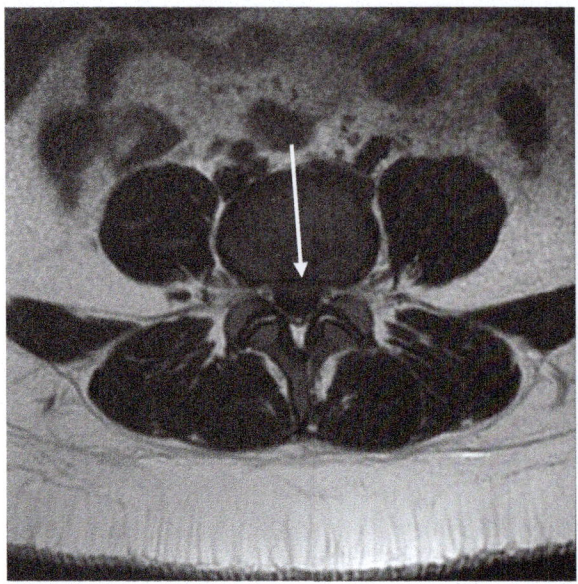 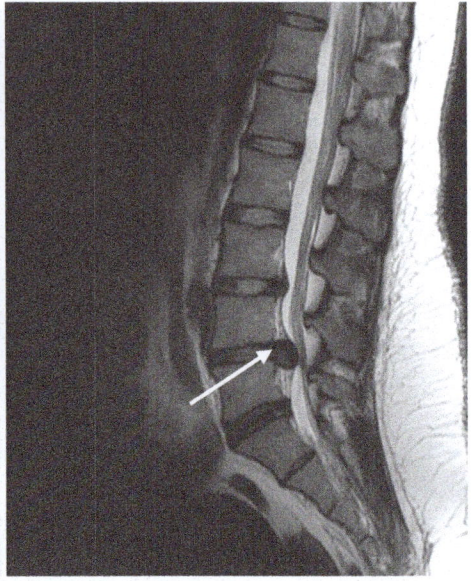

Fig. 10.10 Herniated disc at L4–5 causing severe compression of the cauda equina. Pain is confined chiefly to the buttocks and the back of the thighs and legs. Numbness is widespread from the buttocks to the soles of the feet. Motor weakness or loss is present in the legs and feet with loss of muscle mass in the calves. The bladder and bowels are paralyzed. DP, distribution of pain and paresthesia

Table 10.3 Physical and neurologic exam findings of the lumbar spine (physical exam)

Disk level	Nerve root	Sensory	Motor	Reflex
L1–L2	L2	Anteromedial thigh	Hip flexion	None
L2–L3	L3	Anterior thigh to knee	Quadriceps	Patella
L3–L4	L4	Medial calf/ankle	Anterior tibialis	Patella
L4–L5	L5	Lateral ankle, dorsum of foot	Extensor hallucis longus	None
L5–S1	S1	Gastrocnemius, soleus, peroneals	Plantar/lateral foot	Achilles

straight leg-raising test (SLRT). The conventional SLRT is performed with the patient supine. The examiner slowly elevates the leg by the heel with the knee kept straight. This test is positive when the leg pain below the knee is reproduced or intensified; the production of back and/or buttock pain does not constitute a positive finding. The reliability of the SLRT is age-dependent. In a young patient, a negative test most probably excludes the possibility of a herniated disc. After the age of 30, however, a negative SLRT no longer reliably excludes the diagnosis. Additionally, the contralateral straight leg raise test, in which elevating the asymptomatic leg reproduces radicular symptoms in the symptomatic leg, is even more specific than the ipsilateral straight leg raise.

Finally, the physical examination should evaluate some specific problems that can present as low back pain. This includes a peripheral vascular examination, hip joint evaluation, and abdominal examination. Many patients will present with self-described low back pain that is vague and nonspecific, with physical exam findings not correlating to a particular distribution or localized to the lower back. Waddell signs can be used to differentiate between non-organic or non-dermatomal pain, and pain stemming from the lumbar spine. These signs include broad areas of superficial tenderness crossing multiple dermatomes, sensory changes in a non-dermatomal distribution, regional weakness not associated with a particular myotome, and exaggerated pain response to mild stimuli. Patients with underlying hip pathology such as femoroacetabular impingement will have pain located primarily in the groin that is worsened with knee flexion, adduction, and internal rotation (FADIR test), and should have dedicated hip imaging performed to further assess the nature of their disease.

Diagnostic Studies

As in the cervical spine, diagnostic tests should be used to confirm the core of information gathered from a thorough history and physical examination. Several lumbosacral imaging modalities are currently available including plain films, CT, and MRI.

To evaluate the true clinical value of any diagnostic study, one must know its sensitivity (false-negatives) and specificity (false-positives). The specificity, or false-positive rate, is usually measured in a population of symptomatic patients who have undergone surgery; however, often there is a much higher rate of false positives when an asymptomatic group is studied. The accuracy of any single test increases when it is combined with a second or third diagnostic study. The physician's challenge is to select diagnostic tests on the basis of their performance characteristics so that the correct diagnosis is obtained with the least cost and morbidity. The studies most frequently utilized in the diagnostic assessment of

low back pain will be described and critically analyzed with this in mind.

Plain Radiographs

The diagnosis of disc herniation/radiculopathy can usually be made on the basis of a history and physical examination. Plain radiographs of the lumbosacral spine must be obtained in the appropriate setting to rule out other pathologic conditions such as infection or tumor. Plain radiographs are valuable for seeking the diagnosis of spinal stenosis, spondylolisthesis, gross segmental instability, or fracture.

The radiograph must be of excellent quality and taken with attention to detail. In general, three views are all that are required to assess the lumbosacral spine: an AP view, a lateral view, and a coned-down lateral view of the lower two interspaces. On occasion, two oblique views are also taken to identify subtle spondylolysis or pars interarticularis defects. However, oblique views provide limited information and should not be routinely included. As in the cervical spine, flexion and extension X-rays should be obtained to evaluate for instability and spondylolisthesis (Fig. 10.11). Although plain films are useful for surveying the bony elements of the spine and paraspinal soft tissues, the contents of the spinal

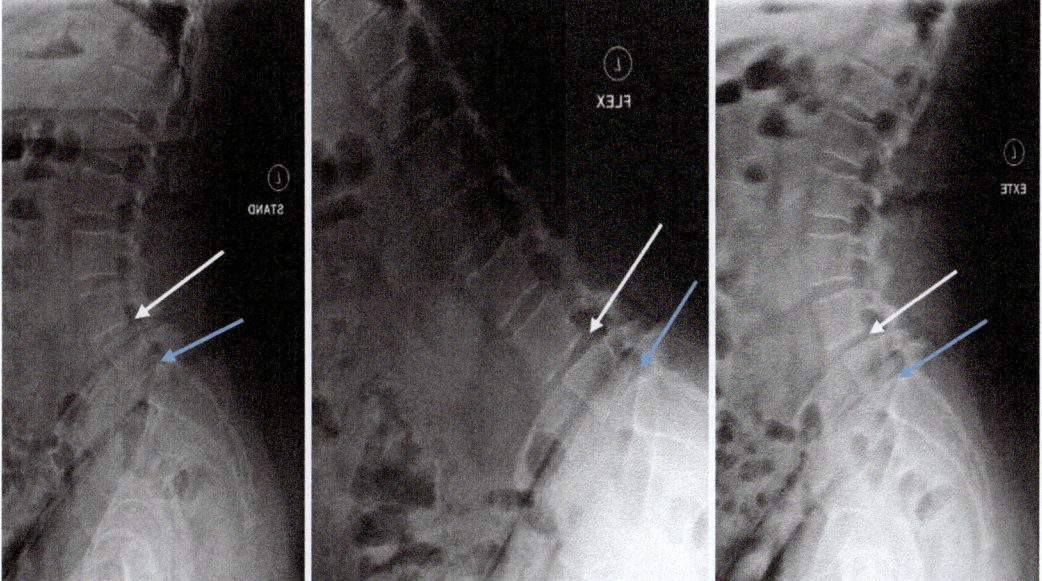

Fig. 10.11   Lateral flexion/extension and standing X-rays of the lumbar spine demonstrating dynamic spondylolisthesis at the L4–L5 level (white arrows). This patient also has severe degenerative disc disease at L5–S1 (blue arrows)

canal, including cord, dura, ligaments, and encroaching disc, are not visualized. In addition, bony lesions may not be apparent until 50% of the cancellous bone has been destroyed.

Finally, degenerative changes such as disc space narrowing, traction osteophytes, vacuum disc phenomenon, and end-plate sclerosis are quite prevalent in older individuals. Unfortunately, these radiographic findings have been shown to correlate poorly with clinical symptoms.

Magnetic Resonance Imaging

Magnetic resonance imaging is the diagnostic modality of choice when trying to evaluate the different tissues in the spine (Fig. 10.12). It is especially good for observing disc pathology. MRI with gadolinium-diethylenetriaminepentaacetic acid (DTPA) contrast enhancement is superb for demonstrating intraspinal tumors and for distinguishing recurrent disc herniation from scar tissue. As discussed with other diagnostic imaging modalities, MRI also has been shown to have a significant clinical false-positive rate in asymptomatic individuals. In one prospective and blinded study, 22% of the asymptomatic subjects under age 60 and 57% of those over age 60 had significantly abnormal scans. In addition, the prevalence

of disc degeneration on the T2-weighted MRI scans was found to approach 98% in subjects over the age of 60.

Computed Tomography

Computed tomography is a very versatile and widely available noninvasive modality for evaluating abnormalities of the lumbosacral spine. Multiple cross-sectional (axial) images of the spine are made at various levels and, with reformatting, coronal, sagittal, and three-dimensional images may be created. The CT scan demonstrates not only the bony spinal configuration, but also the soft tissue in graded shading, so that ligaments, nerve roots, free fat, and intervertebral disc protrusions can be evaluated as they relate to their bony environment (Figs. 10.13 and 10.14).

The CT scan is an extremely valuable diagnostic tool when it is used appropriately to confirm the patient's clinical findings. However, recent studies reveal the pitfalls of making clinical decisions on the basis of isolated CT scan findings. Despite many reports in the literature indicating that CT scanning has a mean accuracy of 90% in symptomatic patients, 34% of asymptomatic patients had abnormal CT scans when reviewed by three independent expert interpreters. The

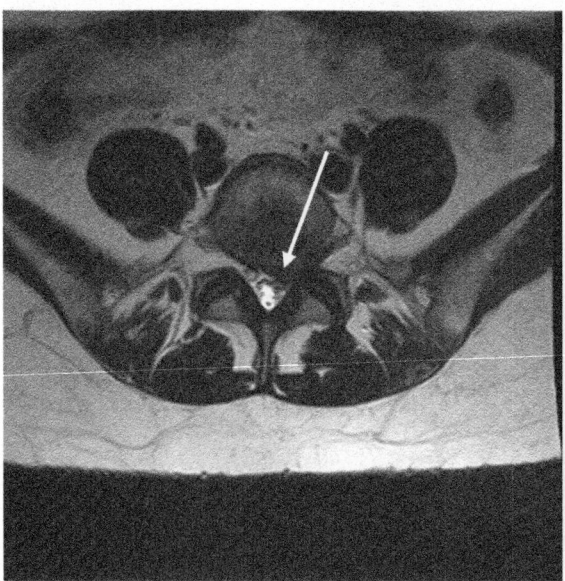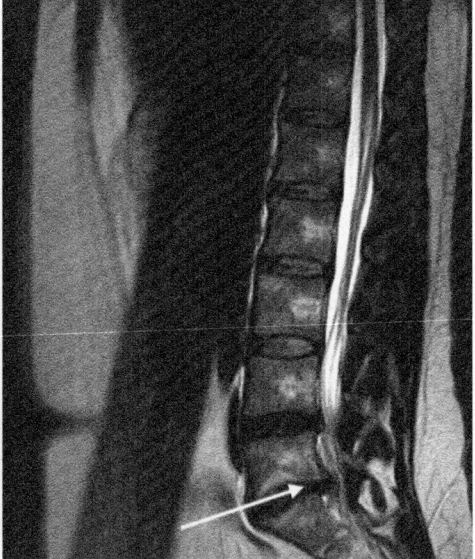

Fig. 10.12 Axial sagittal images of a T2-weighted MRI demonstrating left 5-S1 paracentral disc herniation

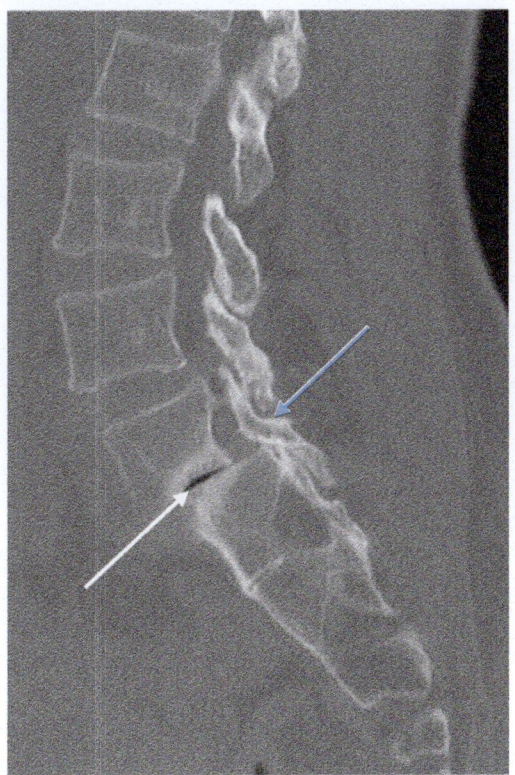

Fig. 10.13 Sagittal CT scan demonstrating degenerative changes (end-plate sclerosis and vacuum disc phenomenon: white arrow) and isthmic spondylolisthesis at L5–S1 with elongated pars and no evidence of a pars defect (blue arrow)

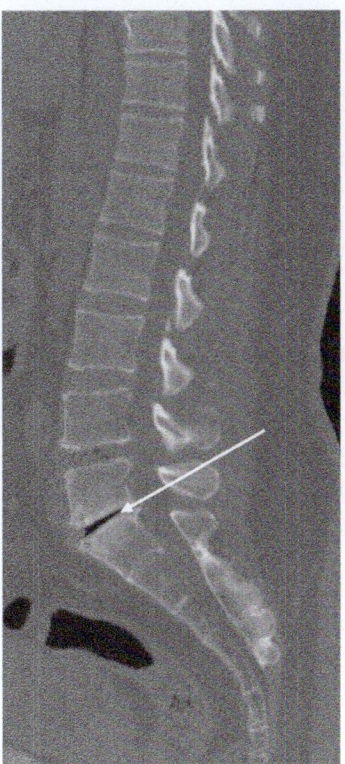

Fig. 10.14 Sagittal CT scan demonstrating chronic degenerative changes including loss of disc height, osteophyte formation, and vacuum disc phenomenon at the L5–S1 level

implication is that a patient with a negative history and physical examination for a spinal lesion has a one in three chance of having an abnormal CT scan. If the decision for surgery is based only on scan results, there is a 30% chance that the patient will undergo an unnecessary and unsuccessful operation. However, if the patient's clinical picture correlates with the CT scan abnormalities, CT scan can be a useful confirmatory diagnostic tool. CT scan can additionally be useful for pre-operative planning in the form of pedicle measurements, deformity assessment, and alignment.

Electrodiagnostic Testing

The EMG is performed by placing needles into muscles to determine if there is an intact nerve supply to that muscle. An abnormal EMG can demonstrate impaired nerve transmission to a specific muscle and isolate the nerve root

involved. Initially, the EMG will be negative in spite of nerve entrapment and will only show muscle irritability. After 3 weeks of significant pressure on a nerve root, signs of denervation with fibrillation can be observed.

The EMG, like all the other confirmatory tests already discussed, is not a screening tool. In fact, when dealing with the average low back problem, the EMG rarely provides any information that cannot be derived from a careful physical examination. It may even confuse the picture, since an EMG may be abnormal from diabetic neuropathy, previous peripheral nerve entrapment, or trauma. In cases in which the correlation of clinical signs and imaging is equivocal, especially with chronic unexpected sciatica, nerve conduction studies and EMG may be helpful. Electromyography can also detect the involvement of a secondary nerve root in cases of complex back injury preoperatively, sometimes prompting a more extensive operation.

Clinical Conditions

There are a number of conditions that can present as low back pain in any particular individual. However, the following four are the most common of those typically evaluated by orthopedic surgeons and will be discussed in detail: back strain, herniated disc, spinal stenosis, and spondylolisthesis.

Back Strain-Lumbago

The vast majority of people who have low back discomfort suffer from a nonradiating type of low back pain called back sprain or lumbago. The etiology is not always clear but is probably a ligamentous or muscular strain secondary to either a specific traumatic episode or the continuous mechanical stress of a postural inadequacy. These may also include patients with a small tear in the annulus fibrosus, which would account for the frequent prior history of low back pain in patients with a ruptured disc transmitted by nociceptors found within the annulus.

These patients' main complaint is back pain, and it can be limited to one spot or cover a diffuse area of the lumbosacral spine. At times, there may be a referral of pain to the buttocks or posterior thigh since the lower back, buttocks, and posterior thigh all originate from the same embryonic tissue, or mesoderm. Such referral of pain does not necessarily connote any mechanical compression of the neural elements and should not be called sciatica.

The usual findings are limited to local tenderness over the involved area and muscle spasm; however, the attacks will vary in intensity and can conveniently be divided into three categories: mild, moderate, and severe. Those placed in the mild group have subjective pain without objective findings and should be able to return to customary activity in less than a week. The moderate group is characterized by a limited range of spinal motion and paravertebral muscle spasm as well as pain and these patients should be able to resume full activity in less than 2 weeks. The severe group includes those patients who are tilted forward or to the side. They have trouble ambulating and can take up to 3 weeks to become functional again.

Since a normal X-ray is a standard occurrence with a patient complaining of back strain, a radiographic study is usually not necessary on the first visit if the physician feels comfortable with the diagnosis; however, if the response to treatment does not proceed as expected, films should be taken to rule out other more serious problems such as spondylolisthesis or tumor. The authors' usual recommendation is that if a patient fails to respond to conservative treatment for an acute attack of low back pain after a period of 2 weeks, then a routine lumbosacral spine X-ray series is clinically indicated.

The authors' preferred treatment for low back strain is the functional restoration approach. The mainstay of treatment is controlled physical activity, with the judicious use of trunk flexibility and strengthening exercises as the acute phase subsides. Often, particularly in the obese patient with weak abdominal muscles, a lightweight lumbosacral corset is useful in helping to mobilize those encumbered by low back strain.

Osteoporosis and Vertebral Compression Fractures

Osteoporosis, defined as a T-score at or below −2.5 standard deviations below the mean on a dexa scan, is a common occurrence in the elderly population, particularly in females. These patients are susceptible to osteoporotic fragility fractures, including fractures of the proximal humerus, distal radius, hip, and vertebral body. Compression fractures of the vertebrae most commonly occur at transitional zone from T11–L1. As the thoracic kyphosis transitions to lumbar lordosis, this area bears a significant amount of axial load with little associated motion.

Plain radiographs will most often demonstrate focal deformity at the vertebral body, including loss of height and occasionally angular deformity. Patients will have tenderness to palpation over the affected area as well as pain with motion. It is important to obtain a detailed physical exam to rule out neurologic deficit, as fracture fragments can be retropulsed into the spinal canal in rare cases.

Treatment of vertebral compression fractures without neurologic deficit consists of rest, analgesics, and gradual mobilization. Kyphoplasty and vertebroplasty, which involve injection of cement into the vertebral body, can prevent further collapse and improve functional pain in some cases. It is important that patients be counseled on osteoporosis and referred to an endocrinologist for bone health evaluation and medication management including bisphosphonates and PTH-analogs.

Herniated Disc

A herniated disc can be defined as the herniation of the nucleus pulposus through the torn fibers of the annulus fibrosus. Most disc ruptures occur during the third and fourth decades of life while the nucleus pulposus is still gelatinous. The perforations usually arise through a defect just lateral to the posterior midline where the posterior longitudinal ligament is weakest. The two most common levels for disc herniation are L4–L5 and L5–S1. These two discs account for 95% of all lumbar disc herniations; pathology at the L2–L3 and L3–L4 levels can occur but is relatively uncommon.

Disc herniations at L5–S1 will usually compromise the first sacral nerve root. A lesion at the L4–L5 level will most often compress the fifth lumbar root, while a herniation at the L3–L4

more commonly involves the fourth lumbar root. It should be pointed out, however, that variations in root configuration as well as in the position of the herniation itself can modify these relationships. An L4–L5 disc rupture can at times affect the first sacral as well as the fifth lumbar root and, in extreme lateral herniations, the nerve ending exiting at the same level as the disc will be involved (Figs. 10.15 and 10.16).

Not everyone with a disc herniation has significant discomfort. A large herniation in a capacious canal may not be clinically significant since there is no compression of the neural elements, while a minor protrusion in a small canal may be crippling since there is not enough room to accommodate both the disc and the nerve root.

Clinically, the patient's major complaint is pain. Although there may be a prior history of intermittent episodes of localized low back pain, this is not always the case. The pain is not only present in the back, but also radiates down the leg in the distribution of the affected nerve root. It will usually be described as sharp or lancinating, progressing from the top downward in the involved leg. Its onset may be insidious or sudden and associated with a tearing or snapping sensation in the spine. Occasionally, when sciatica develops, the back pain may resolve since once

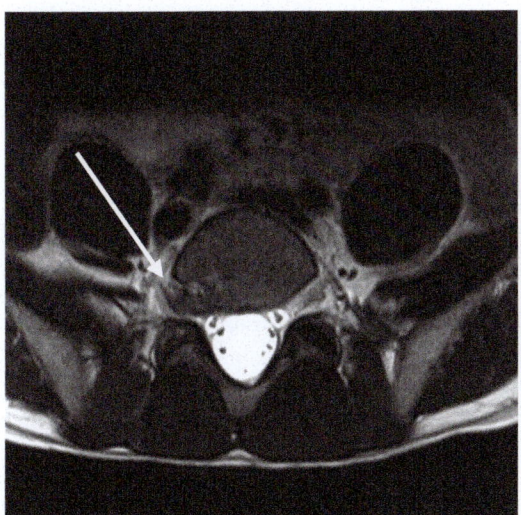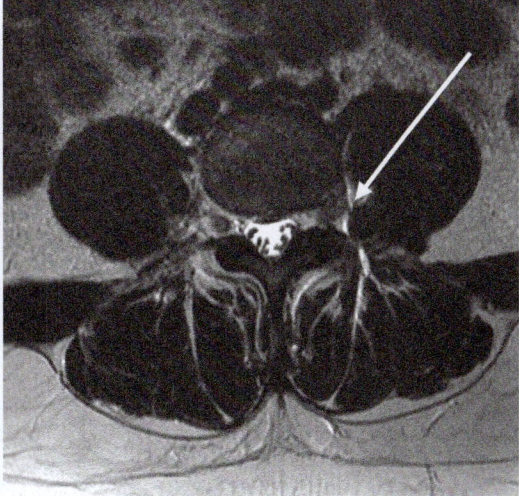

Fig. 10.15 Axial T2-weighted MRI cuts of the lumbar spine demonstrating right foraminal disc herniation causing foraminal stenosis (**a**) and a left-sided far lateral disc herniation (**b**)

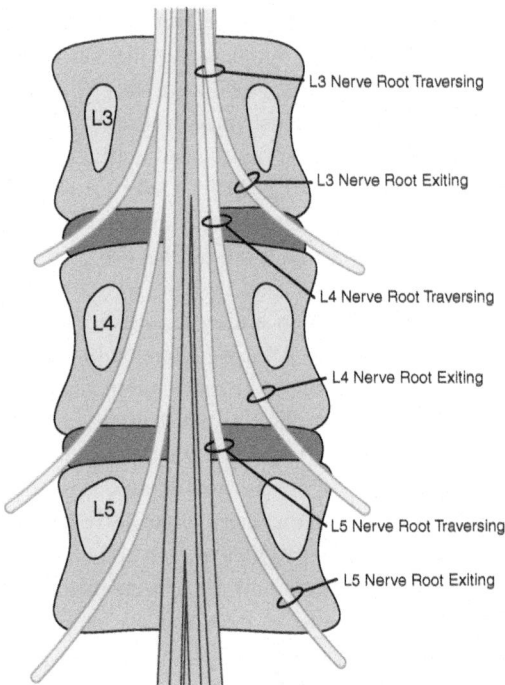

L3 Nerve Root Traversing

L3 Nerve Root Exiting

L4 Nerve Root Traversing

L4 Nerve Root Exiting

L5 Nerve Root Traversing

L5 Nerve Root Exiting

Fig. 10.16 Schematic demonstrating the traversing and exiting nerve roots in the lumbar spine

the annulus has ruptured, it may no longer be under tension. Finally, sciatica may vary in intensity; it may be so severe that patients will be unable to ambulate and will feel that their back is "locked." Conversely, the pain may be limited to a dull ache that increases in intensity with ambulation.

On physical examination, there is usually a decreased range of motion in flexion, and patients will tend to drift away from the involved side as they bend. On ambulation, the patient walks with an antalgic gait, holding the involved leg flexed so as to put as little weight as possible on the extremity.

Although neurologic examination may yield objective evidence of nerve root compression, these findings are often undependable since the involved nerve is often still functional. In addition, such deficit may have little temporal relevance since it may relate to a prior attack at a different level. To be significant, reflex changes, weakness, atrophy, or sensory loss must conform to the rest of the clinical picture.

When the first sacral root is compressed, the patient may have gastrocnemius-soleus weakness and be unable to repeatedly rise up on the toes of that foot. Atrophy of the calf may be apparent and the ankle (Achilles) reflex is often diminished or absent. Sensory loss, if any, is usually confined to the posterior aspect of the calf and lateral side of the foot.

Involvement of the fifth lumbar nerve root can lead to weakness in extension of the great toe and, less often, to weakness of the evertors and dorsiflexors of the foot. An associated sensory deficit can appear over the anterior leg and the dorsomedial aspect of the foot down to the great toe. There are usually no primary reflex changes, but, on occasion, a diminution in the posterior tibial reflex can be elicited. The absence of this reflex, however, must be asymmetrical for it to have any clinical significance.

With compression of the fourth lumbar nerve root, the quadriceps muscle is affected. The patient may note weakness in knee extension, and it is often associated with instability. Atrophy of the thigh musculature can be marked. A sensory loss may be apparent over the anteromedial aspect of the thigh and the patellar tendon reflex is usually diminished. Precise assessment of the fourth and fifth lumbar nerve roots can be difficult given the high degree of crossover in both sensory and motor innervation.

Nerve root sensitivity can be elicited by any method that creates tension; however, the SLRT is the one most commonly employed. As discussed before, a positive test reproduces the patient's pain down the leg. The reproduction of back pain is not considered positive.

The initial diagnosis of a herniated disc is ordinarily made on the basis of the history and physical examination. Plain X-rays of the lumbosacral spine will rarely add to the diagnosis but should be obtained to help rule out other causes of pain, such as infection or tumor. Other tests such as the EMG, CT scan, and MRI are confirmatory by nature and can be misinformative when they are used as screening devices.

The treatment for most patients with a herniated disc is nonoperative since 80% of them will respond to conservative therapy when followed over a period of 5 years. The efficacy of nonoperative treatment, however, depends upon a healthy relationship between a capable physician and a well-informed patient. If a patient has insight into the rationale for the prescribed treatment and follows instructions, the chances of success are greatly increased.

One of the most important elements in the nonoperative treatment is controlled physical activity, best when guided by a physical therapist. Patients should markedly decrease their activity, but bed rest is not indicated. An acute herniation usually takes at least 2 weeks before the pain substantially eases.

Drug therapy is another important part of the treatment and three categories of pharmacological agents are commonly used: anti-inflammatory drugs, analgesics, and muscle relaxants. As mentioned previously, oral steroids can also play an important role in decreasing the inflammation that causes back pain and nerve root irritation after an acute injury. Muscle relaxants such as methocarbamol, cyclobenzaprine, and tizanidine are the current drugs of choice in clinical practice. Inasmuch as the symptoms of low back pain and sciatica result from an inflammatory reaction as well as mechanical compression, the authors feel that anti-inflammatory medication should be taken in conjunction with rest. The patient's pain generally will be relieved once the inflammation is brought under control. There may be some numbness or tingling in the involved extremity, but this is usually tolerable.

Eighty percent of those who follow the above regimen will be markedly improved, but it requires patience since frequently at least 6 weeks will have passed before any additional therapy is indicated. Although the noninvasive treatment of a herniated disc can be quite gratifying, it generally takes a significant period of rest and the patient must be aware of the time constraints from the beginning in order to understand the rationale behind the measures employed. If nonoperative management fails, surgical intervention is very effective in the form of microdiscectomy.

The long-term prognosis for patients with disc herniation is quite good. It has been shown that between 85% and 90% of surgically treated and non-surgically treated patients were asymptomatic at 4 years. Less than 2% of both groups were symptomatic at 10 years.

Spinal Stenosis

Spinal stenosis can be defined as a narrowing of the spinal canal and the mechanical pressure on the neural structures within will depend upon the degree of narrowing. In the lumbar spine there are three main structures that cause spinal stenosis: (1) intervertebral discs, (2) facet joints, and (3) the ligamentum flavum. Acute disc herniations or disc bulges can protrude posteriorly into the spinal canal, decreasing the AP space allowed for the nerve roots. Facet joints become hypertrophic in degenerative cases and can cause stenosis centrally and foraminally. As do the facet joints, the ligamentum flavum can hypertrophy and "buckle" in degenerative cases which further contributes to the degree of stenosis. Every person's spine, however, becomes narrower with age due to osteoarthritis. Not everyone with a narrowed spinal canal, however, will have symptoms.

For those who do suffer, the discomfort can vary from mild annoyance to an inability to walk. The symptom complex is well documented. Patients of either sex, usually not before their fifth decade, will first complain of vague pains, dysesthesias, and paresthesias with ambulation, but will typically have excellent relief of their symptoms when they are sitting or lying supine. The increased lordotic stance assumed when walking, and particularly walking down grades, is most likely the inciting cause. The hyperextension further narrows the spinal canal and increases the symptoms.

With maturation of the syndrome, symptoms may even occur at rest. Muscle weakness, atrophy, and asymmetrical reflex changes may then appear; however, as long as the symptoms are only aggravated dynamically, neurological changes will occur only after the patient is stressed. The following stress tests can be used in an outpatient clinic: after a neurological examination has been performed on the patient, he or she is asked to walk up and down the corridor until symptoms occur or the patient has walked 300 ft. A repeat examination is then done and, in many cases, the second examination will be positive for a focal neurologic deficit when the first was negative. Plain X-rays are often helpful in visualizing spinal stenosis, particularly degenerative spinal stenosis. One can see intervertebral disc degeneration, decreased interpedicular distance, a decreased sagittal canal diameter, and facet degeneration. If a patient fails conservative treatment and becomes a surgical candidate, the location and degree of neurological compression can be assessed with MRI or CT-myelogram.

The majority of patients with spinal stenosis, especially the degenerative and combined variety, can be treated non-surgically with anti-inflammatory medication and physical therapy.

Finally, a lumbosacral corset is often helpful in reminding the patient to avoid excessive motion. This bracing serves as a reminder for patients to engage their core muscles and relieve pressure on the lumbar spine. However, when used for a prolonged period this brace can become compensatory and lead to weakening of the core muscles (Fig. 10.17).

Spondylolisthesis

Spondylolisthesis is a spinal condition where all or part of a vertebra has slipped forward on another. The word is derived from the Greek *spondylos*, meaning "vertebra," and *olisthesis*, meaning "to slip." There are several different types of spondylolisthesis, but the most common is that in which the lesion is in the isthmus or pars interarticularis. If a defect can be identified, but no slipping has occurred, the condition is termed spondylolysis; if one vertebra has slipped forward on another (horizontal translation), it is referred to as spondylolisthesis.

The etiology of the defect in spondylolysis is not clear. Although there may be a hereditary component, the lesion is seldom seen in patients under the age of 5 and is found in 5% of people over the age of 17. The most attractive explanation is that although these children inherit a potential deficiency in the pars, they are not born with any identifiable defect. Between the ages of 5 and 17, however, they become more active and a stress fracture, caused by repetitive hyperextension stresses, can develop into a spondylolysis. It is likely that most of these fractures occur during the period of rapid growth known as the adolescent growth spurt and they are particularly prevalent in gymnasts and football players.

Spondylolisthesis has several characteristic features, but the forward displacement is easily recognized radiographically on the lateral projection (Figs. 10.18 and 10.19). The degree of slip

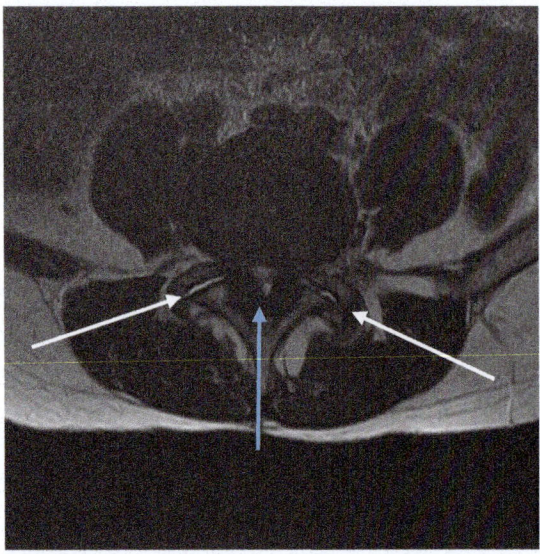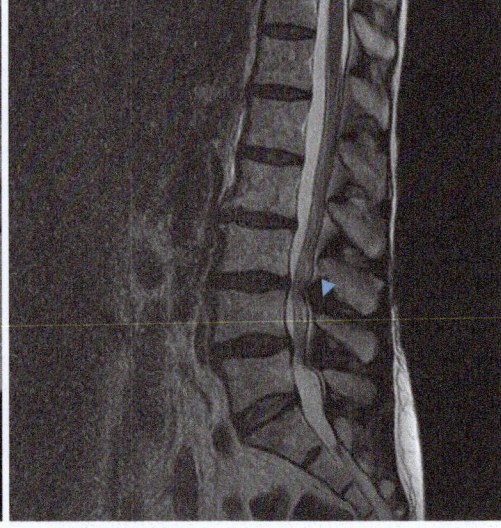

Fig. 10.17 Axial and sagittal T2-Weighted MRI imaging demonstrating severe stenosis as the L3–L4 level due to facet and ligamentum flavum hypertrophy (white and blue lines, respectively)

Fig. 10.18 Meyerding classification system for spondylolisthesis

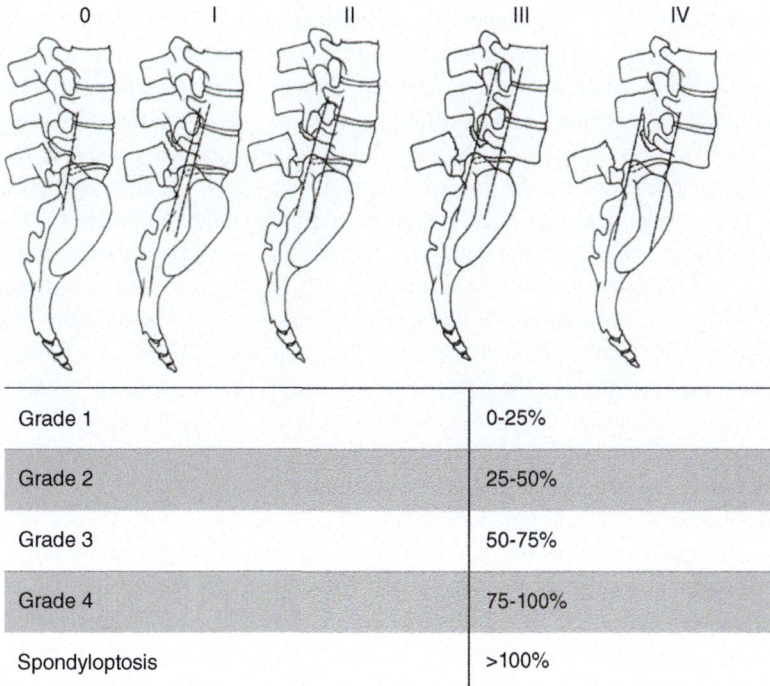

Grade 1	0-25%
Grade 2	25-50%
Grade 3	50-75%
Grade 4	75-100%
Spondyloptosis	>100%

Type	Description	Exampe
I	Dysplastic	Congenital defect in neural arch
II	Isthmic	Defect in the pars interarticularis
-IIA		Spondylolysis (stress fracture of the pars)
-IIB		Elongation of pars via repeated microtrauma (gymnasts, offensive linemen)
-IIC		Acute fracture
III	Degenerative	Facet joint degeneration
IV	Posttraumatic	Acute fracture of posterior column, but not pars
V	Pathologic	Infection, tumor, etc.
VI	Iatrogenic	Post-surgical instability (over-resection of pars intra-operatively)

Fig. 10.19 Wiltse classification system for spondylolisthesis

varies from patient to patient and can range from minimal displacement to complete dislocation of the vertebral body. Increased slipping rarely occurs after the age of 20 unless there has been a severe superimposed injury or surgical intervention. The period of most rapid progression coincides with the rapid growth spurt between the ages of 9 and 15.

The most common clinical manifestation of spondylolisthesis is low back pain. Although the cause of this type of back pain in the adult has been studied extensively, its origin is still not clear. There is no clear understanding of how so many patients develop this lesion between the ages of 5 and 17, but still have no back complaints until perhaps age 35, when a sudden twisting or lifting motion will precipitate an acute episode of back and leg pain. Other patients with significant degrees of slipping, however, will go through life with no discomfort.

Although 50% of patients overall normally cannot associate an injury with the onset of the symptoms of those working in industry, almost all report an associated incident. It is possible to sustain an acute fracture of the pars, but it is a very rare occurrence. If the acuity of a pars defect is in question, it can be documented by a bone scan within 3 months of the injury; if the defect is long-standing, the scan will be negative.

There is also frequently a buildup of a fibro-cartilaginous mass at the defect, and this can cause pain by irritating the nerve root as it exits. It is thus not unusual in spondylolisthesis to have the patient first complain of back pain, but over time have leg pain develop as the most troubling symptom.

Once the symptoms begin, the patient usually has constant low-grade back discomfort that is aggravated by activity and relieved by rest. There are some periods during which the pain is more intense than others, but unless the picture is complicated by severe leg pain, total incapacitation is rare. The patients are seldom aware of any sensory or motor deficit. At this point, it should be reemphasized that in some people even severe displacement is asymptomatic and gives rise to no disability. It is not uncommon to pick up a previously unrecognized spondylolisthesis on a routine gastrointestinal radiological study of a 50-year-old patient.

The physical findings of this syndrome are fairly characteristic. In the absence of any radicular pain, the patient exhibits no postural scoliosis; but there is usually an exaggeration of the lumbar lordosis and a palpable "stepoff" with a dimple at the side of the abnormality. Occasionally, mild muscle spasm is demonstrable, and in most instances, some local tenderness can be elicited. Although the range of motion is usually complete, some pain can be expected on hyperextension.

Radiographs, particularly the lateral views, confirm the diagnosis. Even the slightest amount of forward slipping of the body of the involved vertebra is readily discernible and the oblique views will disclose the actual defect in the pars. Flexion and extension ("dynamic") views may show instability, noted with translation or angulation of the upper vertebra on the lower.

The nonoperative treatment of the adult with spondylolisthesis is much the same as that used for backache from other causes. When the symptoms are acute, rest is indicated. If leg pain is a significant problem, then anti-inflammatory medication can be quite beneficial. Exercises, usually a flexion-extension program, should be started once patients are in remission and they are usually advised to own a corset for use during occasional strenuous activity. Epidural steroid injections may be useful in calming down an acute radicular attack. If conservative treatment is not successful, an operative approach can be considered and would include a spinal fusion.

Lumbar Spine Algorithm

As with patients with neck pain, the task of the physician when confronted with low back pain patients is to integrate their complaints into an accurate diagnosis and to prescribe appropriate therapy. This problem (universe of low back pain patients) has been formatted into an algorithm (Fig. 10.20), the aim of which is to select the correct diagnostic category and proper treatment avenues for each patient with low back pain. A specific patient may fall outside the limits of the algorithm and require a different approach and the physician must constantly be on the alert for exceptions. The algorithm can be followed in sequence and is also presented in table form (Table 10.4).

The information necessary to use the algorithm is initially obtained through the history and physical examination. The key points in the history are differentiation of back pain that is mechanical in nature from nonmechanical pain that is present at rest, detecting changes in bowel or bladder function and defining the precise location and quality of the pain. The physical examination must be oriented toward ruling out other medical causes of low back pain, assessing neurologic function, and evaluating for the presence of tension signs.

Following the low back pain algorithm, the first major decision is to make a ruling on the presence or absence of CEC syndrome. Mechanical compression of the cauda equina is a

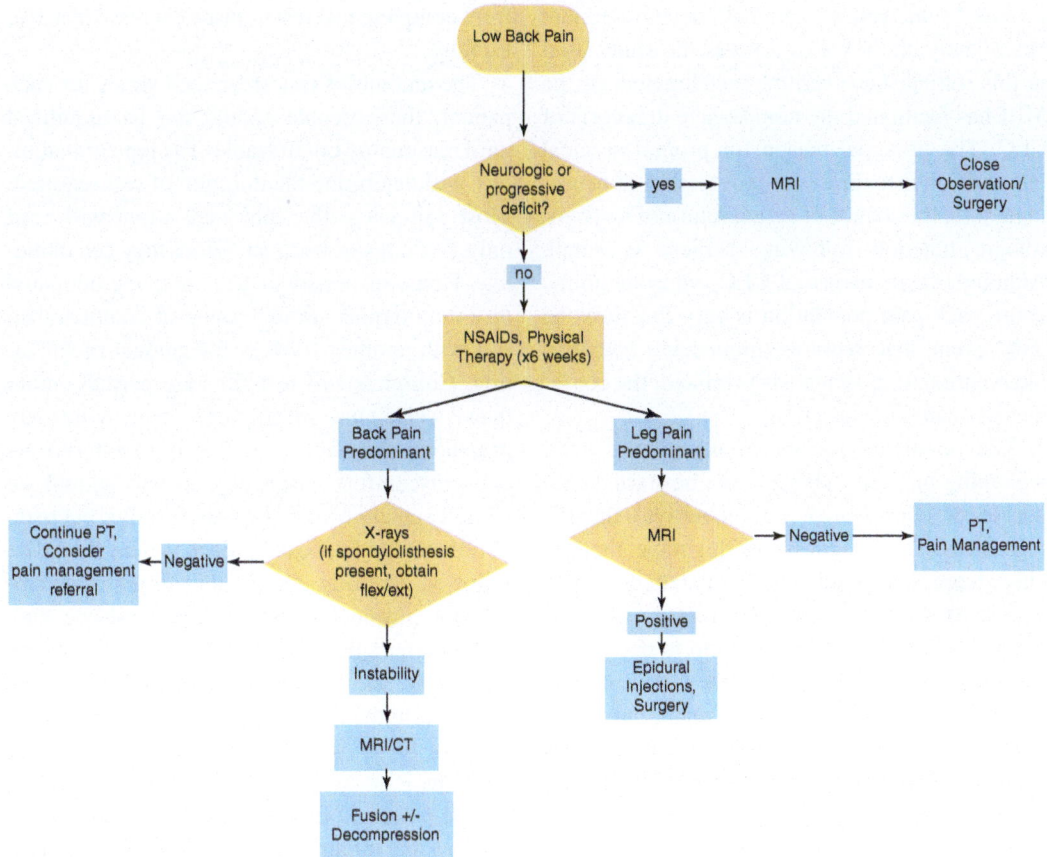

Fig. 10.20 Algorithm for the differential diagnosis of low back pain

Table 10.4 Differential diagnosis and features of common causes of low back pain

	Predominant pain	Constitutional symptoms	Neurologic exam	Plain X-rays	Dynamic X-rays	CT/ MRI
Back strain	Back	–	–	–	–	–
Disc herniation	Leg	–	+/–	–	–	+
Spinal stenosis	Back/leg	–	+/–	+	–	+
Spondylolisthesis	Back	–	–	+	+	+
Spondyloarthropathy	Back	+	–	+	–	–

surgical emergency, much like myelopathy. Once cauda equina is ruled out, further evaluation of low back pain can be undertaken.

Cauda equina, with truly progressive motor weakness, is the only surgical emergency in lumbar spine disease. This compression from a massive rupture of the L4–L5 disc in the midline is usually due to pressure on the caudal sac, through which pass the nerves to the lower extremities, bowel, and bladder.

The signs and symptoms of CEC are a complex mixture of low back pain, bilateral motor weakness of the lower extremities, bilateral sciatica, saddle anesthesia, and even frank paraplegia with bowel and bladder incontinence or urinary retention. Cauda equina compression can be caused by either bone or soft tissue damage, the latter generally a ruptured or herniated disc in the midline. These patients should undergo an immediate definitive diagnostic test and, if it is positive, emergency surgical decompression. Historically, the myelogram was the study used in this setting; however, the development of the MRI has facilitated the noninvasive diagnosis of CEC. The principal reason for prompt surgical intervention is to arrest the progression of neurologic loss; the chance of actual return of lost neurologic function following surgery is small. Although the incidence of CEC syndrome in the entire back pain population is very low, it is the only event that requires immediate operative intervention; if its diagnosis is missed, the consequences can be devastating.

The remaining patients make up the overwhelming majority. They should be started on a course of conservative (nonoperative) therapy regardless of the diagnosis. At this stage, the specific diagnosis, whether a herniated disc or a simple back strain, is not important to the therapy because the entire population is treated the same way. A few of these patients will eventually need an invasive procedure (surgery), but at this point there is no way to predict which individuals will respond to conservative therapy and which will not.

Conservative Treatment Modalities

As the algorithm indicates, all low back pain patients, regardless of diagnosis (except those with CEC syndrome), require an initial period of conservative therapy. At present, there are many modalities available, but few have been scientifically validated because of the difficulty in performing a prospective double-blind study in this field. Each treatment plan in popular use today is surrounded by conflicting claims for its indications and efficacy. The purpose of this section is to discuss the rationale behind the use of some of the more common therapeutic measures.

Controlled Physical Activity

Decreased activity has evolved over the years as one of the most important elements in the treatment of low back pain. The degree of rest depends on the severity of the symptoms and can vary from complete bed rest to just a decrease in active exercise.

The amount of rest prescribed varies for each patient; these people should not be mobilized until reasonably comfortable. The type of pathology will determine the duration of rest required. Most patients with acute back strain will need only 2–7 days of bed rest before they can ambulate. However, a patient with an acute herniated disc may require up to 1 week of complete bed rest with another 10 days for gradual mobilization. Complete bed rest for long periods (more than 2 weeks) has a deleterious effect on the body in general and should be closely monitored. As their discomfort eases, the patient should be strongly encouraged to take short walks, but to do as little sitting as possible. Each patient should be followed carefully and given a formal prescription for physical therapy. Close guidance with physical therapists can allow for controlled return to activity, activity modification and education, core strengthening, and stretching to allow patients to return to their previous levels of function.

The purpose of controlled physical activity is to allow any inflammatory reaction that is present to subside. Bed rest will not result in the disc's return to its original position. However, as the disc herniates, it causes a secondary inflammatory process responsible for the patient's pain; if this reaction can be brought under control, the patient's symptoms will disappear. This relief may or may not be permanent.

Drug Therapy

The judicious use of drug therapy is an important adjunct in the treatment of low back pain. As in the cervical spine, there are three main categories of drugs in common use: anti-inflammatories, analgesics, and muscle relaxants.

Anti-inflammatory agents are employed because of the belief that inflammation within the affected tissues is a major cause of pain in the low back. This is especially true for those patients with symptoms secondary to a herniated disc.

There are a variety of NSAIDs available. Based on several scientific studies, none of these appear to be superior to the others. Most patients will get significant relief. Again, all anti-inflammatory medications are utilized in conjunction with controlled physical activity to relieve pain; they do not replace adequate rest. Occasionally, after an initial recovery, a patient will experience intermittent recurrent attacks or complain of a chronic low backache; in some instances these patients will be helped by a maintenance dose of an anti-inflammatory drug.

Analgesic medication is very important during the acute phase of low back pain. The goal is to keep the patient comfortable while in bed. Most of the anti-inflammatory agents also have analgesic properties. In more severe cases, patients may require narcotic medications. However this should be monitored closely (usually by a pain management specialist) and these medications are only to be used sparingly.

The biggest mistake seen is treatment with very strong narcotics such as oxycodone or hydromorphone on an outpatient basis. Many of these patients become addicted to the medication. In other cases, patients try to shortcut the controlled physical activity and use analgesic medication instead. This, of course, will not work and when the patient tries to stop the drug, the back pain returns.

Muscle relaxants generally are not recommended for the treatment of low back pain. In most cases, the muscle spasm is secondary to a primary problem such as a herniated disc. If the pain from the ruptured disc can be controlled, the muscle spasm will usually subside.

Occasionally, muscle spasm will be so severe that some type of treatment is required. Tizanidine (zanaflex), methocarbamol (Robaxin), or cyclobenzaprine (Flexeril) are the drugs recommended. Diazepam (Valium) should be discouraged since it is actually a physiological depressant and depression is often an integral feature of back pain syndromes. Administering diazepam to depressed patients only increases their problems. If anxiety is prominent and a sedative is needed, phenobarbital will alleviate the symptoms.

In summary, drug therapy for low back pain should be viewed as an adjunct to adequately controlled physical activity. Anti-inflammatory medication should be the primary agent employed. Analgesic medication should be used selectively in a controlled environment and not for extended periods. Muscle relaxants are generally not recommended and, if employed, should be carefully monitored.

Trigger-Point Injection

Trigger-point therapy is indicated for nonradiating low back pain when a point of maximal tenderness can be identified. This procedure involves the injection of steroids and Xylocaine at an area of maximal tenderness in the low back. The precise mechanism of action is not clear but may be related to modulation of peripheral nerve stimulation as it affects the afferent input perceived as pain.

Trigger-point therapy is easy to perform, has a negligible risk, and may help certain patients. Further controlled research is required to delineate the true value of this modality in the treatment of low back pain.

Epidural Steroid Injection

Epidural steroid injections are indicated for severe lumbar radiculopathy, not, in most cases, for nonradiating low back pain. They have generally been viewed as an intermediate form of treatment between conservative and surgical management. It is a more aggressive attempt at pain relief after conservative therapy has failed, yet avoids the disadvantages of surgery. The rationale for this therapy is that lumbar radiculopathy (in the early phase) involves a significant inflammatory component, evoked by chemical or mechanical irritation or an autoimmune response—all of which should be amenable to treatment with corticosteroid drugs in the early stages.

Unfortunately, few studies have systematically and accurately studied the efficacy of this treatment modality. Poorly controlled, nonrandomized studies have yielded controversial results with a range of success rates from 25% to 75%. Another problem is that some studies have attempted to determine the efficacy of epidural steroids compared to epidural saline injection, while others have compared their results to a true placebo.

Despite the lack of optimally designed investigations, upon review of the literature, certain trends seem to be evident. Epidural steroids appear to be more beneficial in acute rather than chronic radiculopathy, especially when no neurologic deficit is present. Improvement may not be noted until 3–6 days after injection and may be only temporary. No neurotoxicity has been reported in humans or animal models; complications stem from the technique of epidural injection and are rare. Suppression of plasma corticosteroid concentration may occur up to 3 weeks following the injection.

The authors maintain that epidural steroids may be helpful in relieving some component of radicular pain in 40% of patients. Until controlled investigations indicate otherwise, this is a treatment worth trying in patients who have failed 6 weeks of conservative management in an effort to avoid a major invasive procedure.

Traction

The application of traction to the lumbar spine is a popular treatment for patients with herniated discs. The theory is that stretching the lumbar spine distracts the vertebrae so that the protruded disc is allowed to return to a more normal anatomic position. In fact, the disc material probably does not change position at all. Scientific evidence indicates that a traction force equal to 60% of body weight is needed just to reduce the intradiscal pressure at the third lumbar vertebra by 25%. Such a force could not practically be applied to a patient. Furthermore, there has never been any proof that disc material returns to its normal position following herniation.

Traction can be applied as gravity lumbar traction, autotraction, and through motorized techniques. None of these methods has been proven to be more effective than the others. While a few studies have shown traction to have a short-lived benefit on sciatica patients, most double-blind studies have not demonstrated any positive effect. In one study, two groups of patients with proven herniated discs (by myelogram) were treated by applying traction apparatuses to each group in the hospital. However, for one group there were weights in the traction bag; for the other, no weights. There was no statistically significant difference between the two groups in terms of relief of symptoms. Traction had no effect on spinal mobility, tension signs, deep tendon reflexes, paresis, or sensory deficit and although it usually was well tolerated, it made some patients worse.

Manipulation

Spinal manipulation is another popular conservative modality in treating low back pain. In the USA, it is somewhat controversial because it is performed mostly by chiropractors. The principle involved is that any malalignment of the spinal structures can be corrected by manipulation; the assumption here is that the malalignment is the etiology of the patient's pain. Unfortunately, there is no scientific proof for or against either the efficacy of this therapy or its pathophysiological foundation.

The authors' experience is that some patients do have short periods of symptomatic relief after manipulation, but must keep returning for repeated sessions to maintain it, substantially increasing the cost of treatment. Some patients, in fact, may be harmed if pathologic bone disease such as a tumor or osteopenia is present when manipulation is performed. At present, it is felt that manipulation is not indicated for the routine treatment of chronic low back pain. There is not adequate scientific evidence to justify its routine use.

Braces and Corsets

External support of the lumbar spine with a corset or brace is indicated for only a short period in the average patient's recovery process, and even then only rarely. As the acute symptoms subside, a properly fitted corset or brace will aid the patient in regaining mobility sooner. As the recovery progresses, the patient usually should abandon the brace in favor of an exercise program. With continued long-term use of a brace, soft tissue contractures and muscle atrophy will occur. The young patient should rely on a brace only to hasten ambulation. In theory, strong, flexible lumbar and abdominal muscles function as an excellent internal brace because they are adjacent to the structures (vertebrae) that they are supporting.

Physical Therapy

Some form of exercise is probably the most commonly prescribed therapy for patients recovering from low back pain. There are two regimens commonly advocated: isometric flexion exercises and hyperextension exercises. These programs are purported to reduce the frequency and intensity of low back pain episodes, although there is no scientific evidence to support this contention.

The isometric flexion exercises are the most popular. They are based on the theory that by reducing the lumbar lordosis, back pain is decreased. This goal is achieved by strengthening both the abdominal and lumbar muscles, thereby creating a corset of muscles to support the lumbar spine. Flexion exercises are commonly utilized in patients with spondylolisthesis or spinal stenosis.

Hyperextension exercises are the other form of therapy. They are purported to strengthen the paravertebral muscles. These exercises generally are used after a patient has satisfactorily performed a course of isometric flexion exercises. The goal is to have the paravertebral muscles act as an internal support for the lumbar spine.

The authors believe that an exercise regimen is very important for the rehabilitation of low back patients. This regimen should not be instituted while the patient is experiencing acute pain, but may be started after his symptoms have subsided to the point where no list or paravertebral muscle spasm is present. The number of repetitions is increased gradually; if the patient has any recurrence of acute symptoms, the exercises are stopped. The patient is then closely monitored; when his symptoms again decrease, the exercises can be resumed.

There are many other treatment modalities used for low back pain. These include hot packs, cold packs, light massage, ultrasound, transcutaneous electrical nerve stimulation, and diathermy. They are all well tolerated and pleasant. Most patients experience some immediate relief of symptoms, but unfortunately, there is not a long-lasting impact on the disease process. There is no evidence that any of these treatment modalities offers any long-term benefit or even adds to the efficacy of decreased physical activity alone.

The utility of physical therapy cannot be overstated in its importance in the nonoperative management of lumbar pain. Guided exercises, stretching, and alternative modalities are a critical tool in managing patients.

Operative Management

When patients fail extensive conservative management and advanced imaging supports the diagnosis, operative intervention must be considered. In the lumbar spine, there are two basic techniques used both separately and in conjunction to treat lumbar and radicular pain: decompression and fusion.

Decompression

In patients with minimal back pain whose symptoms are primarily radicular in nature, including weakness and pain. Surgical decompression without fusion can be considered. In the setting of an acutely herniated disc, a microdiscectomy can be considered and performed in a minimally invasive fashion. This involves removing herniated disc material and decompressing the affected nerve root under direct visualization. Laminectomy is another procedure used for decompression that involved surgically removing the lamina causing stenosis at the affected levels. This allows more room for the thecal sac and nerve roots posteriorly. Other procedures such as facetectomy and foraminotomy involve decompressing specific areas of the spine and allowing more room for the exiting nerve roots.

Fusion

While decompression is a viable surgical option for many patients, in patients who have severe back pain, imbalance, or instability seen on imaging, fusion must also be performed to best alleviate their symptoms. Another situation where fusion is indicated is when the decompression procedure will require removing a significant portion (>50%) of the facet joints, thereby destabilizing the operative level. If fusion is not performed in this case, the patient may develop iatrogenic instability, usually as a result of a pars defect created by a wide decompression.

There are a number of procedures available to spine surgeons in order to perform fusion, but the mainstay is the pedicle screw and rod construct used in a posterolateral fusion. This involves placing pedicle screws posteriorly to achieve three column fixation and then securing those screws with bilateral rods that span all levels. The transverse processes, facet joints, pars, and remaining lamina are then decorticated and bone graft products are placed with the goal of achieving a fusion mass in approximately 3–6 months. The previously unstable levels now act as one single construct with the goal of improved alignment and reduced pain from prior instability.

Summary and Conclusion

Neck and low back pain affects the majority of adults at some time during the course of their lives. Every physician should have a working knowledge of the common pathologic conditions and be able to differentiate a serious problem from the more common benign types. In both the cervical spine (myelopathy) and the lumbar spine (cauda equina compression), disastrous sequelae such as paralysis or loss of bowel and bladder control can occur if these serious conditions are not recognized in a timely fashion.

To help in the decision-making process, algorithms for both the cervical and lumbar spine were described. This will allow the physician to make the right diagnosis using the indicated diagnostic procedures at the correct time.

Further Reading

Kane PM, Daniels AH, Akelman E. Double crush syndrome. J Am Acad Orthop Surg. 2015;23(9):558–62. https://doi.org/10.5435/JAAOS-D-14-00176.

Borenstein DG, Wiesel SW, Boden SD. Low back and neck pain. 3rd ed. Philadelphia, PA: WB Saunders; 2004.

Frymoyer JW, Wiesel SW. The adult & pediatric spine. 3rd ed. Philadelphia, PA: Lippincott Williams & Wilkins; 2004.

Wiesel SW, Delahay JN. Principles of orthopaedic medicine and surgery. Philadelphia, PA: WB Saunders; 2001.

The Elbow

Kyle W. Zittel and Michael W. Kessler

Introduction

When elbow and forearm function are compromised by pain, injury, or loss of motion, significant disability can result. The goals of this chapter are to present the elbow's functional anatomy, describe how to clinically evaluate this region, and how to approach diagnosis and treatment of common elbow problems.

We discuss presentations of elbow pathology encountered in outpatient clinic, chronic atraumatic settings, while incorporating management principles and sequelae of acute traumatic injury, with a general focus on adult and adolescent patient populations. An in-depth review of pediatric elbow anatomy, injuries, and treatment is out of the scope of this text.

Anatomy

Skeletal

The elbow joint contains three osteochondral (bone-cartilage) articulations between the proximal forearm and distal humerus: the ulnar-humeral, radiohumeral, and radioulnar joints. The ulnar-humeral and radiohumeral joints are uniquely oriented side by side at the distal humerus. These articulations allow hinge-type motion in the flexion–extension plane, and rotatory motion in the pronation–supination plane, and can be performed throughout their full arcs of motion simultaneously. The elbow's bony anatomy starts several centimeters proximal to the joint itself, as the humeral shaft flares into medial and lateral columns which end in medial and lateral condyles. These form two distinctly shaped articular surfaces at the joint line called the trochlea and capitellum, and two, medial and lateral, epicondyles (Fig. 11.1).

The lateral column consists of the lateral epicondyle and the capitellum, a hemispherical structure that articulates with the concave, disk shaped, proximal surface of the radial head to create the radial-humeral joint (radiocapitellar joint). In the proximal forearm, the radial head articulates medially with the ulna in a shallow recess called the lesser sigmoid notch, located on the radial (lateral) and volar-distal aspect of the olecranon. The sides of the radial head articulating with the proximal ulna are covered in a 240° arc of cartilage allowing smooth rotatory motion. Distally, the head narrows to become the radial neck and angulates itself medially on average 10–20° to the radial shaft (160–170° neck shaft angle). At the radial neck shaft junction, a prominent tuberosity is present medially for the attachment of the biceps tendon (radial/bicipital tuberosity).

K. W. Zittel · M. W. Kessler (✉)
MedStar Georgetown Orthopedic Institute,
Georgetown University School of Medicine,
Washington, DC, USA

Department of Orthopedics, MedStar Georgetown
University Hospital, Washington, DC, USA
e-mail: Michael.W.Kessler@gunet.georgetown.edu

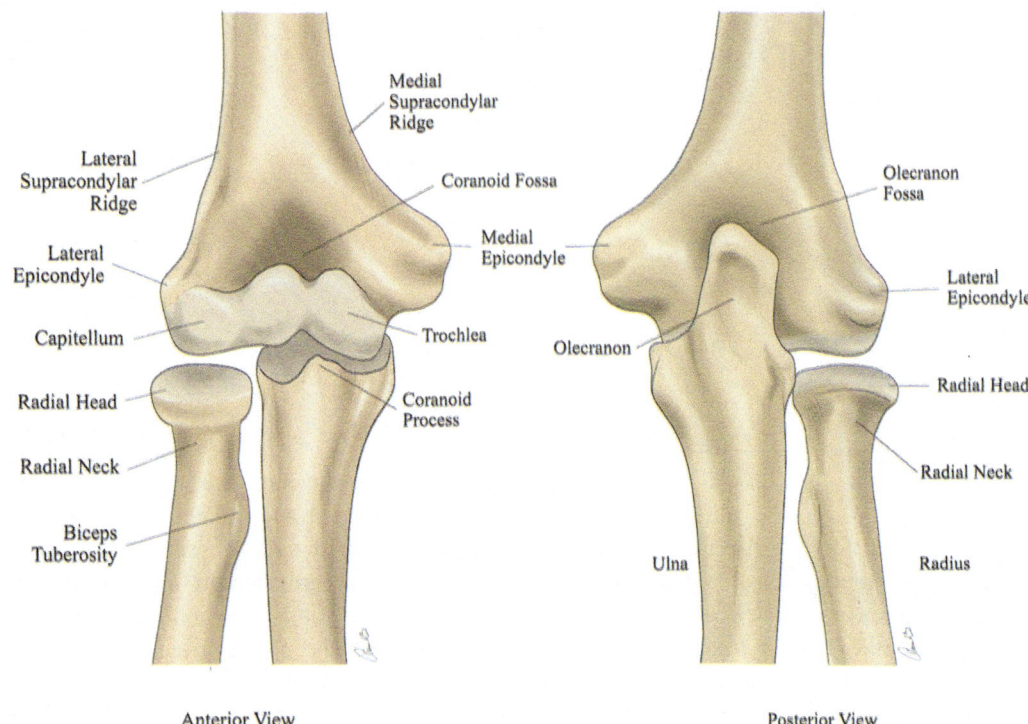

Fig. 11.1 Anterior and posterior views of a right elbow joint demonstrate the three articulations, including the ulnotrochlear joint, the radiocapitellar joint, and the proximal radioulnar joint

The medial column develops a broad outcropping called the medial epicondyle and is bridged laterally to the capitellum by the trochlea, a spool-shaped articular segment with a 300° arc of cartilage. The trochlea is cradled by the sigmoid notch of the olecranon, creating the ulnar-humeral joint (or ulnotrochlear joint). The sigmoid notch is a deep, semilunar shaped recess, with anterior and posterior prominences called the coronoid and olecranon processes, respectively.

Proximal to the trochlea, medial and lateral humeral columns converge centrally to create two fossae on the volar and dorsal aspects of the distal humerus. The volar coronoid and dorsal olecranon fossae are depressions that allow the tip of the coronoid and posterior olecranon processes to recess beyond the cortical width of the humerus at terminal flexion and extension.

The ulnar-humeral joint is considered the most important static stabilizer in the elbow.

In the sagittal plane, the trochlea is flexed ~30° anteriorly, and sits within the reciprocally oriented (posterior angled) sigmoid notch; framed and deepened by its coronoid and olecranon processes (Fig. 11.2). The reciprocal alignment and complementary ulnar-humeral relationship are why the elbow is often referred to as "highly constrained" and "inherently stable," all the while allowing a tremendous flexion–extension arc of motion.

Unlike the shoulder whose stability is dependent on surrounding soft tissues, the osseous anatomy of the elbow renders its stability. Yet, the elbow is capable of rapid changes in position and at extreme ranges of motion, subjecting it to large and repetitive static/dynamic forces. To maintain its stability and articular congruence during flexion/extension, rotatory motion, and varus/valgus directed stress, the elbow is supplemented by two important ligamentous structures. The medial collateral ligament complex (MCL) and lateral collateral ligament complex (LCL). Both of these structures are considered to be primary static stabilizers of the elbow.

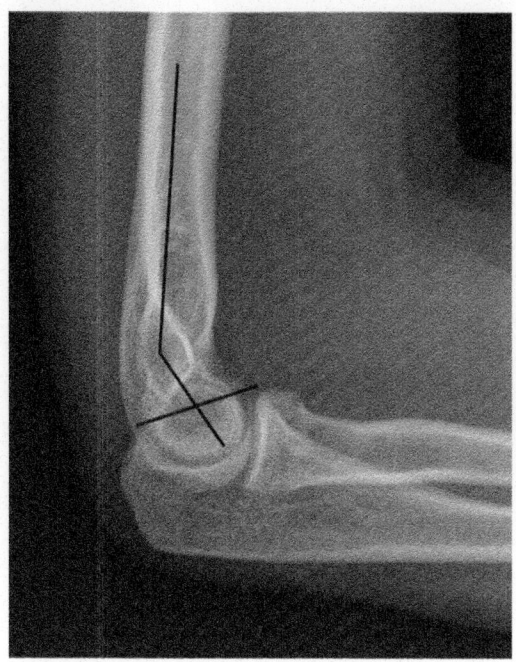

Fig. 11.2 Lateral X-ray of the elbow

The MCL has three segments; the most important for stability is the anterior bundle. It primarily resists against valgus directed stress. It attaches the medial epicondyle to the medial ulna at the sublime tubercle (Fig. 11.3).

On the lateral side of the elbow, the LCL consists of the lateral ulnar collateral ligament (LUCL), which attaches the lateral epicondyle to the lateral ulna, at the tubercle of the supinator crest. In addition to the LUCL, included in the LCL is the annular ligament (surrounding the radial head and helps to stabilize the ulnar and humeral articulation), the radial collateral ligament, and the accessory lateral collateral ligament. Of its four components, the lateral ulnar collateral ligament is the most important primary static stabilizer of the elbow to varus and external rotational stresses (Fig. 11.4).

Anteriorly and posteriorly the elbow joint is lined by a single-cell layer of synovium and covered by a relatively thick fibrous capsule. Beneath the capsule, within the olecranon and coronoid fossae, a fatty layer of tissue is present between the synovium and the surrounding capsule (Fig. 11.5). This layer is of significance in radiographic evaluation of elbows in which intra-articular (intracap-sular) effusion (fluid) or hemarthrosis (bleeding into the joint) causes capsular distention. Subsequently, the displacement of these fat pads is either anterior or posterior to their usual position.

Muscles

The muscles surrounding or crossing the elbow can be divided into separate groups based on their location in the arm or forearm (anterior, posterior) and function (flexion, extension). They originate in the upper arm, on the epicondyles, or proximal forearm. They can be thought of as four groups including the wrist/finger flexor and extensor compartments; and the elbow flexor and extensor compartments.

The extensor compartment of the elbow (posterior) consists of the triceps/triceps brachii (Long, medial, lateral heads). It inserts as one triceps tendon on the olecranon process to provide a powerful extension moment.

The elbow flexor muscles specifically can be found at the anterior aspect of the distal humerus and consists of the brachioradialis, brachialis, and biceps/biceps brachii (long and short heads). The brachioradialis is the most superficial lateral elbow muscle, arising from the anterior lateral aspect of the distal humerus, crosses the elbow joint and helps elbow flexion via its insertion on the radial styloid (lateral distal radius at the wrist). The brachialis, deep to the biceps, is the elbow's primary flexor. It originates broadly along the anterior humeral shaft and inserts distal to the coronoid of the proximal ulna on the ulnar tuberosity. The biceps, with two heads (long-lateral, short-medial), crosses the elbow and has two insertions that blend on the proximal radius.

1. The short head of the biceps (medial side of arm) inserts on to the distal and apex of the radial tuberosity, providing flexion strength (20% compared to brachialis giving 80% of elbows flexion strength).
2. The long head of the biceps (lateral side of arm) inserts on to the oval footprint of the radial tuberosity more medial and is a strong forearm supinator.

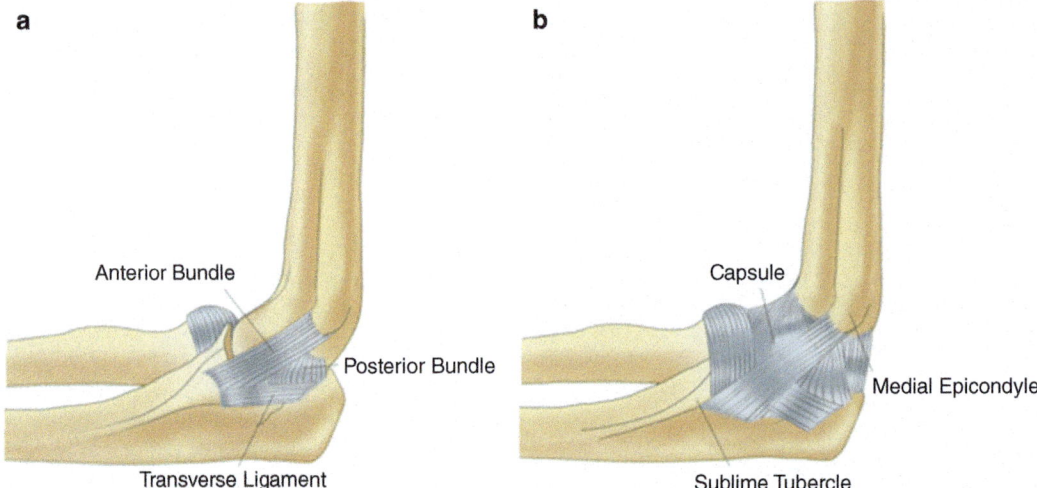

Fig. 11.3 (**a**) A schematic view of a right elbow demonstrating the three bundles or bands of the Medial Collateral Ligament complex. The anterior bundle is most important in elbow stability and attaches at the sublime tubercle of the ulna. (**b**) Grossly, these ligaments are seen as thickenings, blending with the joint capsule as depicted in **b**

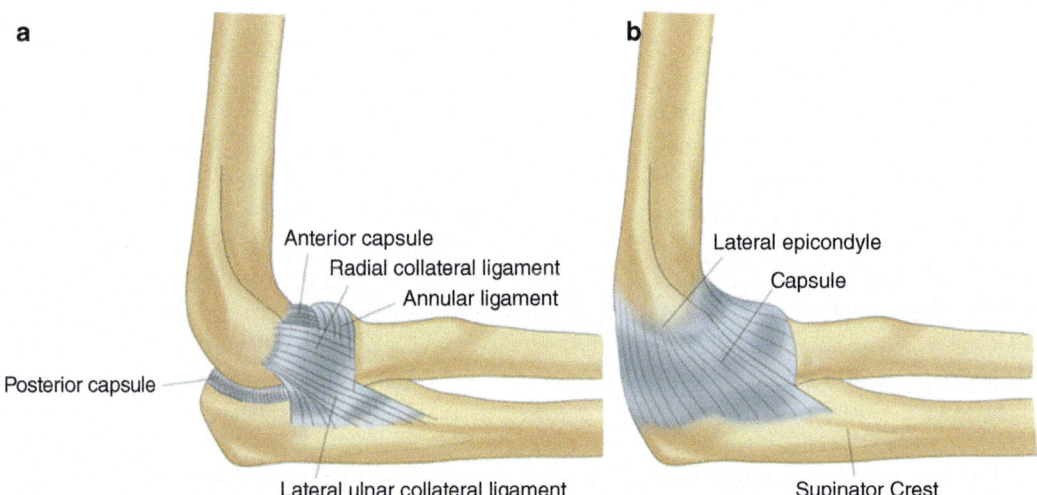

Fig. 11.4 (**a**) A lateral view of a right elbow demonstrating the lateral collateral ligament complex (LCL) consisting of the annular ligament, radial collateral ligament, and lateral ulnar collateral ligament (LUCL). The LUCL is the most important in stability and attaches at the supinator crest of the ulna (**b**)

Just distal to the elbow crease as the two heads become tendinous, the short head of the biceps tendon gives off a bicipital aponeurosis (fascia) called the lacertus fibrosus. This structure travels obliquely, medially, and distally to envelop the forearm flexor muscle bellies (wrist flexors) and helps to protect the underlying brachial artery and median nerve.

The wrist/finger flexor and extensor muscle groups originating around the elbow include the extensor mass and the flexor-pronator mass. The extensor mass muscles arise from the lateral epicondyle and include the extensor carpi radialis longus and brevis, which insert on the 2nd and 3rd metacarpal, respectively (extends the wrist); and extensor carpi ulnaris, inserting on the 5th metacarpal (extends the wrist); the extensor digitorum

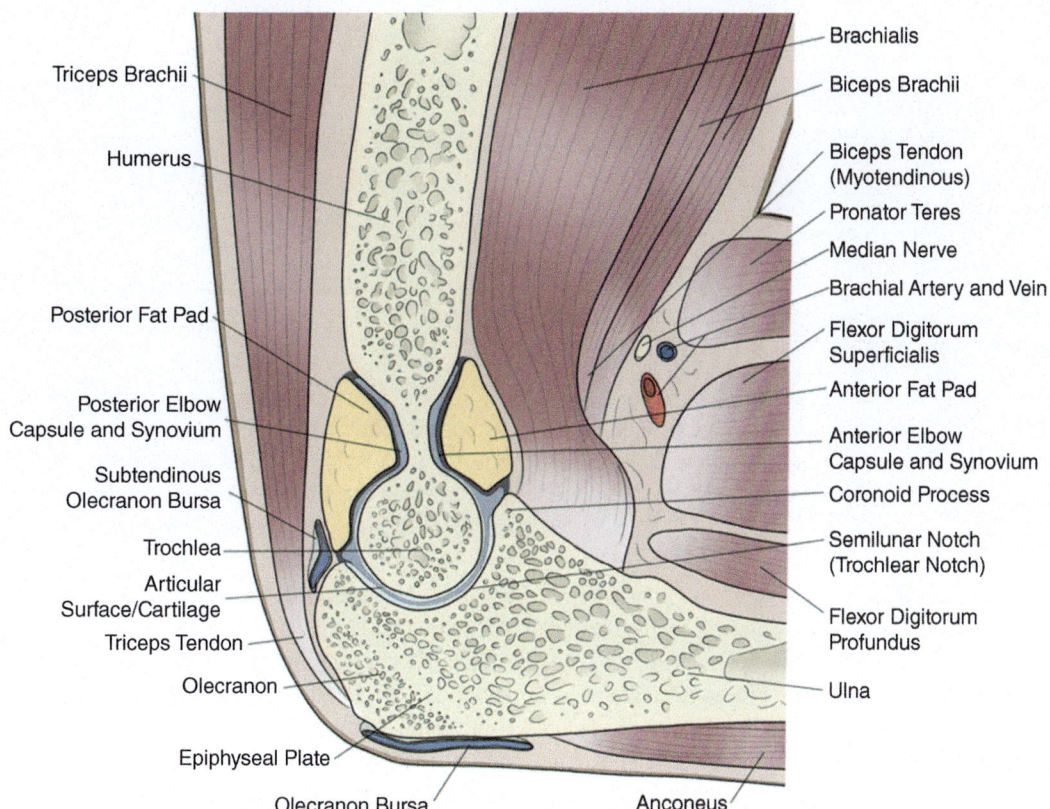

Triceps Brachii
Humerus
Posterior Fat Pad
Posterior Elbow Capsule and Synovium
Subtendinous Olecranon Bursa
Trochlea
Articular Surface/Cartilage
Triceps Tendon
Olecranon
Epiphyseal Plate
Olecranon Bursa

Brachialis
Biceps Brachii
Biceps Tendon (Myotendinous)
Pronator Teres
Median Nerve
Brachial Artery and Vein
Flexor Digitorum Superficialis
Anterior Fat Pad
Anterior Elbow Capsule and Synovium
Coronoid Process
Semilunar Notch (Trochlear Notch)
Flexor Digitorum Profundus
Ulna
Anconeus

Fig. 11.5 Sagittal illustration of the elbow joint demonstrates the normal skeletal and soft tissue anatomy. Note the presence of fat pads both anteriorly and posteriorly, directly outside the joint capsule. Intra-articular swelling can lead to displacement out of the olecranon (posterior) or coronoid (anterior) fossae, leading to the appearance of "positive fat pad sign(s)" on lateral X-rays. An anterior fat pad can be normal; a posterior fat pad if seen is always abnormal and indicates elbow effusion

communis and extensor digiti mini (extend the fingers). Deep to these posterior muscles lies the supinator muscle which originates on the proximal ulna and inserts on the proximal radius. It assists the biceps with supination of the forearm. In addition, the anconeus is a small triangular muscle that originates on the lateral epicondyle and inserts on the lateral aspect of the olecranon, it is thought to assist with elbow extension and lateral stability of the elbow (Fig. 11.6).

The flexor-pronator mass takes its origin from the medial epicondyle, the medial ulna, and the interosseous membrane. From proximal to distal on the medial epicondyle, it consists of the pronator teres, inserting on mid lateral radius (forearm pronation); flexor carpi radialis, inserting on 2nd metacarpal (wrist flexion); palmaris longus, inserting on flexor retinaculum (weak wrist flexor/

absent in ~30% of population); flexor digitorum superficialis, inserting on middle phalanges 2–5 (finger flexion at PIP and MCP joints); and the flexor carpi ulnaris, inserting on the pisiform, hook of hamate, 5th metacarpal (wrist flexion). Occasionally, there is an accessory muscle present superficially at the medial elbow called the anconeus epitrochlearis. It is present in approximately 15% of the population and can be a source of compression of the ulnar nerve at the cubital tunnel.

Neurovascular

In contrast to deeper-seated neurovascular structures of other extremities, those about the elbow are both tightly concentrated and superficial, making them uniquely vulnerable to both direct

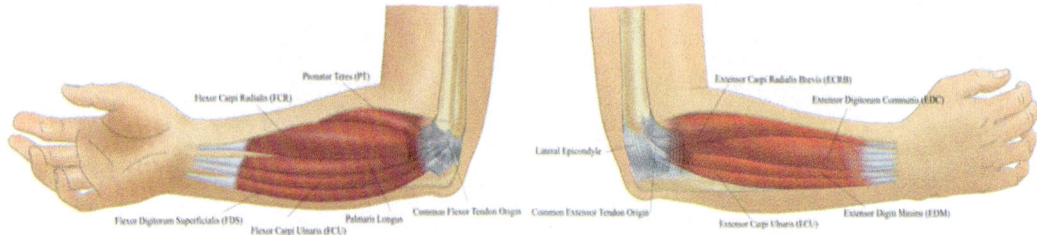

Fig. 11.6 Medial view of forearm demonstrating the flexor-pronator muscle mass and lateral view showing extensor mass. Note the common tendon origins on the medial and lateral columns of the distal humerus over lie the elbow capsule, medial and lateral ligamentous complexes

and indirect injury. Injuries or symptoms due to nerve involvement around the elbow make familiarization with normal neurovascular anatomy crucial.

Brachial Artery

The brachial artery lies anterior to the medial aspect of the brachialis muscle, entering the antecubital space medial to the biceps tendon and lateral to the median nerve. At the level of the radial head, it divides into its terminal branches, the ulnar and radial arteries.

Musculocutaneous Nerve

Continuing from the lateral cord of the brachial plexus and composed of fibers from the C5–C8 nerve roots, this nerve travels through (and innervates) the biceps and brachialis. Injury to the musculocutaneous nerve results in inability to flex the elbow and loss of sensation to the lateral forearm from its terminal sensory branch, the lateral antebrachial cutaneous nerve (LABCN). The LABCN is vulnerable to injury during anterior approaches to the elbow, especially during distal biceps repair.

Median Nerve

Arising from C5–T1 nerve roots, combined from the upper and lower cords, the median nerve travels along anterior to the brachialis muscle, enters the antecubital fossa, then passes medial to the biceps tendon and the brachial artery. It then passes through the pronator teres and gives off the anterior interosseous nerve (AIN), a branch which supplies motor innervation to the flexor pollicis longus, the index and middle flexor digitorum profundus, and the pronator quadratus. Injury to the AIN results in the inability to flex the thumb at the IP joint. The remainder continues distally in the forearm under the flexor digitorum superficialis. The median nerve provides sensory innervation to the volar radial aspect of the hand, including the thumb, index, middle, and radial half of ring finger; dorsally its sensory contribution is isolated, present only distal to the IP joint of the thumb and the PIP joints of the index, middle, and radial half of the ring finger. Sensory testing is commonly performed at the volar index or middle finger.

Radial Nerve

Originating from C6–8 nerve roots, the radial nerve is a continuation of the posterior cord and travels in the spiral (radial) groove of the proximal humerus until its encountered laterally at the distal 1/3 of the humerus, entering the anterior compartment between the brachialis and brachioradialis. It innervates the triceps, brachioradialis, and extensor carpi radialis longus and brevis muscles. In the antecubital fossa, anterior to the lateral epicondyle, the nerve divides into a deep motor branch, or posterior interosseous nerve (PIN); and a superficial sensory branch continues underneath the brachioradialis to provide sensation to the dorsal radial aspect of the wrist and hand to the level of the IP joint of the thumb, and PIP joints of the index, middle, and radial half of the ring finger. Check radial sensory function over the dorsal thumb–index web space. The PIN is found on the posterolateral surface of the radius after it pierces the supinator muscle entering the posterior compartment. The PIN innervates the supinator, extensor carpi radialis brevis, extensor digitorum communis, extensor carpi ulnaris, extensor pollicis longus and brevis, extensor indicis, and abductor pollicis longus. Injury to PIN results in inability to extend the wrist or fingers.

Ulnar Nerve

Derived from roots C8 and T1, the ulnar nerve continues from the medial cord of the brachial plexus until passing posteriorly through the intermuscular septum at the level of the mid-humerus. It then travels through the cubital tunnel of the medial elbow, where pathologic compression, traction, or irritation commonly can occur. In the forearm, the ulnar nerve innervates the flexor carpi ulnaris and the ulnar half of the flexor digitorum profundus. Distally, it continues to provide motor function to many of the intrinsic hand muscles and sensation to the skin of the ulnar wrist/hand (palmar cutaneous branch), little finger and ulnar half of ring finger both volarly (superficial cutaneous branch), and dorsally (dorsal cutaneous branch). Sensory testing commonly occurs at the ulnar border of the little finger. Injury to the ulnar nerve can result in a loss of finger abduction; test by crossing the index and middle finger.

Extrinsic muscles (located in the forearm) innervated by the ulnar nerve include flexor carpi ulnaris, medial half of flexor digitorum profundus (4th and 5th digit). Intrinsic muscles (located in the hand) innervated by the ulnar nerve include: 1 thenar muscle (adductor pollicis—oblique and transverse heads), 3 hypothenar muscles (flexor digiti minimi, abductor digiti minimi, opponens digiti minimi), the 3rd and 4th (ulnar/medial two) lumbricals, all 7 interossei muscles (three volar interossei and four dorsal interossei), and palmaris brevis.

"FOAL" Mnemonic for the four intrinsic hand muscles, *not* innervated by the ulnar nerve. Instead, are innervated by the median nerve:

F: flexor pollicis brevis
O: opponens pollicis
A: abductor pollicis brevis
L: lateral/radial two (1st and 2nd) lumbricals

Evaluation of Elbow Problems

The evaluation of elbow problems relies on a thorough history, physical, and radiographic examination, supplemented by other pertinent clinical or diagnostic tests when indicated.

History

Elbow problems can be divided into two major categories: (1) acute traumatic injuries and (2) chronic elbow problems which tend to be more atraumatic in nature, though can present as post-traumatic sequelae. In the situation of acute trauma, a detailed history of the event must be obtained. The mechanism of injury including the position of the arm, initial treatment, and subsequent symptoms are all very important in guiding further evaluation and management. For chronic elbow conditions, the most common complaint is pain. Stiffness or other mechanical symptoms such as locking, catching, or instability may accompany pain or become the primary problem. Determine what treatments the patient has had including specifics of previous surgery, and if anything has been effective.

The nature of the pain and any zone to which they radiate is important. For example, is it burning or radiating (nerve) or is it an aching related only to activity (tendinitis)? Does it hurt at rest or at night (tumor, infection)? Establish the exact location of the symptoms and if there is a relationship to the patient's activity. In a throwing athlete, when during the pitch or throw does the pain occur? Medial elbow pain when the arm is in the cocking position suggests medial collateral ligament pathology, whereas medial pain during follow-through suggests involvement of the flexor-pronator group or impingement in the posterior ulnar-humeral joint.

Is it associated with any other symptoms, such as neck pain (cervical radiculopathy) or wrist pain (distal radioulnar joint problem)? Numbness, tingling, and weakness may be obvious clues to neurologic involvement, but sometimes nerve entrapment syndromes in the arm or neck present with pain only. In addition to inquiring about tingling or numbness, ask about weakness or loss of dexterity.

The elbow is commonly involved (and sometimes one of the first joints affected) in inflammatory arthritides, so it is important to elicit a history of other joint complaints, known arthritis, and family history. Is there a history of skin problems (lupus, dermatitis, psoriasis) or gastrointestinal problems (colitis)? Have there been any systemic symptoms of illness (malaise, fevers), suggesting septic arthritis?

Perhaps the most important part of the history is determining how the symptoms interfere with function and is the patient's dominant extremity affected. This can direct treatment strategies more than any other factors. For example, a functional arc of motion, 30–130° flexion/extension, 50° pronation, 50° supination, is typically relied upon for most activities of daily living. The inability to flex the elbow completely is generally well tolerated by most patients. However, considering a patient with rheumatoid arthritis, shoulder motion may already be compromised, thus, a seemingly mild degree of elbow restriction actually may interfere with independence, and/or their ability to feed or clean themselves.

Physical Examination

The examination of the elbow begins with inspection, palpation, passive/active range of motion assessments, evaluation for strength, and neurovascular integrity. These maneuvers are then followed by special tests, designed to evaluate specific conditions based on the examiner's differential diagnosis. A thorough physical exam should also include a directed evaluation of the shoulder, wrist and hand, including the cervical spine when relevant.

Inspection begins with careful observation of elbow, forearm, and hand use as soon as one begins interaction with the patient. Does the patient extend the elbow to shake hands with the examiner? Are there obvious adaptive maneuvers that the patient uses to avoid pain or compensate for functional loss?

A more formal visual exam is then performed. One should evaluate the elbow alignment (neutral, varus, and valgus) in flexion/extension, and the "valgus carrying angle." The carrying angle is formed between the longitudinal axis of the humerus/forearm with the elbow in extension (normally 10–15° valgus). With the elbow flexed 90°, note that the normal bony prominences (medial/lateral epicondyles/olecranon) form an equilateral triangle. In dislocations, this normal relationship is often distorted. Look for evidence of joint swelling laterally by inspection of the soft tissue triangle bordered by the radial head, olecranon tip, and lateral epicondyle.

Palpate the anterior, medial, lateral, and posterior elbow in a systematic fashion, noting its anatomic structures: the medial epicondyle, lateral epicondyle, olecranon, radio capitellar joint, biceps, triceps, forearm muscle masses and their respective origins. Be specific in trying to identify the exact area of tenderness.

Note the location and timing of pain during motion. Check both active and passive motion, noting any difference between them. Comparing the ROM to the unaffected side can serve as a reference. Normal flexion values are on average between 130 and 154° and extension between −6 and 11°; pronation from 75 to 85° and supination from 80 to 104°. If passive motion is greater than active motion, consider pain, muscle, or nerve injury as possible causes.

Check for sensation to light touch and motor function in the distribution of the ulnar, median, radial nerves, and specific branches (AIN, PIN, cutaneous). A positive *Tinel sign* is useful in the assessment of peripheral entrapment problems. Gently tapping in the vicinity of suspected pathology reproduces the symptoms, causing numbness, tingling, or pain in the nerves distribution indicating a positive test.

Vascular assessment is mandatory after any acute elbow trauma or suspected vascular compromise from pathology at the elbow. It includes palpation of the radial and ulnar arteries at the wrist, and the brachial artery in the antecubital fossa. If an extremity appears warm, pink, and well perfused, but there is delayed capillary refill (>2 s), a nonpalpable, "thready" or weak pulse, compared to the unaffected side, a portable ultrasound-Doppler should be used to confirm the presence or absence of an arterial pulse. Doppler is commonly used for objective exam trending or clinical confirmation when examination is limited by factors such as patients body habitus, acute traumatic/post-operative swelling, overlying wounds, overlying splint/bandages, vascular disease. Specific physical examination tests and signs are useful depending on the condition suspected.

Radiographic Evaluation

Anteroposterior (AP) and lateral X-rays are the minimum views necessary to evaluate the elbow joint. Following trauma, additional views are often necessary, including oblique elbow and radiocapitellar joint / radial head views (Figs. 11.7 and 11.8). Obtain full forearm/wrist and humerus/shoulder series if concomitant injury is suspected or for preoperative planning. After any fracture manipulation or reduction maneuvers with application of an immobilizing split, it is prudent to obtain repeat "post-reduction" X-rays to assure

adequate osseous alignment, soft tissue integrity, and splint mold or position as it relates.

Alignment: On a lateral XR of the elbow, alignment should be assessed by the anterior humeral line (AHL) and radiocapitellar line (RCL). The AHL is drawn down the anterior cortex of the humerus and should intersect the middle 1/3rd of the capitellum. If it does not, consider a distal humerus fracture. On AP and lateral XR, the RCL is drawn along the radial neck and should always intersect the capitellum. If it does not, consider radial head dislocation or subluxation, and check for accompanying fracture, especially at the proximal ulna (Monteggia fracture).

Bones: Trace the cortex of each bone, the distal humerus, radial head-neck-shaft, olecranon, coronoid process, and ulnar shaft. Evaluate the joint surfaces and space. Look for lucency, erosions, osteophytes, cortical irregularity, and common fractures: radial head and neck, capitellum, coronoid, olecranon, epicondyles, distal humerus.

Effusion: On a lateral elbow X-ray, the presence of a posterior fat pad (usually deeply contained in olecranon fossa) indicates an elbow effusion. Think occult intra-articular fracture not well visualized on XR; commonly radial head/

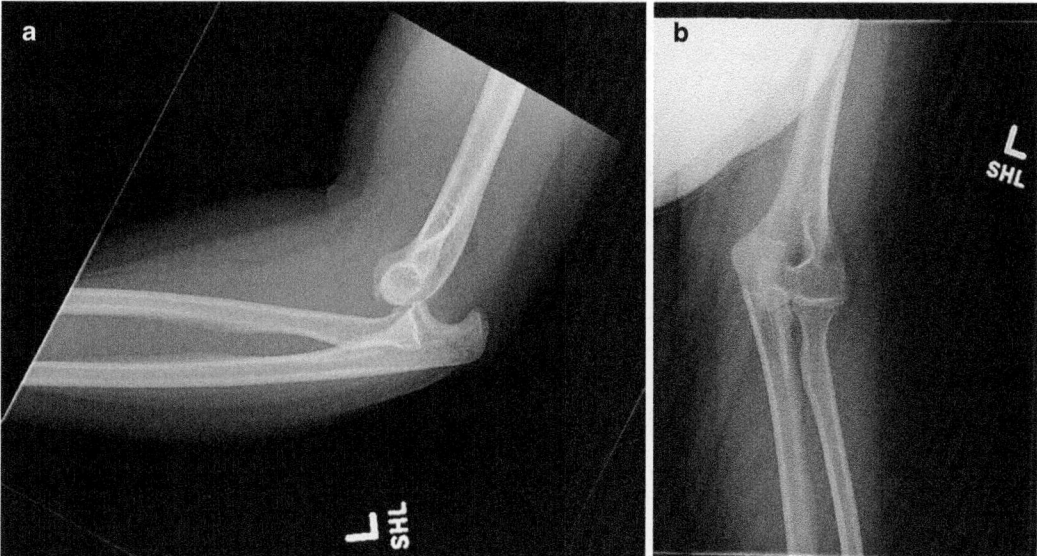

Fig. 11.7 (**a**) Lateral X-ray view demonstrating a posterior elbow fracture dislocation with an osseous fragment anteriorly and irregular radial head contour with cortical step off at the articular surface. Findings indicate a displaced intra-articular radial head fracture and possible coronoid process fracture. (**b**) Attempted AP view redemonstrates a postero-lateral dislocation and radial head fracture. In addition to the above elbow X-ray series, two views (AP and Lateral) of the wrist, forearm, and humerus is recommended, three views if concern for concomitant injury or fracture

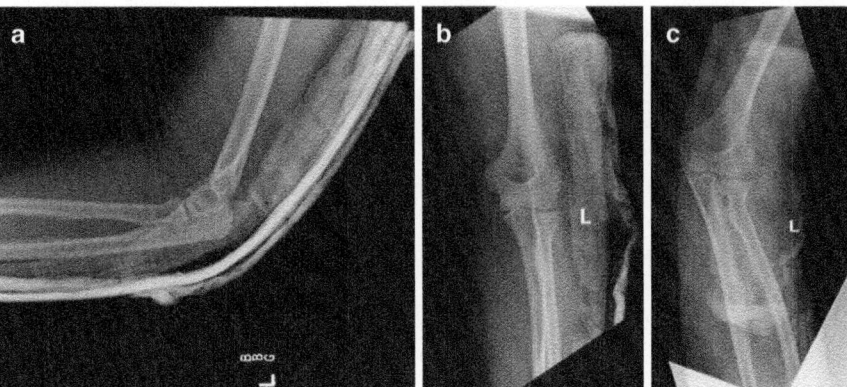

Fig. 11.8 Elbow fracture dislocation status post-reduction and splinting. After reduction, the next step in management of this injury is to obtain a CT scan of the elbow to further evaluate the fracture patterns and for preoperative planning. The presence of a coronoid fracture, known dislocation (LUCL injury), and radial head fracture is often referred to as the "Terrible Triad" because of its frequency of persistent instability if not surgically treated. (**a**) Lateral view of left elbow demonstrating a concentrically reduced ulnotrochlear joint; a well reduced radiocapitellar joint with alignment confirmed by the straight radiocapitellar line intersecting the radial head and capitellum. Re-demonstrated is the radial head fracture and small coronoid process fracture. Note the presence of a posterior slab plaster splint with cotton (webril) padded soft tissue protection. Elbow reduction held by the splint in 70–80° of flexion to diminished risk of compartment syndrome from an increase in antebrachial soft tissue pressure seen with excessive elbow flexion past 90°. (**b**) Anterior–Posterior view and (**c**) External Oblique X-ray views demonstrating appropriate reduction

neck in an adult or supracondylar fracture in a child. A small anterior fat pad can be seen in patients and considered normal, though it may be significant with a history of trauma or if massively raised.

Beyond X-rays, the following special radiographic tests can be helpful.

Stress X-Rays

Stress views may be helpful in evaluating the patient with a suspected tear of the medial or lateral collateral ligament complexes. This is achieved through manual stress, during which the clinician applies a valgus or varus stress to the elbow to open the contralateral side, with 2 mm of gapping usually indicating pathology.

Traction X-Rays

In the case of a severely shortened or comminuted distal humerus or proximal ulna/radius fractures, traction X-rays can be performed, utilizing a principle called *ligamentotaxis*. The is defined as the molding fracture fragments into alignment because of tension applied across a fracture by the surrounding intact soft tissues and can help to discern seemingly unidentifiable elbow anatomy sometimes encountered on initial injury XRs.

Computed Tomography

Computed tomography (CT) scans without contrast enhancement are effective in preoperative planning of complex elbow trauma, assessment of bone fracture morphology and joint deformity, and occasionally for the evaluation of loose bodies of the elbow. A CT with intravenous contrast can be obtained to evaluate the presence of infection/abscesses within the surrounding soft tissue. A CT angiogram (CTA), using arterial contrast, can help identify locations of vascular injury, occlusion, or compression.

Magnetic Resonance Imaging

Magnetic resonance imaging (MRI) without contrast provides superior soft tissue imaging and allows visualization of cartilage, marrow and vascularity changes in bone. Its current use about the elbow includes imaging occult fractures, tumors, infections, synovitis or other causes of joint effusion, and osteochondritis dissecans. It also can be repeated after time to compare and evaluate stages of osteochondral healing. It is occasionally useful in evaluating ligament disruptions, but it is usually unnecessary in diagnosing medial or lateral epicondylitis and rarely helpful in nerve entrapment syndromes. MRI with contrast enhancement is generally reserved for infectious or oncologic pathology.

Electrodiagnostic Tests

Electromyography (EMG) and nerve conduction velocity (NCV) testing have definite indications in the patient with suspected nerve entrapment or injury. Such testing may indicate the site of the compression or injury. However, failure to demonstrate specific neurologic findings by electrodiagnostic testing does not rule out their presence.

Treatment of Elbow Problems: Introduction to Nonoperative and Operative Principles

Treatment of elbow problems is algorithmic, dividing conditions into either traumatic or atraumatic causes. One general principle of treatment in the elbow is to minimize the length of immobilization. The adult elbow has a high propensity for developing stiffness with prolonged immobilization (>2 weeks), especially after fracture or dislocation. The resultant loss of motion can be disabling, and treatment for it can be prolonged and difficult. Because of this, in the adult population, casting with circumferentially wrapped fiberglass for the treatment of upper arm/elbow injuries or fractures is uncommon. Occasionally, after initial management/immobilization, casting for definitive management is indicated in adults if they are nonsurgical candidates or in specific circumstances such as cognitive impairment or compliance concerns. This is a different treatment strategy than in adolescent or pediatric elbow/arm injuries which often are casted. The developing elbow in children can tolerate longer periods of immobilization. Therefore, circumferential fiberglass casting, with or without bi-

valving (splitting/cutting the fiberglass with a cast saw and loose overwrap), commonly is used as a primary means of treatment.

In adults, when immobilization is indicated acutely, noncircumferential fiberglass or plaster splints or a brace is often placed with the elbow positioned in 90° of flexion and neutral pronation/supination. This allows for maintenance of the most useful arc of function and a position of maximal capsular volume (less pain/intracapsular pressure/stretch from effusion). After an initial treatment such as closed reduction, casting, splinting, external fixation, internal fixation, one should carefully assess and sometimes trend the patient's neurovascular exam. Swelling commonly increases up to 24 h after an acute injury and the multiple confined fascial compartments of the forearm leave patients vulnerable to compartment syndrome or other severe compromise. Avoidable iatrogenic causes (caused by treatment), include circumferential casting or excessively tight wrapping of an acutely swollen extremity, and elbow immobilization in exaggerated flexion (>90–100°) increasing anterior antecubital pressure. Occasionally, splinting of the arm in varying degrees of extension, pronation, supination is necessary for elbow stability after reduction, unstable fractures, anatomic considerations, or comfort.

Nonoperative Treatment

Rehabilitation and Pain Management
Rehabilitation through either a patient self-guided program or formal occupational/physical therapy plays an important role in the treatment of elbow problems. The goals should include (1) reduction of pain and inflammation, (2) restoration of motion, (3) rebuilding strength, and (4) return to normal function and activity. These goals, often accomplished with help of hand/elbow therapists, should be carefully monitored by the treating physician until the patient is discharged or alternative management is instituted.

Elbow stiffness is best treated by prevention. Restoration of motion lost is done through careful stretching exercises and takes much longer to regain than to lose. Once lost, motion return is best achieved through active work done by the patient, rather than simple passive stretching by the therapist. Motion loss is usually in extension (inability to completely straighten the elbow). A characteristic of the elbow, like that of the hip, is its propensity to develop heterotopic ossification (HO) bone formation within the soft tissues, after trauma or surgery. This is particularly common anteriorly because of the presence of the brachialis muscle belly immediately anterior to the elbow capsule. The risk of ossification is increased with passive stretching, and for this reason, aggressive passive motion is often discouraged. Some specially designed splints which exert a dynamic force across the elbow can be effective in restoring motion.

Injections

Generally, corticosteroid or protein rich plasma (PRP) injections are reserved for specific diagnoses and conditions which fail initial activity modification, anti-inflammatories, and therapy. The exact timing and number of injections is controversial, but in general, no more than three injections should be given over a 6-month time frame.

The use of corticosteroids injections about the elbow facilitates treatment of inflammatory or degenerative arthritis by decreasing pain and potentiating motion. Because corticosteroid injections can lead to cartilage and tendon damage, dermal depigmentation, and infection, they should not be used arbitrarily or excessively.

PRP injections are now utilized more commonly for medial and lateral epicondylitis with moderate results. For epicondylitis, corticosteroids have fallen out of favor and are now infrequently used since published outcomes versus saline placebo have been shown to be similar. In addition, authors have argued against its use for epicondylitis, citing that the disease pathology does not involve inflammation, but rather histological changes called *angiofibroblastic hyperplasia.*

Operative Treatment

Surgery for the elbow is for patients in whom nonoperative management has failed or inappropriate. Surgery can be performed via open

approaches or arthroscopic methods. Common open elbow procedures include open reduction internal fixation (ORIF) for fracture fixation, anatomical restoration of length, alignment, rotation, bone healing, joint restoration, and allows for early elbow ROM. In addition to ORIF, open dissections are used for ulnar nerve decompressions and elbow instability requiring ligamentous repair, augmentations, auto and allograft reconstructions. Common open approaches to the elbow include lateral (Kaplan, Kocher, EDC split), medial, posterior, and anterior.

Elbow arthroscopy has proven to be very effective for specific elbow pathologies; however, it should only be done by surgeons who are comfortable with the surrounding anatomy. Even then, should be approached cautiously. Because of the very tight concentration of nerves and blood vessels in the area, the depth of the joint capsule under the musculature, and tight articular constraint, the procedure is technically difficult and involves more risk than arthroscopy at most other joints. Therapeutically, it has been used effectively for the removal of inflammation, synovectomy, debridement of the capsule and/or extensor carpi radialis brevis (ECRB) origin for lateral epicondylitis, radial head resections, release of soft tissue contractures, excision of painful or motion limiting osteophytes and/or intra-articular loose bodies. Occasionally, it is used in osteochondral reconstruction (osteochondritis dissecans). Interestingly, in other joints of the body, arthroscopy is not generally indicated or employed for the treatment of osteoarthritis. The elbow's ulnohumeral joint is an exception and has shown to have mild/moderate results for motion and pain. Relative contraindications to arthroscopy include severe contracture, previous ulnar nerve transposition or open elbow surgery, significant bone or joint distortion.

Evaluation and Treatment of Common Elbow Problems

The following discussion highlights selected examples of common chronic and acute traumatic elbow problems.

Chronic: Atraumatic, Post-Traumatic, Overuse Injuries of the Elbow

Lateral and Medial Epicondylitis

Lateral Epicondylitis: "Tennis Elbow"

Lateral epicondylitis is popularly known as tennis elbow, even though only 5% of these patients play tennis. Conversely, nearly 50% of tennis players will develop some degree of the condition during their sports careers. It affects men and women equally, most commonly between the age of 30 and 50 years of age, and those engaged in backhanded sporting activity, repetitive gripping or lifting tasks.

In skeletally mature adults, strains to the medial and lateral structures at the epicondyle can result in epicondylitis and are the most common elbow pathologies seen in clinical practice. These conditions can result from a single, particularly strenuous action, or with any repetitive stress such as sports (especially racket sports, golf, and baseball), labor intensive jobs, carrying heavy bags, typing and cleaning activities. The tendon origin is thought to undergo microtears, degeneration, replacement with abnormal scar and granulation tissue called angiofibroblastic hyperplasia (microscopic appearance). This occurs within the extensor carpi radialis brevis (ECRB) on the lateral side (Fig. 11.9) or the flexor carpi radialis (FCR) and pronator teres (PT) muscle origins on the medial side (Fig. 11.10).

Patients complain of weakened grip strength, pain over the lateral epicondyle with activity or at night, often with some radiation into the forearm. Symptoms develop gradually over a period of weeks to months, typically without a specific injury. The key physical exam finding is focal tenderness over the lateral epicondyle or myotendinous attachment just anterior to it. Tenderness more distal to the lateral condyle in the proximal forearm, may instead suggest pain from posterior interosseous nerve (PIN) entrapment.

Differential diagnosis for lateral elbow pain includes radial tunnel syndrome/PIN entrapment (which can coexist in 5% of patients), posterolateral plica (space occupying capsular involutions/hypertrophy), posteromedial and posterolateral rotatory instability, occult fracture (radial neck, head, lateral column/distal humerus), cervical radiculopathy, triceps tendinitis, capitellar osteochondritis dissecans, radiocapitellar arthritis, and varicella-zoster (shingles).

XR imaging is non-diagnostic and usually normal, though it may reveal calcifications in the extensor muscle mass (up to 20%). MRI is not necessary for diagnosis, though it may show increased signal intensity, thickening, edema, degeneration at the ECRB tendon origin. Ultrasound is a useful diagnostic tool in experi-

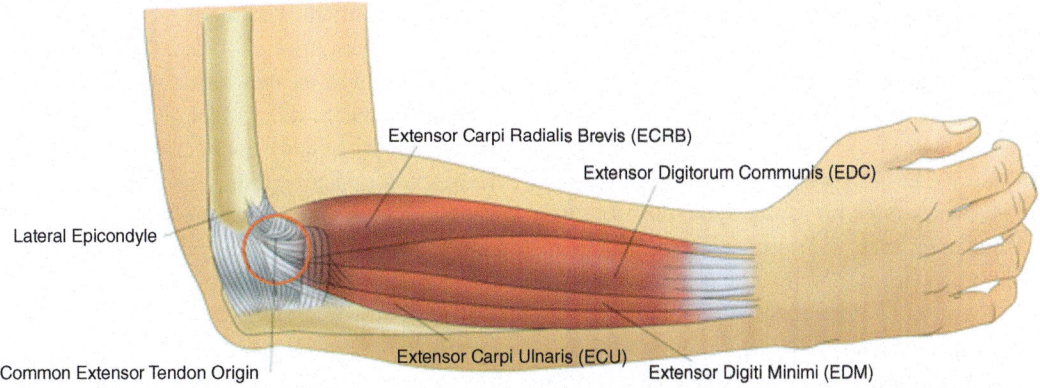

Fig. 11.9 Lateral view of a right elbow illustrating the common extensor origin, extensor muscle mass, site of pain and point of maximal tenderness in lateral epicondy- litis. Most commonly occurring within the extensor capri radialis brevis. Other lateral muscle origins not imaged: brachioradialis, extensor carpi radialis longus, anconeus

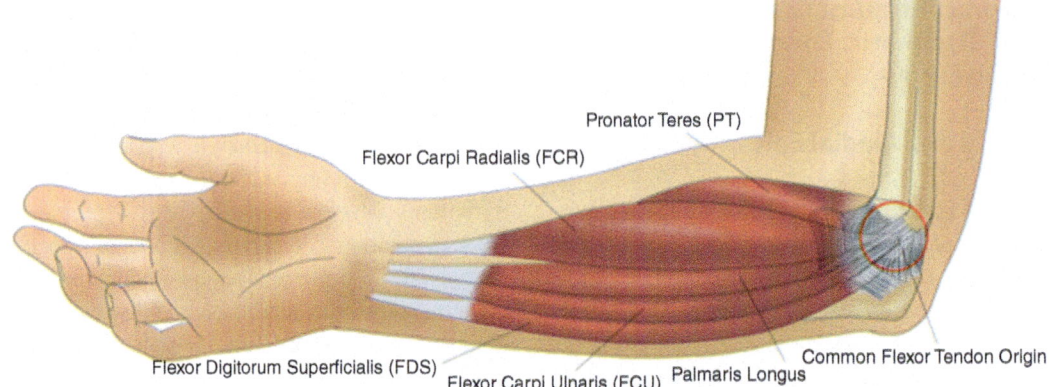

Pronator Teres (PT)

Flexor Carpi Radialis (FCR)

Flexor Digitorum Superficialis (FDS)

Flexor Carpi Ulnaris (FCU)   Palmaris Longus

Common Flexor Tendon Origin

Fig. 11.10 Medial view of a right elbow showing the flexor-pronator muscle mass and common flexor tendon origin. Point of maximal tenderness and site of pain in medial epicondylitis, most commonly occurring within the pronator teres and flexor carpi radialis

enced operators and can reveal a thickened and hypoechoic ECRB tendon or used to aid in placement of injections.

Treatment is almost always conservative and based on pain modulation, emphasizing rest, ice, avoidance of provocative activities. In addition, identification and correction of sporting techniques is important; common tennis modifications include slower playing surfaces, more flexible racquets, lower string tension, or larger grips. Nonsteroidal anti-inflammatory drugs (NSAIDs) do not treat the pathology (not an inflammatory reaction) but are effective for pain control. Wrist bracing during the night primarily, and daytime with activity, is often utilized and helpful by decreasing the need to fire wrist extensor muscles. Structured physical therapy programs once pain levels have decreased, <2 out of 10 on visual analog scale (VAS), can be helpful in treatment and prevention. PRP injections (up to three/one every 2 weeks) are used in those unresponsive to conservative management or those presenting with severe symptoms. In clinical practice, even with proper use of nonoperative strategies, symptoms can persist for up to 12–18 months before complete resolution.

Therefore, surgery for lateral epicondylitis is only indicated in patients who fail an appropriate conservative trial (considered 2 years of duration), and in those compliant with the recommended nonsurgical treatment. Surgery is necessary for less than 10% of patients. Open or arthroscopic procedures involve identification and debridement of the pathologic tissue, usually located within the substance of the extensor carpi radialis brevis. Advocates of arthroscopic technique report advantages in visualization and ability to address intra-articular pathology and faster return to work following surgery. Albeit is associated with risk of neurovascular injury that accompanies arthroscopy.

Complications of surgical management include excessive resection of the LUCL leading to posterolateral rotatory instability (PLRI), iatrogenic radial nerve injury, heterotopic ossification, infection, and missed concomitant pathology.

Medial Epicondylitis: "Golfer's Elbow"

Medial epicondylitis is often called golfer's elbow because of its association with forehanded sporting activities like golf, bowling, throwing, racquet sports, that require repetitive wrist flexion, forearm pronation, and valgus force on the elbow. It is seen in patients with jobs requiring forceful gripping, lifting, or exposure to constant vibration at the elbow (plumbers, carpenters, construction workers). It affects men and women equally, commonly between the ages of 30 and 60, and involves the dominant extremity in 75% of cases. It is 5–10 times less common than lateral epicondylitis.

Patients typically complain of pain over the medial epicondyle (Fig. 11.10), with or without numbness and/or tingling in the ulnar digits. Pain is generally an insidious onset but may be associated with history of an acute traumatic blow to the elbow. Pain may also be worse in overhead throwers during late cocking/early acceleration phases. Physical exam is positive for point tenderness to the medial epicondyle or just anterior to it. When more distal, it may be due to medial ulnar collateral ligament (MCL) insufficiency or tears. Soft tissue swelling and warmth may be present. Occasionally, in more chronic cases, a flexion contracture may be observed. It is important to examine the patient for associated conditions such as valgus instability and MCL insufficiency/injury or ulnar neuritis/neuropathy looking for hypothenar bulk and positive Tinel signs.

The differential diagnosis for medial sided elbow pain includes MCL injury, cubital tunnel syndrome, ulnar-humeral arthritis, fracture, cervical radiculopathy, triceps tendonitis, and shingles.

X-rays are not needed for diagnosis and usually unremarkable, but can identify posterior medial osteophytes or degenerative changes, and 25% of patients may have calcification of the common flexor tendon or ulnar collateral ligament. Stress XRs are useful to evaluate for valgus instability if it is a concern. MRI is standard of care to evaluate for concomitant pathology (UCL injury/trochlear osteochondral lesions in overhead thrower), evaluate for loose bodies, rule out rupture of flexor-pronator origin, or if there is an unclear source of medial elbow pain. Ultrasound is effective to evaluate hypoechoic/anechoic areas of focal degeneration and allows for dynamic examinations or direct visualization of injections. EMG/NCS may be used to evaluate for ulnar nerve compression if symptoms are identified on history or physical exam.

Like lateral epicondylitis, treatment for medial epicondylitis is almost always conservative, emphasizing rest, ice, avoidance of provocative activities, and NSAIDs/Acetaminophen. It is important to emphasize strict activity modification and a stop to all throwing for 6–12 weeks (about 3 months) in overhead athletes. Use of a wrist brace (day and/or night), and structured therapy with passive wrist extension stretching (once pain <2/10 on VAS), can be helpful. PRP injections into peritendinous tissue may be beneficial, however, must be performed carefully to avoid ulnar nerve injury.

Surgery should be considered only after a prolonged trial of appropriate conservative management (2 years in duration). As symptom resolution can take up to 12–18 months and due to less predictable success, operative treatment is often avoided. Only 80% of patients report good to excellent outcomes (less than lateral epicondylitis). Worse outcomes tend to occur when ulnar nerve symptoms are present preoperatively. A clear diagnosis, appropriate conservative management, and severe symptoms affecting quality of life are an indication for surgical management of medial epicondylitis. It involves an open medial approach to the elbow to excise or debride pathological tissue near the flexor-pronator mass. This is done in conjunction with repair or reattachment, if the proximal tendon origin is involved. Cubital tunnel release and ulnar nerve transposition can also be performed if nerve symptoms are present.

Complications after surgical management include medial collateral ligament complex injury (posterior medial rotatory or valgus instability), medial antebrachial cutaneous nerve neuropathy, ulnar nerve injury, and infection.

Elbow Arthritis

Arthritis (degenerative joint disease) is much less commonly seen in the elbow than encountered in the hip or knee, generally, because it is a nonweight bearing joint. The three major types are primary osteoarthritis (OA), post-traumatic arthritis, and inflammatory arthritis (rheumatoid, psoriatic, systemic lupus erythematosus, pigmented villonodular synovitis).

Clinically symptomatic primary osteoarthritis of the elbow is rare (2%). It is characterized by widespread osteophyte and loose body formation, capsular contraction, with relative preservation of articular cartilage in some areas. It typically occurs in middle aged males with a history of manual labor, from 20 to 70 years of age (avg. 50). Post-traumatic elbow arthritis is more common in younger patients, seen after nonoperatively treated radial head fractures, simple elbow dislocations with instability, elbow fracture dislocations, and other general trauma. In either circumstance, primary OA or post-traumatic OA, patients typically present with progressive elbow pain at end ranges of motion secondary to osteophytes and impingement, associated with painful locking and clicking, worsened with activity. Midrange motion pain and night pain are less common complaints. Loss of terminal extension is common with pronation/supination motion preserved early. Ulnar neuropathy is commonly observed in up to 50% of patients.

In patients with inflammatory (especially rheumatoid) arthritis, 20–50% have elbow involvement. Elbow inflammatory arthritis may present with hand and wrist involvement preceding the elbow. In some cases, rheumatoid disease first presents in the elbow and should be considered in patients with an atypical history on presentation. They will complain of elbow pain and loss of range of motion often without an inciting incident or without a manual labor history. On physical exam, a fixed flexion contracture, ligamentous incompetence, and ulnar nerve symptoms may be seen. It is important to include cervical spine evaluation in all RA patients. If undiagnosed or in first time presenters with suspected elbow pain secondary to RA, patients require appropriate lab tests for evaluation of systemic arthritis including erythrocyte sedimentation rate (ESR), C-reactive protein (CRP), antinuclear antibody (ANA) test, rheumatoid factor (RF) test, and complete blood count (CBC). Additional rheumatologic tests should be determined in consultation and referral to a rheumatologist. Prevention is key as treatment with disease modifying anti-rheumatic drugs (DMARDs) has significantly decreased the incidence of inflammatory arthritis and need for operative treatment.

The differential diagnosis includes infection/septic arthritis, gout (uric acid crystallization), chondrocalcinosis or pseudogout (calcium pyrophosphate deposition) crystalline arthropathy, osteoarthritis versus inflammatory arthritis. To aid in the diagnosis and treatment planning, aspiration of the elbow joint synovial fluid, and analysis of cell count, differential, gram stain, and crystals, can often be performed.

AP and lateral X-rays of the elbow can confirm the presence of osteoarthritis. XR findings include joint space narrowing (<2 mm), with the ulnohumeral joint space relatively preserved. Osteophytes at the coronoid process and fossa, radial head and fossa, olecranon tip and posteromedial olecranon fossa are common (Fig. 11.11). In RA, XR findings are more diffuse and range from periarticular osteopenia in early disease to subchondral erosions, destructive appearing joint collapse, and ultimately bony ankylosis (fusion) as untreated disease progresses. Including a cervical spine XR in patients with RA is necessary prior to surgery because of the risks of cervical manipulation while under anesthesia. CT scan, although not often necessary, can be used for surgical planning and useful to define osteophytes and loose bodies.

First line treatment of primary and post-traumatic elbow osteoarthritis is nonoperative with NSAIDS, cortisone injections, resting splints, and activity modification. Treatment of the rheumatoid elbow varies with the stage of presentation. Early in the course, anti-inflammatory and anti-rheumatoid medication, analgesics, and activity modification may be sufficient treatment and slow the progression. Initial goals are to decrease pain and inflammation, maintain motion, and avoid further destructive changes.

Late stage efforts to relieve pain and improve function may rely on surgical treatment such as arthroscopic or open debridement, synovectomy with or without radial head resection. In end-stage disease, a total elbow replacement (TEA) may be the only viable or functional option. Total elbow replacement is indicated in low demand patients, generally older than 65 years of age, with severe osteoarthritis or post-traumatic

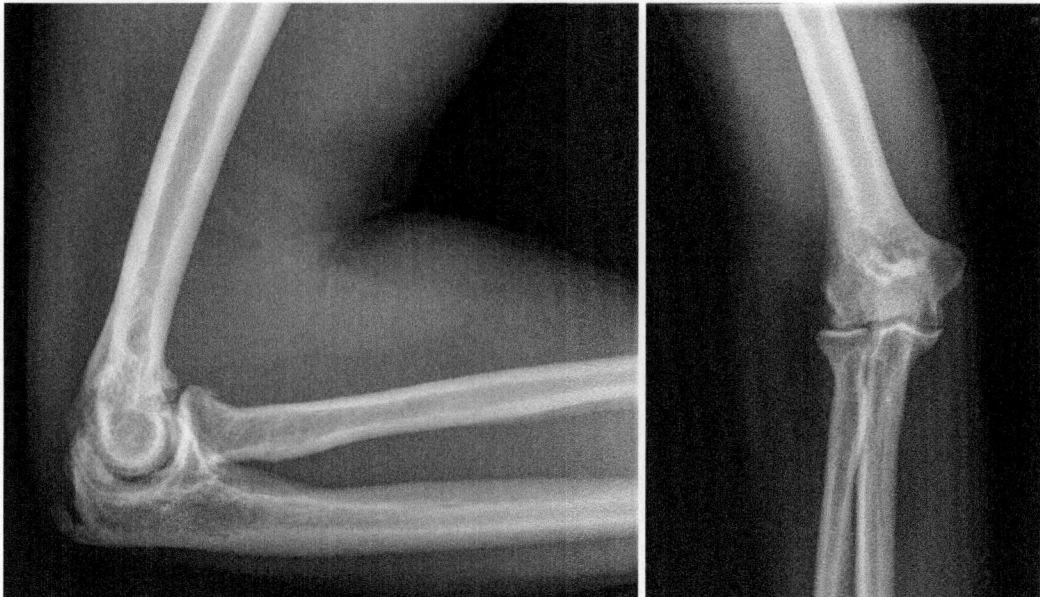

Fig. 11.11 Elbow Arthritis

arthritis, and OA secondary to distal humerus nonunion/malunions in the elderly. The procedure involves a hinged type metal prosthesis that replaces the distal humerus and proximal ulna at the ulnar-humeral joint and spares the radial head articulation. After TEA, patients are restricted to a 5-pound weight restriction to the operative extremity for life. TEA is contraindicated in another variant of OA called Charcot joint arthropathy, and in active patients with high demand because overuse is known to lead to failure.

Cubital Tunnel Syndrome (Ulnar Nerve Compression)

Cubital tunnel syndrome is a compressive neuropathy of the ulnar nerve caused by entrapment amongst the structures of the medial elbow. The position of the ulnar nerve at the medial elbow renders it susceptible to compression, traction, and direct trauma. There are five major sites of compression of the ulnar nerve in the region of the medial elbow: the arcade of Struthers (a fascial band of the triceps 5–10 cm proximal to the medial epicondyle), the medial intermuscular septum, the medial epicondyle groove, the ligament of Osborne (between the medial epicondyle and olecranon) and the humeral and ulnar heads of the flexor carpi ulnaris muscle (FCU). Up to 16% of patients are further predisposed to symptoms by having "instability," with either subluxation or frank dislocation out of the groove. Cubital tunnel syndrome can occur in isolation or be associated with chronic elbow deformity such as cubitus varus or valgus, medial epicondylitis, burns, or elbow contractures.

Patients with cubital tunnel syndrome present with complaints of numbness and tingling in the distribution of the ulnar nerve in the hand (ring, little finger, ulnar dorsal hand). They often have isolated elbow pain with or without radiation; usually worse during long periods of elbow flexion such as in sleep or repetitive flexion activities. The patient may feel clumsy or weak in grasping or throwing (ulnar nerve—hand intrinsic muscles). He or she may note actual "snapping" in cases in which the ulnar nerve is unstable and contributory.

In early disease, there is usually no sensory or motor deficit, although a Tinel sign over the cubital tunnel may be positive. Check for nerve instability by flexing and extending the elbow while feeling the ulnar nerve at its recess below the medial epicondyle. As compression progresses, patients can lose sensation over the ulnar border of the ring finger and all of the small finger. Weakness to finger abduction and eventually intrinsic atrophy of the interosseous muscles and first webspace (adductor pollicis) can develop. Moreover, in advanced cases with chronic ulnar denervation, 4th and 5th digit claw deformities can occur.

The differential for Cubital tunnel syndrome includes Guyon canal syndrome (ulnar nerve compression at wrist), C8 radiculopathy (commonly compression in cervical spine), concomitant medial elbow pathology associated with ulnar neuropathy such as arthritis, MCL injury, epicondylitis.

Differentiation between ulnar nerve compression at Guyon canal (wrist) vs. the cubital tunnel (elbow) can be done by testing the strength of intrinsic (hand) vs. extrinsic (forearm) muscles supplied by the ulnar nerve, respectively. Weakness in both intrinsic and extrinsic groups points toward Cubital tunnel syndrome (compression proximal to muscle innervation loss). Spared extrinsic strength (FCU/4–5th FDP) in the presence of weak intrinsics, and/or spared light touch of the dorsal surface of ulnar dermatome (dorsal medial hand and 4th and 5th fingers), points to more Guyon canal syndrome and distal nerve compression. The anatomy of Guyon canal and its three common sites of ulnar nerve compression (via cysts, lipomas, hamate fracture), are out of the scope of this chapter. Signs and symptoms can be purely motor, purely sensory, or mixed depending on the zone.

X-rays are almost always negative although they may reveal deformity or structural compression. Electrodiagnostic tests, nerve conduction study/electromyography (NCS/EMG), are helpful to establish diagnosis and prognosis. Often negative in early disease, a conduction velocity <50 m/s across the elbow is diagnostic for cubital tunnel syndrome.

Treatment is initially nonoperative, with rest, ice, NSAIDs, night-time arm position education and modification versus extension splinting with the elbow in 45° extension and forearm in neutral rotation. The goal of treatment is to halt the progression and resolution of symptoms. For patients with continued symptoms or significant denervation on NCS/EMG, surgery involves in situ nerve decompression and anterior transposition of the ulnar nerve via an open medial elbow approach.

The most common post-operative complications include recurrence of symptoms, neuroma, or hematoma formation.

Olecranon Bursitis

Olecranon bursitis (OB) is inflammation around and fluid collection within the bursa of the olecranon and is the most common superficial bursitis (Fig. 11.12). It is caused by aseptic, inflammatory, and infectious processes (occurring in 20% of acute cases). The olecranon bursa is anatomically present after 7 years of age, covering the dorsal aspect of the olecranon to the distal insertion of the triceps and proximal subcutaneous border of the ulna. Pressure from the bony olecranon and shearing forces applied to the skin contributing to fluid filled bursa formation.

Patients with olecranon bursitis present with unilateral swelling over the proximal olecranon (acutely up to 7 cm long × 3 cm wide), commonly with a history of repetitive micro trauma (desk jobs/chronic elbow positioning/pressure). Aseptic OB is characterized as a compressible, fluctuant mass, with or without tenderness. In sterile bursitis up to 45% of these patients report

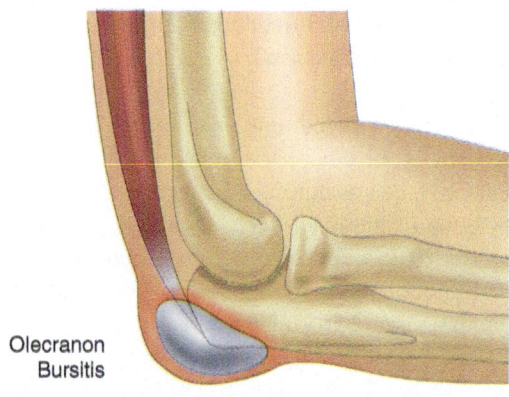

Olecranon Bursitis

Fig. 11.12 Olecranon Bursitis

tenderness depending on the level of acute inflammation and may have hyperemia of the skin (increased blood flow, warmth, color change), with edema extending into the forearm. Septic olecranon bursitis is associated with greater tenderness and may also have a visible cellulitis component. Elbow effusions can be seen in severe cases with elbow ROM limited by the degree of swelling and pain. These factors make olecranon bursitis often indistinguishable on initial exam.

The differential includes idiopathic, infection, and inflammatory when associated with systemic conditions such as rheumatoid arthritis, gout, chondrocalcinosis (pseudo gout), and pigmented villonodular synovitis.

Imaging including XR is generally not indicated unless there is concern for concomitant pathology, ruling out inoculating or foreign bodies, or history of acute trauma. Instead, aspiration of the fluid collection can be performed with analysis of gram stain, culture, white blood cell (WBC) count, and glucose level, to aid in the diagnosis and treatment. A positive Gram stain and culture, most commonly gram-positive staphylococcus species, definitively diagnoses a septic process. However, gram stains are positive in only 50% to 60% of cases, and it may take several days to obtain the results of culture. A WBC count $<1000/mm^3$, is consistent with aseptic bursitis, and a WBC count $>10,000/mm^3$ is generally consistent with septic bursitis. With counts between these levels, the predominant cell type may be used to distinguish septic from aseptic bursitis. A preponderance of polynuclear cells is indicative of septic bursitis, whereas predominance of mononuclear leukocytes is indicative of aseptic bursitis. Bursal fluid glucose levels indicate infection when values are <50% of serum levels.

Proper recognition and medical management of inflammatory systemic conditions, in addition to nonoperative principles (RICE), generally provides adequate treatment and prevents recurrence of inflammatory olecranon bursitis,

Treatment of acute atraumatic or idiopathic olecranon bursitis is also generally nonoperative with ice, compression, avoidance of aggravating activity. In patients with bothersome aseptic atraumatic bursitis or failed conservative management, aspiration has shown patient recovery of 90% at 6 months. Patients should be aware of the risk of infection via direct inoculation when utilizing aspiration injection as a form of treatment for aseptic bursitis. Septic bursitis is managed with aspiration sent for culture/analysis, RICE, and oral or intravenous systemic antibiotics. Surgical management with open bursectomy is rarely necessary and reserved for failed nonoperative management, advanced or uncontrolled infection.

Postoperative complications can include infection, recurrence, and hematoma formation.

Osteochondritis Dissecans and Panner's Disease

Osteochondritis dissecans (OCD) of the elbow and Panner's disease are considered two separate disease processes with different etiologies. Despite having nearly identical pathology and characteristics, it should be recognized that alternative treatment strategies for each are employed.

Panner's disease is the presence of a subchondral defect or lesion in the capitellum of preadolescent aged children. Commonly occurring before the age of 10, it is diagnosed with the absence of overhead throwing or a history of repetitive elbow stress. Thought to be caused by an interference in blood supply to the growing epiphysis, the natural history of this process is most commonly a period of symptomatic subchondral resorption with eventual self-limited repair and resolution of pain if properly treated.

Osteochondritis dissecans of the elbow occurs in adolescent aged patients and is an osteochondral injury that can persist or worsen if not addressed. It has been described as the leading cause of permanent disability in the young throwing athlete. It is characterized by localized stress to the immature capitellum, resulting in subsequent separation of articular cartilage and subchondral bone, possibly as a result of avascular necrosis (AVN) of the capitellum. OCD is particularly common among adolescent throwing athletes and gymnasts (particularly vaulting, balance beam, uneven parallel bars, floor exercises). Patients predictably present with a history of these activities, overuse, and mild to moderate associated pain. In throwing, enormous valgus stresses are imparted to the elbow joint, absorbed primarily by the medial collateral ligament. The second line of defense is the radiocapitellar buttress, which in turn is subjected to significant repetitive compression and shear stress, even with an intact or normally functioning MCL.

The most common presenting symptom is that of activity-related lateral elbow pain with insidious onset in the dominant or throwing arm. On physical exam, there is often pain and a restriction in motion, loss of extension up 20–30° in more advanced cases and/or crepitus on supination/pronation. There may be associated tenderness over the radiocapitellar joint and presence of swelling or effusion. Catching, locking, or grinding episodes with mechanical blocks to motion can occur later in the disease process if loose bodies are present.

AP and lateral X-rays are recommended and are initially often normal, although there may be early signs of lucency or irregular ossification of the capitellum upon presentation. This is often a subtle and easily missed finding on XR, thus a high level of suspicion should be present when the history and physical exam is positive. In Panner's disease, XRs exhibit an irregular epiphysis, while in OCD, a well-defined subchondral lesion is visible. In later stages, there may be a crescent sign, fragmentation, or loose body formation. MRI is often obtained and is the best method of establishing the diagnosis and assessing the degree of articular involvement. It is also useful in assessing subchondral involvement, loose bodies, and extent of disease. MRI is often repeated after treatment is undertaken to view the status and healing of the lesion.

In the treatment of Panner's disease, without the presence of the loose body, surgery is contraindicated. 3–4 weeks of long arm cast may be necessary to reduce elbow activities until pain, swelling, and tenderness subsides. Elbow immobilization in this pre-adolescent age group is generally well tolerated with low concern for persistent ROM deficits. Repeat MRI is often obtained to ensure healing and typically self-resolution of the lesion is seen without lasting sequelae.

In OCD of the elbow, goals of treatment include painless elbow function and return to activity or prior level of sport. Articular involvement and lesion characterization as stable or unstable is an important treatment consideration. The characterization of lesions remains under considerable debate. Generally, in stable lesions, there is formation of an osteochondral fragment without separation from its bed, in unstable lesions, there is separation with loose body formation. In addition, lesions are described as with or without articular involvement. Treatment depends on lesion characteristics, clinical and radiographic findings. Nonoperative treatment for extra articular and stable fragments includes rest, ice, NSAIDs, extension splinting, and physical therapy with modalities for 3–6 weeks (about 1 and a half months). Because the healing process is slow, the area must be protected against overzealous activity (i.e., hard throwing or weight-bearing), with gradual return to activities over a period of 6–12 weeks (about 3 months). This results in about a 90% success rate. Treatment of articular, stable or unstable lesions is generally nonoperative initially but operative treatment is frequently required. Surgical treatment includes arthroscopic micro-fracture or drilling of the capitellum, fixation of the lesion, debridement, and loose body excision, or osteochondral autograft or allograft transplantation (OATS). In unstable extra-articular or stable intra-articular lesions, micro-fracture or subchondral drilling of defects has shown success. In contrast, large unstable lesions that require fixation have highly variable outcomes. In unstable articular lesions, arthroscopic debridement with loose body excision is indicated. If large lesions engage the radial head, OATS can be indicated. OATS commonly is performed with autologous osteochondral graft harvest from the ipsilateral knee.

Complications after surgery include elbow stiffness, pain, and arthritis. Returning to sport at the same level after surgery is highly variable with a wide range of potential future disability.

Little Leaguer's Elbow

In the skeletally immature athlete, injury to the medial epicondylar apophyseal structures is known as little leaguer's elbow because of its high incidence in young baseball players. It is caused by repetitive stresses to the vulnerable epicondylar origin of the flexor-pronator group and MCL, during both acceleration and follow-through phases of throwing (Fig. 11.13). This results in abnormalities in secondary ossification and physeal plate structures. Younger patients are more likely to have apophysitis or avulsion injuries rather than UCL sprains or tears because the cartilaginous growth plate is weaker than the bone or ligament. These children present with medial elbow pain, diminished throwing effectiveness, and distance. On examination, there is focal tenderness over the medial epicondyle and pain on attempting active wrist flexion or forearm pronation, especially against resistance.

X-ray findings vary and include apophyseal fragmentation, irregularity or widening of the physis, or avulsion of the medial epicondyle. The medial epicondyle physis typically is no longer visible (fused) by the age of 15 years in females and up to 18 years in males. Valgus stress views are useful; even an innocent appearing minimally displaced fracture may be unstable. MRI will show edema of the medial epicondyle apophysis and can rule out UCL insufficiency.

Fortunately, treatment is rarely operative and includes rest, ice, physical therapy, and gradual return to activity as pain resolves. Immobilizing the elbow is not usually recommended. Educating coaches and parents is critical for treatment, after recovery, and in prevention, as restricting the number of innings pitched in Little League has led to a reduction in the incidence of elbow complaints. Surgery is reserved for those with displaced (>2 mm), unstable avulsion injuries or symptomatic nonunions via open reduction internal fixation of the medial epicondyle. Ulnar collateral reconstruction is indicated for UCL disruption and insufficiency, instability.

Complications after surgery include ulnar nerve neuropathy, continued pain/instability, loss of motion, and inability to return to the same level of play.

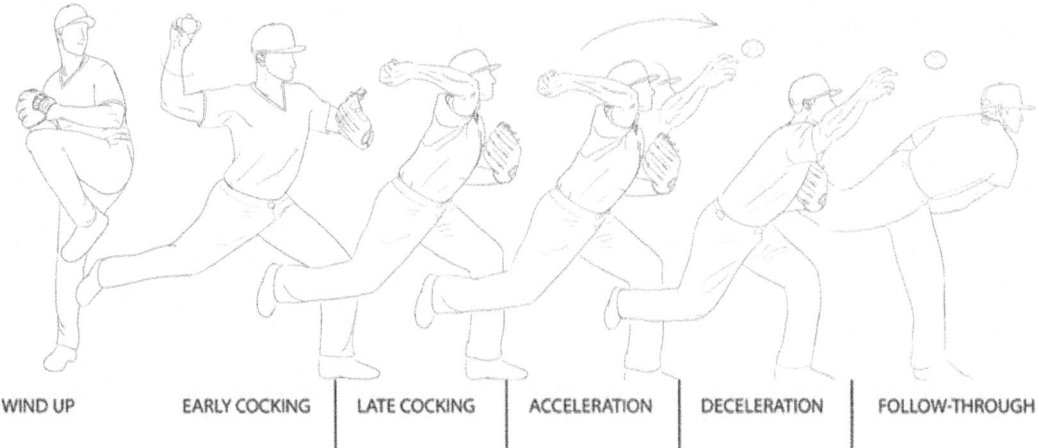

WIND UP   EARLY COCKING   LATE COCKING   ACCELERATION   DECELERATION   FOLLOW-THROUGH

Fig. 11.13 Phases of throwing

Acute: Traumatic Common Tendon, Ligament, Fracture, Dislocation Injuries

Thorough examination, knowledge of injury patterns and elbow anatomy, with a proper work up after an elbow trauma is necessary for management and the best possible patient outcomes. Acute traumatic elbow injuries can present as an array of mild simple soft tissue injuries such as contusion, sprains, strains, avulsions, ruptures, to more significant soft tissue-based injuries requiring acute clinical or surgical attention like deep penetrating lacerations or gunshot wounds (GSWs) resulting in traumatic arthrotomies. Higher energy mechanisms can result in more complex elbow injuries that manifest in combination with neurovascular injury, fractures, ligament disruption, dislocations (with or without associated fracture).

In the adult patient, most acute elbow trauma occurs during high energy mechanisms such as falls from height or motor vehicle crashes. Elderly osteoporotic patients are at risk for elbow injuries and traumatic fractures following even low-energy falls. Acute elbow injury in young adults commonly occurs in sports such as weightlifting (tendon rupture, avulsion injuries). Likewise, fracture and dislocations present after a direct blow to the elbow or fall on outstretched hand (FOOSH) during skateboarding, skiing, football, or soccer, to name a few.

Treatment of acute traumatic injuries to the elbow can be nonoperative with a short period of immobilization and controlled early range of motion, plus or minus bracing. Acute treatment can also include operative management, using temporary stabilization techniques like external fixation, internal fixation, or sometimes both. Temporary immobilization via a splint, limited ORIF, percutaneous fixation, and external fixators are often utilized in the acute setting with a plan for further surgery. This allows for pain control, swelling reduction/soft tissue rest, and time that is sometimes needed to carry out a safe and effective definitive treatment plan. During the acute phase of treatment, it is always important to consider and plan for the subacute/chronic sequelae of traumatic elbow injury. Additionally, identify associated or untreated clinical pathology after the initial evaluation and early management is complete.

Tendon Ruptures

Distal Biceps Rupture

Ruptures of the distal biceps tendon represent about 10% of all biceps ruptures. They commonly occur in the dominant elbow of muscular men aged 30–60 years. They can occur as partial tears at the insertion or the musculotendinous junction, but they are most commonly complete insertional detachments from the biceps tuberosity of the radius. They almost always occur during a heavy eccentric load to the biceps (from flexion to extension). Patients usually feel a "pop" and sharp pain in the antecubital space at the time. Patients may have visual change in muscle contour proximally depending on the level of retraction, ecchymosis, and a palpable defect at the biceps' attachment. Patients are tender anteriorly and have weakness with elbow flexion and primarily with supination.

XR imaging of the elbow is usually normal though can show avulsed bone from the radial tuberosity. If the diagnosis is unclear, an MRI can be helpful in differentiating complete versus partial tears, tendon versus muscle tear, and degree of retraction, but is rarely needed to make a diagnosis.

Nonoperative, supportive treatment and physical therapy can be considered in older low demand patients who are okay with sacrificing some level of strength in supination (40%), flexion (20%). Generally, complete ruptures should be surgically reattached within 10–14 days to prevent future weakness. Surgery involves finding the ruptured tendon via an incision over the antecubital fossa and then reattaching it to the biceps tuberosity. This can be done using bone tunnels placed via a second incision over the posterior lateral elbow (two incision technique) or with suture anchors or suture button placed from the anterior incision (one incision technique). In chronic presentations, patients can be treated with graft reconstructions or just observed if their functional losses are tolerated. Light activities can begin soon after surgery, but heavy lifting and vigorous activity should be avoided for several months.

Complications after surgical management include injury to the lateral antebrachial cutaneous nerve, radial or posterior interosseous nerves, synostosis, and heterotopic ossification.

Triceps Tendon Rupture

Triceps tendon ruptures are more uncommon. Patients again present after an eccentric load, sometimes after a fall onto an outstretched hand. It more commonly occurs in male, ages 30–50, engaging in competitive weightlifting or can be seen in patients with systemic diseases. Patients can note a painful pop and a defect in the triceps tendon at the olecranon fossa is often palpable. Elbow extension against resistance or gravity is commonly weak though with a partially intact triceps or compensating anconeus, but the patient may be able to still extend. Complete tears are generally unable to extend against gravity.

Diagnosis can be made clinically, however, XR and/or MRI can be useful if a patient is too painful to examine or a partial tear is suspected. XR imaging can show an avulsion of the olecranon tip and is pathognomonic for a triceps rupture.

Nonoperative management is reserved for low demand patients or partial tears and able to extend versus gravity by immobilizing the elbow in 30° of flexion for 4 weeks. Acute surgical management is indicated in complete tears or partial tears >50% with significant weakness. These injuries should be treated with reattachment of the tendon or fixation of an osseous avulsion to the olecranon process with transosseous tunnels or suture anchors. Occasionally delayed reconstruction may need tendon graft. Post-operative patients are immobilized for about two weeks in a safe degree of flexion (30–60°), so as to not stress the repair tested intraoperatively. Active ROM is initiated at 4 weeks and resistance training avoided for 4–6 months.

Complications after surgical management can include elbow stiffness/weakness, ulnar nerve injury, re-rupture or failure of repair.

Dislocations

The elbow is second only to the shoulder in frequency for major joint dislocations. They usually occur after a fall on an outstretched hand. By far the most common type is posterolateral, in which the radius and ulna dislocate posteriorly and laterally relative to the humerus. The overall forces involved in creating the dislocation include axial compression, valgus stress, and supination (Fig. 11.14). The LUCL is torn and more variably the MCL is torn. Associated injuries are common, such as radial head and neck fractures

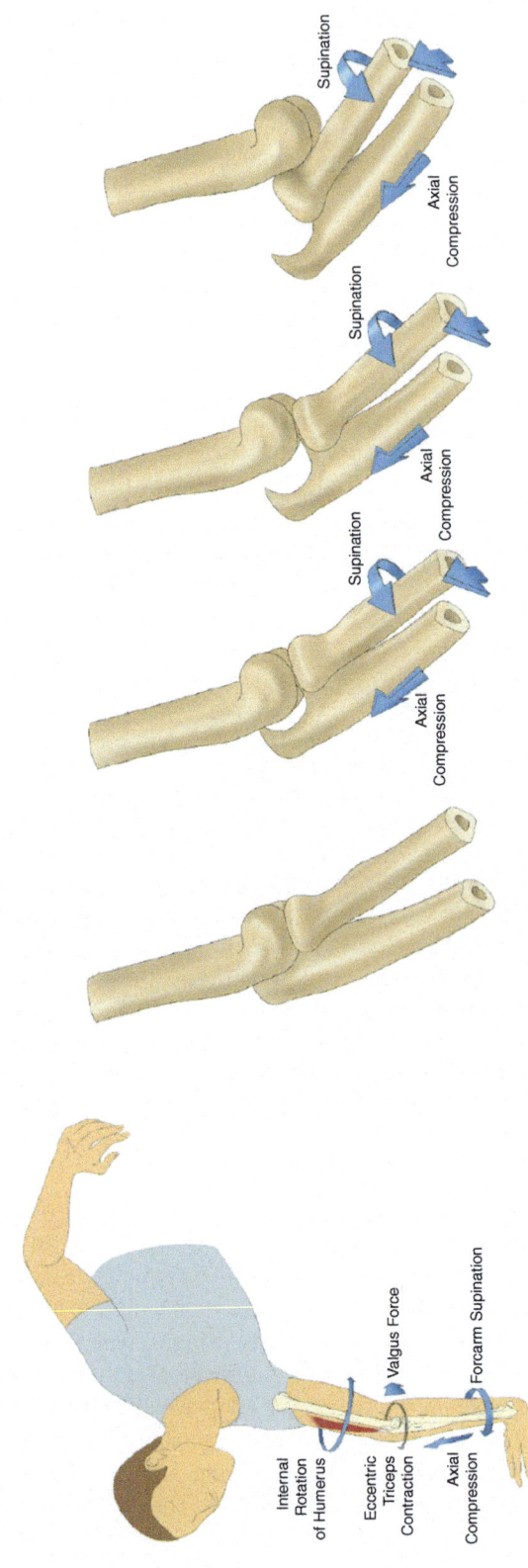

Fig. 11.14 Proposed mechanism of an elbow dislocation: humerus internal rotation, eccentric triceps contraction, valgus force at the elbow, axial loading, and forearm supination. This can be thought of in stages. A resulting spontaneous reduction and joint relocation may occur (mechanism concerning for ligamentous injury though not identifiable on X-ray). Subluxation or complete dislocation seen on physical exam and X-ray (expected ligamentous injury, possible fracture identifiable on XR)

(5–10%), avulsion fractures from the medial or lateral epicondyle (12%), and fractures of the coronoid process (10%).

Simple elbow dislocation, by definition, is without an associated fracture. A complex elbow dislocation is associated with fracture. The term elbow fracture dislocation is commonly used and typically fractures with known described patterns.

Simple Elbow Dislocation

Upon physical examination, there is visible deformity, with loss of the normal bony equilateral triangle, significant swelling, and loss of motion. A careful neurologic exam is mandated; the ulnar nerve is the most injured nerve. Significant antebrachial ecchymosis and swelling anteriorly can lead to and raise concern for compartment syndrome of the forearm.

An AP and lateral X-ray are sufficient to make the diagnosis. The radial head should line up with the capitellum on both views using the RCL. Failure to do so suggests residual subluxation. Advanced imaging such as a CT scan is rarely necessary to diagnose simple elbow dislocation. In the patient with median nerve injuries, one must consider arterial injury because of the median nerve's proximity to the brachial artery. If there is any question, arteriography is appropriate via CT angiogram or fluoroscopic angiogram (less commonly used/performed intraoperatively).

Initial neurovascular and radiographic assessment is followed by prompt reduction with pain control or under conscious sedation in the emergency department. Reduction is affected through manual forearm traction and brachial counter traction. The elbow is assessed for stability following reduction. If it is stable throughout the range of motion, application of a splint and sling, followed by early range of motion exercises, is indicated. If the elbow starts to subluxate or dislocate, immobilization at 90° is appropriate for a longer period, but usually not more than 3 weeks to minimize the risk of permanent stiffness. Rarely, the elbow will remain unstable, even at 90° of flexion, in which case acute surgical repair of the lateral and possible medial collateral liga-

ments is indicated. Likewise, if closed concentric reduction cannot be obtained, open reduction in the operating room is indicated. Common blocks to closed reduction include intra-articular fragments and/or interposed soft tissue structures such as the medial epicondyle and collateral ligaments.

Common Elbow Fractures

Common fractures about the elbow in adults occur at the distal humerus, radial head/neck, and proximal ulna. They occur through a wide variety of mechanisms, can be isolated or in combination, and are often with recognizable or named patterns. Fracture patterns can be described as transverse/oblique/spiral, displaced or nondisplaced, extra-articular or intra-articular (involving ulnohumeral joint or proximal radiohumeral joint) with articular split, depression, impaction, etc. Proximal radius and ulna fractures can range from simple olecranon or radial head fracture to more complex fractures and patterns like a proximal ulna shaft fracture with radial head dislocation, commonly referred to as a Monteggia fracture. Elbow subluxation and dislocation injuries can be associated with fractures. Generally referred to as an elbow fracture dislocation, if encountered, one must consider elbow stability and standard fracture care in their workup, diagnosis, and treatment plan. Both osseous avulsions and fractures in this setting can be indicative of a ligamentous injury, leading to elbow instability and/or potentially the primary treatable problem. Distal humerus fractures are common after high energy events or falls in the elderly. They can be supracondylar, single column, medial and lateral column, or coronal shear fractures. Treatment goals are complete healing of the fracture with pain-free motion and good function. One must be vigilant for associated acute soft tissue injury (compartment syndrome, neurovascular injury, ligamentous/tendinous injury).

Unless there is concern for an open fracture, neurovascular deficits, after appropriate reduction and immobilization, patients are commonly discharged from the emergency department.

Outpatient follow-up with an orthopedic surgeon within 1 week of injury is generally an appropriate time to reassess the patient after an elbow fracture. This allows for timely repeat X-ray imaging to identify any changes in alignment; reevaluation of soft tissue swelling and skin integrity; transitioning to more definitive types of immobilization or bracing if nonoperative treatment in indicated; and appropriately timed scheduling if there is need for operative repair or reconstruction. With nonoperative or operative management, associated elbow problems are common and can present in the post-traumatic, subacute and chronic setting (ligamentous instability, malunion, nonunion, arthritis). If missed or unrecognized, these associated problems can have lasting detrimental impacts on function, pain, and quality of life.

Olecranon Fractures

After XR imaging is obtained and a simple olecranon fracture is diagnosed, patients are typically immobilized in a well-padded, long arm posterior slab/ulnar gutter splint with the forearm and wrist in neutral position, loosely over wrapped with an ace. Before molding a splint and immobilizing the elbow in a usual position of 90° of elbow flexion, consider the fracture morphology and fragment displacement, as some olecranon fractures are best treated with the elbow in an extended position. For example, an acute transverse intra-articular olecranon fracture likely has an intact triceps tendon attachment to an unstable proximal fracture fragment. Thus, flexing the elbow and tensioning the triceps may create a distracting force at the fracture site and further displace the fracture. To decrease triceps tension when temporarily stabilizing a minimally displaced olecranon fracture or to help reestablish ulnar trochlear joint congruency in a displaced fracture, splinting the elbow in a slightly extended position (60–70° flexion) is appropriate.

Operative treatment strategies for olecranon fractures are dependent on fracture morphology, joint involvement, and patient specific demands. Open reduction and internal fixation (ORIF) with plates and or screws is common. The priority in surgical management besides stability and

bone healing is to anatomically restore the articular surface of the sigmoid notch, thereby diminishing risk of post-traumatic arthritis. In simple transverse fracture patterns without the presence of comminution, *Tension-band wiring, intramedullary screw fixation, and plate osteosynthesis (plate and screw fixation)* are effective strategies to achieve a stable reduction suitable for early ROM, appropriate fragment apposition and compression for bone healing. In simple oblique fracture patterns, after fracture reduction and lag screw fixation, a pre contoured plate can be applied, acting to protect the screw fixation by neutralizing bending and rotational forces across the fracture site. These techniques have shown excellent results when used with the right indication.

In the case of comminuted fractures, a dorsally positioned, single or double contoured plate and screw fixation is an effective and safe strategy yielding good functional results. Locking compression plates (LCP) are now more commonly used because they are pre-contoured and allow variable angle locking screw placement for effective articular surface buttressing and bridging of the fracture comminution. LCPs have recently replaced the "classic" low contact dynamic compression plate (LCDCP) for olecranon fractures. After nonoperative or operative treatment, gentle range of motion is typically initiated within the first week after injury or surgical fixation.

Common postoperative complications after ORIF using plates or tension-band wiring techniques include posterior elbow impingement, soft tissue irritation, and symptomatic hardware/prominence. This often requires a return to the operating room for hardware removal after the fracture is fully healed.

Radial Head and Neck Fractures

Fractures of the radial head are common (20–30% of all elbow fractures), occurring by a FOOSH mechanism with the arm extended and forearm pronated, transmitting a longitudinal force from the wrist to the radial head. Radial neck fractures (at the metaphysis) are more commonly seen in isolation in the pediatric elbow population. While radial neck fractures are less common in adults, when occurring with or without a radial head fracture, general fracture fixation and treatment principles are applied.

Radial head fractures are intra-articular fractures. They can be associated with scaphoid fracture, distal radioulnar joint (DRUJ) injury, DRUJ subluxation/dislocation with interosseous membrane disruption (Essex-Lopresti injury: DRUJ + IOL + radial head fracture), elbow dislocations, LCL and MCL injury, instability, and additional elbow fractures such as the olecranon or coronoid.

Patients will have pain and tenderness along the lateral elbow, difficulty with pronation/supination motion, and potentially a mechanical block to elbow motion. When examining a patient with a radial head fracture identified, it is important to approach a physical exam with a high level of suspicion for concomitant ipsilateral hand, wrist, forearm, and elbow injury as approximately 30% have associated soft tissue or osseous injury. Ligamentous injury is particularly common as radial head fractures often occur in conjunction with elbow subluxation or dislocation. Physical exam maneuvers testing the ligaments about the elbow (Table 11.1) are key in determining the integrity of these structures. Patients often are unable to tolerate these maneuvers acutely after injury and therefore the exam is performed under anesthesia before or after a planned radial head surgery. Otherwise, if treating a radial head fracture nonoperatively, elbow stability should be questioned, and physical exam testing performed when tolerable with a healed fracture. If there is persistent ligamentous injury, instability can result, and have subsequent implications on treatment strategy.

X-ray imaging of the elbow and forearm/wrist should be obtained, and is all that is needed to diagnose a radial head or neck fracture. When there is clinical suspicion but an absence of an identifiable fracture on XR, look for a fat pad sign. It can be assumed that a nondisplaced fracture is present if a positive fat pad sign is seen. The elbow should be re-imaged with X-ray upon 1–2 week-follow-up and a fracture line or subtle irregularity will often be identifiable. CT of the elbow without contrast can be helpful in fracture dislocations or comminuted fracture patterns for surgical planning or to identify intra-articular fragments. MRI to evaluate soft tissue, ligamentous, or cartilage injury is not necessary prior to surgical treatment, though one must be prepared to evaluate for such problems intraoperatively and address any additional injury. MRI can be helpful to identify location of ligamentous tears and used in diagnosis for chronic cases when there is recurrent instability.

The treatment of radial head fractures depends on fracture morphology and concomitant injury. Isolated radial head fractures can be successfully treated nonoperatively with good outcomes if there is a no mechanical block to motion and the fracture is minimally displaced. Key factors in nonoperative treatment are short period of immobilization (commonly patient self-limitation and/or an arm sling for comfort), and appropriate oral pain control allowing for early elbow range of motion. Elbow stiffness is a serious complication that can become permanent if patients are not properly counseled and educated or if they are immobilized with subsequent delay or lost to follow-up.

The goal of surgical treatment is stable anatomic reduction and restoration of the joint surface. Surgical strategies for radial head fractures are broad. A useful and common classification system used to guide treatment of radial head fractures is the Mason Classification. Minimally displaced fractures (<2 mm) with no mechanical block to motion/rotation (Type I) are most common and are treated with a sling and early motion (within 3 days). Displaced fractures (>2 mm) with one fragment (Type II) and block to motion are often managed with ORIF. Fragments less than ~30% of the articular surface may be excised, if there is no concern for instability. Displaced, multi-fragmentary fractures (Type III) are usually managed with radial head arthroplasty but may be treated with ORIF in young patients with less than three fragments (>3 fragment ORIF has shown poorer outcomes). Hotchkiss modified the Mason classification to add radial head fracture with an elbow dislocation (Type IV), to include instability patterns such as LUCL avulsion and coronoid fractures (terrible triad).

Table 11.1 Provocative physical exam maneuvers and signs

Lateral epicondylitis	Pain with grip testing; resisted wrist extension with elbow fully extended; resisted extension of the long finger, maximal flexion of the wrist, and passive wrist flexion in pronation. Radial Tunnel Syndrome (PIN) is implied by pain with resisted middle finger extension or forearm supination
Medial epicondylitis	Pain with resisted wrist flexion and resisted forearm pronation
Cubital Tunnel Syndrome	Tinel's test over the cubital tunnel, elbow flexion test (holding elbow flexed for >60 s), direct cubital compression *Froment's sign*—the patient is asked to strongly pinch paper between the thumb and index finger, and the thumb IP joint collapses into flexion, is an important diagnostic exam maneuver (compensating FPL via AIN and weak adductor pollicis seen in ulnar nerve palsy) *Wartenberg sign*—when the fifth digit is observed in an over abducted position at rest and seen because of ulnar denervation of the palmar interossei muscles, normally responsible for 5th digit adduction
Medial Collateral Ligament—posterior lateral rotatory instability	Sprain or attenuation is determined by applying a valgus stress to the 15–30° flexed elbow, looking to reproduce pain or joint opening. Provocative tests include the valgus stress test, milking maneuver, and moving valgus stress test
Little Leaguer's Elbow	Pain with resisted wrist flexion and forearm pronation; valgus stress testing where instability or gapping indicates more severe involvement
Distal Biceps Rupture	The hook test is performed with the elbow flexed to 90° and forearm fully supinated, the examiner's index finger is used to "hook" the lateral edge of the tendon. The biceps tendon will be absent in a complete tear, and if intact/partially torn, will be palpable and the finger able to be inserted approx. 1 cm beneath the tendon. Biceps squeeze test performed with the elbow in 60–80° of flexion, forearm pronated, the examiner squeezes across the biceps muscle belly and tendon distally. A positive test is failure to observe supination of the wrist or forearm
Triceps Rupture	Modified Thompson squeeze test performed with the patient lying prone with their forearm hanging from the end of the table. The triceps is squeezed firmly, and the test is positive if the arm is unable to extend against gravity
Lateral ulnar collateral ligament—Posterior Lateral Rotary Instability	Lateral pivot shift test, posterior drawer test, apprehension test, chair rise test, table top relocation test, or floor push-up test. Patients often are unable to tolerate clinical exam maneuvers, in which case they are frequently performed, and instability confirmed, intraoperatively

Partial radial head fragment excision (fragments <25–30% of radial head surface area) or complete radial head resection (severely comminuted fractures) is not commonly indicated but can be utilized if there is no ligamentous injury or concern for instability. It is typically reserved for low demand, elderly patients. Commonly, even a small fragment excision decreases available radial head area and results in elbow instability, as this joint sees 60% of axial load transfers across the elbow. After partial resection, new increased stresses are imparted on the medial elbow ligamentous complex if the elbow is subjected to repetitive valgus loads (radial head acts as a secondary static stabilizer to valgus stress). This potentially can lead to chronic attenuation of the MCL (primary stabilizer to valgus stress) and is an important consideration for treatment when the MCL is deficient.

Open reduction and internal fixation or ORIF with Mini-frag screws (buried), headless compression screws, or a periarticular locking plate (plate and screws within the safe zone), are frequently used in Mason Type II fractures. The safe zone is an arc of approximately 110°, contains thin to no articular cartilage, and does not contact the proximal ulna at the PRUJ during pronosupination. Its arc is typically identified at the radial head with the forearm in a neutral position, between the tip of radial styloid and Lister's tubercle at the wrist.

Radial head arthroplasty with a metal prosthesis (radial head and stem) is performed in Mason Type II and III fractures when fragments are significantly displaced, 3 or more, nonsalvageable, or require fixation outside of the safe zone that would impinge motion.

The surgical approach most commonly used for radial head treatment is the Kocher approach, at the lateral elbow, between the anconeus and ECU. The forearm should be pronated to avoid nerve damage to the PIN. More anterior and often used for radial neck/proximal shaft ORIF, the Kaplan approach is used between the ECRB and EDC, with a greater risk to the PIN due to its more anterior position.

Complications after surgical treatment include PIN injury, iatrogenic LUCL damage, articular damage or mechanical block to motion from hardware, heterotopic ossification. Decreased strength, elbow stiffness, OA (~30%) are not uncommon. After arthroplasty, stem loosening can occur and overstuffing the radial capitellar joint with too large of a prosthesis leads to capitellar wear and malalignment instability.

Distal Humerus Fractures

Treatment includes bracing, casting, traction, percutaneous pin fixation, rigid internal fixation, resection, reconstruction, replacement arthroplasty, or fusions. Stable, nondisplaced injuries such as simple condylar fractures can be treated with a brief period (1–2 weeks) of splinting followed by gentle range of motion. Most other fractures, however, require operative management with rigid internal fixation (Fig. 11.16) and early motion to avoid stiffness, nonunion, and other complications. Severely comminuted, intra-articular fractures of the distal humerus in elderly or rheumatoid patients are sometimes best treated with a total elbow arthroplasty.

Coronoid Fractures

Coronoid fractures after elbow trauma are generally pathognomonic for an episode of elbow instability. XR and CT help in diagnosis and surgical planning. They can be seen at the tip of the coronoid process, treated nonoperatively if stable. Also the anterior medial facet can be fractured, generally treated with surgery from a medially approached ORIF. Coronoid fractures can be treated with ORIF or suture augmented

fixation of the anterior capsule to the ulna (Fig. 11.15).

Monteggia Fracture

A Monteggia fracture is defined as a proximal 3rd ulnar fracture with an associated radial head dislocation (radiocapitellar joint dislocation). Treatment is either nonoperative with a closed reduction and immobilization in children (uncommonly in adults) or operative with ORIF of the ulna shaft and possibly open reduction of the radial head.

Ligamentous Injuries

Ligamentous injuries leading to chronic elbow instability can be difficult to diagnose and treat. Addressing the source of pathology usually leads to a stable elbow. Anterior or posterior instabilities are usually due to displaced olecranon or coronoid fractures or, more rarely, anterior capsule and brachialis disruptions. Other types include varus, valgus, posteromedial and posterolateral rotatory instabilities. They can all result from a single traumatic event such as a dislocation or subluxation, but they can also come from repetitive stresses, malalignment and malunion after fracture, or iatrogenic injuries such as excessive removal of epicondyles for ulnar nerve decompression or in the treatment of epicondylitis.

Lateral Ulnar Collateral Ligament Injury

Injury to the lateral collateral ligament is usually associated with posterolateral rotatory instability. It occurs most often after a traumatic elbow dislocation (Figs. 11.6 and 11.17b) but can occur after iatrogenic injury to the LUCL or from chronic attenuation. Patients usually present with lateral elbow pain and often a mild flexion contracture. They have varus instability with clicking and may report recurrent symptoms of popping or subluxation of the elbow. In subtle cases, the patient may not report gross instability, but instead, apprehension to various elbow positions or activity. Physical exam maneuvers (Table 11.1)

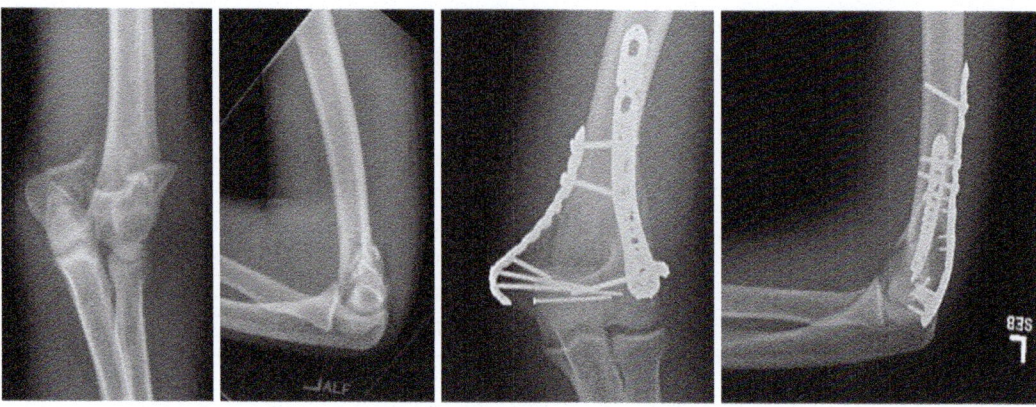

Fig. 11.16 Intra-articular distal humerus fracture involving both the medial and lateral columns

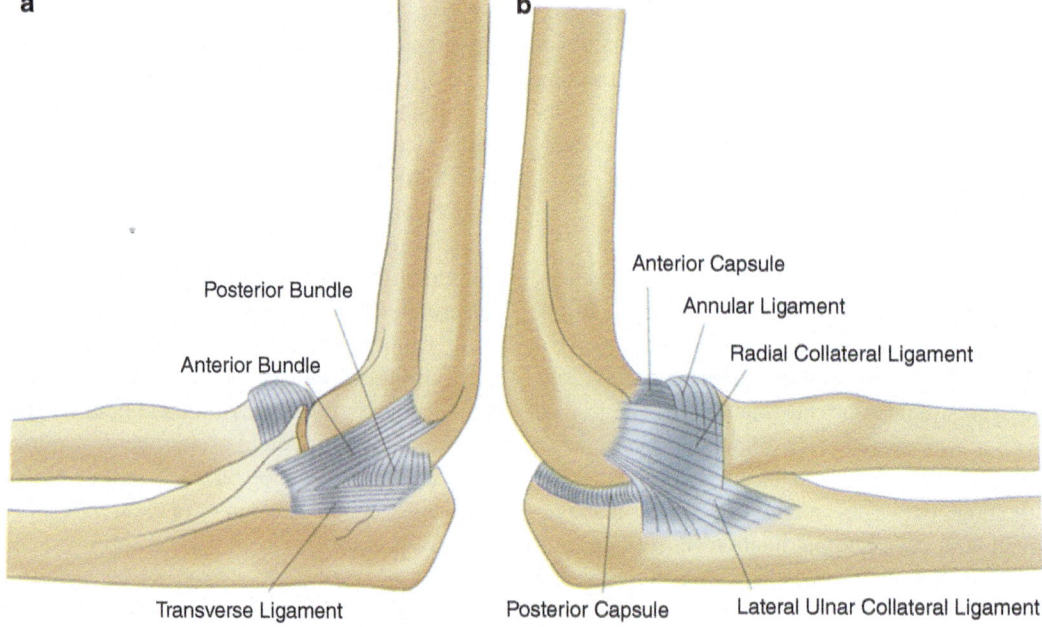

Fig. 11.17 (a) Medial and (b) Lateral views of the elbow ligaments

can indicate posterolateral rotatory instability (PLRI).

X-rays are usually negative, although in cases of chronic instability, arthritic changes can be appreciated. Stress views can also be helpful but are not well tolerated. MRI may be helpful in acute cases to identify avulsion, and less useful in chronic cases with ligament attenuation difficult to visualize.

Treatment involves reconstruction of the lateral ligamentous structures via the lateral Kocher approach; this often requires a tendon graft and or suture augments. When a terrible triad injury, elbow dislocation with LUCL tear (or radial head fracture) and coronoid fracture is diagnosed, the LUCL is generally fixed first. This alone typically renders the elbow stable, though is assessed with attention to the anterior and medial structures if still unstable. Hinged elbow braces are effective to immobilize patients post operatively with progressive to ROM. In rare cases, after all soft tissue procedures, the elbow remains grossly unstable or with joint subluxation, and an external fixator is surgically applied to immobilize the elbow until healing of the repairs and range of motion is warranted.

Complications include recurrent instability, infection, decreased range of motion (Fig. 11.18).

Medial Ulnar Collateral Ligament Injury

Isolated Injuries to the medial collateral ligament (MCL) cause valgus instability. It can be seen after acute trauma or chronic attenuation. It ranges from the sprain with microscopic hemorrhage causing chronic pain to complete disruption and true instability to valgus stress. The problem is particularly common in throwing athletes. Patients have a sense of "giving way" of the medial elbow. They have medial elbow pain and tenderness, especially with throwing. Pain typically occurs when the arm is in the "late cocking position" of throwing, that is, with the shoulder maximally abducted and externally rotated (Figs. 11.13 and 11.17a).

Occasionally, the patient has sudden onset of symptoms with one event such as in javelin throwing, but more commonly, prodromal symptoms precede the "final event" when the ligament completely tears.

Physical examination shows focal tenderness over the MCL or its coronoid insertion. Evaluate the integrity of the flexor-pronator mass and presence of palmaris longus tendon (for preoperative planning). Look for signs of ulnar nerve irritability, which commonly accompanies MCL pathology. When patients have varus posterior medial rotatory instability (VPMRI) on physical exam (Table 11.1), the MCL could be ruptured. The differential for VPMRI includes coronoid fracture of anterior medial facet and LCL complex injury.

The most difficult differential diagnosis is that of medial epicondylitis versus MCL pathology. Valgus stress may cause pain in this condition as well because of stress on the medial epicondylar tendinous origin. However, in the isolated MCL sprain, forearm pronation or wrist flexion against resistance (common in epicondylitis) should not cause pain. Other causes of medial elbow pain in this setting can be flexor-pronator strain, ulnar neuropathy, or valgus extension overload seen in overhead throwing athletes.

X-rays may show ossification or the "spur" sign at the ulnar insertion of the ligament, loose bodies or calcifications of the MCL. Special stress X-rays may be helpful to document subtle instability. By flexing the elbow 30°, thereby unlocking the olecranon from its fossa, either gravity or manual force can apply a valgus stress. Any opening is likely of some significance, although it is appropriate to compare it with the other side. When positive, these stress views are confirmatory. When negative, however, they do not exclude MCL insufficiency. MRI and MRI arthrogram can be used to evaluate partial versus full thickness tears and the location of the tear. Likewise dynamic ultrasound is helpful to evaluate laxity with valgus stress dynamically.

In almost all sprained or partially torn MCL ligaments without instability, symptomatic treatment, including rest, ice, compression, and strengthening, allows return to activity. Complete or unstable partial tears, especially in throwing

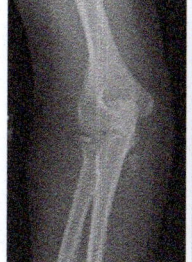 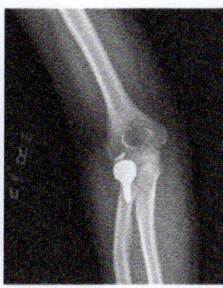 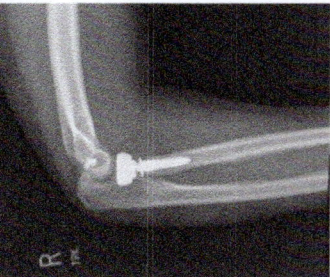 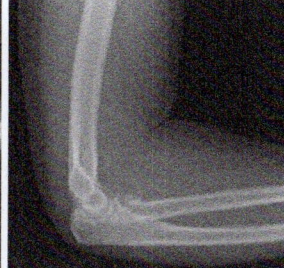

Fig. 11.15 Radial head fracture and LUCL avulsion injury after elbow dislocation treated with radial head arthroplasty and LUCL repair with suture and anchor

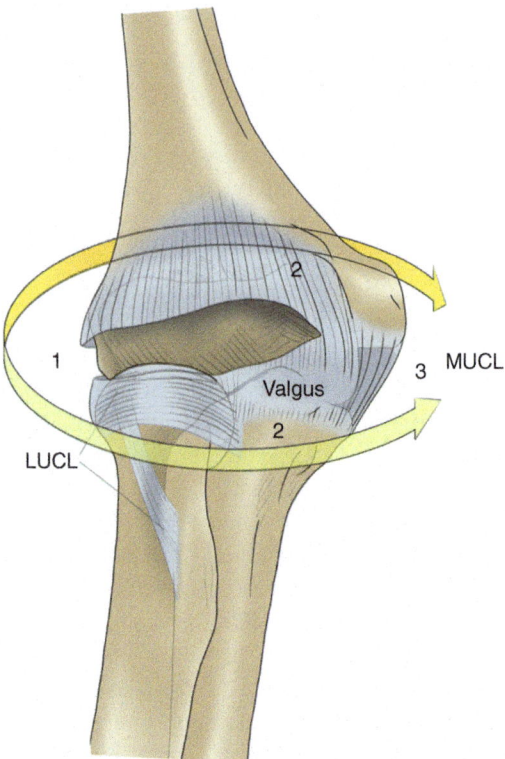

Fig. 11.18 Proposed order of ligamentous tearing from lateral to medial during a traumatic elbow subluxation or dislocation, also termed "Horii Circle." Injury can be thought of as a spectrum of involvement and severity, typically starting with the 1. Lateral structures (LUCL); 2. Anterior capsule structures (coronoid avulsion) /Posterior capsule; followed by 3. Medial structures (MCL- anterior bundle). Depending on the mechanism of injury, tearing can be seen in any combined pattern, location, or in isolation

athletes, often require surgical reconstruction, in which a tendon graft (palmaris longus or gracilis autograft/allograft) is used to reconstruct the MCL (tommy john surgery). In selected patients, where there is a small avulsion injury of the medial epicondyle, MCL repair with suture aug-

mentation is a viable alternative with promising results utilizing newer augmented techniques.

Complications after surgical management include ulnar neuropraxia, medial antebrachial cutaneous nerve injury, fracture of ulna or medial epicondyle, elbow stiffness, and inability to regain pre-injury level of activity.

Summary and Conclusions

The elbow is the critical link between the highly mobile shoulder joint and the precisely coordinated wrist and hand. Conditions that interfere with the elbow's normal motion can significantly compromise a patient's ability to feed, dress, and clean himself or herself. In the athlete, compromise in function often precludes the ability to participate. Fortunately, most conditions affecting the elbow do not result in significant limitations. The majority of elbow problems can be readily diagnosed with a thorough history, physical, and basic radiographic examination. An algorithmic approach to treatment facilitates resolution of most problems of the elbow.

Further Reading

Morrey BF, editor. The elbow and its disorders. 3rd ed. WB Saunders: Philadelphia, PA; 2000.
Galatz LM, editor. Orthopaedic knowledge update: shoulder and elbow. 3rd ed. Rosemont, IL: Journal of the American Academy of Orthopaedic Surgeons; 2008.
Cheung EV, Steinmann SP. Surgical approaches to the elbow. J Am Acad Orthop Surg. 2009;17(5):325–33.
Karbach LE, Elfar J. Elbow instability: anatomy, biomechanics, diagnostic maneuvers, and testing. J Hand Surg Am. 2017;42(2):118–26. https://doi.org/10.1016/j.jhsa.2016.11.025. PMID: 28160902; PMCID: PMC5821063.

The Hand

12

Edward Fakhre and Curtis M. Henn

Introduction

The human hand is perhaps the most important interface of a person's body with the outside world. It allows us to touch, feel, manipulate, and modify our environment. Its cortical representation in the brain is nearly as large as the rest of the musculoskeletal system combined. Loss of hand function can have devastating effects on a person's ability to work or perform activities of daily living. Unfortunately, because of its constant use and its position at the forefront of human activity, it is frequently affected by trauma and other disease processes. Nearly all physicians, regardless of specialty or subspecialty, will encounter a wide variety of hand pathology. Hand problems will affect their patients, their family members, their friends, and their colleagues. Therefore, familiarity with the basic hand evaluation, hand pathology, and basic treatment is crucial.

E. Fakhre · C. M. Henn (✉)
Georgetown University School of Medicine, Washington, DC, USA

Department of Orthopedics, MedStar Georgetown University Hospital, Washington, DC, USA
e-mail: Curtis.M.Henn@gunet.georgetown.edu

History

As in all fields of medicine, the history begins by determining the patient's chief complaint, which at times can be surprisingly difficult. Asking the patient to locate the point of maximal pain or what is the primary reason they came to see you is often helpful. Obtaining a detailed history of the present illness should then follow. Supplemental information specific to hand function should be obtained, including hand dominance, occupation, sports involvement, and hobbies.

The history of present illness is tailored to the patient's chief complaint and requires an understanding of various pathologic processes in the hand and upper extremity. For instance, in patients with congenital hand differences or birth-related injuries, one should obtain a careful understanding of the gestational and birth history. One must inquire about gestational diabetes, pre-eclampsia, and other maternal and fetal health problems, including exposure to teratogens. A family history of similar anomalies should also be determined. This information allows for the prediction and detection of other associated anomalies and conditions. The physician should also inquire if improvement in the condition has occurred and seek to understand the parental goals and expectations of treatment.

In nontraumatic situations, one should have the patient focus closely on the exact site of the problem and detail the history of onset, progression, and interventions. An understanding of what helps relieve symptoms and what aggravates them can aid in determining the diagnosis and tailoring the treatment. In patients who attribute their problems to repetitive activities, it is further important to understand the length of time it takes before symptoms begin, how long the patient had been doing this activity before this problem developed, and whether symptoms are now present when the patient is not involved in these activities.

When a traumatic injury is present, the exact nature of the injury and the surrounding circumstances under which it occurred should be carefully noted and documented; this includes the environment in which the injury occurred, whether it was clean or dirty, and whether the patient perceives that the injury was caused by another person's fault, their own error, or an unavoidable circumstance. These injuries often entail worker's compensation claims or other medicolegal litigation. By carefully determining and recording the events that occurred, the treating physician can give the most accurate representation of the injury and avoid later difficulties in trying to reconstruct events from memory.

Often patients present late after having been treated elsewhere or having avoided treatment altogether. This was particularly true during the COVID-19 pandemic. In these cases, one should note the evolution of the patient's problems, what treatments have occurred, and the current functional limitations of the patient.

The remainder of the patient's medical history should be elicited. An understanding of the patient's diseases including the presence of diabetes, hypothyroidism, heart disease, or other problems can help determine factors contributing to a hand problem. Previous surgical history, including complications of anesthetics, is also very important in the treatment process. Medications and allergies have obvious implications in the treatment. Social history should include the patient's occupation and hobbies, as well as tobacco, alcohol, and illicit drug use. Family history and review of systems then complete a thorough evaluation of the patient's history.

Physical Examination

When examining the hand and upper extremity, it is important to develop a systematic approach that evaluates all joints and sensory and motor function of all peripheral nerves. The exam is then completed with specific provocative tests tailored to the patient's complaints. It is important to compare the injured or affected extremity with the contralateral extremity, because there is a wide variation in normal exams from person to person.

One begins the evaluation with the observation of both upper extremities, noting atrophy, deformity, or any other lesions. Active range of motion is then assessed, including of the shoulders, elbows, forearms, wrists, and digits. If there is limited or asymmetric active range of motion, passive range of motion should then be assessed. Motor function and strength can then be evaluated. Typically, the extensor digitorum communis, the first dorsal interosseous, and the abductor pollicis brevis muscles are tested to evaluate the radial, ulnar, and median nerve motor function. Adding strength testing of wrist extension, extensor pollicis longus, flexor digitorum profundus to the small and/or index finger can further localize the lesion. Sensation is then tested. The radial aspect of the index finger tip, ulnar aspect of the small fingertip and first dorsal webspace are the best places to test for radial nerve, ulnar nerve, and median nerve sensation. In evaluating the sensory function, it is often helpful to obtain some measured data, such as two-point discrimination or Semmes–Weinstein monofilament threshold testing. For young children, assessment of wrinkling after immersion under water or the presence or absence of sweating can be helpful, as they are functions of the autonomic nervous system and cease when a peripheral nerve function is absent. Finally, vascular supply should be assessed by palpating the radial artery at the wrist and/or assessing capillary refill in the finger(s). A Doppler ultrasound can also be used if a radial pulse is not palpable or there is question about distal perfusion.

Palpation of the general area of the chief complaint should be performed next. In this section, one should localize the patient's pain or symptoms as anatomically as possible, but it is also important to start your palpation away from the point of maximal pain. The hand is unique in that many of the affected structures are easily palpated and distinguished from other structures, which often allows the examiner to make the diagnosis by determining the precise anatomic structure that is symptomatic. Thus, an understanding of surface anatomy is critical. For example, one must know that the scaphoid waist underlies the anatomic snuff box and that the A-1 pulley of the flexor tendon sheath is at the level of the metacarpophalangeal joint.

Specialized testing for specific injuries or problems can help confirm a diagnosis, and these tests are addressed under the sections describing those specific disease processes. In the setting of traumatic injury and or open wounds, strength testing is often deferred and the examination then seeks to determine if the function of the peripheral nerve or digital nerve is present or absent and seeks to determine if a partial or complete tendon laceration is present. Flexor and extensor tendon function can be determined by evaluation of active range of motion as well as the tenodesis effect of the wrist. Normally, the digits should flex upon passive wrist extension and extend with passive wrist flexion, and a digit not doing so indicates a possible flexor or extensor tendon injury. Pain with resisted tendon function may indicate a partial tendon injury. Following a thorough history and physical exam typically is imaging of the hand. The exam may then be repeated or further tailored following evaluation of the imaging findings.

Imaging

Imaging of the hand and upper extremity starts with radiographs. The standard views of the hand and wrist include anteroposterior (AP), lateral, and oblique views, and further views can be added depending on the specific area of concern (Fig. 12.1). For example, an AP of the wrist in ulnar deviation, also called a scaphoid view, provides an excellent view of the scaphoid in profile. All physicians who will evaluate the hand should have familiarity with the basic normal radiographic anatomy of the carpals, metacarpals, and phalanges. The physician should evaluate the overall alignment and relative relationships of the carpal bones to avoid missing a dislocation in an emergency room setting, such as commonly

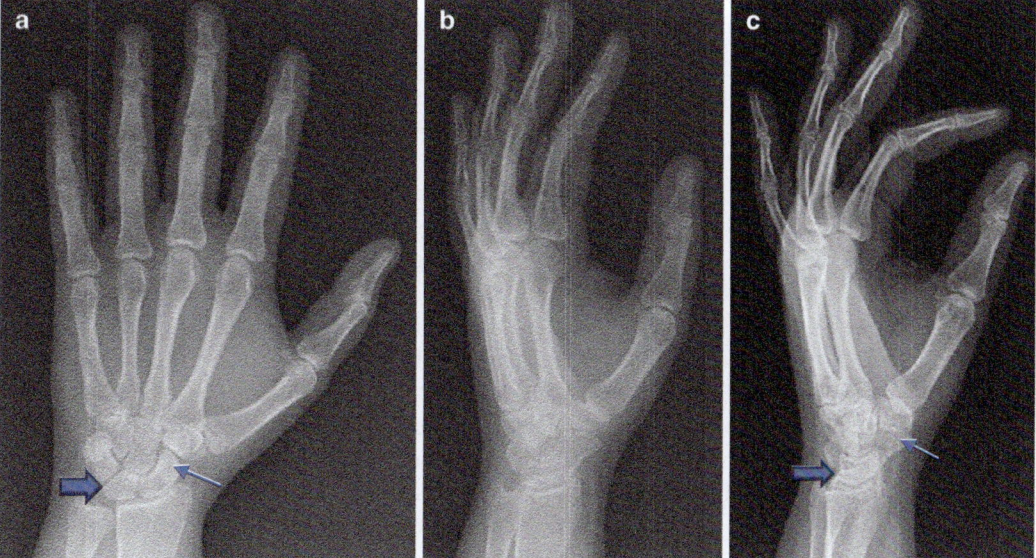

Fig. 12.1 AP (**a**), oblique (**b**), and lateral (**c**) radiographs of a normal wrist without any evident pathology or abnormality. The line arrow on the AP and lateral views points to the scaphoid bone and the block arrow in both points to the lunate

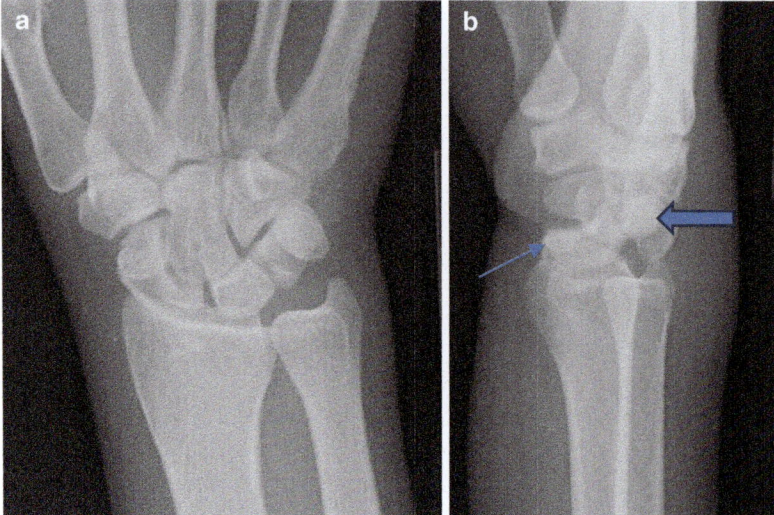

Fig. 12.2 AP (**a**) and lateral (**b**) radiographs of a perilunate dislocation that was missed in the emergency department. Evaluation of the PA show subtle abnormalities of the carpal alignment, and the lateral then shows the dorsal dislocation of the capitate from the lunate. The line arrow points to the volar aspect of the lunate. Note that the lunate is no longer articulating with the capitate, which is dorsal and signified by the block arrow

occurs in the setting of a perilunate dislocation (Fig. 12.2). Any detection of abnormality should prompt further three-dimensional imaging or immediate evaluation by a hand surgeon.

Advanced imaging modalities are used for disease or injury processes that present with normal radiographs and the diagnosis remains uncertain, such as an occult scaphoid fracture. Advanced imaging may also be used to further characterize a known abnormality, such as further evaluation of a soft tissue tumor. Computed tomography (CT) scans can evaluate precise bony anatomy and are useful in defining fracture presence, fracture displacement, fracture healing, and bony lesions. Magnetic resonance imaging (MRI) is the modality of choice for soft tissue lesions and has become the modality of choice for occult fractures of the scaphoid. MRI can also be used to diagnose ligamentous injuries of the wrist such as scapholunate or lunotriquetral ligament injuries. Ultrasound is rapidly becoming a useful imaging technique, especially to define soft tissue lesions, bony abnormalities, and ligamentous injuries. It can be particularly helpful in differentiating between rupture or scarring of a tendon repair and for visualizing foreign bodies that are not radiopaque. Ultrasound allows for a dynamic study in which tendons or other soft tissue structures can be evaluated while they are moving. It is a cost-effective imaging modality but is highly operator dependent in terms of performance and interpretation of the study. Bone scans can also be useful for helping define infection, reflex sympathetic dystrophy, and occult fractures, but utilization of bone scan has largely been replaced by MRI, except in unique situations.

Arthroscopy

Arthroscopy has become a common and important treatment modality in treating wrist pathology. Wrist arthroscopy has significant diagnostic value and is the gold standard for diagnosis of ligamentous injury, chondral damage, and capsular tears. As a treatment modality, arthroscopic debridement or repair is frequently employed in the treatment of triangular fibrocartilage complex (TFCC) tears, and arthroscopically assisted procedures are becoming more common (Fig. 12.3). As indications and technique are refined, arthroscopy will likely play an increasingly important role in the treatment of other bony, ligamentous, and chondral injuries.

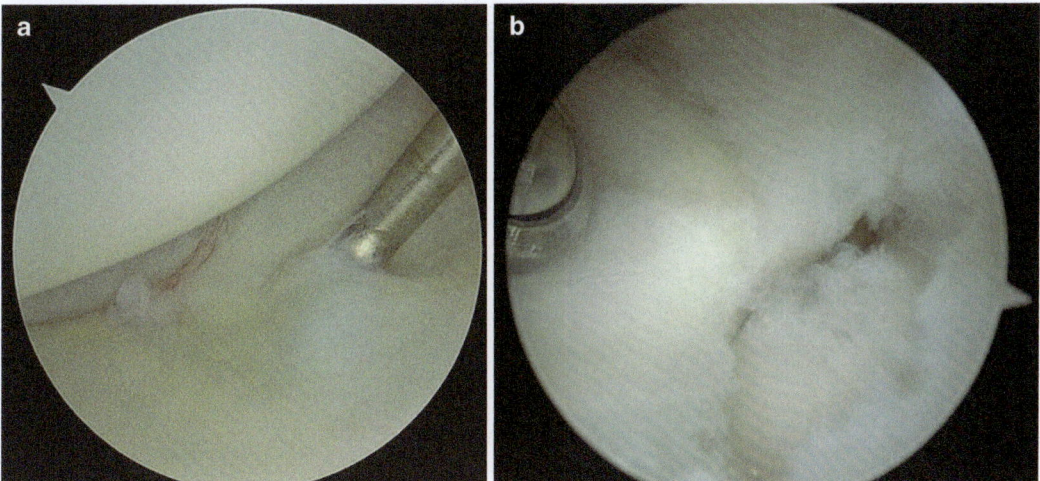

Fig. 12.3 (a) Arthroscopic image demonstrating a central tear of the TFCC. The probe is inserted into the tear. These tears generally require debridement. (**b**) Arthroscopic image demonstrating a complete tear of the TFCC with the ulnar head visible through the torn TFCC on the right side of the image. The shaver probe on the left of the image is radial to the tear and resting on the lunate facet of the radius

Pathophysiology

Hand problems can be grouped into seven major categories of disease: congenital, developmental/acquired, infectious, traumatic, metabolic, vascular, and neoplastic. There is tremendous overlap between these divisions, and a given disease process may have origins in more than one category. However, keeping these categories in mind and eliminating those that do not fit a patient's complaint can help focus one's differential diagnosis, leading to the proper diagnosis and treatment protocol. The remainder of this section reviews the most common disease entities within each category.

Congenital Hand Differences

In the human embryo, the upper extremity begins to develop as a limb bud at 4 weeks after fertilization when a segment of mesoderm outgrows and protrudes into the overlying ectoderm. A small segment of ectoderm then condenses and forms the apical ectodermal ridge, which guides further longitudinal growth of the limb. A second area, named the zone of polarizing activity, forms in the posterior margin of the limb bud and controls

radial and ulnar growth and differentiation. A third area in the dorsal ectoderm helps control formation of volar and dorsal characteristics of the limb. From weeks 4–8 after fertilization, this small outgrowth of mesoderm becomes a fully differentiated upper extremity with separate joints and digits. It is during this time that most congenital upper extremity anomalies originate.

Failure of Formation

Failures of formation may be transverse or longitudinal. Transverse failures are caused by injuries to the apical ectodermal ridge. They result in complete congenital amputation distal to the site of injury, which can vary from loss of fingertips to complete absence of the arm. The most common presentation is a congenital below-elbow absence of the hand and distal two thirds of the forearm. Depending on the level of the congenital absence, it is often treated by observation and parental reassurance or prosthetic replacement.

Longitudinal failures of formation involve loss of only part of the distal segment. They can be divided into radial (preaxial), central, and ulnar (postaxial). The most common of these are

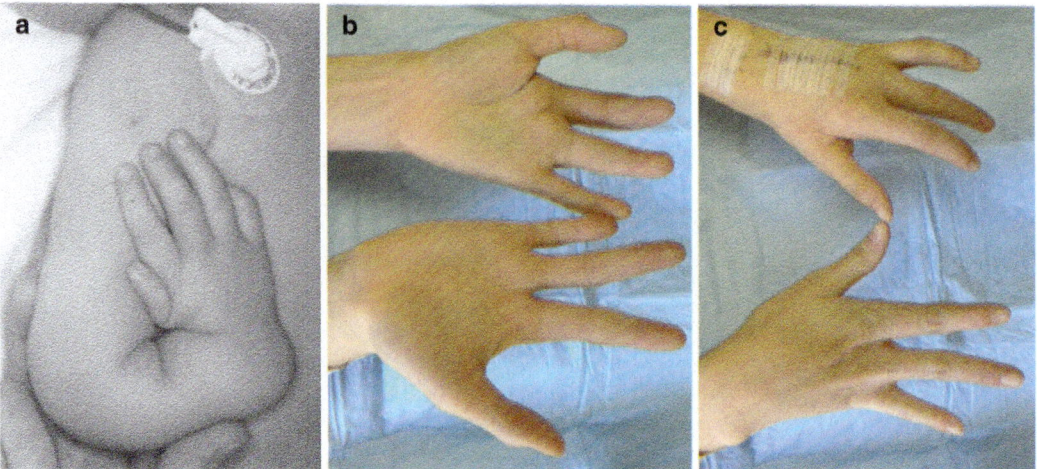

Fig. 12.4 Congenital malformations. (**a**) Radial club-hand produced by longitudinal absence of radius. (**b** and **c**) Bilateral cleft hand with failure of formation of the cen- tral digit. The patient has undergone a derotational oste- otomy of the left middle metacarpal

the radial-sided deficiencies such as congenital absence of the thumb or radial clubhand (Fig. 12.4a). These problems are often associated with visceral and bone marrow abnormalities such as Holt–Oram (cardiac septal defects); Fanconi anemia; thrombocytopenia absent radius (TAR); and vertebral, anal, cardiac, tracheo-esophageal, renal, and limb abnormalities (VACTRL). These patients should undergo eval- uation by the appropriate pediatric subspecialists. Central defects are much less common and pri- marily include the cleft hand (Fig. 12.4b, c). Ulnar-sided deficiencies include ulnar clubhand and its variations; these are often associated with other orthopedic anomalies. A very uncommon form of longitudinal growth arrest involves intra- segmental losses such as phocomelia, in which a relatively normal hand is attached to either the trunk or a very short segment of arm. Treatment of longitudinal failures of formation varies widely, as the severity and functional limitations vary widely from patient to patient.

Failure of Differentiation (Separation of Parts)

Failure of differentiation occurs when the normal programmed cell death between tissues fails to occur and bones, joints, or individual digits fail to form. The most common manifestation of this is syndactyly, in which individual digits are still linked together either by webs of skin or some- times by continued fusion of the bones (Fig. 12.5a, b). These parts often require surgical separation when the patient reaches the appropriate age. Other common failures of separation include the congenital lunotriquetral coalition; this is rarely symptomatic and is often an incidental finding. Synostosis, particularly of the proximal radius and ulna, which restricts pronation and supina- tion, and symphalangism, in which there is con- genital fusion of the proximal interphalangeal (PIP) joint, are other manifestations that can be more functionally limiting and symptomatic.

Duplication

Duplication or polydactyly, another fairly com- mon congenital hand difference, can range in scope from a simple skin tag attached to the small finger to a complete mirror hand. The very small skin tags formed on the ulnar aspect of the hand can sometimes be treated with suture ligation in the nursery, but more complex polydactylies require formal surgical resection and reconstruc- tion (Fig. 12.6). This is particularly true when a joint is involved, as osteotomy to allow the joint surfaces to maintain normal congruity and liga-

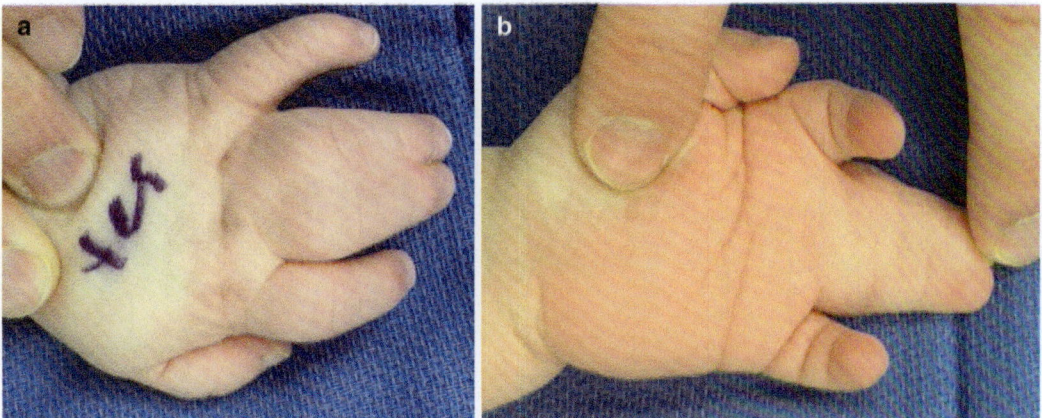

Fig. 12.5 (**a** and **b**) Syndactyly in an infant

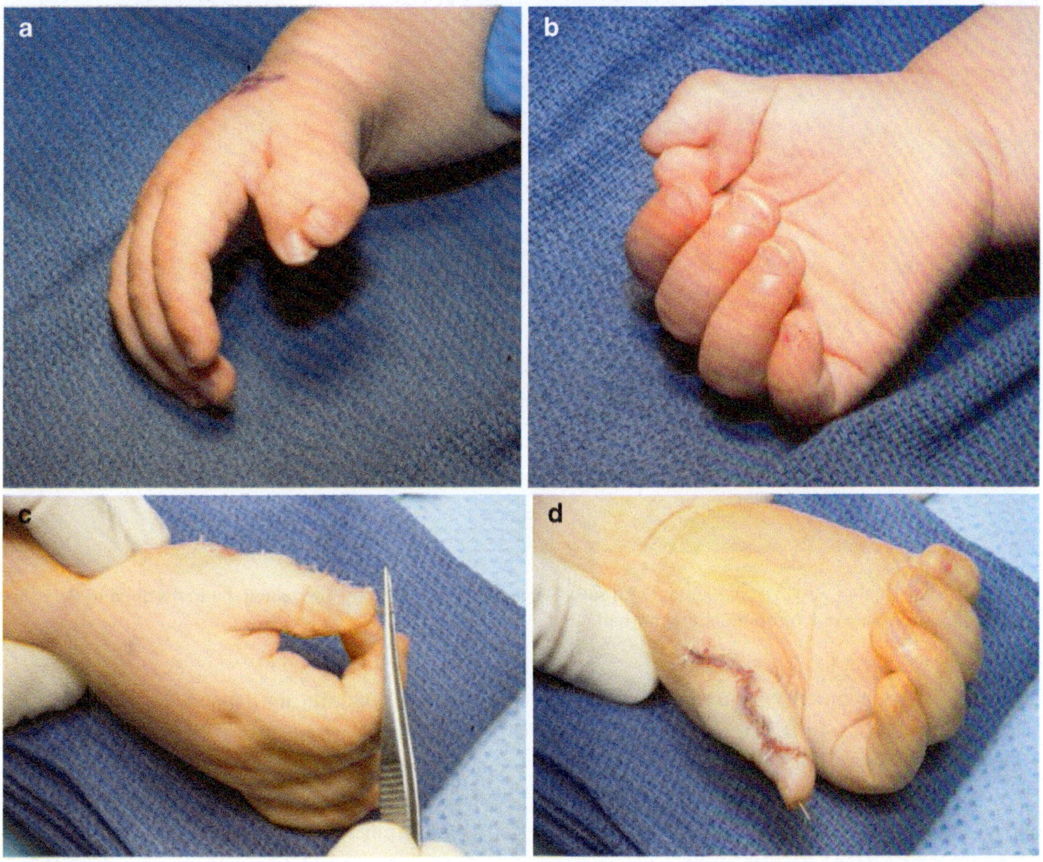

Fig. 12.6 (**a** and **b**) Thumb polydactyly at the level of the metacarpophalangeal joint requiring removal of the duplicate radial digit and reconstruction of the radial soft tissue (**c** and **d**)

ment reconstruction to reestablish stability may be required. Often the individual duplicated segments are not equal in size to a normal part, and function may not be completely normal after reconstruction. Many of the thumb reconstructions, in particular, require later secondary operations to fine-tune the result or to make adjustments for growth-induced deformities. Occasionally

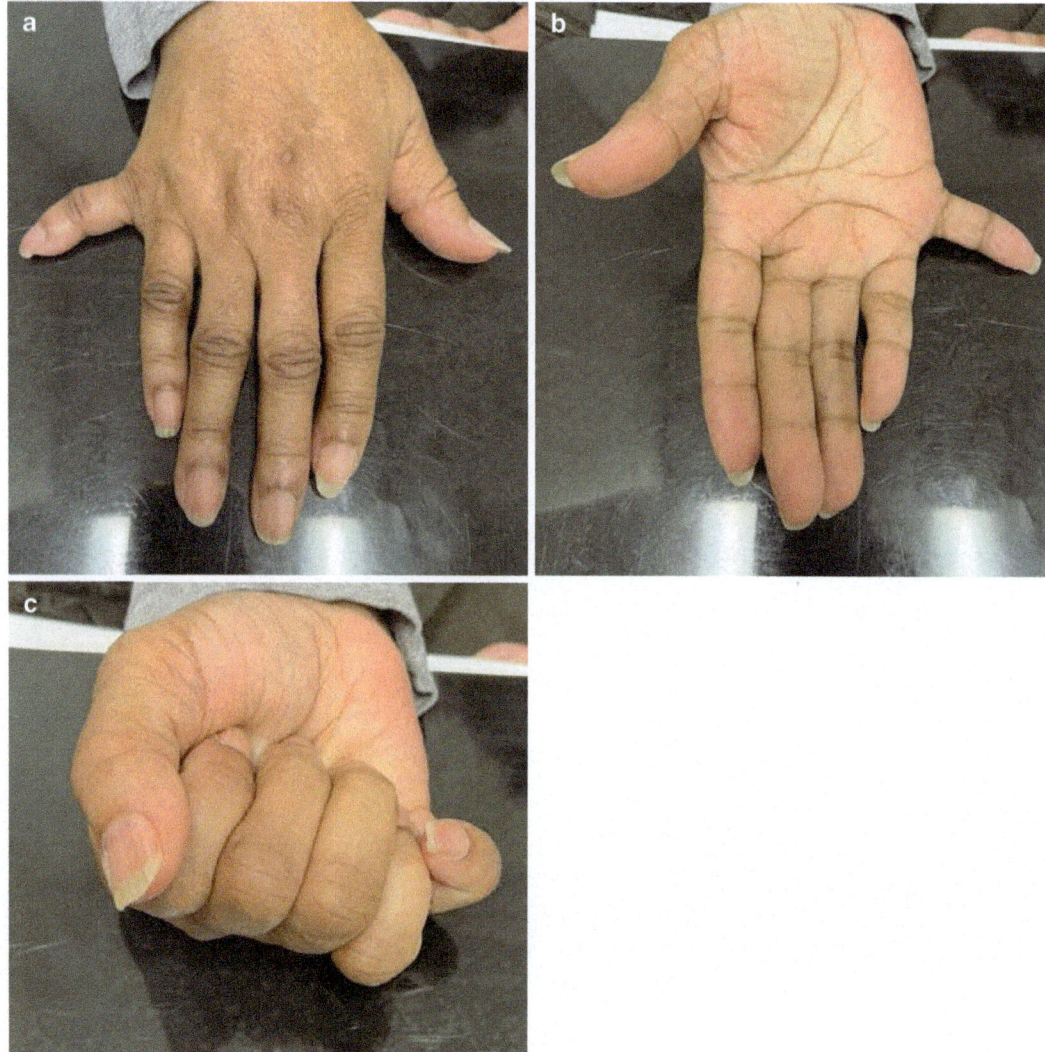

Fig. 12.7 (**a**, **b**, and **c**) 75-year-old woman with fully functioning polydactyly. The patient had presented to the office with complaints related to the contralateral normal hand

patients and their parents forgo surgical correction and can live a normal life with an extra digit (Fig. 12.7).

Other Congenital Anomalies

The remaining categories of congenital hand differences are less common. Overgrowth is a condition that can affect either an entire limb or an individual digit or section of the upper extremity. When this is encountered, the physician should look for an underlying cause such as a vascular malformation or neurofibromatosis. The problem can be exceedingly difficult to treat, and when debulking procedures fail, ray amputation of affected digits often is required.

Undergrowth or hypoplasia also includes a wide spectrum of problems including such minor differences as brachymetacarpia (short metacarpals) or involving significant hypoplasias of the entire upper extremity. It is sometimes associated with other syndromic conditions such as Poland syndrome (pectus excavatum and other chest wall abnormalities, hypoplasia of the hand, syndactyly, and other associated abnormalities). The treatment is patient specific, and often supportive care is all that is needed.

Congenital constriction band syndrome is a process in which it is thought that amniotic bands form around segments of the extremities, causing deep circumferential bands, fusions of distal parts, and even amputation. In rare instances, surgery very soon after birth is required to prevent neurovascular compromise, but most cases the bands can be treated in a delayed fashion. Treatment often involves excision of the deep constriction band and multiple Z-plasties for reconstruction. In some situations, a separation of distal syndactyly of the digits can be required.

Developmental or Acquired Disease

Arthritides

Arthritis of the hand and wrist is a common problem, and as it becomes progressively more severe, patients can experience marked limitation in hand function due to pain, deformity, or loss of range of motion.

Nearly all types of arthritis affect the hand, but osteoarthritis is by far the most common. The distal interphalangeal (DIP) joints of the fingers and interphalangeal (IP) joints of the thumbs are the most common joint in the hand affected, and patients often notice painless nodules early in the disease process. Mucous cysts, which are ganglion cysts arising from the arthritic distal interphalangeal joints, can develop at these joints as well. The PIP joints can also become involved and can develop significant stiffness and/or angular deformity. The thumb carpometacarpal (CMC) joint, also known as the basilar joint or trapeziometacarpal joint, is a common site of involvement as well, and it is the joint that most commonly requires surgical intervention for osteoarthritis in the hand. Arthritis in the basal joint can be extremely painful and cause debilitating loss of pinch and grasp function. In the carpus itself, the scaphotrapeziotrapezoid (STT)

joint also has high rates of involvement and often accompanies thumb CMC arthritis.

The diagnosis can often be made by the patient's description of their symptoms alone. Patients will complain of pain at the base of the thumb, particularly with opening jars or pinching with any force. Physical examination often shows a characteristic deformity with swelling about the basal joint with or without adduction of the thumb metacarpal and hyperextension of the thumb metacarpophalangeal joint. The patient will also have significant tenderness at the affected joint. Thumb CMC arthritis can further be diagnosed by a positive thumb CMC grind test. The thumb metacarpal is carefully grasped between the examiner's thumb and index finger. The remainder of the wrist is stabilized with the other hand, and an axial load and circumduction force are applied to the thumb metacarpal. This procedure usually results in severe pain for patients who have arthritis of this joint. Plain radiographs confirm the diagnosis in nearly all cases and advanced imaging is rarely needed. Classic radiographic findings are joint space narrowing, subchondral sclerosis, subchondral cyst formation, and osteophyte formation (Fig. 12.8).

Treatment is dictated by the patient's level of symptoms and their radiographic staging. For moderate pain and earlier radiographic stages, simple rest and anti-inflammatories can often provide significant relief. Splinting is often an adjunct, particularly for the thumb CMC and STT joints. Corticosteroid injections are a second-line treatment that provides significant short to medium term relief, particularly at the thumb CMC joint and the STT joint. If patients have developed mucous cysts at the DIP joint causing pain, skin breakdown, or nail deformities, surgical treatment with resection of the mucous cysts and the underlying osteophytes is indicated. Symptomatic PIP and DIP joint osteoarthritis refractory to conservative management is usually treated by fusion. Arthroplasty is an option for the treatment of MCP osteoarthritis as well as select cases of PIP involvement. Isolated STT joint arthritis can be treated with fusion or resection arthroplasty by removing the trapezium and proximal trapezoid. Arthritis of the CMC

Fig. 12.8 (a and b) Thumb carpometacarpal arthritis with accompanying STT arthritis; arrows point to the CMC joint composed of the trapezium proximally and metacarpal distally. Joint space narrowing, osteophyte formation, and subchondral sclerosis are present. (c and d) The patient underwent trapeziectomy and resection of the proximal half of the trapezoid to treat the arthritis in both joints. Arrows point to the void left by the removal of the trapezium and part of the trapezoid

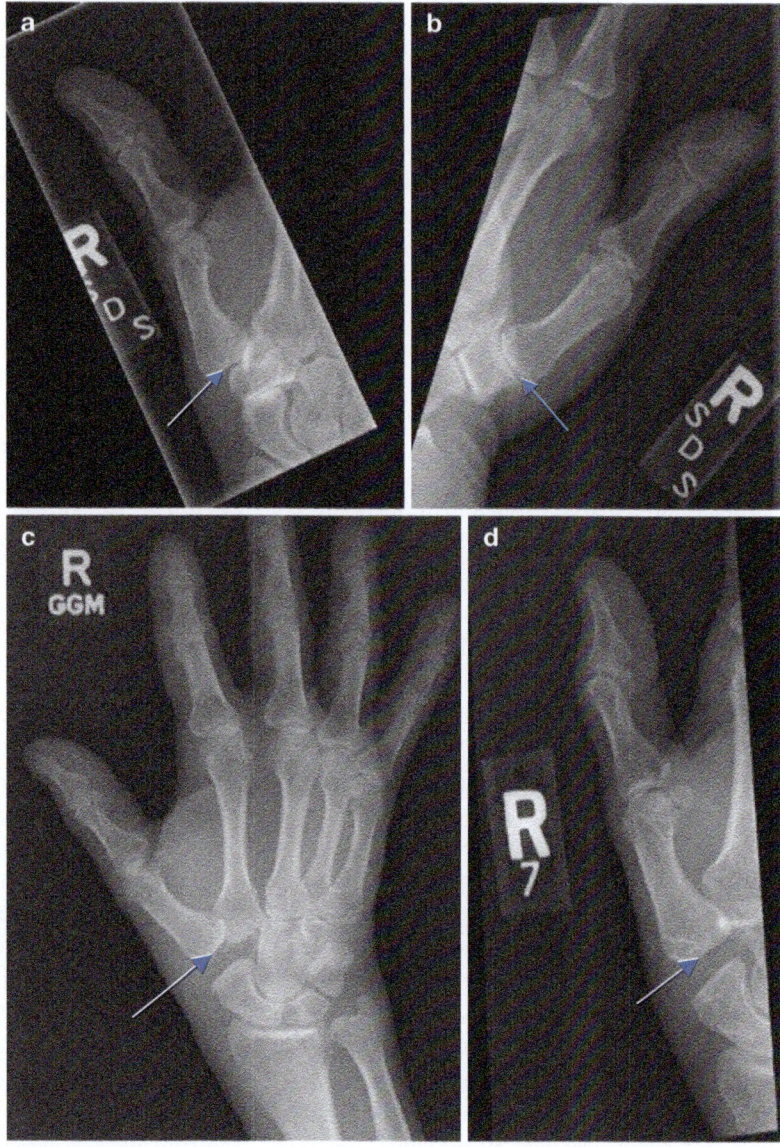

joint is treated primarily by trapeziectomy, typically with addition of surgical adjuncts such as ligament reconstruction, tendon interposition, or suture suspension. None of these adjuncts have shown any benefit beyond that of trapeziectomy and a complete trapeziectomy is a key to achieving resolution of symptoms (Fig. 12.8). CMC fusion can be considered for younger, highly active patients.

Carpal instability, most often a result of a torn scapholunate ligament, causes abnormal carpal motion and loading which can lead to character-istic patterns of arthritis in the wrist. The most frequently seen form is the scapholunate advanced collapse pattern or SLAC wrist. The sequence begins with a rupture of the scapholunate interosseous ligament causing uncoupling of the scaphoid and lunate. The scaphoid assumes a flexed posture and rotates within the scaphoid facet of the radius, which leads to altered loading and subsequently arthritis in the radioscaphoid joint initially. This process classically starts in the radial styloid region (Stage I), then extends to the entire scaphoid fossa (Stage II), and then to the midcarpal joint with proximal migration of the capitate (Stage III) (Fig. 12.9). Eventually pan-carpal arthritis (Stage IV) develops, though the radiolunate joint is classically spared, likely due to the highly congruent lunate and distal radius. Treatment options depend upon the stage and include symptomatic treatment initially with wrist braces, NSAIDs, activity modification, and steroid injections. After failure of conservative treatment, Stage II wrists may be treated with either scaphoid excision and capitate-hamate-triquetral-lunate fusion (four corner fusion) or proximal row carpectomy, which involves excision of the scaphoid, lunate, and triquetrum. Stage III can be treated with four corner fusion as above as well as wrist fusion. Stage IV requires wrist fusion for symptomatic relief.

Rheumatoid arthritis extensively affects the hand and wrist. This disease is a systemic inflammatory problem affecting nearly all tissues in the hand including bone, joint, tendon, and vascular tissues. Despite the advent of disease-modifying antirheumatic drugs (DMARDs) and the reduc-tion in the prevalence of severe disease, patients still often present to a hand surgeon with complaints regarding pain, function, and deformity.

The extensor and flexor tendons are often involved and tenosynovitis, inflammation of the tendon and its sheath, is common. Patients often present with pain as their chief complaint, but occasionally patients present with acute loss of function related to extensor or flexor tendon rupture. Other than institution of DMARDs, treatment often includes bracing, NSAIDs and steroid injections. If pain, swelling, and stiffness persists, tenosynovectomy may improve symptoms as well as prevent tendon rupture. The distal radioulnar joint is frequently involved, which can cause instability and dorsally prominent distal ulna. The prominent ulnar head can then abrade the overlying extensor tendons and lead to extensor tendon rupture(s). This is called a Vaughn–Jackson Syndrome. Surgical treatment of this problem includes resection or fusion of the distal ulna with removal of overlying osteophytes in addition to reconstruction of the affected tendons.

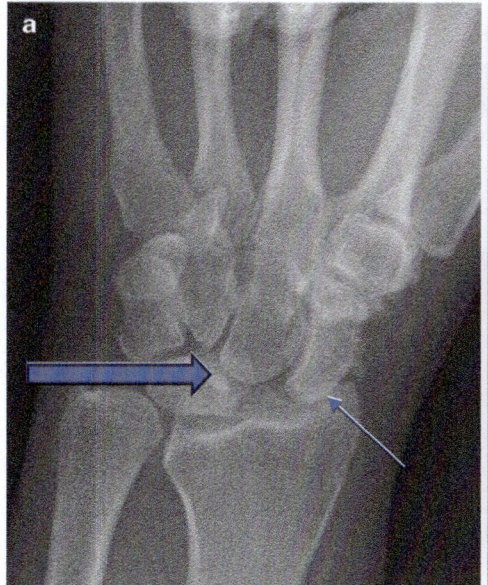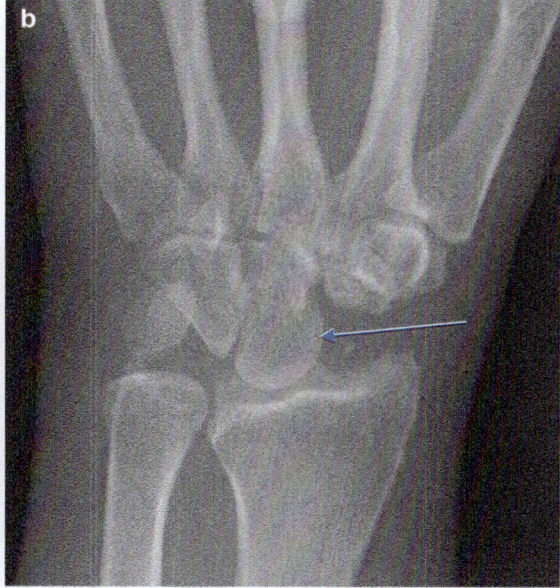

Fig. 12.9 (a) AP radiograph of the wrist demonstrating a Stage II SLAC wrist with involvement of the entire radioscaphoid joint signified by the line arrow. Note that the cartilage of the capitate is maintained as indicated by the normal capitolunate joint (designated by the block arrow). If this joint were involved this would be a Stage III SLAC wrist. (b) AP radiograph of the same wrist after treatment with a proximal row carpectomy. After removal of the scaphoid, lunate, and triquetrum the capitate migrates proximally to articulate with the lunate facet of the radius as shown in the radiograph. The capitate is designated by the arrow

Osteophytes on the distal pole of the scaphoid volarly can cause attritional rupture of the flexor pollicis longus tendon within the carpal tunnel; this is called a Mannerfelt lesion. The remainder of the carpus can develop extensive erosions, frequently causing volar and ulnar subluxation of the carpus on the radius and a radial deviation deformity of the wrist. The thumb CMC joint often erodes and dislocates, pushing the thumb into an adduction deformity. The metacarpophalangeal (MP) joint of the thumb is also frequently involved. The MP joints of the remaining digits usually drift into an ulnar deviation deformity, further compromising hand function. The PIP joints develop severe synovitis that can lead to either a boutonnière or swan-neck deformity. The DIP joints are usually spared (Fig. 12.10).

In the early phases of the disease, treatment is focused on medical management. Accompanying therapy and splinting can be useful adjuncts for maintaining strength and slowing the progress of deformity. As the disease progresses, the individual problems that develop must be addressed. Rheumatoid destruction of the wrist itself is usually addressed with a wrist fusion. Wrist arthroplasty is also an option and newer versions have shown promise as reliable long-term solutions that maintain some wrist range of motion. The thumb CMC joint is usually addressed with a trapeziectomy with or without ligament reconstruction. The

MP joint of the thumb is usually fused when necessary, and MP joints of the other digits are either fused or replaced with Silastic or other implant arthroplasties. Fusions and replacements are available for the PIP joints, and DIP joints are typically fused. Complex and diverse pathology caused by rheumatoid arthritis requires an experienced hand surgeon who understands how various interventions and pathologic processes interact in affecting function, comfort, and deformity.

Nerve Compression Syndromes

Compressive neuropathies of the upper extremity are common problems that can cause significant disability and pain. Carpal tunnel syndrome is by far the most common of these problems. Carpal tunnel syndrome is caused by compression of the median nerve at the wrist underneath the transverse carpal ligament. The hallmark symptoms include numbness, tingling, and paresthesias in the median nerve distribution (the thumb, index, middle and radial half of the ring finger), loss of dexterity in the hand, and discomfort. Symptoms are typically worse at night, during prolonged wrist flexion or extension, or gripping for long periods of time. In more-advanced stages, patients may develop weakness of the hand and dropping of objects, pain radiating to the elbow

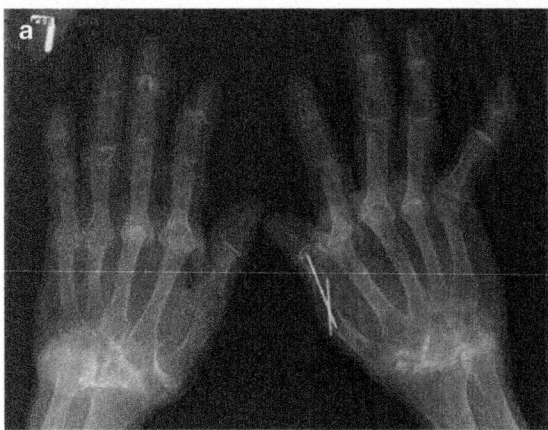
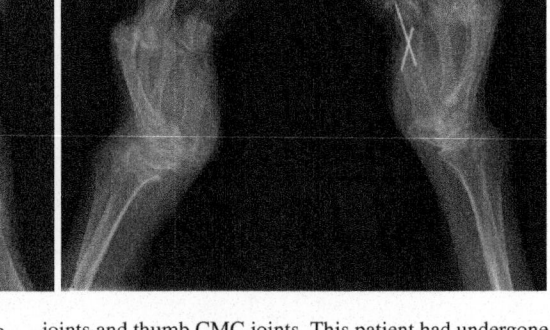

Fig. 12.10 Rheumatoid arthritis. (**a** and **b**) Severe erosive destruction of carpal bones with dorsal dislocation of distal radioulnar joint. Severe involvement of the MCP joints and thumb CMC joints. This patient had undergone a fusion of the right thumb MCP and a silicone arthroplasty of the right small finger MCP

or even the shoulder, or atrophy of the thenar musculature.

The underlying cause of carpal tunnel syndrome is often unknown in most patients. Patients with metabolic diseases such as hypothyroidism, diabetes, and renal failure are at much higher risk for developing this disease than patients without these diseases. The relationship of repetitive motion tasks, especially keyboarding, with carpal tunnel syndrome is controversial, but most patients attribute their symptoms to computer or smartphone use. However, carpal tunnel syndrome was very common prior to the development and widespread use of computers and smart phones, so a direct causal relationship is unlikely.

Physical examination findings include a positive Tinel's sign, in which tapping over the median nerve at the wrist crease elicits paresthesias in the median nerve distribution. A positive Phalen's sign occurs when symptoms are reproduced by holding maximal flexion of the wrist for a minute or less. The carpal tunnel compression test is positive if pressure directly over the carpal tunnel applied by the examiner elicits symptoms within 30 s or less. Thumb palmar abduction strength should be tested, and a sensory evaluation should be documented. When patients have an atypical presentation or physical examination, an electromyograph (EMG) and a nerve conduction study as well as X-rays can be very helpful to look for other causes of the patient's symptoms, including proximal nerve compression, cervical radiculopathy, or peripheral neuropathy.

Carpal tunnel syndrome can be treated initially by splinting the wrist in neutral position. Anti-inflammatory medications may also be helpful if patient's have acute flares of symptoms. If this does not help, a corticosteroid injection into the carpal tunnel gives relief in nearly 80% of patients with carpal tunnel syndrome, but only 22% of patients will still have symptom relief 1 year following the injection. When conservative measures have failed and the patient has persistent symptoms, surgical release of the transverse carpal ligament is indicated. This operation can be done through an open technique or through an endoscopic technique. Overall results are excellent with both methods.

Cubital tunnel syndrome, or compression of the ulnar nerve at the elbow, is the second-most common compressive neuropathy. Patients present with numbness and tingling in the small finger and the ulnar half of the ring finger and frequently complain of medial elbow pain. Symptoms are often worse at night or after long periods in which the elbow has been flexed. Physical examination findings include a positive Tinel's sign over the ulnar nerve behind the medial epicondyle, a positive elbow flexion test in which full flexion of the elbow for more than 30 seconds reproduces symptoms, and in some cases subluxation of the ulnar nerve over the medial epicondyle when flexing the elbow. There is often decreased sensation in an ulnar nerve distribution in the ring and small fingers. In advanced cases, weakness to finger abduction or even intrinsic atrophy can be present. Froment's test, in which the patient is asked to pinch a card between the thumb and index finger, is positive when the patient either cannot strongly pinch the card or collapses into a flexed IP joint position and hyperextended MP joint position of the thumb (Fig. 12.11). The main differential diagnosis includes cervical radiculopathy, thoracic outlet syndrome (i.e., brachial plexus compression in the region from the scalenes to the clavicle), and ulnar nerve compression at the

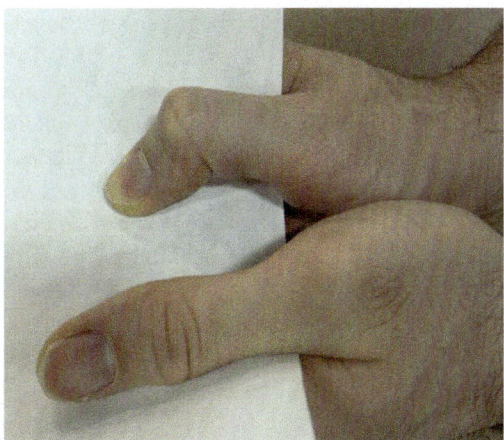

Fig. 12.11 Clinical photograph demonstrating Froment's test. Weakness with thumb adduction leads to flexion of the thumb when trying to grip. The right thumb is the affected thumb in this case while the left demonstrates normal ulnar nerve function

wrist. An EMG and nerve conduction study can be helpful to differentiate between these sites, but these are often negative even in moderately advanced stages of cubital tunnel syndrome. Treatment usually starts with extension splinting, activity modification, and anti-inflammatory medication. If symptoms do not resolve with conservative management or patients develop constant numbness or significant atrophy, operative treatment is indicated. Surgical options primarily include in situ ulnar nerve decompression versus decompression with nerve transposition. Outcomes are equivalent between the two techniques; however, a subluxating ulnar nerve on preoperative examination would be an indication to perform transposition.

Tendon Disorders

Stenosing tenosynovitis is the most common acquired tendon disorder affecting the hand and wrist. As the name implies, the underlying pathology is characterized by narrowing of the tunnel the tendons normally glide through, which then leads to inflammation and thickening of the tendon and its sheath. The inflammation and thickening then exacerbates the mismatch in size of the tendon and the tunnel it glides through. Once the tendon cannot glide smoothly within the sheath, the patient then experiences frank catching, or triggering, of the tendon as it passes through its retinacular housing. As the disorder worsens, then the patient cannot pull the tendon through its tunnel, which leads to flexion contractures and/or inability to fully extend the digit. The underlying etiology is frequently unknown but diabetes and renal failure are associated with these disorders. Occasionally there is an inciting event, such as trauma or overuse, that can create initial swelling of the tendon or its sheath. This can then initiate a viscous cycle of the swelling causing a mismatch in size of the tendon and its tunnel leading to more tendon inflammation and swelling, resulting in worsening of the mismatch.

The most common of these tendon disorders is trigger finger, in which the flexor tendons of the fingers or thumb become entrapped underneath the A-1 pulley of the flexor tendon sheath. Patients initially develop pain over the A1 pulley, which can then progress to triggering of the digit with flexion and extension. As the disorder progresses, patient can then experience locking of the finger in full flexion, necessitating manual passive extension of the digit, which is often associated with a palpable pop as the finger fully extends. The problem is typically worse in the morning, as swelling in the hand from lack of movement overnight can exacerbate the problem. Then as the day progresses and swelling subsides, the problem and symptoms improve. Patients will often be able to demonstrate the triggering and nearly all will exhibit tenderness over the A1 pulley. Initial treatment with corticosteroid injections has very high success rates, and often leads to permanent resolution of the problem. If symptoms recur or do not resolve, a surgical release of the A-1 pulley is indicated, which also has a very high success rate. Prompt recognition and treatment of this disorder prevents the primary complication from it, which would be the development of stiffness in the interphalangeal joints as a result of untreated trigger finger.

Another very common stenosing tenosynovitis is de Quervain's tenosynovitis, in which the abductor pollicis longus and extensor pollicis brevis tendons become constricted under the extensor retinaculum at the first dorsal compartment of the wrist. Patients with this disorder can often develop significant pain over the first dorsal compartment at the radial styloid and can reliably point directly at the first dorsal compartment as the source of the problem. The etiology is also often unclear, but this disorder is particularly prevalent in new mothers, and especially nursing mothers. Triggering or locking is much less common in de Quervain's than in trigger finger. Hallmark physical findings are significant tenderness over the first dorsal compartment at the radial styloid and lack of tenderness over the remainder of the wrist or thumb. Finkelstein's or Eichoff's test can be used to confirm the diagnosis and involves forcefully maneuvering the patient's thumb and wrist into adduction and ulnar deviation, respectively (Fig. 12.12). A posi-

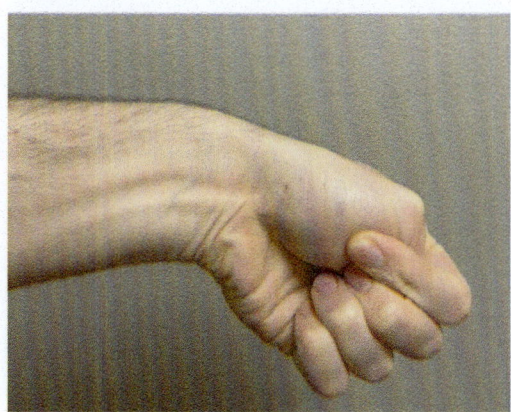

Fig. 12.12 Clinical photograph demonstrating Eichoff's test involving wrapping the digits around the thumb and forceful ulnar deviation of the wrist. A positive test is pain at the radial aspect of the wrist in the area of the first dorsal compartment indicating Dequervain's tenosynovitis

tive test reproduces the patient's pain. Treatment of de Quervain's tenosynovitis begins with nonsteroidal anti-inflammatory medications, bracing (which must include the thumb and wrist), and corticosteroid injections. If pain persists or recurs, surgical release of the first dorsal compartment reliably resolves the pain.

Tenosynovitis can also develop in other less common locations in the wrist, including the flexor carpi radialis (FCR), extensor carpi ulnaris (ECU), and extensor pollicis longus (EPL). Intersection syndrome is stenosing tenosynovitis of the second dorsal compartment tendons, the extensor carpi radialis brevis (ECRB) and extensor carpi radialis longus (ECRL), where the first dorsal compartment musculature crosses over them five centimeters proximal to the radiocarpal joint. Treatment of these conditions proceeds in a similar fashion to that of de Quervain's tenosynovitis.

Dupuytren's Contracture

Dupuytren's contracture is characterized by the gradual development of typically painless nodules and cords in the palm and digits that can then prevent full digital extension. It is a disease of the palmar fascia, which normally serves to tether the palmar skin to the underlying skeleton, facili-

tating grasp. As the disease progresses the normal fascial bands become thickened nodules and cords, which pull the digits into flexion and cause web space narrowing. The diseased tissue can also pathologically tether the skin, leading to visible pits, which are pathognomonic of Dupuytren's contracture. As the disease progress, the contractures can lead to significant functional impairment, including making glove wear impossible or preventing the patient from putting their hand in a pocket. The disease can affect one or both hands and can also involve thickening of the plantar fascia in the foot and/or of the fascia of the penis, which is called Peyronie's Disease. The underlying etiology is not known, but the disease is particularly common in older men of Celtic and Scandinavian origins, suggesting a hereditary component to the process, but disease severity within families is variable.

Surgical excision of the diseased tissue does not prevent development of further disease either in the same digit or other digits, and conservative treatment, including therapy and splinting, has not been shown to alter disease progression. Therefore, the treatment of Dupuytren's contracture is aimed at correcting functionally limiting contractures. Patients typically present initially with minimal or no contracture, so initial treatment is often reassurance and observation. As contractures worsen, though, there are three main treatment options to correct the contracture. Needle aponeurotomy is a procedure to percutaneously cut the specific cord causing the contracture, and can be an excellent, minimally invasive option, especially in very prominent cords in the palm. Clostridial collagenase is an enzyme that breaks down the diseased tissue and can be injected into the specific areas of maximal disease. 24–48 h after the injection a manipulation is then performed to manually disrupt the cord and passively extend the digit. Perhaps the most definitive treatment is surgical excision of the diseased tissue (Fig. 12.13). All three treatment options have advantages and disadvantages, and the decision of which procedure to use depends on many factors, including surgeon and patient preference, the location and severity of disease, and previous treatment successes or failures. No

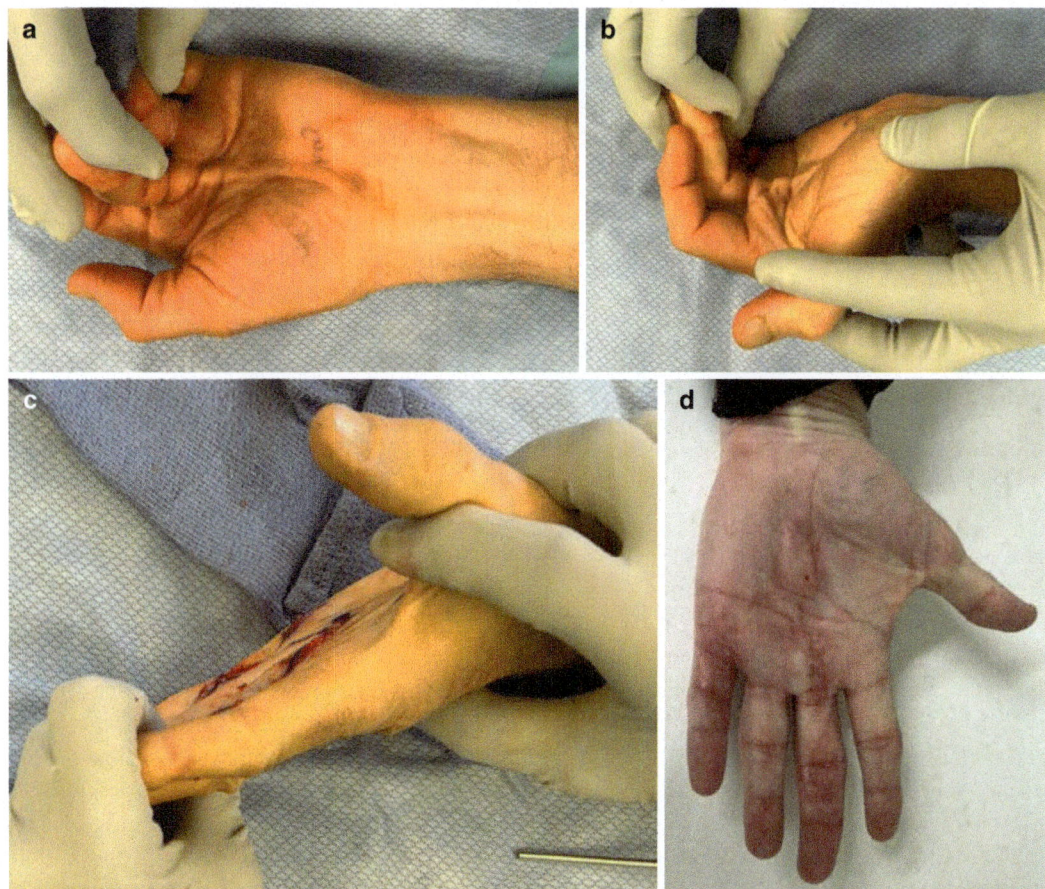

Fig. 12.13 (**a** and **b**) Dupuytren's contracture. Preoperative photographs of significant Dupuytren's contracture with a prominent pretendinous cord causing a significant flexion contracture of the middle finger. (**c**) Intraoperative photograph following excision of the cord, allowing full passive extension. (**d**) 6 weeks postoperatively demonstrating full active extension

treatment, though, can fully eradicate the disease and patients often require multiple treatments throughout their lives.

Kienböck's Disease

Kienbock's disease is idiopathic osteonecrosis of the lunate. As the osteonecrosis progresses, the lunate collapses and fragments, often leading to collapse of the carpus and wrist arthritis. Patients experience pain, which can be severe, loss of wrist range of motion and weakness. The disease most commonly occurs in the second through fourth decades of life. The underlying etiology is unclear, but patients with ulnar negative variance

(the radius is longer than the ulna) may be more likely to get the disease, leading to the theory that altered loading on the lunate leads to osteonecrosis. Early in the disease, radiographs are normal, but an MRI clearly shows the abnormality in the lunate (Fig. 12.14). As the disease progresses, it can be diagnosed with plain radiographs, which will show a sclerotic lunate with or without fragmentation, collapse, or arthritis. Initial treatment is typically conservative, including immobilization with either a brace or cast, anti-inflammatories, and activity modification. Optimal surgical treatment is debatable, but potential surgical treatments are determined by the presence or absence of carpal collapse and the relative ulnar variance. In patients with ulnar

Fig. 12.14 Kienbock's Disease (**a**) PA radiograph showing subtle sclerosis of the lunate. The arrow points to the area of sclerosis (increased density or "whiteness") in the lunate. (**b**) Coronal MRI scan of the same wrist showing obvious avascular necrosis of the lunate. This is designated by the arrow pointing at the lunate which appears hypointense or "dark" on T1 sequence MRI

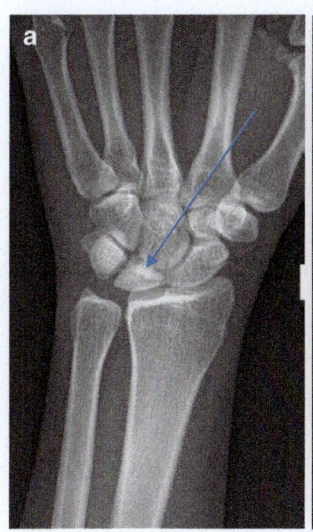
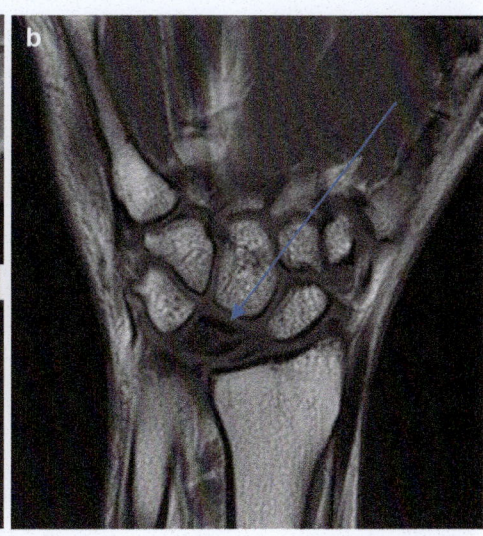

negative variance and early disease, radial shortening osteotomy is often performed in an attempt to alter the loading on the lunate and perhaps prevent progression of the disease. Other options for early disease include drilling of the radius (distal radial core decompression) or vascularized bone grafting to the lunate. Once carpal collapse and/or wrist arthritis has developed salvage surgical options include intercarpal fusion, proximal row carpectomy, and, in the case of pan-carpal arthritis, total wrist fusion.

Infection

The hand is relatively resistant to infection because of its robust blood supply. However, hand infections are relatively common due to its frequent exposure to trauma, particularly lacerations, open fractures, puncture wounds, foreign body penetration, and paronychial or cuticle injuries. Hand infections can also become severe, particularly in diabetics and immunocompromised patients, necessitating intravenous antibiotics and often surgical drainage.

Hand cellulitis involves infection of the subcutaneous tissue in the hand without development of a deep space infection or abscess. It typically develops after an often innocuous skin injury to the hand. Patients will exhibit classic signs of cellulitis with erythema, impressive

swelling throughout the hand, and occasionally streaking erythema up the forearm. Treatment involves prompt administration of antibiotics, splinting, and elevation. Localized cellulitis in immunocompetent hosts typically responds to oral antibiotics. Advanced cellulitis, spreading erythema up the arm, immunocompromised hosts, or failed oral antibiotics all require admission, IV antibiotics, and close observation to rule out the development of a deep space infection.

Perhaps the most common infection in the hand is a paronychia, which is an infection that affects the soft tissues overlying the proximal nail fold or the lateral edges of the nail. It is usually caused by Staphylococcus and presents as red, painful swelling overlying the nail fold. Mild cases in immunocompetent hosts typically resolve with warm water soaks with or without oral antibiotics. In more-advanced stages, and especially when purulence is visible, surgical drainage is required. This is typically done in the emergency department, urgent care or the office, and a subsequent course of oral antibiotics resolves the infection.

A felon is an infection of the pulp of the fingertip. Due to the many fibrous septae that connect the skin to the underlying skeleton in the finger pulp, infections generally create abscesses in the finger pulp. Patients present with a very swollen, tense, and painful finger pulp (Fig. 12.15). Treatment is prompt surgical drain-

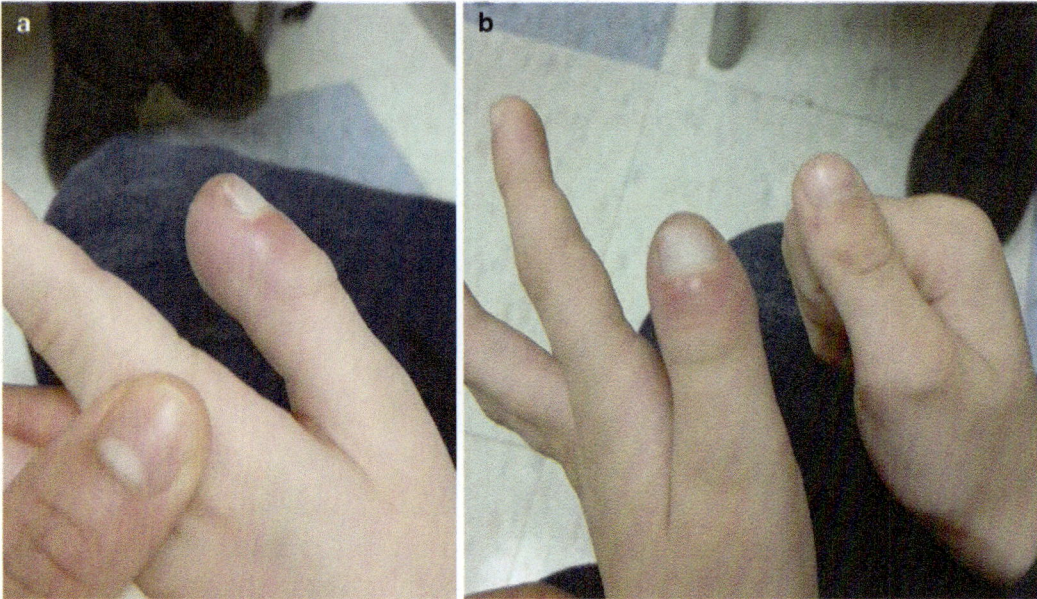

Fig. 12.15 (**a** and **b**) Clinical photograph of a 10-year-old patient with a felon

age of the abscess, which must include releasing all of the septae to fully drain the infection. Oral or IV antibiotics then supplement surgical drainage in clearing the infection. Delay in surgical drainage and/or antibiotics, especially in immunocompromised patients, leads to local spread of the infection to the adjacent distal phalanx, flexor tendon sheath, and/or distal interphalangeal joint.

Infection within the flexor tendon sheath is called purulent or septic flexor tenosynovitis. This is an extremely serious infection that can result in amputation if not treated emergently and aggressively. Infection typically is the result of a penetrating injury to the volar digit, inoculating bacteria directly into the tendon sheath. The bacteria can then proliferate within the tendon sheath unchecked by the body's immune system due to lack of blood supply within the sheath. As the infection worsens, the tendons can become ischemic and rupture. If left untreated, it can also lead directly to digital ischemia and/or spread into the thenar space, the palmar space, or even the carpal tunnel, causing a more severe and widespread infection. The four classic physical exam findings in patients with flexor sheath infections are called Kanavel's signs (Fig. 12.16). They include fusiform swelling of the digit, severe tenderness

Kanavel's Signs
Fusiform swelling of the digit
Tenderness along the flexor tendon sheath
Digit held in slight flexion
Pain with passive extension

Fig. 12.16 Table of the Four Kanavel's Signs for diagnosis of flexor tenosynovitis

over the flexor tendon sheath, semi-flexed posture of the digit, and severe pain with passive extension of the digit. The more of these signs the patient exbibits, the more likely a flexor sheath infection is present. Treatment of this problem includes urgent surgical drainage of the flexor tendon sheath and culture-directed prolonged IV followed by oral antibiotics.

Septic arthritis in the IP and MCP joints also typically arises from direct inoculation from penetrating injuries. Treatment is prompt surgical drainage and prolonged IV antibiotics in order to preserve the articular cartilage, which is rapidly destroyed in the setting of infection. Infections caused by penetration of a human tooth, such as when a patient punches another person in the mouth, deserve special attention. These injuries, termed clenched-fist injuries lead to direct inoculation of the MCP joint with human mouth flora and subsequent immediate closure of the wound to the outside air when the patient extends the digit. An abscess within the joint then rapidly develops and can cause extensive damage to the joint. As a result, these wounds should be urgently surgically opened and drained, and the joint should be left open to allow continued drainage. Prolonged IV antibiotics are then often required and should cover Eikenella corrodens, a common pathogen found in the human mouth.

Dog and cat bite wounds can also cause significant hand infections including septic flexor tenosynovitis and septic arthritis. Appropriate debridement should be performed when necessary and antibiotics should cover Pasteurella multocida, a pathogen commonly found in these infections. Infections to the hand and wrist from fungi, mycobacteria, and other atypical flora are relatively rare, but should considered in subacute cases, cases that do not respond appropriately to routine surgical and medical treatment, and in immunocompromised patients. A history of exposure to soil, rose thorn injury, birds, shellfish, or seawater should also raise the clinician's suspicion of an atypical infection. These infections often require multiple extensive surgical debridements and long periods of antibiotic therapy.

Trauma

The hand is often the human body's primary and initial contact point with the environment and thus subject to high rates of traumatic injuries. These injuries may include soft tissue injuries, involving the skin, subcutaneous tissue, tendons, and neurovascular structures; or they may include isolated bone or joint injuries; or a combination of any and all of these structures. They range from very minor injuries that recover to normal function with or without treatment, to devastating mangling injuries, to traumatic amputation. Many traumatic hand injuries require urgent hand surgical treatment to optimize functional outcome of the hand, and so basic knowledge of

hand injuries and their treatment are important for all physicians.

Lacerations

Large, complex lacerations, crush injuries, and penetrating injuries with obvious tendon, bone, or neurovascular injury require emergent hand surgical evaluation and treatment. Simple, isolated lacerations, though, generally can be evaluated and initially or definitively treated in the emergency room or urgent care. Direct exploration or probing of these wounds is not necessary but noting obvious tendon injury in the wound prior to closure can be helpful. A thorough physical exam of the digit before or after closure can often reliably identify complete injury to the tendons or nerves. Pain with resisted tendon function or any numbness should raise suspicion that a partial tendon or nerve injury exists, and surgical exploration should be recommended to assess the extent of the presumed partial injury. Capillary refill should be checked to insure maintenance of blood supply to the digit. A pale digit without capillary refill requires emergent hand surgical evaluation and revascularization. Radiographs should be obtained in all cases to ensure that no fracture or residual foreign body is present. Appropriate tetanus and antibiotic coverage should be instituted.

If the decision is made to take a wound to the operating room urgently due to gross contamination, vascular compromise, or severity of the injury, the wound can be irrigated, dressed, and splinted to await passage to surgery. If the external wound is minor, but the patient has an obvious tendon or nerve injury that will require repair, a loose closure can be performed in the emergency room. Splinting is usually initiated, and the patient can follow-up with the hand surgeon on an elective basis. Minor lacerations that are clean and do not have deep tissue involvement should be definitively closed and dressed in the emergency room. It is important to recognize, though, that even very small lacerations or puncture wounds can disrupt tendons and/or nerves and lead to permanent hand or finger disfunction if

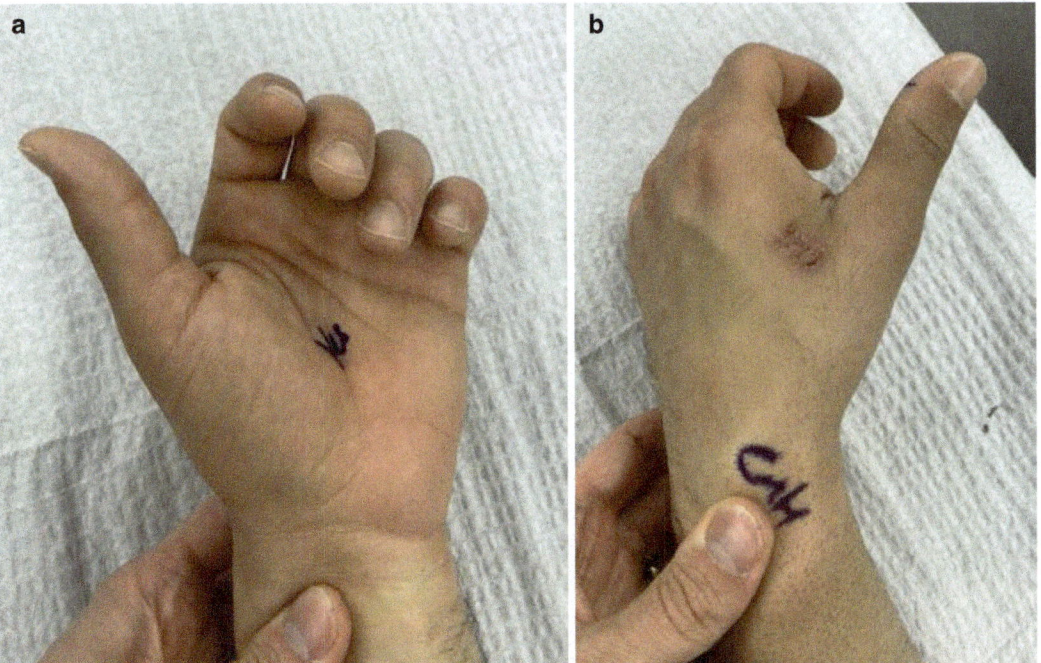

Fig. 12.17 (**a** and **b**) Photograph of a patient who sustained a puncture wound to the dorsal webspace seen in **b**. The patient lost the ability to flex the thumb IP joint due to a complete FPL laceration through this wound. Note the resting posture of the extended IP joint, due to the complete FPL laceration

not managed urgently by a hand surgeon (Fig. 12.17). Therefore, it is important to contact the hand surgeon who will eventually and definitively treat the patient so that appropriate care and follow-up can be arranged. Nerve and flexor tendon injuries ideally are addressed within a week or two to avoid permanent loss of function.

Fractures and Dislocations

Fractures and dislocations of the hand and wrist can occur through a variety of mechanisms including falls on an outstretched wrist or hand, crush injuries, or direct blows. They range from minor, inconsequential nondisplaced fracture, to highly comminuted, unreconstructable fractures from high-energy injuries. Most fractures in the hand and wrist are diagnosed with appropriate radiographs, including orthogonal views of the affected bone and often an oblique view. In the case of normal radiographs and high clinical sus-

picion of a fracture, MRI or interval radiographs may be required to confirm or rule out fractures. Initial evaluation of hand fracture should assess for associated soft tissue injuries, including open fracture and/or nerve, tendon, or vessel injury.

Fractures of the phalanges range from simple distal phalangeal tuft fractures to extensive intraarticular fractures with significant comminution and associated joint instability (Fig. 12.18). The fractures must be assessed for stability, angular deformity, rotational malalignment, and shortening. If these factors are all found to be acceptable, the fracture can be treated conservatively with 3–4 weeks of immobilization or protected early range of motion until healing occurs. If these factors are not acceptable, surgical management should be considered to restore alignment and/or stability and facilitate healing of the fracture and optimal function. Fracture healing is often weighed against stiffness caused by fracture treatment. Reduction of phalangeal fractures can often be accomplished with manipulation under anesthesia and then percutaneous wires or screws

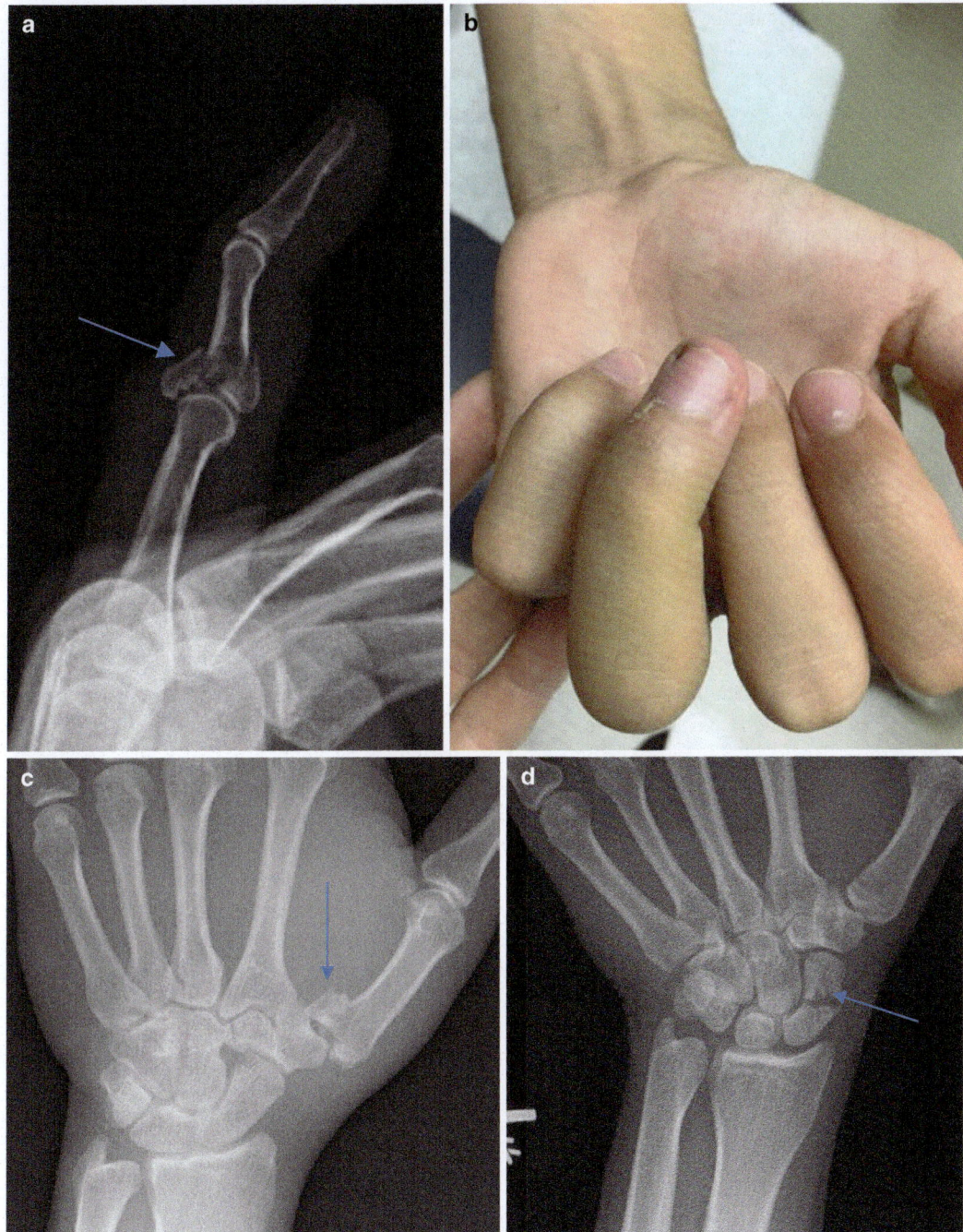

Fig. 12.18 (**a**) Comminuted middle phalangeal base fracture with articular impaction and displacement. (**b**) Rotational deformity from a middle phalangeal fracture. (**c**) Bennett's fracture dislocation of the first metacarpal base. The arrow points to the volar ulnar fragment of the metacarpal. Note that the volar ulnar fragment remains reduced to the trapezium while the rest of the metacarpal has dislocated. (**d**) Scaphoid waist fracture designated by the arrow

can be used to maintain the reduction until fracture healing. Occasionally an incision must be made to restore phalangeal alignment because manipulation was unsuccessful, and fixation with a plate-and-screw construct may be chosen to facilitate earlier return to function or may be required to stabilize a complex fractures. Goals of surgery include restoring joint congruency, articular reduction, and overall alignment of the digit.

The vast majority of metacarpal fractures can be treated nonoperatively with casting, bracing, or buddy taping. Exceptions to this include fractures with rotational malalignment, excessive angular deformity, or intraarticular displacement—especially of the first metacarpal base. Fractures of the first metacarpal base often occur in a pattern in which the ulnar segment of the base stays attached to the trapezium and index metacarpal through their ligamentous connections. The remainder of the metacarpal base and shaft then subluxates or dislocates dorsally (Fig. 12.18c). This pattern is called a Bennett's fracture and routinely requires fixation to restore the metacarpal base articular surface and CMC joint stability. Boxer's fractures are fifth metacarpal neck fractures that are extremely common. As the eponym implies, the mechanism is from punching a hard object. Rotational deformity, and subsequent surgical intervention, is rare, and up to even 70° of apex dorsal angulation can be treated nonoperatively in most cases. Angular deformity in the second and third metacarpal neck fractures is less well tolerated due to the relative lack of compensatory motion at the second and third CMC compared to the fourth and fifth CMC joints.

The most commonly injured carpal bone is the scaphoid (Fig. 12.18d). When patients are tender over the anatomical snuff box or the scaphoid tubercle, one should maintain a high index of suspicion for this fracture, because initial radiographs are often normal. If initial X-rays are negative, and suspicion of a scaphoid fracture is high, treatment should be initiated with a brace or cast. Confirmation of the fracture can be obtained immediately with an MRI, or follow-up radiographs can be obtained at weekly intervals to identify a healing scaphoid fracture, which

becomes more obvious radiographically. Due to its tenuous blood supply, scaphoid fractures have high rates of nonunion and avascular necrosis, and treatment delay increases the risk of both of these complications. Scaphoid nonunion and avascular necrosis can then lead to a well-defined progression of carpal collapse and arthritis, resulting in permanent wrist disfunction. Nondisplaced fractures that are treated early heal reliably with prolonged immobilization. Displaced fractures or fractures that have been missed are treated surgically to improve the rates of union and decrease the chance of avascular necrosis. Another common carpal fracture is the dorsal triquetral avulsion fracture, which often occurs after a fall on an outstretched wrist. This is best seen on lateral radiographic view where a small fleck of bone is noted dorsal to the triquetral region. Patients with these fractures reliably heal with immobilization in a cast or brace for 4–6 weeks and return to normal function with no residual effects.

Dislocations of the interphalangeal joints are quite common and can usually be reduced by manipulation with or without anesthesia. Radiographs should be obtained following reduction to ensure concentric joint reduction and to evaluate for commonly associated volar plate avulsion fractures. In the case of isolated dislocations or if the fracture fragment is small and the joint is concentric, the treatment is immediate range of motion to prevent significant stiffness, which sets in rapidly with any immobilization. Irreducible dislocations or larger fracture fragments require urgent surgical intervention. DIP and MP joint dislocations are rarer and more commonly are irreducible due to interposition of soft tissue. MP dislocations require special attention because attempted reduction by traction alone can cause interposition of the volar plate and turn a reducible dislocation into an irreducible dislocation. Therefore, emergent hand surgical consultation is recommended to avoid this complication. Irreducible dislocations in the DIP and MP joints also require surgical intervention. Early range of motion following these injuries is also required to combat inevitable stiffness that results from the dislocation and surgery.

Injuries to the collateral ligaments of the PIP and MP joints are common. MP collateral ligament injuries, except for the index radial collateral ligament and the thumb MP joint, are treated successfully with buddy taping the digit to the adjacent digit. PIP collateral ligament injuries are treated similarly without surgery, but these injuries can result in prolonged and often permanent swelling and stiffness of the joint. Index RCL and thumb MP collateral ligament injuries are often treated surgically. An injury to the thumb MP joint ulnar collateral ligament is called a skier's thumb and is a frequent athletic injury. Patients who have tenderness over the ligament, but good stability, should be immobilized for 3–4 weeks and then range of motion should be initiated. If the examination demonstrates obvious instability, significantly increased deviation on stress radiographs, or has a palpable Stener's lesion (a completely ruptured ulnar collateral ligament that is displaced dorsal to the adductor pollicis apponeurosis), surgical repair of the ligament is indicated.

Severe and Complex Upper Extremity Injuries

Amputations of portions of the upper limb, especially the fingers, are very common, especially in industrial and agricultural environments. Modern microvascular surgical techniques allow reimplantation of the amputated parts in many situations. The severed part should be wrapped in a gauze dressing soaked in sterile saline and placed in a container or sealed plastic bag that can be immersed in ice and transported to a treating facility. The part should never be placed directly on ice, and dry ice should never be used. An experienced hand surgeon should be consulted emergently to assess whether the part is a good candidate for reattachment. Relative indications for replantation include any amputated part in a child, the thumb at any level, multiple digits, or an amputation through the mid palm or proximally. Relative contraindications to replantation include severe contamination, crush injury, avulsion mechanism, segmental injury, broad area of vascular damage. Replantation also requires a

lengthy surgery, prolonged hospitalization, and specialized hand therapy to restore function. Older patients, laborers, and medically complicated patients may elect to undergo revision amputation rather than replantation. Extensive mangling injuries must be treated by an experienced hand surgeon emergently. The extent of the injury and what structures are salvageable and what structures are primarily amputated are often determined once the patient is under anesthesia. Therefore, it is important to discuss with the patient and/or the patient's family the possibility of amputation following such an injury.

Compartment syndrome in the hand or forearm occurs when significant swelling causes increased pressure in the muscle compartments, preventing flow through the venules and capillaries leading to ischemia of soft tissues of the compartment. If the pressure is not emergently alleviated, permanent and profound disability ensues. Acute carpal tunnel syndrome is, in effect, a compartment syndrome in the carpal tunnel. Profound swelling leads to direct pressure on the median nerve in the carpal tunnel and will lead to permanent median nerve dysfunction if not emergently surgically decompressed. The mechanism of injury should raise suspicion for these problems, including crush injuries and high-energy trauma, such as a fall from significant height or a car accident. Conscious patients with these injuries should be closely monitored for the signs of compartment syndrome, which include the five P's: pain out of proportion to the injury, severe pain with passive stretch, later paresthesias, pallor, and pulselessness. One should not wait for the development of the last three P's, as these develop following muscle and nerve necrosis and it is too late. If the index of suspicion is high due to increasing pain and the mechanism of injury, the compartment pressure can be directly measured to confirm the diagnosis. When the diagnosis is confirmed or when the suspicion is high, the compartment should be emergently and fully decompressed. In the case of an obtunded or intubated patient, the clinical threshold may be lower to proceed with fasciotomy.

Thermal, chemical, or electrical injuries cause widely variable degrees of soft tissue issue. The degree of injury depends on many factors, including the mechanism, magnitude, and duration of the exposure. The skin is the initial point of contact and may show first-degree (redness), second-degree (blistering), or third-degree (full-thickness or charring) injuries, particularly with thermal burns. Early care of the second-degree injury can minimize the chance of infection, which would exacerbate tissue loss. Early referral to a hand therapist for exercise and splinting may minimize contractures. Third-degree burns should be treated by early surgical excision of the eschar and skin grafting. Chemical injuries should be treated in a facility that has experience in managing these conditions as specific antidotes can be used to neutralize many chemicals and minimize damage.

Cold injury varies from minor frostbite to extensive freezing of tissues and peripheral parts. The initial treatment should involve rapid rewarming of the area of frostbite followed by observation. Blisters should be debrided to limit soft tissue damage from the inflammatory mediators found within the blisters. Early amputation is not necessary in the absence of infection, and observation until the injury and necrosis has fully demarcated is the treatment of choice. Electrical burns can be quite deceptive as to the extent in damage and require repeated evaluation.

Other Common Injuries

Mallet finger is rupture of the terminal extensor tendon's attachment to the distal phalanx, often following trivial injury. Fracture of the dorsal lip of the distal phalanx may be seen on X-ray in some cases. Full passive extension is present, but active extension is not, leading to the classic mallet deformity. Treatment usually involves full time splinting of the DIP joint in full extension for 6–8 weeks.

Boutonnière deformities occur from disruption of the central slip of the extensor tendon over the PIP joint by blunt trauma or laceration. Patients may often exhibit full range of motion immediately after the injury due to intact pull of the terminal extensor through the lateral bands. However, if the injury is untreated, the lateral bands subluxate volar to the axis of rotation of the PIP joint. Once

this happens, the patient can no longer actively extend the PIP joint and develops a flexion deformity at the PIP joint and compensatory hyperextension at the DIP joint. When diagnosed early, this can be treated by splinting the PIP joint in full extension for 6 weeks. It is important to allow DIP flexion and extension in the splint to prevent DIP stiffness and prevent volar subluxation of the lateral bands. If initial treatment is delayed or fails, surgical treatment can be considered.

Metabolic Disease

Many metabolic illnesses such as diabetes, hyperthyroidism, hyperparathyroidism, and renal failure can predispose patients to the development of many of the hand problems discussed in this chapter, such as carpal tunnel syndrome. Several metabolic diseases can directly affect the hand, though. Perhaps the most common is crystalline arthropathy. Gout is a common metabolic illness in which uric acid forms crystals of monosodium urate, which can then accumulate in joints or soft tissues and cause impressive inflammation. Although it is most common in the first MTP joint of the foot, it can occur in the joints and soft tissues of the hand. Often, it presents as a warm, tender, swollen, erythematous region and can mimic infection. In fact, when gout flares within one or two joints in the hand or wrist, it can cause profound swelling throughout the entire hand. Aspiration of an involved joint and visualization of negatively birefringent crystals under polarized light microscopy confirms the diagnosis. Treatment options include rest, immobilization, anti-inflammatory medications, corticosteroids (injections or oral steroids), and other antigout medications. Rarely gout can progress to severe tophaceous gout in one or more locations in the hands, which can cause extensive destruction of tendons or joints. Surgery in the form of debulking, joint fusion, and amputation can sometimes be indicated for severe erosive gout.

Calcium pyrophosphate dihydrate deposition disease (or pseudogout) is another crystalline arthropathy in which calcium pyrophosphate crystals accumulate in joints and around tendons, leading to significant inflammation. This, too, causes significant redness, swelling, and warmth over a joint and, again, aspiration and visualization of crystals in the fluid can be diagnostic for the problem. Treatment includes corticosteroid injections, nonsteroidal anti-inflammatories, oral steroids for acute flareups, and surgery in severe, chronic cases.

Vascular

Arterial occlusion and small vessel disease in the hand can cause severe pain and occasionally necrosis of the fingers. These can result from scleroderma, peripheral vascular disease, embolic phenomena, and Buerger's disease. Ulnar artery occlusion, which usually occurs at the level of the hook of the hamate, can cause significant ulnar nerve symptoms in addition to ischemia in the ulnar digits. When this occurs after a repetitive trauma, it is called hypothenar hammer syndrome, and it is most often seen in manual laborers. A vascular ultrasound or angiogram may confirm the diagnosis. The treatment depends on the degree of ischemia in the digits and symptoms. Surgical treatment involves decompression of the nerve and artery, and reconstruction of the thrombosed segment of the artery.

Vascular deficiencies secondary to other underlying diseases can be a significant problem in the hand, particularly in diabetes and scleroderma. In earlier stages of scleroderma, a digital sympathectomy or removal of the vascular adventitia can decrease the amount of vascular spasm that occurs, improve pain, and limit the damage done to the digits. As the disease progresses, though, digital ulcers can progress into gangrene, leading to autoamputation or surgical amputation of the digit.

Patients who have severe loss of flow to the hands due to shock can also develop gangrene of the digits. This is particularly common in patients who are in shock and require vasopressors, which redirect blood flow from the extremities to the vital organs, further decreasing the blood flow to the digits. Treatment in these instances involves warming the digits and occasionally applying nitro paste to the digits. The primary treatment, though, is treating the underlying cause of shock and then

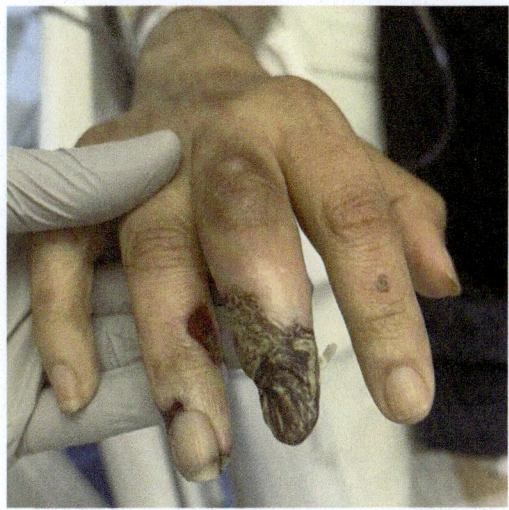

Fig. 12.19 Clinical photograph demonstrating a gangrenous long finger developed after a prolonged exposure to vasopressors. The extent of the necrosis demarcates the extent of amputation necessary

reducing the vasopressors. Often, though, the digits have developed irreversible ischemia that progresses to gangrene. Treatment then involves observation until the area of gangrene is clearly demarcated, and then surgical amputation or autoamputation follows (Fig. 12.19).

True aneurysms of the wrist and hand are relatively uncommon, but they occasionally occur in the ulnar artery at Guyon's canal. These aneurysms cause symptoms very similar to hypothenar hammer syndrome and can be treated the same way. Pseudoaneurysms are more common and can occur anywhere in the hand. They result of from direct trauma to an artery, typically from an arterial line placement, blood gas draw or ganglion cyst aspiration attempt. Symptomatic aneurysms are usually treated by ligating or reconstructing the artery involved, depending on the collateral circulation.

Neoplasms

Skin Cancer

Skin cancers (squamous cell carcinoma, basal cell carcinomas, and melanoma) are relatively common, especially in the elderly or those with predisposing factors (Fig. 12.20). These factors

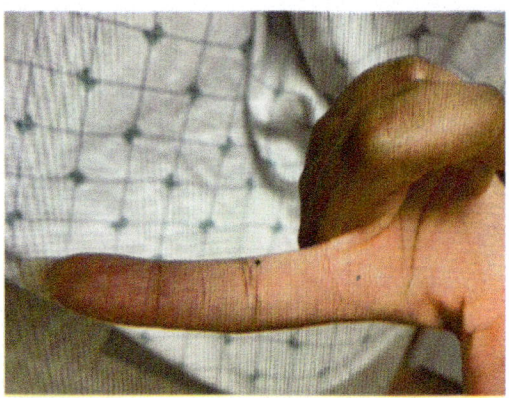

Fig. 12.20 Clinical photograph of melanoma on the volar aspect of the index finger of a 37-year-old patient. This was treated with wide excision and full-thickness skin grafting to the site

include prolonged exposure to the sun in farmers and other outdoor workers, and excessive exposure to X-rays, arsenicals, or other chemicals. Squamous and basal cell carcinomas can usually be cured by wide excision if they have not already metastasized. Melanomas and Merkel cell carcinomas are much more likely to recur and/or metastasize. As such, a multidisciplinary approach to these patients is vital to optimizing survival. Treatment typically involves surgical excision, reconstruction of the soft tissue, lymph node biopsies, staging studies, chemotherapy, and occasionally radiation.

Other Soft Tissue Masses

Benign soft tissue masses are very common in the hand and wrist and can arise from nerves, vessels, fat, or fascia. The most common "tumors" of the hand include ganglion cysts and giant cell tumors of the tendon sheath. Ganglion cysts are fluid filled sacks that arise from synovial lined structures, such as joints and tendon sheaths. Ganglion cysts occur in four common locations in the hand and wrist: on the dorsum of the wrist from the scapholunate ligament, on the volar radial aspect of the wrist adjacent to the radial artery from the radioscaphoid or scapho-trapezial-trapezoid (STT) joint, from the flexor tendon sheath at the base of the finger, and over

the dorsum of the DIP joint (mucous cyst). Treatment options for ganglion cysts include observation, aspiration or surgical excision. Cysts on the dorsum of the wrist or over the flexor tendon sheath are easily amenable to aspiration, although rates of recurrence are fairly high. Aspiration of a volar wrist ganglion should be approached cautiously, if at all, due to the proximity of the radial artery and risk of causing a pseudoaneurym. Surgical resection is a more definitive option, but recurrence following surgical excision is still 5–10%.

Giant cell tumors of the tendon sheath are solid tumors that present as slowly growing, painless, firm masses. Malignant etiologies are often in the differential, so an MRI with and without contrast can help point toward giant cell tumor of the tendon sheath. These tumors can extend into the joint, into the tendon sheath, and even circumferentially around the tendon. They also create mass effect and erosion into the adjacent phalanx. Treatment involves simple marginal excision which is typically curative. Local recurrence is possible, though, and the rate of recurrence increases for tumors that have invaded into adjacent joints.

Other common benign soft tissue masses include foreign body granulomas, epidermal inclusion cysts, arteriovenous malformations and hemangiomas, neurilemmoma, and glomus tumors. Surgical excision is diagnostic and typically curative for these benign lesions.

Malignant soft tissue tumors in the hand are very rare outside of skin cancers. The most common are epithelioid sarcoma, synovial cell sarcoma, and malignant fibrous histiocytoma. Delay in diagnosis is a common problem due to the extreme rarity of the diagnoses and relatively common benign lesions. Preoperatively, if there is any question that the lesion may be a soft tissue sarcoma, the patient should be referred immediately to a tertiary medical center for treatment. Similar to the treatment of melanoma and Merkel cell carcinoma, treatment of malignant soft tissue tumors of the hand requires a multidisciplinary team experienced the care of these complex patients to optimize outcomes and survival.

Tumors of Bone

Benign bone tumors of the hand are often diagnosed incidentally on radiographic examination for trauma. The most common is the enchondroma, which is a benign cartilage tumor of the bone. Treatment of incidentally found enchondromas is controversial and often involves radiographic and clinical follow-up. There is a small risk of malignant transformation into chondrosarcoma, and there is also a risk of pathologic fracture, which may lead the patient and/or surgeon to choose surgical resection over observation. If a pathologic fracture has occurred through the lesion or is impending, surgical treatment is typically the treatment of choice. Simple curettage, with or without bone grafting, often suffices. This may be done concurrently with fracture fixation or following complete healing of the fracture.

Osteochondromas, fibrous dysplasia, and giant cell tumor of bone can also present in the small hand bones and may require surgery for diagnosis or treatment. Malignant tumors of the hand skeleton are very rare. Partial or total hand amputation may be required along with adjuvant radiation therapy or chemotherapy. Metastatic tumors of the hand seldom occur as isolated metastases, but are not uncommon during widespread metastatic disease, especially from lung or breast cancers.

Management Protocols

A wide variety of problems can affect the hand and wrist, which range from self-limiting and inconsequential to devastating functional problems, to potentially life-threatening problems. It is, therefore, important to have in mind a standardized approach to patients with these problems to help arrive at the correct diagnosis and management options. The physician should begin with a thorough problem-focused history. With a differential diagnosis in mind, the physician should then perform a directed, but thorough physical examination. Plain radiographs are usually, but not always, useful adjuncts to confirm the diagnosis.

Nearly all patients with a history of an injury should obtain radiographs. If the initial radiographs show a fracture, dislocation, or carpal instability pattern, appropriate operative or nonoperative treatment should be initiated. When X-rays are negative, a soft tissue injury may have occurred, or an occult fracture may be present. When a specific soft tissue injury is noted, appropriate treatment should be initiated. If none is found and the patient's symptoms cannot be explained, either further imaging should be performed or splinting or casting for a period of time followed by reevaluation should be considered.

In patients who have had no specific history of trauma or injury, radiographs are often unnecessary, especially if the patient has a classic history and physical examination for a soft tissue process, such as trigger finger or de Quervain's tenosynovitis. If the diagnosis is unclear after the history and physical, radiographs should be obtained. If radiographs demonstrate arthritis, tumor, or occult bony injury, appropriate operative or nonoperative management should be undertaken. If they are negative, further evaluation and/or indicated treatment should be initiated.

Due to the significant variability in hand and wrist conditions and associated variability in urgency of treatment, early referral or consultation with a hand surgeon is often the best course of action when dealing with hand and wrist complaints. However, it is equally important that all physicians who manage patients with hand complaints have a basic understanding of the hand pathology and treatment options described in this chapter.

Further Reading

Weiss APC, editor. The American Society for Surgery of the hand textbook of hand & upper extremity surgery. 2nd ed. Chicago, IL: American Society for Surgery of the Hand; 2019.

Wolfe SW, Pederson WC, Kozin SH, Cohen MS, editors. Green's operative hand surgery. 8th ed. Amsterdam: Elsevier; 2021.

Hip Osteoarthritis and Arthroplasty

13

Gregory Perraut, Brian G. Evans, and Kevin W. Park

Anatomy

Development

The hip joint is a ball and socket joint with the round femoral head articulating within the matching acetabular socket. The acetabulum is formed from the confluence of three bones: the ischium, ilium, and pubis. In skeletally immature patients, these three bones are joined in the medial acetabulum by the triradiate cartilage, which is a growth plate for the acetabulum. There is also appositional growth from the edges of the acetabulum and pelvis resulting in increased depth of the acetabulum and size of the pelvis. Normal development of the acetabulum requires the femoral head to articulate with the acetabular cartilage. The acetabular socket will not develop normally if the femoral head is chronically dislocated or subluxated out of the acetabular fossa. This often results in a shallow and malformed acetabulum and is termed developmental dysplasia of the hip (DDH). The severity of this condition is determined by the degree of subluxation of the femo-

ral head. If DDH is identified at birth or soon thereafter, the hip can be reduced with either casting or surgery. This treatment can allow the hip to grow and develop almost normally. If the hip is left subluxated or dislocated, the acetabulum will be shallow and predispose the patient to develop osteoarthritis as an adult. This is reviewed in greater detail in the chapter on pediatric orthopedic conditions.

Osteology and Musculature

The innominate bone consists of the ilium, ischium, and pubis, which are joined in the area of the acetabulum (Fig. 13.1). The ilium is a large flat bone providing broad surfaces for muscular attachment. The ischium extends posteriorly and forms the posterior aspect of the acetabulum. The ischium joins the ilium superiorly and the pubis inferiorly through the inferior pubic ramus. The ischium also serves as the origin of the hamstring and short external rotator muscles of the hip. The pubis consists of the superior pubic ramus, inferior pubic ramus, and the pubic symphysis.

The superior pubic ramus joins the pubic symphysis with the ilium and the inferior pubic ramus connects the pubic symphysis with the ischium. The pubis serves as the site of insertion of the musculature of the abdominal wall as well as the site of origin for the adductor muscles of the thigh.

G. Perraut (✉) · B. G. Evans · K. W. Park
MedStar Georgetown Orthopedic Institute,
Georgetown University School of Medicine,
Washington, DC, USA

Department of Orthopedics, MedStar Georgetown
University Hospital, Washington, DC, USA
e-mail: Gregory.T.Perraut@medstar.net;
Kevin.W.Park@medstar.net

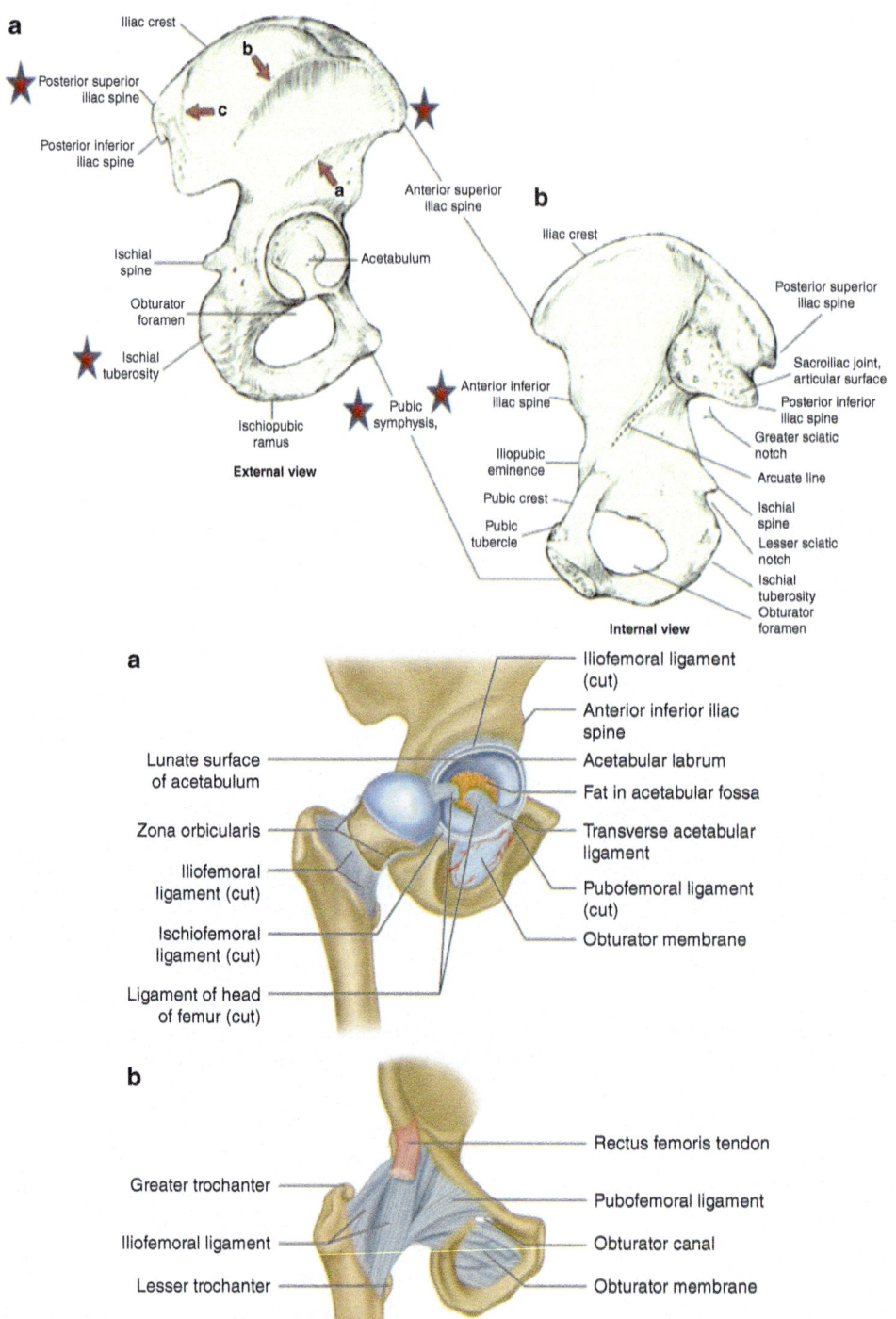

Fig. 13.1 (a) Lateral aspect of left hip bone. (b) Ligamentous attachments are shown. (From Mayer, S.W., Spahn, K.M., Griffith, R. (2020). Hip Joint. In: Khodaee, M., Waterbrook, A., Gammons, M. (eds) Sports-related Fractures, Dislocations and Trauma. Springer, Cham. https://doi.org/10.1007/978-3-030-36790-9_22. From Weber, A.E., Ross, J.R., Kelly, B.T., Bedi, A. (2015). Layered Concept of the Hip and Pelvis. In: Nho, S., Leunig, M., Larson, C., Bedi, A., Kelly, B. (eds) Hip Arthroscopy and Hip Joint Preservation Surgery. Springer, New York, NY. https://doi.org/10.1007/978-1-4614-6965-0_10)

The acetabulum is formed at the junction of the ilium, ischium, and pubis. The ilium forms the superior dome of the acetabulum. The ischium forms the posterior acetabulum and the pubis the anterior acetabulum. The lateral opening of the acetabulum forms a circular horseshoe with the open end directed inferiorly. The medial base of the acetabulum contains a depression called the acetabular fossa. This is filled with a fatty tissue called the pulvinar and the ligamentum teres. The ligamentum teres is a ligament that extends from the acetabular fovea and the fovea of the femoral head. The artery of the ligamentum teres is a branch of the obturator artery and supplies approximately 10–20% of the bone of the femoral head.

The fovea of the femur is a depression on the femoral head, which serves as the site of attachment of the ligamentum teres. Attached to the rim of the horseshoe is a fibro-cartilaginous labrum, which is similar to the meniscus in the knee. This serves to improve stability and more importantly cushion and distribute force more evenly across the acetabulum. The hip joint capsule is a dense fibrous structure extending from the base of the intertrochanteric region of the femur to the acetabular rim. Thickenings within the capsule are the iliofemoral and pubofemoral ligaments anteriorly and the ischiofemoral ligament posteriorly. These ligaments as well as the ligamentum teres and the labrum augment the stability of the hip joint.

The femoral head is essentially spherical in geometry (Figs. 13.2 and 13.3). The spherical portion of the femoral head is covered by articular cartilage. The sphere is altered in two areas, laterally where the femoral neck begins and medially at the fovea of the femoral head. The femoral neck joins the femur at approximately 125° angle. The neck is also rotated anteriorly (anteverted) 12–15° relative to the axis represented by the posterior femoral condyles (Fig. 13.4). The femoral neck flares laterally to join the proximal femur in between the greater and lesser trochanters. The greater trochanter, a large osseous prominence at the proximal lateral aspect of the femur, serves as the site of attachment of the abductor musculature. Between the greater and lesser trochanters is an osseous ridge, which serves as the site of attachment of the short external rotators. The lesser trochanter is the site of attachment of the iliopsosas tendon. This exits the pelvis over the anterior column and superior pubic ramus and then travels over the anterior femoral neck to insert on the lesser trochanter, which lies on the posterior inferior aspect of the intertrochanteric ridge. Within the proximal femur and femoral neck is a large and dense trabeculation known as the calcar. The calcar provides increased strength to the proximal femur. Frequently the proximal posteromedial femur from the base of the femoral neck including the lesser trochanter is also referred to as the calcar. If the medial calcar region of the proximal femur is a separate fragment of a proximal femur fracture, the fracture is considered unstable.

The muscles of the hip form several distinct groups. The anterior muscles are the hip flexors. These consist of the iliopsoas and rectus femoris and sartorius muscles. The femoral nerve innervates the rectus and sartorius muscles. Motor branches from spinal roots L2, L3, and L4 innervate the iliopsosas. The lateral group consists of the abductors: the gluteus medius, minimus, and tensor fascia lata. These muscles are essential for normal gait. They stabilize the pelvis in single limb stance phase of normal gait. The anterior one-third of the gluteus medius muscle is also the principle internal rotator of the hip. The superior gluteal nerve innervates the gluteus medius, minimus, and tensor fascia lata. Surgical dissection that extends greater than 5 cm proximal to the greater trochanter can disrupt the nerve and will result in a limp, referred to as a Trendelenburg gait. Due to the inability of the muscles to stabilize the pelvis during gait from denervation, the pelvis will tilt away from the weakened side while the torso will lurch toward the affected side to compensate (Fig. 13.5).

The posterior muscles are in two layers. The superficial layer consists of the gluteus maximus, the primary extensor of the hip, which is innervated by the inferior gluteal nerve. The deep layer consists of the short external rotators of the hip: the piriformis, superior gemellus, obturator internus, inferior gemellus, obturator externus, and

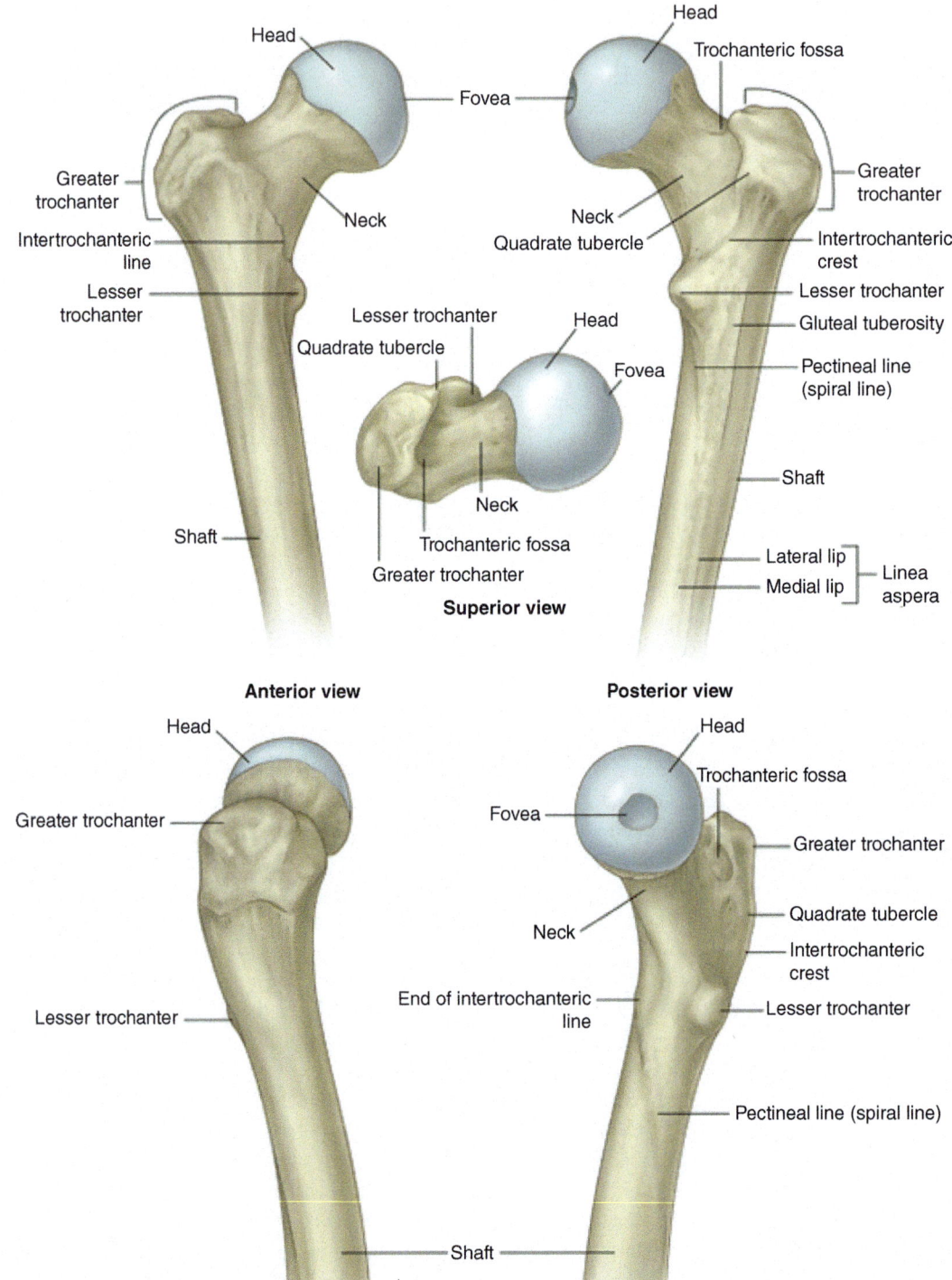

Fig. 13.2 Bony anatomy of proximal right femur. (From Battista, C. (2022 Aug 10). Hip Anatomy. Retrieved from https://www.orthobullets.com/recon/12769/hip-anatomy)

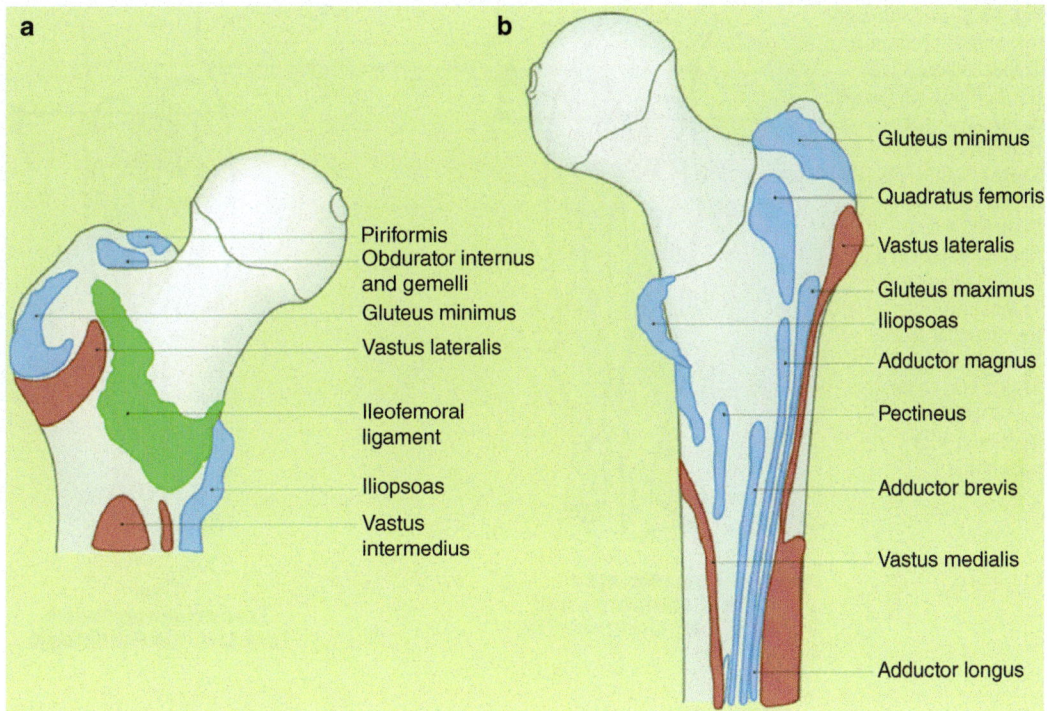

Fig. 13.3 (**a**) Muscular attachments of proximal right femur. (From Mokawem, Michael & Bobak, Peter & Aderinto, Joseph. (2012). (**b**) The management of pertro-chanteric fractures of the hip. Orthopaedics and Trauma. 26. 112–123. 10.1016/j.mporth.2012.04.001. Reprinted by permission)

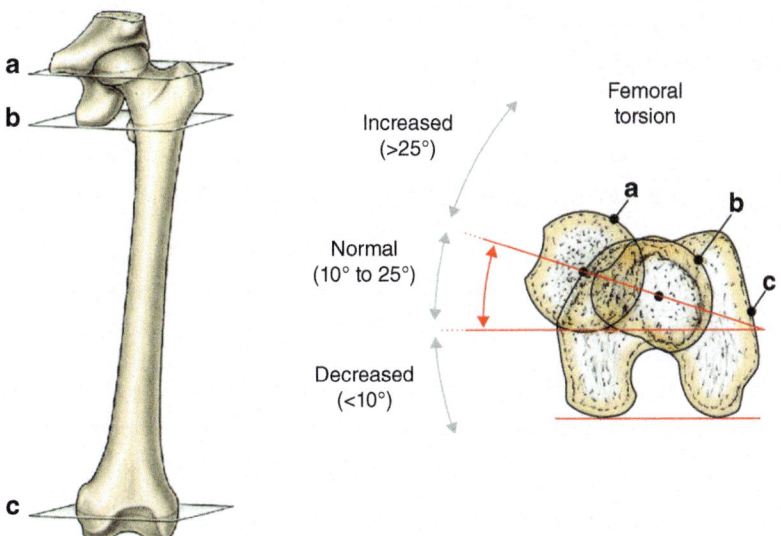

Fig. 13.4 Average rotary, or torsion, angle of the femur. Three transverse CT slices are used: one through the femoral head center (**a**), one just above the lesser trochanter (**b**), and one through the distal femoral condyles (**c**). On a superimposed image of these three slices, the femoral torsion angle is defined by the femoral condyles and a line connecting the femoral head center with the centroid of the femoral neck. (From Lerch, Till & Eichelberger, Patric & Baur, Heiner & Schmaranzer, Florian & Liechti, Emanuel & Schwab, Joe & Siebenrock, Klaus & Tannast, Moritz. (2019). Prevalence and diagnostic accuracy of in-toeing and out-toeing of the foot for patients with abnormal femoral torsion and femoro-acetabular impingement: implications for hip arthroscopy and femoral derotation osteotomy. The bone & joint journal. 101-B. 1218–1229. 10.1302/0301-620X.101B10.BJJ-2019-0248.R1. Reprinted by permission)

Fig. 13.5 Depiction of true and compensated Trendelenburg's gait. (From Elumalai, Ganesh & Jha, Ameet & Kanagarajan, Palani & Sanyal, Sanjoy. (2016). Soccer Syndrome—3: Common Sacral Malalignments and Its Manual Diagnostic Techniques. International Journal of Sports Science. 4. 25–37. 10.11648/j.ajss.20160402.12. Reprinted with permission)

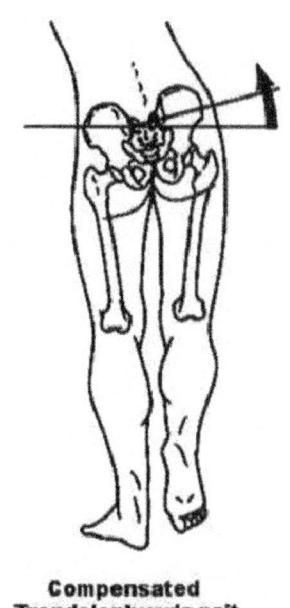
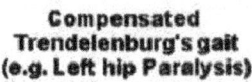
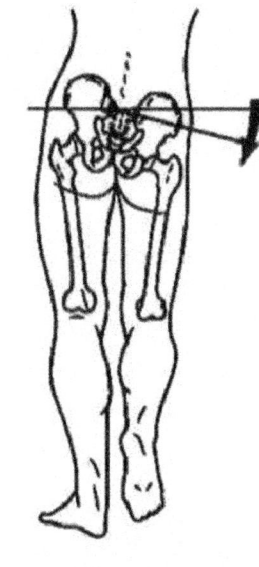

Compensated Trendelenburg's gait (e.g. Left hip Paralysis)

True Trendelenburg's gait (e.g. Left hip Pathology)

the quadratus femoris, and the gluteus minimus and medius. These muscles externally rotate the femur and provide abduction. Small branches from the sacral plexus innervate the short external rotators. The medial muscle group consists of the pectineus, adductor brevis, longus, and magnus, and the gracilis. The adductors and gracilis are supplied by the obturator nerve, with the posterior portion of the adductor magnus also receiving innervation from the tibial division of the sciatic nerve. The femoral nerve innervates the pectineus.

The sciatic nerve crosses the hip joint posteriorly. It exits the pelvis through the superior sciatic notch, under the piriformis muscle, and lies superficial to the short external rotators. The nerve has two distinct divisions within the single nerve sheath, the tibial and peroneal divisions. The peroneal division is more susceptible to injury, compared to the tibial division, at all levels along the course of the sciatic nerve. The increased susceptibility is due to the more lateral location and a more tenuous blood supply. Therefore, a partial injury to the sciatic nerve, such as one that can occur with a stretch injury during total hip replacement surgery, will commonly result in a foot drop, clinically similar to

the deficits seen in an isolated injury to the common peroneal nerve injury at the level of the fibular neck. One anatomic point with important clinical relevance is that the peroneal division of the sciatic nerve has only one motor branch in the posterior thigh supplying the short head of the biceps femoris. Determining if the short head of the biceps is normally innervated can assist in determining the level of peroneal nerve injury clinically (i.e., the hip or knee).

Vascular Anatomy of the Proximal Femur and Femoral Head

The medial and lateral femoral circumflex vessels in conjunction with the artery of the ligamentum teres provide the vascular supply to proximal femur and femoral head (Fig. 13.6). The medial femoral circumflex artery, which is the dominant supply of the femoral head, extends posteriorly and ascends proximally deep to the quadratus femoris muscle. At the level of the hip, it joins an arterial ring at the base of the femoral neck. The lateral femoral circumflex artery extends anteriorly and gives off an ascending branch, which also joins the arterial ring at the base of the femo-

Fig. 13.6 Arterial supply to the head and neck of the posterior aspect of the left proximal femur. Note the extracapsular arterial ring on the surface of the capsule, the ascending cervical arteries on the neck of the femur, and the intra-articular sub-synovial arterial ring at the articular cartilage margin. (From Elumalai, Ganesh & Jha, Ameet & Kanagarajan, Palani & Sanyal, Sanjoy. (2016). Soccer Syndrome—3: Common Sacral Malalignments and Its Manual Diagnostic Techniques. International Journal of Sports Science. 4. 25–37. 10.11648/j.ajss.20160402.12)

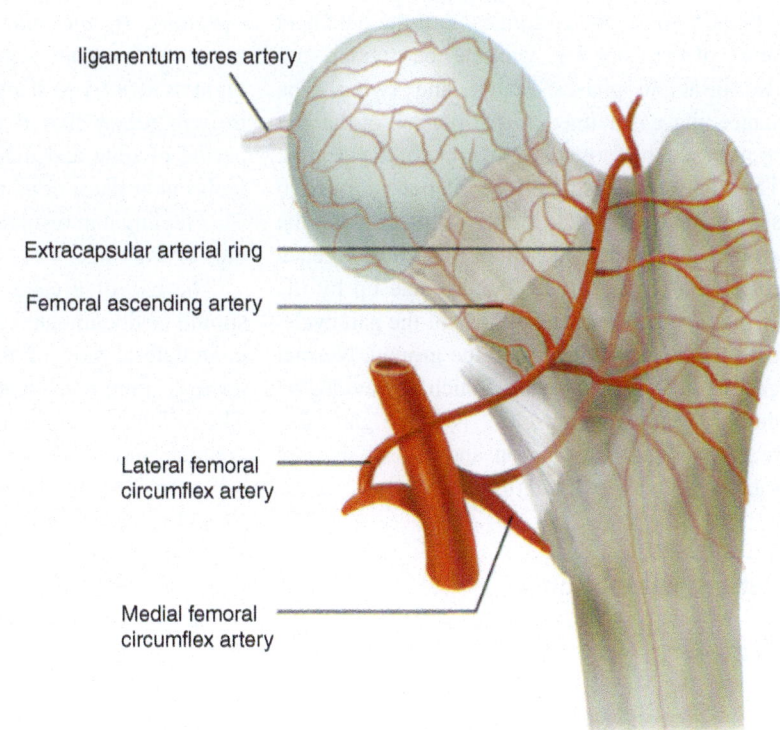

ligamentum teres artery

Extracapsular arterial ring

Femoral ascending artery

Lateral femoral circumflex artery

Medial femoral circumflex artery

ral neck. This vascular ring gives rise to a group of vessels which run in the retinacular tissue inside the capsule to enter the femoral head at the base of the articular surface. These vessels provide 80–90% of the blood supply to the femoral head. The artery of the ligamentum teres, a branch of the obturator artery, travels within the ligamentum teres and supplies only 10–20% of the blood supply to the femoral head.

Biomechanics

The joint reaction force is the sum of all forces that cross a joint. This includes components from gravity, body weight, and muscle forces acting upon the joint. In two-legged stance with both feet on the ground and static conditions, a joint reaction force of approximately 1.3–1.5 times body weight will cross each hip joint. However, in single limb stance, this force will increase to 2.5–3 times body weight across the hip joint. The primary contribution to the increase is the force generated by the abductor muscles to maintain balance and to keep the pelvis level. If the system is in motion, such as with walking, the joint reaction forces can be as high as 4 times body weight.

Several studies have measured the actual joint reaction forces during rehabilitation using an implanted-instrumented prosthesis. The greatest joint reaction force was noted when the patients arose from a low chair or during stair climbing. However, even non-weight-bearing activities, such as getting onto a bedpan, were found to have a joint reaction force of 1.5–1.8 times body weight. The lowest joint reaction forces with ambulation were recorded when patients used touch-down weight-bearing. Touch-down weight-bearing allows the patient to rest the foot on the ground to balance the weight of the leg, but not to step down or weight bear on the involved lower extremity.

Gait

As mentioned previously, the principle function of the lower extremities is ambulation. In gait analysis, a gait cycle examines one leg, beginning with heel strike and continues until the next heel strike of the same leg. Gait can be divided into two principle phases: stance and swing. The stance phase is defined as that portion of the gait cycle when the foot is in contact with the ground. The swing phase is therefore the portion of each step when the foot is not in contact with the ground. The stance phase makes up 60% of each step, with the remainder being made up by the swing phase. Therefore, in 20% of the gait cycle, both feet are in contact with the ground. Normal gait requires a stable pelvis, which is provided by the hip abductor muscles. Normal gait also requires 40° of hip flexion and 10° of internal rotation and external rotation.

Patient Evaluation

History

The evaluation of a patient with hip pain requires careful attention to the history, physical examination, and radiographic studies. The character, nature, and duration of the patient's pain should be documented. Acute or recent onset pain will more commonly be associated with trauma or infection. Chronic and gradually progressive pain is associated with arthritic conditions. Intra-articular pain is usually described as a deep, aching pain. Pain from the hip joint will commonly be noted anteriorly in the groin or posterior to the greater trochanter. Hip pain can radiate down the inner and anterior thigh to the knee with little or no pain in the area of the hip. Only rarely will hip pain radiate distal to the knee. In adolescent patients, it is not uncommon for hip pathology to present as knee pain. Therefore, a thorough physical and radiographic evaluation of the hips is necessary to identify the pathology in these patients. Posterior pain and buttock pain is more commonly associated with lumbar spine pathology. Spine pain also will more commonly radiate down the posterior thigh and below the knee.

Hip pain is commonly aggravated by activity and relieved by rest. Patients will report difficulty donning and doffing their shoes and socks and difficulty with toenail care on the involved

extremity. As the pain progresses, patients will begin to have pain with prolonged sitting and at night as they try to sleep. Patients with hip arthritis will report that if they sit for a prolonged period of time and then get up to walk, the hip feels out of place or painful for the first few steps. This feeling can resolve quickly after a few minutes of walking.

The use of a cane, walking stick, or crutch should be documented. A cane is best used on the contralateral side of the patient's pain to help decrease joint reactive forces of the affected joint. The patient may also have begun to take over-the-counter anti-inflammatory medication or pain relievers. The medication and the amount the patient is taking, as well as the level of relief that is provided, need to be recorded. The patient's walking tolerance can be measured in terms of blocks the patient can walk, or in terms of how many minutes the patient can be ambulatory doing activities, such as grocery shopping or walking in a mall. Documentation of the above data will give a detailed picture of the degree of pain and the patient's functional limitations.

Patients should also be questioned about past problems with the hip such as hip subluxation or dislocation at birth, delays in ambulation as an infant, and any bracing as a child. If previous surgery or trauma to the hips has occurred, this should be explored in detail. The past medical history and any medications the patient is taking should be noted. This information can have implications for the patient's hip problems and may have an impact upon what treatment may be instituted.

Physical Examination

The most important aspect of the physical exam in patients with hip disease is to evaluate their gait pattern. This will reveal important information about the patient's ambulatory status and their pain. Patients with significant hip pain will manifest a coxalgic gait. This gait pattern is represented by a reduced stance phase on the painful leg and the shoulders lurch laterally over the affected hip. Patients with mild pain or weakness in the abductor muscles may have a stance phase equal to the opposite leg, but the shoulders will continue to lurch over the affected leg. This lurch results in moving the center of gravity closer to the center of rotation of the hip, which in turn reduces the force necessary to stabilize the pelvis in stance phase. This gait is referred to as a Trendelenburg gait (equal stance phase and the shoulders lurching over the affected hip).

The hip should be inspected for previous scars, swelling, bruises, or abrasions. The region then should be palpated to identify areas of focal tenderness such as over the greater trochanter, sciatic nerve, or anterior hip capsule. The range of motion of the hip should then be determined. Normal range of motion of the hip is flexion to 130°, extension to 20°, adduction to 30°, abduction to 40°, internal rotation to 30°, and external rotation to 70°. When assessing the range of motion of the hip, it is important to stabilize the lumbar spine. Motion in the lumbar spine may be attributed to the hip if the examiner is not careful. The Thomas test will stabilize the lumbar spine to measure for a flexion contracture of the hip (Fig. 13.7). Movement of the pelvis with abduction and adduction can be accurately assessed by placing a hand on the opposite anterior superior iliac spine and recording the patient's motion as the amount of motion prior to pelvic abduction.

To assess the function of the hip abductor muscles, the patient should be standing and the involved leg lifted off the floor. The patient should stand on the uninvolved leg and the pelvis should remain level. The patient then stands on the involved leg and lifts the uninvolved leg off the floor. If the pelvis is level, the patient has normal strength of the abductor muscles. If the pelvis is noted to be lower on the elevated leg, the abductor muscles are weak or the hip which is weight bearing is painful. This is referred to as the Trendelenburg sign.

A careful neurologic exam and lumbar spine exam are essential to assessing the possibility of spine pathology producing pain radiating to the hip. Patients with significant arthritic disease in the hip will also commonly have spine pathology as well. Hip arthritis and restriction in hip range of motion can exacerbate spine pathology. The limited range of motion of the hip will result in increased motion at the lumbo-sacral junction. This can aggravate degenerative facet arthropathy and lumbar stenosis. Replacement of the hip and improvement in the range of motion in the hip, however, can relieve stress from the lumbosacral junction and subsequently relieve the patient's pain.

In addition, the pulses should be palpated in the foot and ankle. Significant reduction may indicate vascular insufficiency and may require further evaluation. Vascular compromise may impair wound healing or may lead to acute vascular crisis in the early post-operative period if this is not recognized and treated prior to any elective hip procedure. In addition, if any significant vascular reconstruction has been done in the area of the involved hip, care needs to be taken at the time of surgery to avoid damage to the previous reconstruction.

Radiographic Evaluation

Routine radiography of the pelvis and hips is the most useful study in evaluating hip pathology. Standard anteroposterior (AP) radiography of the pelvis will reveal the lower lumbar spine, sacroiliac joints, innominate bone, pubic symphysis, hip joint, and proximal femurs. Frequently, in unilateral disease, the normal side can be used for comparison (Fig. 13.7). Lateral views of the proximal femurs can also be helpful in defining pathology and in determining the size and location of a pathologic lesion. Weight-bearing X-rays are crucial to obtain an accurate depiction of the joint space during ambulation and movement. Four pelvic oblique views can be obtained to further evaluate the pelvis and acetabulum, particularly in cases of trauma; these are the inlet, outlet, and Judet views. Judet views are 45° pelvic oblique views. They are useful for examination of the acetabulum, including the anterior and posterior columns (Figs. 13.8, 13.9, 13.10, and 13.11). The inlet and outlet views are useful for patients with pelvic trauma in order to evaluate for any superior/inferior or anterior/posterior translation of the hemipelvis.

Fig. 13.7 (a, b, c)
Diagrammatic
representation of the
Thomas test to assess
hip flexion contracture.
(Adapted from von Lanz
T, Wachsmith W:
Praktische Anatomic.
Berlin, Julius Springer,
1938, p 157.) (From
Tachdjian MO: Pediatric
Orthopaedics, ed. 2.
Philadelphia, WB
Saunders Company,
1990, p 28. Reprinted by
permission)

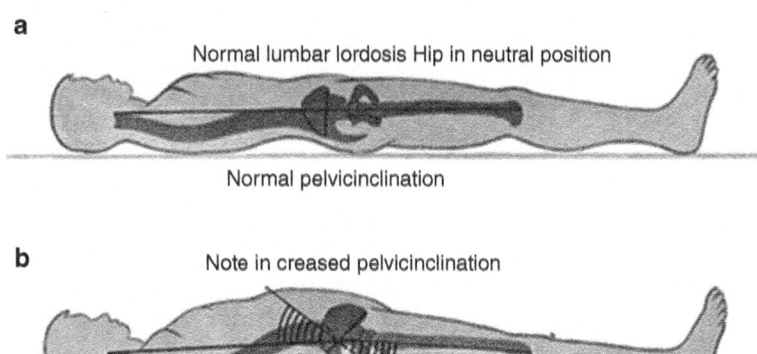

a

Normal lumbar lordosis Hip in neutral position

Normal pelvicinclination

b

Note in creased pelvicinclination

Compensatory lumbar lordosis in flexion contracture of the hip

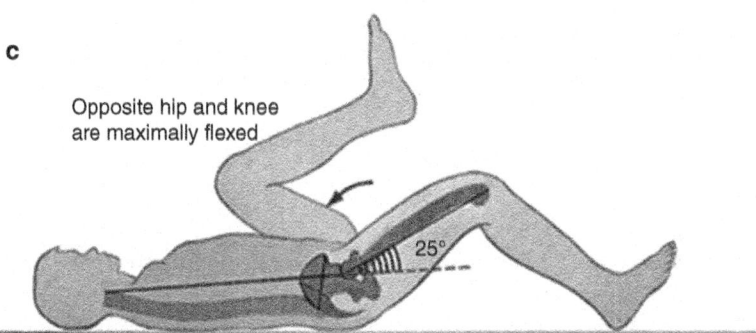

c

Opposite hip and knee
are maximally flexed

25°

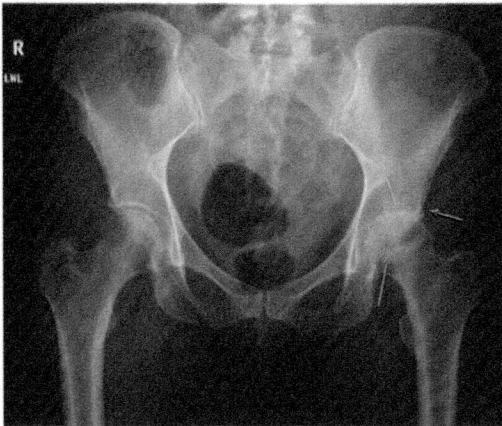

Fig. 13.8 This is a 75-year-old patient with severe left hip pain. The radiograph reveals a normal right hip and advanced arthritic changes in the left hip. The left hip demonstrates an acetabular osteophyte (red arrow), subchondral sclerosis (green arrow) of the subchondral bone, and a subchondral cyst (blue arrow) in the femoral head

Computerized tomography (CT) of the pelvis is most helpful in evaluating trauma. In some centers, this modality has replaced and certainly augments the use of oblique pelvic radiography. CT imaging is particularly helpful in demonstrating fractures in the posterior pelvis and sacrum, which may be poorly visualized in routine radiography. Fractures to the acetabulum are well visualized on CT scan images (Figs. 13.12 and 13.13). CT images can clearly delineate the extent of the fracture as well as demonstrate any intra-articular fragments, which may be present. The CT can also be converted into a three-dimensional image to more clearly demonstrate the fracture pattern. CT imaging can also be utilized to demonstrate other non-traumatic pathology. For example, anterior osteoarthritis, which may be subtle on the plain radiographs, can readily be appreciated on CT images.

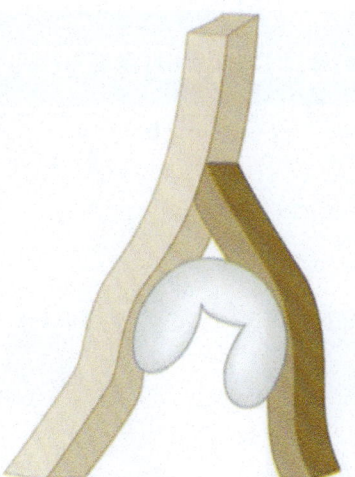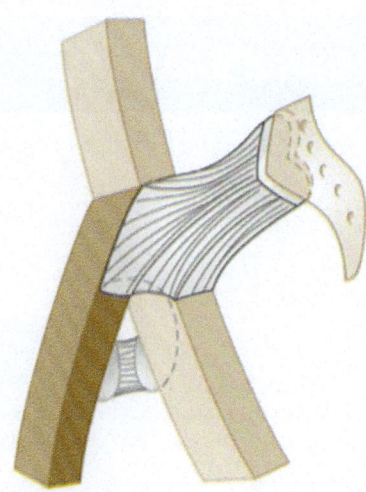

Fig. 13.9 Graphic depiction of the anterior and posterior columns of the acetabulum. Left, diagram of left acetabulum viewed from outside. Note that the anterior column (light) is larger than the posterior column (dark) and that both columns support the horseshoe-shaped articular surface. Right, view of the left acetabulum viewed from inside the pelvis. The sciatic buttress (stippled) connects both columns to the axial skeleton through the sacroiliac joint (From Brandser E. Fractures. Diagnosis and Treatment. In: David Moehring H, Greenspan A, eds. ©2000 Current Medicine Group LLC)

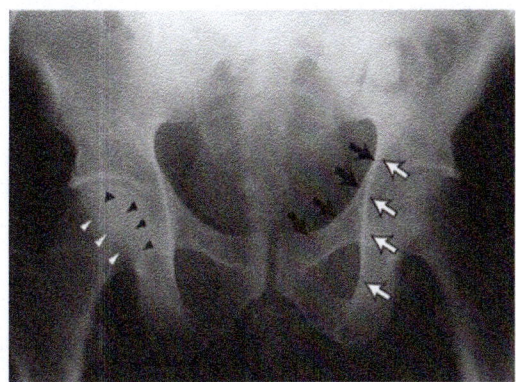

Fig. 13.10 Anteroposterior radiograph with arrows depicting the anterior and posterior wall of the right hip (black and white arrows, respectively). The left hip demonstrates the iliopectineal line of the anterior column (black arrows) and the ilioischial line of the posterior column (white arrows) (Brandser E. Fractures: Diagnosis and Treatment. In: David Moehring H, Greenspan A, eds. ©2000 Current Medicine Group LLC)

Magnetic resonance imaging (MRI) of the hips is indicated in patients where a peri-articular lesion is suspected, labral pathology is suspected, or to evaluate for the presence of avascular necrosis (AVN) of the femoral heads (Fig. 13.14). MRI is a very sensitive and specific tool for the evaluation of AVN. It can readily demonstrate the avascular segment prior to changes on the plain radiographs. MRI can also be helpful in demonstrating a tear in the acetabular labrum. This is best demonstrated by the use of MR arthrography. MR contrast material is injected intra-articularly and an MR of the hip is obtained. The contrast will outline the labrum and any defect in labrum can be identified.

The Tc99-MDP bone scan can be used as a sensitive indicator of osseous pathology in the pelvis. Metastatic disease, occult fractures, infection, or osteomyelitis can be identified. The bone scan is most helpful as a general skeletal screening tool for metastatic disease. The bone scan is very sensitive but is not specific. Therefore, other studies such as MRI or CT may be necessary to fully evaluate the nature and extent of any identified the pathology.

Hip aspiration and arthrography can be helpful in the evaluation of pathology. Aspiration can be helpful in evaluating hip sepsis in both a native hip and after hip arthroplasty. Aspiration is best performed under fluoroscopic guidance to ensure proper entry into the small joint space of the hip. An arthrogram can then be utilized to confirm the intra-articular position of the needle.

LINES (LANDMARKS) – OBLIQUE (JUDET VIEW)

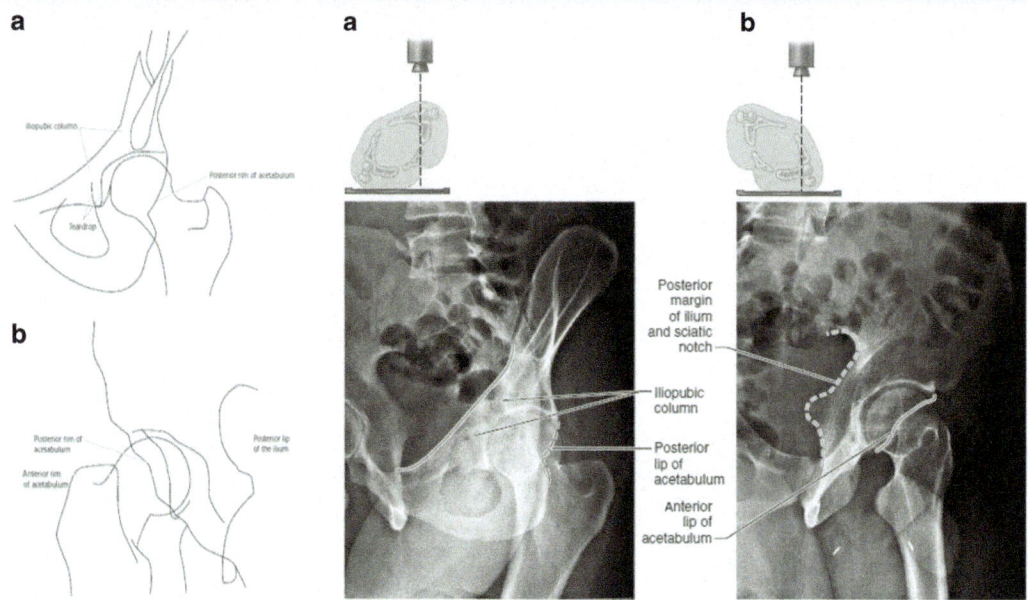

Fig. 13.11 Depiction and angles of the (**a**) obturator oblique and (**b**) iliac oblique radiographs (From Epomedicine. Pelvis X-ray: Simplified Approach [Internet]. Epomedicine; 2020 Nov 17 [cited 2023 Jul 29]. Available from: https://epomedicine.com/medical-students/pelvis-x-ray/)

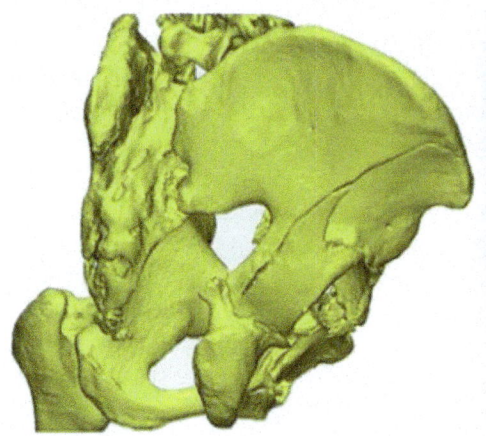
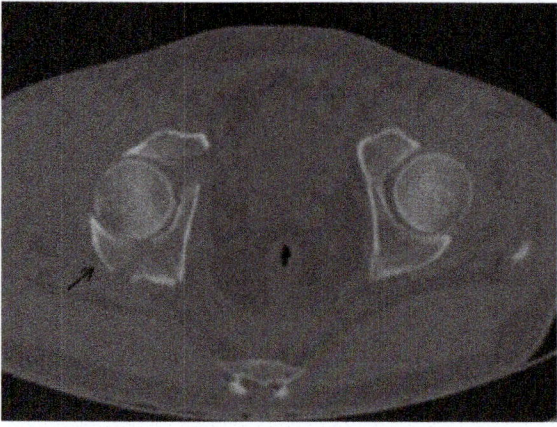

Fig. 13.12 CT images of a both column acetabular fracture in 3D reconstruction and the axial plane. (From Tian, S., Chen, Y., Yin, Y. et al. Morphological Characteristics of Posterior Wall Fragments Associated with Acetabular Both-column Fracture. Sci Rep 9, 20164 (2019). https://doi.org/10.1038/s41598-019-56838-5)

Commonly, patients will present with a history of both hip and spine pathology. Injection of local anesthetic, with or without a corticosteroid medication, into the hip under fluoroscopic guidance can be helpful in differentiating the pain coming from the hip with that coming from the spine. If the intra-articular local anesthetic results in significant relief of pain, the pain is most likely intra-articular in origin. If the local anesthetic agent does not alter the pain, extra-articular pathology or spine disease should be investigated.

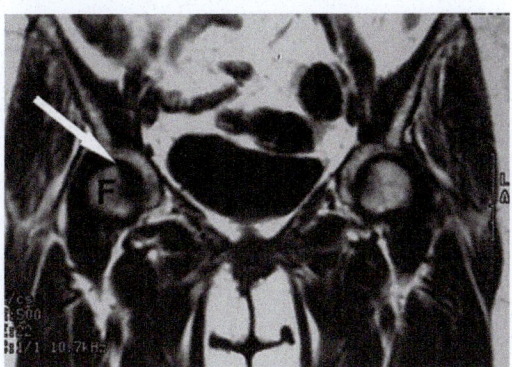

Fig. 13.13 Coronal section of magnetic resonance imaging (MRI) of a patient with steroid-induced osteonecrosis of the right femoral head. Note the loss of signal within the superior region of the head. (From Mabrey J. Current Orthopedic Diagnosis and Treatment. In: Heckman JD, Schenck RC, Agarwal A. ©2002 Current Medicine Group LLC)

The patient's history and physical examination direct the use of these radiographic techniques. The appropriate use of these diagnostic tests can result in cost-effective and accurate diagnosis and properly directed treatment.

Hip Pathology

A variety of soft tissue conditions can affect the hip. These are not uniformly associated with trauma or injury; however, an injury can be the inciting event. Trochanteric bursitis is a common condition of the hip. The pain results from inflammation within the trochanteric bursa. This is located over the lateral aspect of the greater trochanter under the fascia lata. It is associated with pain over the lateral aspect of the hip in the region of the greater trochanter. The pain is a deep ache centered over the greater trochanter with radiation both proximally to the pelvic brim and distally, occasionally down to the knee. Patients often complain of pain while seated, or upon arising from a chair, as well as pain that awakens them from sleep when lying on the involved side. The pain is exacerbated by adduction of the hip with the knee extended. No pathologic changes are noted on either plain radiographs or MRI. The treatment consists of stretching the fascia lata and the iliotibial band,

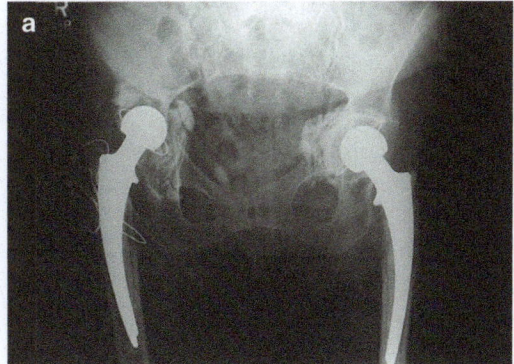

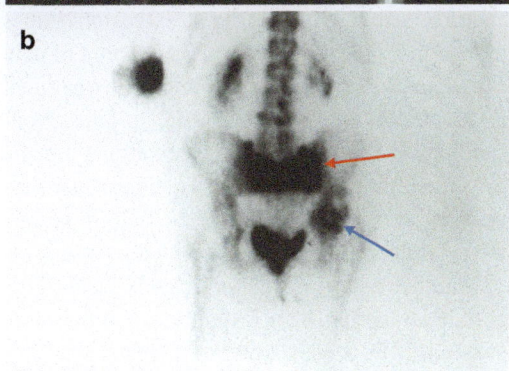

Fig. 13.14 This 84-year-old woman presented with severe hip pain after a car ride. The patient had bilateral hip replacement approximately 15 years before presentation. (**a**) AP pelvic radiograph demonstrates a patient with significant diffuse osteopenia and two hip replacements. Both hips appear to have some loosening of the acetabular components but demonstrate no acute changes. (**b**) Delayed image from a Tc 99-MDP bone scan demonstrates significant uptake in the left acetabulum (blue arrow). However, there is diffuse marked increase uptake throughout the sacrum (red arrow). This pattern of uptake is consistent with a sacral insufficiency fracture

and non-steroidal anti-inflammatory medications. If these conservative measures are unsuccessful, the patient may benefit from physical therapy with the use of local modalities such as ultrasound and iontophoresis. These modalities can be augmented with a corticosteroid injection into the bursa. If these non-operative modalities fail to relieve the pain, the bursa can be surgically excised. However, this option is rarely required and is not routinely successful. There is a push to rename this condition to greater trochanteric pain syndrome as oftentimes there is not a true bursitis or swelling within the bursa, but rather pain centered around the bursa.

The iliotibial band and the trochanteric bursa can also be involved in the snapping hip (coxa saltans). The iliotibial band snapping over the trochanteric bursa and the greater trochanter causes this condition and is known as external snapping hip. This is not always painful. The treatment is like that for trochanteric bursitis. Snapping in the hip can also occur anteriorly as the iliopsoas tendon can snap over the anterior aspect of the hip where the tendon exits the pelvis over the anterior pelvic brim. This results in an anterior snap with flexion and extension and is termed internal snapping hip. The amount of pain associated with the snap is variable. The treatment is directed toward alleviation of the pain. Nonsteroidal anti-inflammatory medications can be helpful at alleviating pain. Stretching of the iliopsoas with hip extension can also help to reduce the symptoms.

Another cause of a snapping hip is a tear in the acetabular labrum. This is typically a more subtle snapping. The acetabular labrum is a dense, fibrocartilaginous structure that is attached to the acetabular rim. This structure can be injured similar to a meniscal injury in the knee. The labrum is more prone to injury in patients with acetabular dysplasia and with femoroacetabular impingement (FAI). In acetabular dysplasia, the acetabulum is shallow which places more stress across the labrum with subsequent tearing over time. In FAI, there is a mismatch in the shapes of the acetabulum and femoral head thus causing shearing or compression of the labrum. A tear in the acetabular labrum presents clinically with pain in the hip anteriorly, particularly with internal rotation. This is also commonly associated with a click noted when the hip is flexed and extended. The diagnosis can be confirmed with an MRI obtained after the injection of intra-articular contrast dye.

Intra-articular loose bodies can occur either as a result of trauma or as a result of synovial chondromatosis. In synovial chondromatosis, the synovium will develop osteochondral loose bodies that will be free in the articular space. In the knee, these loose bodies cause a great deal of mechanical symptoms such as locking. In the hip, there is not enough free space for the loose body to cause locking. However, these loose bod-

ies can restrict motion and cause pain. Synovial chondromatosis can be difficult to diagnose. The plain radiographs are usually normal or will demonstrate the very subtle stippled calcifications of the osteochondral fragments. An MRI or CT scan can be helpful in demonstrating the loose bodies and the expansion of the synovial space and effusion. The treatment is surgical. An open arthrotomy is performed and the fragments removed. Synovectomy can be performed although care should be taken to preserve the vascularity of the femoral head. Arthroscopy typically is inadequate to remove all of the loose bodies.

Avascular necrosis is a condition that most commonly affects the femoral head. However, this condition can also affect the proximal humerus, knee, and talus. The specific mechanism causing AVN is unclear. Several factors have been associated with the increased risk of developing this condition. The most common factors are trauma to the femoral head or neck, systemic corticosteroid administration, and excessive alcohol intake. In addition to these factors, there is a long list of other less common factors such as hemoglobinopathies, metabolic conditions, and inflammatory conditions, which can cause AVN. However, in as many as one-third of patients with non-traumatic AVN, no specific etiology can be identified, and thus these cases are identified as idiopathic AVN.

In all cases of AVN, there is compromise of the blood supply of the femoral head. This most commonly occurs in the anterior, superior portion of the femoral head, leading to necrosis of a portion of the subchondral bone. If the avascular segment is large and in a weight-bearing area, the stability of the subchondral bone will be compromised as the necrotic trabeculae weaken. While an MRI or Tc99-MDP bone scan can demonstrate the lesion early (see Fig. 13.14), the plain radiographs are frequently normal after the segment becomes avascular. Over time the round femoral head will weaken and then develop an area of collapse. At this point, the joint is no longer round and congruent and will progress to degenerative arthritis.

The lesion of AVN has a very typical pathologic and radiographic pattern. The lesion is most commonly in the anterior and superior subchondral bone of the femoral head. There are several distinct zones to the lesion. The outer zone is an area of increased vascularity and inflammation that is in response to the necrotic segment. The next layer is a dense area of sclerotic bone, which is laid down around the necrotic segment in an attempt to heal the lesion. However, this simply serves to wall off the lesion and prevents vascular invasion and healing of the lesion. Inside the sclerotic bone is the necrotic bone with the trabecular structure that is relatively intact. Histologically, the necrosis of the bone is demonstrated by trabecular bone with empty lacunae. Closer to the subchondral bone is the area of collapse of the trabecular bone. The outer layer is composed of the subchondral bone and articular cartilage. Radiographically, a subchondral radiolucent line that is referred to as a crescent sign demonstrates this region. Frequently, after collapse of the subchondral region, there will be a defect through the cartilage and the subchondral bone that will allow articular fluid to enter the necrotic area. This will further impair healing of the lesion.

In early cases prior to collapse of the femoral head, attempts can be made to save the femoral head and restore viability to the necrotic bone. There are several surgical variations; all involve drilling a core tract into the avascular portion of the femoral head in an attempt to restore vascularity to the necrotic bone and possibly heal the lesion. Several techniques have been described to augment this procedure. These include the use of autologous cancellous bone grafting, bone marrow aspirate, bone graft substitutes, allograft cortical or cancellous bone, or one of the patient's fibulae on a vascular pedicle to place vascularized bone into the lesion. These procedures do not work once collapse, evidenced by the crescent sign or loss of sphericity, has occurred.

Of patients who have documented AVN that is untreated, 70% will require a total hip replacement within 5 years. Patients who have had a core decompression type procedure will require a total hip replacement in 30–35% of cases by 5 years. The results are improved compared to the natural history; however, the success rate is less than optimal. Vascularized fibular grafting has demonstrated an improvement in the survivorship of the involved hip in a few centers. However, this requires highly specialized surgical technique and can lead to significant weakness in foot and ankle function on the involved side after harvesting the fibula.

For patients with small lesions that have already undergone subchondral collapse, an osteotomy may be done to rotate the necrotic collapsed segment out from under the weight-bearing area of the hip. However, commonly the lesion is extensive and not enough viable bone remains to allow the necrotic segment to be rotated out of the weight-bearing area of the hip. As the AVN progresses and the hip becomes severely degenerated, a hip replacement offers the most reliable means of restoring function and relieving pain and can be considered in even relatively young patients.

Hip Arthritis

A wide variety of arthritic conditions can affect the hip joint. While the medical therapy can vary based upon the specific diagnosis, the operative treatments fall into several broad categories and will be discussed as such. Arthritis is defined as any condition that results in articular cartilage damage with resulting pain and limitation of the motion of a joint. Hip arthritis can be divided into several broad categories (Table 13.1).

The clinical presentation of hip arthritis is a gradual increase in pain and limitation of motion. Frequently patients will complain of a reduction in their ability to walk for distances. Patients will also notice a marked stiffness in the joint when they have been sitting for a period of time and go to stand. The joint may feel out of place or stiff. As the arthritis progresses and the joint begins to lose motion, patients will also notice a reduction in their ability to care for their own toenails and have difficulty with activities such as putting on socks or stockings and tying their shoes. A limp will also commonly occur in patients with hip arthritis, particularly after long walks or at the end of the day.

Table 13.1 Classification of hip arthritis

Category	Examples	Etiology
Osteoarthritis	Primary osteoarthritis	Idiopathic
		Congenital
	Secondary osteoarthritis	Developmental
		Avascular necrosis
		Post-traumatic
Inflammatory arthritis	Rheumatoid arthritis	Immunogenic
	Ankylosing spondylitis	
	Psoriatic arthritis	
	Systemic lupus	
Infectious	Pyogenic	*Staphylococcus aureus, S. epidermidis, gonococcal*
	Lyme disease	*Borrelia*
	Non-pyogenic	*Mycobacterium*
Other	Crystals	Gout, pseudogout
	Hemophilia	Hemosiderin deposition

Table 13.2 Primary interventions in the non-operative management of osteoarthritis

Non-steroidal anti-inflammatory medications
Physical therapy
Intra-articular injection of corticosteroids
Assistive devices
Modification of activities

Radiographic and etiologic criteria can assist in dividing the patients into two broad categories, osteoarthritis and inflammatory arthritis, based upon the history and the radiographic appearance of the hip joints. Osteoarthritis has four classic features on plain radiography: localized joint space narrowing along the weight-bearing surface, subchondral sclerosis, osteophyte formation, and subchondral cysts (see Fig. 13.7). In rheumatoid arthritis, a classic example of an inflammatory arthritis, the radiographic features are peri-articular osteopenia and erosions, diffuse or global joint space narrowing, and occasionally subchondral cysts. In inflammatory arthritis of the hip, protrusio deformity of the femoral head beyond the ilioischial line can be noted as well. In most cases of arthritic disease in the hip, no additional studies other than plain radiography are necessary for the evaluation.

The non-operative treatment will vary based upon the specific diagnosis. Osteoarthritis, whether primary or secondary, is treated in a similar fashion. The initial treatment for the majority of patients with osteoarthritis is non-operative. There are five primary interventions in the non-operative management of the patient with osteo-

arthritis (Table 13.2). These five interventions can be used in isolation or in combination based upon the specific clinical situation in which the patient presents. Non-steroidal anti-inflammatory drugs (NSAIDs) can be very effective in reducing the pain and improving function. However, there is a large individual variation in the efficacy and side effects with each of these agents. Therefore, patients should be tried on several NSAIDs from different chemical classes prior to abandoning this limb of therapy. The principal side effect of NSAID is gastrointestinal (GI) intolerance with the possibility of ulcer formation. NSAIDs can also affect renal and hepatic function; and in the long-term use of these agents, renal and hepatic function test should be followed. In addition, these medications can affect platelet function and may have an adverse effect on bleeding times. These medicines should not be used in patients requiring anticoagulation therapy or within 5–7 days prior to any surgical intervention.

The cyclo-oxygenase-2 (COX-2) inhibitors were thought to offer lower side effects compared to the non-specific cyclo-oxygenase inhibitors which represent the majority of NSAIDs on the market. However, their safety was brought into question in several large clinical trials which suggested an increased rate of cardiac and vascular events after long-term use at high doses although this can be seen with traditional NSAIDs as well. The COX-2 inhibitors do have the advantage of a lesser effect on platelet function and have been shown to be safe for patients on anticoagulation therapy, which allows them to be safely used in the peri-operative setting.

Intra-articular corticosteroid injections are another non-operative treatment option. Intra-articular injections are more common in the treatment of shoulder and knee compared to the hip. They have not been as widely utilized for arthritis of the hip, in part due to the difficulty ensuring the injection is intra-articular but they also do not have the efficacy seen in the knee. Fluoroscopy is helpful in confirming proper placement of the needle. Injection of the hip with local anesthetic can be helpful in differentiating referred back pain from intra-articular hip pathology. Also, there are patients who will have a strong referred pain from the hip to the knee. In these patients, an intra-articular hip injection will relieve the knee pain and confirm the site of origin of the knee pain. However, injections are limited in their ability to provide long-term relief of symptoms. Corticosteroid injection for arthritis should not be done more than three or four times per year. If the patient requires more frequent injections for pain control, other therapeutic measures or surgery should be considered, as obtaining injections too frequently can result in acceleration of the articular cartilage degeneration and increase the risks of complications, such as infection.

Physical therapy can be beneficial in reducing pain and improving range of motion for osteoarthritis (OA) involving the knee or shoulder; however, limited benefit has been found for the treatment of OA involving the hip. If this modality is to be utilized, it should be done early in the course of OA. As the arthritis progresses, therapy will only serve to exacerbate an already painful joint. However, all patients should be encouraged to maintain aerobic fitness to maintain their joint function as well as their general health. Activities such as swimming and cycling have minimal repetitive impact and are excellent for aerobic fitness. Higher impact activities such as running and racquet sports can further damage an arthritic joint and should be discouraged in a patient with hip arthritis. As the arthritis progresses, the patient will be able to do less and become more sedentary. As this occurs, the symptoms will also increase in severity.

Assistive devices, including crutches, cane, and a walker, can be quite effective in the relief of stress across the joint surface during ambulation in patients with OA involving the lower extremities. A cane used in the contralateral hand of a patient with isolated hip arthritis can reduce the joint reaction force by as much as 30%. However,

the use of these devices is associated with a significant change in a patient's perception of themselves and their global health status. So, while this modality can be helpful in relieving symptoms and maintaining mobility, it will commonly meet resistance from the patient.

Modification of activities is one of the most significant aspects in the non-operative management of arthritis. This includes modification in a patient's activities of daily living and self-care. Modification of the patient's parking, as well as obtaining devices to assist in putting on shoes and socks, can be very helpful for patients with limitations due to hip arthritis. The reduction in certain activities such as running or racquet sports can improve the joint symptoms. However, this will result in a gradual progressive decrease in the patient's quality of life. The level of social interaction and activities in which the patient can comfortably participate can become markedly reduced. Modification of activities should also address patients who are overweight. Reduction in weight can significantly improve a patient's symptoms, increase mobility, and improve global health status. In addition, reduction in weight will reduce the stress placed upon the joint replacement if they require surgery.

The non-operative management of a patient with OA involves all of the above therapies. However, as the arthritis progresses, pain and limitation of activities will continue to increase. When the patient fails to achieve acceptable symptomatic relief with the non-operative regimen, joint replacement should be discussed. Rarely is there any significant change in the complexity of the surgery or outcome in patients with hip arthritis who delay operative intervention with non-operative treatment. Therefore, the timing of the surgical intervention is based entirely upon the patient, the patient's pain, and limitations of daily activities.

Surgical Management

Most hip pathology can be managed with one of several options; these include arthroscopy, osteotomy, arthrodesis, hip resurfacing, and arthroplasty (hemiarthroplasty or total hip arthroplasty). Each option has specific indications and contra-indications, which will be discussed in the next few sections.

Arthroscopy

Hip arthroscopy is in its infancy compared to this technique in the knee. The indications for hip arthroscopy are growing and now include the removal of loose bodies from the hip joint, addressing acetabular labral pathology, bone resection procedures for femoral-acetabular impingement, synovial disease, snapping hip syndrome from the iliopsoas tendon or iliotibial band, and identification and treatment of articular cartilage defects. The technique requires the use of special equipment due to the more extensive soft tissue envelope around the hip compared to the knee. The soft tissue envelope also limits the mobility of the arthroscope within the hip. In addition, the hip capsule is quite thick and the articular space quite small. Traction is required to gain visualization of the hip joint. The portals must be opened with care to avoid injury to the neuro-vascular structures surrounding the hip. These issues have presented challenges to the widespread use of this technique, but its application is rapidly expanding.

Arthrotomy

Arthrotomy involves surgical opening of the hip joint. Many of the indications for hip arthroscopy are also indications for hip arthrotomy, such as removing loose bodies or to address acetabular labral lesions. However, hip arthrotomy can also address the drainage of hip sepsis and hip syno-vectomy. The hip joint can be exposed and opened either from the anterior aspect or the pos-terior aspect. Anterior approaches are more com-monly utilized as this approach is less likely to injure the blood supply to the femoral head which predominantly arises from the medial femoral circumflex vessels along the posterior intertro-chanteric line.

The hip joint is normally entered from the acetabular edge, with care taken to preserve the acetabular labrum. If the labrum is torn, it can either be excised or repaired, depending upon the condition and nature of the tear. It may be neces-sary to apply traction to the leg to allow inspec-tion of the hip joint. Any loose bodies or fragments can be removed. If the indication for arthrotomy is synovectomy, it may be necessary to open the hip both from the posterior and from the anterior aspect. This does increase the risk of post-operative avascular necrosis; however, the synovium of the hip cannot be removed from a single approach.

Osteotomy

Osteotomy involves redirecting the articular sur-face to move damaged cartilage away from the weight-bearing areas of the joint and place a less damaged area of the articular surface in the weight-bearing area of the hip joint. Osteotomy can also reduce joint forces by realigning the bone of the pelvis or proximal femur to yield a larger area of contact to distribute the force of weight-bearing. During osteotomy, the bone of the pelvis or femur is transected, redirected, and then fixed rigidly (Fig. 13.15). If the arthritis is localized to only one region of a joint, perform-ing an osteotomy can move the damaged carti-lage away from the weight-bearing area and transfer undamaged articular surfaces into the high-stress area. This may result in reduced pain and prolong the functional life of the patient's native joint. Prerequisites for an osteotomy are that the patient has an adequate range of motion of the joint, that the joint is stable, and that the articular damage involves only a limited area of the joint. If extensive arthritis or an inflammatory arthritis is present, an osteotomy will not be successful.

In properly selected patients, hip osteotomies can have a success of greater than 80% at 8–10 years follow-up. For young patients with focal articular damage, osteotomy can provide an acceptable result and allow them to retain their native hip joint. This can delay or possibly elimi-

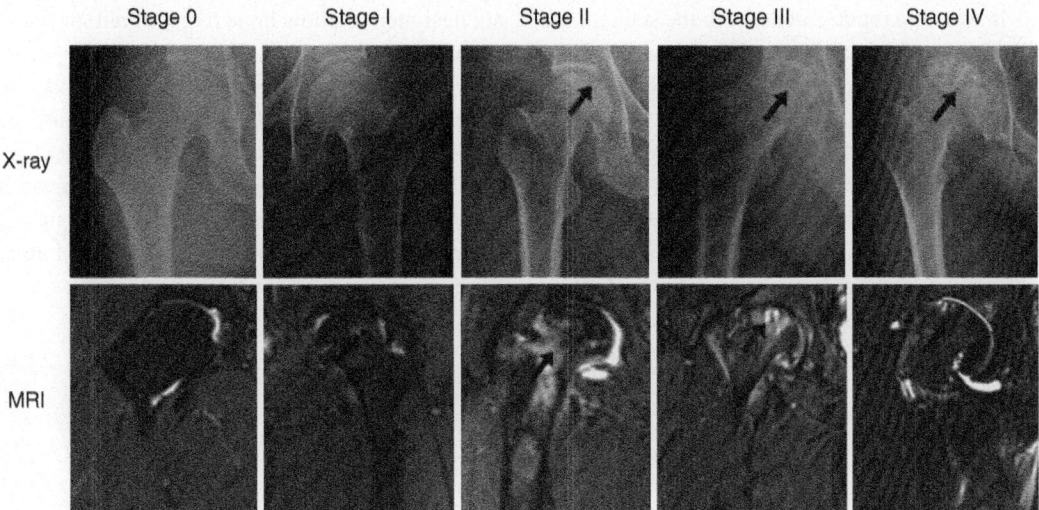

Fig. 13.15 Progressive stages of femoral head AVN displayed. Stage I appears normal on radiographs, however, there may be early findings on MRI. This progresses to femoral head flattening (Stage III) and eventual joint space destruction (Stage IV). (From Xie XH, Wang XL, Yang HL, Zhao DW, Qin L. Steroid-associated osteonecrosis: Epidemiology, pathophysiology, animal model, prevention, and potential treatments (an overview). J Orthop Translat. 2015 Jan 13;3 (2):58–70. doi: 10.1016/j.jot.2014.12.002. PMID: 30035041; PMCID: PMC5982361)

nate the need for replacement with artificial materials that can wear or become loose. Acetabular osteotomy for developmental dysplasia of the hip can make subsequent total hip arthroplasty easier by redirecting the acetabular bone stock and providing better coverage for an acetabular component. However, osteotomy of the proximal femur can make a future hip replacement more difficult by altering the anatomy of the proximal femur. This may require an additional osteotomy to reconstruct the femur at the time of total hip replacement.

Arthrodesis

Arthrodesis involves the fusion of the proximal femur to the pelvis. This can provide a strong, stable, painless lower extremity. The patient can return to even heavy labor without the risk of loosening or damaging the arthrodesis. Arthrodesis is indicated in patients who are young with unilateral hip disease with no symptoms or disease involving the lumbar spine, contralateral hip, or the ipsilateral knee. Patients with an inflammatory arthritis or non-traumatic AVN

are relatively contraindicated for arthrodesis, as these diseases are frequently bilateral. Several studies looking at the long-term results of arthrodesis have found good results lasting greater than 20 years. However, the hip is no longer mobile, and over 15–20 years, the arthrodesis can result in low back pain and pain in the ipsilateral knee due to force transference in those areas. Several reports have noted that between 50 and 60% of patients complain of pain in the back or knee at 25–50 years follow-up. This technique has become less common due to the better options that are now available in total joint bearing surfaces that seem to provide a more durable and functional solution.

Hip Replacement Surgery

Total hip replacement (THR) is a common operation today. Approximately 450,000 replacements are performed each year. The primary goal of hip replacement is to relieve pain and improve mobility. Long-term studies have demonstrated excellent results, with survivorship ranging from 65 to 90% at 30 years of follow-up.

In total hip replacement, both the socket (acetabulum) and the ball (femoral head) are replaced with metal/ceramic and plastic components. The socket is commonly reconstructed with a metal shell impacted into the prepared acetabular space with a modular plastic or metal liner (Figs. 13.16 and 13.17). The ball is replaced by a ceramic or metal ball attached to a stem that fits inside the proximal canal of the femur. Two principle types of implants are used: those inserted with bone cement and those inserted without cement which are designed to allow bone to grow onto or into a porous metal surface. Both techniques have excellent long-term follow-up data supporting their effectiveness. The cemented technique has seen a dramatic decrease in use over recent years due to the successful results of the uncemented (press-fit) designs that can be easier to insert, and also eliminate the possible mode of failure at the cement interface (Fig. 13.18).

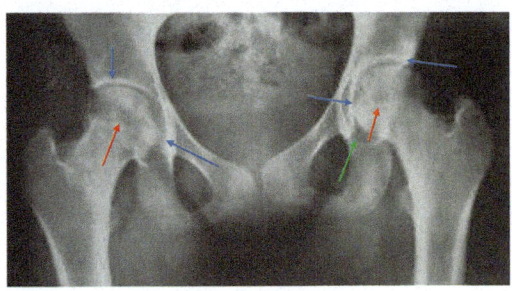

Fig. 13.16 Findings typical of rheumatoid arthritis include concentric joint space narrowing (blue arrows), subchondral cysts (red arrows), as well as peri-articular erosions (green arrow), which may affect bilateral hips. (From GLICK EN, MASON RM, WENLEY WG. RHEUMATOID ARTHRITIS AFFECTING THE HIP JOINT. Ann Rheum Dis. 1963 Nov;22(6):416–23. doi: 10.1136/ard.22.6.416. PMID: 14087252; PMCID: PMC1030881)

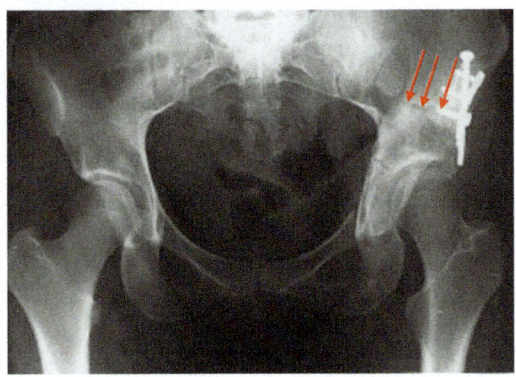

Fig. 13.17 Anteroposterior radiograph of a 26-year-old female 6 months after a left pelvic osteotomy (red arrow) was performed to deepen her acetabulum and improve coverage of the femoral head. Her primary diagnosis was developmental dysplasia of the hip, which left her with a shallow left acetabulum

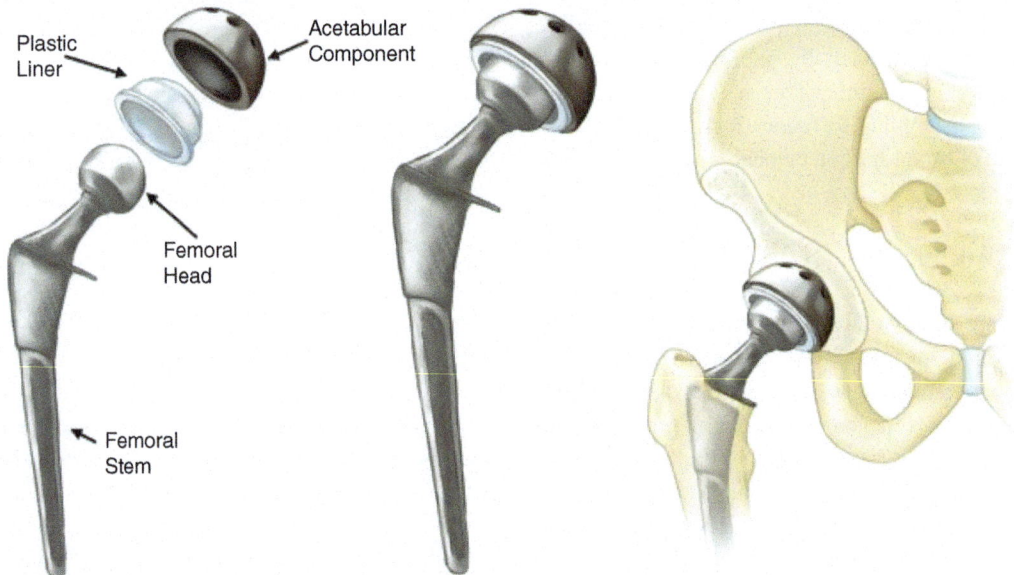

Fig. 13.18 Depiction of a press fit total hip arthroplasty. (From AAOS)

Uncemented stems have a press-fit design which allows for rigid, stable fixation at the time of implantation, since the prosthesis is slightly larger than the bony space which is prepared by broaches, creating a tight wedging effect. Proximal tapered designs have a wedge-shaped taper in the stem, which provides an enhanced level of bony contact in the proximal femur, providing more physiologic loading of the femur with weight-bearing. Longer stems have a cylindrical or conical design of the stem which provides a large area of bony contact in the diaphysis of the femur. This moves the load transfer distally and can stress shield the proximal femur, leading to gradual resorption of the unloaded bone over time. These designs are commonly used in revision cases where the proximal femur is deficient. The key aspect of successful implantation of an uncemented stem is solid fixation at the time of surgery. Initial instability can occur if the stem is undersized or due to improper technique. This leads to micro-motion at the bone–prosthesis interface, causing the creation of a fibrous union. This can produce thigh pain, particularly with the first few steps ("start-up pain") that may or may not resolve with time. Initially, this is treated with limited weight-bearing and NSAIDs. If the pain persists, revising the stem becomes necessary.

Total hip arthroplasty is performed from either an anterior, posterior, or lateral approach. The posterior approaches are commonly used for total hip replacement. The dissection is carried posterior to the trochanter. The short external rotators are released from the femur and the posterior capsule is opened. The hip is dislocated posteriorly by flexion, adduction, and internal rotation. The posterior approach provides an excellent extensile exposure to the pelvis, hip, and femur. In addition, the gluteus medius and minimus are preserved, optimizing the function of the hip abductors post-operatively. However, post-operatively patients are at risk for a posterior dislocation with flexion, adduction, and internal rotation. The dislocation rate after a posterior approach is 1–3% in primary total hip replacement.

Anterior approaches to the hip are also commonly employed for total hip replacement. These approaches enter the hip from the front between sartorius and tensor facia lata superficially, and rectus femoris and gluteus medius deep. The anterior capsule is then opened, and the hip is extended, adducted, and externally rotated to dislocate the femoral head and the arthroplasty completed. This approach can yield extensile exposure proximally and distally. This leaves the posterior capsule intact, protecting the patient from a posterior dislocation. The rate of instability is 1–2% in most series.

Currently, there is a great deal of interest in minimally invasive approaches for hip replacement, which include anterior and posterior approaches. Though there is no defined definition of minimally invasive, the smaller incision and limited soft tissue dissection may reduce perioperative pain and quicken recovery. These techniques, when combined with aggressive pain management protocols, have shown promise in improving the early recovery of the patient. While this is a significant benefit, it must be emphasized that proper surgical placement and technique is required for long-term success. Any short-term benefit from MIS surgery must not come at the expense of long-term results.

The patient is mobilized early after a total hip replacement, often beginning physical therapy on the day of surgery. The best exercise in the post-operative period is walking.

If the posterior approach is used, patients need to be careful to limit hip flexion, adduction, and internal rotation for at least the first 6 weeks to prevent the femoral head from dislocating out of the acetabular component. The rate of instability and the position of greatest instability vary with the approach used for the arthroplasty as outlined above. With anterior approaches, the greatest instability is with extension and external rotation. The patients usually report a dislocation occurring while they are standing and pivoting or while they are supine in bed with the legs adducted and the feet externally rotated. In contrast, posterior instability occurs when the hip is in a flexed, adducted, and internally rotated position. Patients are at risk of instability when they are getting out of a chair, getting off the toilet seat, or getting out of an automobile. The rate of dislocation is greatest in the first 6-weeks post-operatively while the soft tissues are healing. If a dislocation does occur within the first 6 weeks, the rate of recurrent instability is approximately 30%, with the majority having a single event. However, if the first dislocation occurs after the first 6 months, the rate of recurrent instability increases to 60%, with the majority of patients having recurrent instability, often requiring revision surgery to address the problem.

The treatment of a dislocated hip is to first reduce the hip, usually with conscious sedation. If this is unsuccessful, general anesthesia may be required. The patient is often placed into a brace or a knee immobilizer to limit hip flexion for a period of 6 weeks and can weight bear as tolerated. If the patient does have recurrent instability, revision may be necessary. Prior to revision, it is helpful to determine the precise position of the components. Plain radiography can accurately determine the vertical inclination of the acetabular cup; however, it is the degree of version of the component that is typically a greater factor in instability after total hip replacement. Accurate assessment of cup version can be best assessed by the use of CT imaging. If CT scan imaging cuts are also taken through the femoral condyles, the rotation of both the femoral and acetabular components can be determined. This information is important to aid in identifying the cause of the recurrent instability and to plan appropriate revision surgery to correct the problem.

Aseptic loosening of the implant from bone occurs at a low rate with modern techniques and implant materials. Many studies have shown that at 10 years approximately 90–95% of patients retain their original implant. This drops to 80–85% at 20 years, and approximately 65% at 30 years. The rate of loosening of the femoral component is usually less than that of the acetabular component. Acetabular loosening tends to increase over time due to osteolysis or stress shielding of the bone behind the more rigid metallic cups.

The survival of implants in patients less than 50 years of age is less than that noted in older patients. This is related to the higher demands and higher activity level in this younger group of patients. In an attempt to reduce the rate of aseptic loosening after THR in this younger patient population, surgeons have tried to achieve implant fixation directly to bone with increased use of uncemented stems. This can be achieved through the use of porous surfaces. If this surface is closely approximated to bone, and no significant motion occurs at the interface, bone trabeculae will interdigitate and grow into the porous surface and secure the implant. The press-fit designs of current stems help to achieve early stability while bone ingrowth occurs over time. It is also important to have minimal motion between the polyethylene liner and the metal cup. Motion and wear can occur at this interface as well as on the articulating interface. This leads to the development of wear debris which loosens the implant or it can cause a mechanical failure of the polyethylene liner and require revision surgery (Fig. 13.17). In addition, it is important to have high-quality locking mechanisms and sufficiently thick polyethylene liners for acetabular components.

Most designs limit the amount of screw holes in the metal cup which are used for supplementary fixation with screws to fix the cup to bone prior to bone ingrowth. The holes in the cup can provide a direct conduit for wear debris to the implant bone interface. This debris can lead to an osteolytic reaction and subsequent loosening of the acetabular cup. In cases of abnormal anatomy and osteopenic bone, or in revision cases, screws may be needed to supplement early stability.

Loosening appears to be primarily related to the generation of polyethylene wear debris from the articulation. Several new technologies have been developed to reduce wear from the articulation in a total hip replacement. The first new concept was to improve the polyethylene. This was accomplished by cross-linking the polymer strands within the material by means of free radical production using radiation. Think of a polymer as a bowl of cold spaghetti. If a strand of spaghetti is pulled, the whole strand can be teased from the bowl. If some of the strands are cut, and then these shorter strands are linked to other strands, it will be more difficult to pull out a strand and also more difficult to pull out a long strand. This logic applies to cross-linked polyethylene. The wear rate is reduced by tenfold and the debris produced is of much smaller particles (Fig. 13.19).

In order to reduce particle wear seen with polyethylene liners, two other alternatives were developed. These, however, have fallen out of favor given the excellent wear properties of newer highly-cross-linked polyethylene. These are referred to as hard-on-hard interfaces, metal-on-metal and ceramic-on-ceramic. By using much harder materials for the articulation, the wear rate and debris production can be reduced by up to 1000-fold. These articulations, however,

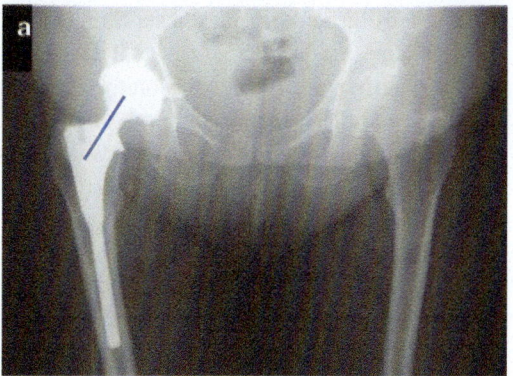

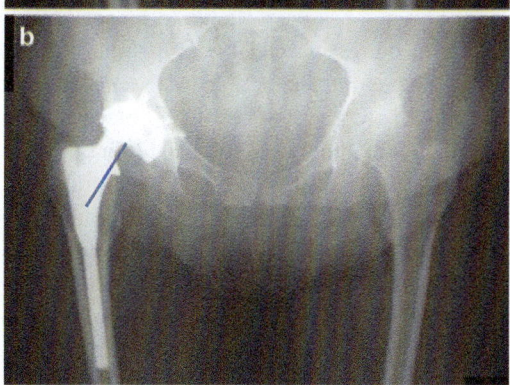

Fig. 13.19 (**a**) Anteroposterior radiograph of the left hip of a patient immediately post-operatively after a noncemented total hip arthroplasty compared to (**b**) 2-year postoperatively demonstrates a markedly eccentric position of the femoral head within the acetabular component. The blue line demonstrates the original center of the femoral neck in relation to the acetabulum from post-op compared to 2 years. (From Knox, D., Hamilton, S.W., Wardlaw, D. et al. Early catastrophic acetabular failure in Furlong total hip replacements. J Orthopaed Traumatol 10, 39–42 (2009). https://doi.org/10.1007/s10195-008-0045-z. Reprinted with permission)

also have some limitations. Metal on metal involves the use of a cobalt–chromium femoral head on a cobalt–chromium acetabular liner. This articulation has been in clinical use for approximately 30 years. Early designs failed early due to design problems. The early heads were made of equal dimension to the acetabular opening, which would result in binding of the head within the acetabulum and the component would loosen. Current designs have slightly reduced the size of the head relative to the acetabulum. This allows for lubrication of the interface and less friction. However, metal debris is produced in the form of small metal ions which are detectable in the blood, lymphatics, and urine of patients with metal-on-metal hip articulations. The long-term effects of this are unknown, but there is a concern since the ions continue to be produced over the entire life of the joint replacement. These implants are contraindicated for women of childbearing age and patients with renal failure for this reason. The metal-on-metal bearing surface also has the advantage of using very large femoral head designs which can improve stability and range of motion by increasing the head to neck ratio and maximizing the jump distance necessary for the head to dislocate. Many surgeons allow patients to participate in higher impact activities with hard-on-hard bearing surface implants. However, recent problems have begun to appear with patients developing painful hips and no evidence of gross loosening. Patients can also develop a pseudotumor in response to metal particles or issues with their abductors. A pseudotumor is a large, solid, or semi-liquid mass of soft tissue that grows around the hip joint. It is thought that some patients develop hypersensitivity to metal debris particles, leading to pain and, in some cases, significant synovitis. Early investigation suggests that a vertical placement of the acetabular component can lead to edge loading and subsequent increase of wear debris. Further studies are needed to help clarify the situation.

Ceramic-on-ceramic is the other hard on hard interface and results in the least amount of wear debris of all the currently used articulations for total hip arthroplasty. However, it is limited by the strength of the ceramic material. Ceramic implants can be prone to fracture and when a ceramic implant fails, it results in a catastrophic failure. The ceramic fragments are very hard and abrasive, resulting in rapid extensive wear of the metallic implants that are attached to the bones. Frequently, the metal components attached to the bones and the ceramic articulation all need to be removed after a fracture. The remaining particles in the soft tissue surrounding the joint lessen the success rates of revision surgery after ceramic fracture. A phenomenon of "squeaking" has also been reported in which patients develop audible squeaking when actively moving their hip replacement. It is thought that improper placement of the components increases the likelihood this problem and can require revision surgery.

Wear and loosening are worrisome complications, which are being addressed by improvements in materials and designs. However, the current devices have such high success rates that determining if new technologies are truly an improvement will need at least 10 years of clinical follow-up. All the new devices need to be evaluated not only for their benefits but also for the real and potential limitations.

Complications

The most frequent complication after THR is thromboembolic disease (TED). This includes deep venous thrombosis (DVT) and pulmonary embolism. Early in the history of THR, the rate of fatal pulmonary embolism was 1–2%. However, at that time patients were kept on bed rest for as long as 2–3 weeks and kept up to 6 weeks in the hospital. Early mobilization of patients has undoubtedly contributed to the significant reduction in the rate of fatal pulmonary embolism. However, significant reduction has also occurred through the use of anticoagulant prophylaxis, regional anesthesia, shorter operating times, and lower blood loss. In the USA, THR is considered a significant risk factor for TED and therefore the routine use of medical and/or mechanical prophylaxis has been recommended. At present, the rate of TED ranges between 5% and 20%. The rate of fatal pulmonary embolism is low, approximately 0.01%. The principal methods of prophylaxis are low-dose Coumadin (warfarin), aspirin, low-molecular weight heparin, and pneumatic compression stockings.

Aspirin has been used for DVT prophylaxis historically and has gained popularity for use after joint replacement. Aspirin irreversibly inhibits platelet function and theoretically will reduce the rate of formation of DVT. Multiple studies have examined the effectiveness of aspirin for DVT prophylaxis after total joint replacement. Aspirin has been demonstrated to be equally as effective as multiple other pharmacologic anti-coagulants, including low-molecular weight heparin, rivaroxaban, and enoxaparin.

Hypotensive epidural anesthesia (HEA) is an excellent anesthesia technique for THR; however, it requires careful patient monitoring and a dedicated anesthesia team. This form of anesthesia results in reduced blood loss while maintaining blood flow in the lower extremities. This reduces the need for transfusion post-operatively, which has been shown to increase the risk of DVT. In addition, the reduction in blood loss results in less activation of the coagulation cascade, again minimizing the risk of DVT. While this technique has been shown to be very effective, it has not been widely applied due to concerns about the reduction of mean arterial pressure in elderly patients, which may result in stroke, renal failure, or myocardial infarction.

Dislocation of the prosthetic femoral head from the acetabular component occurs in 1–3% of patients after THR. Post-operatively patients are instructed to not bend their replaced hip beyond 90°, to keep their legs abducted and in neutral rotation. These restrictions should be followed closely for the first 6 weeks following surgery. After this time, the patient should have formed a sufficient pseudocapsule to protect against dislocation. However, a replaced hip is always at greater risk for dislocation compared to a native hip joint. The majority of patients who dislocate their hip in the early post-operative period can be reduced without additional surgery and protected with a hip abduction brace or knee immobilizer for 6 weeks to allow healing of the pseudocapsule. In addition to patient compliance, the other etiologies for dislocation are component malposition, excessive soft tissue laxity, and impingement of the prosthetic or osseous structures resulting in levering of the femoral head out of the acetabulum. If a patient recurrently dislocates, revision surgery may be indicated.

The most devastating complication after THR is prosthetic joint infection. Early post-operative infection occurs in approximately 0.3–0.5% of cases after primary THR. Late infection resulting from hematogenous spread can occur in 1–2% of patients. If detected within the first 6 weeks post-operatively, aggressive open debridement and modular component exchange combined with intravenous antibiotics may be successful. However, if the infection recurs after debridement or is detected beyond 6 weeks of symptoms, treatment typically consists of a two-stage procedure. This involves the removal of the prosthetic components and all cement if present. An antibiotic impregnated spacer is placed at the time of explant, which provides a local depot of antibiotics at the site of the infection and improves mobility and maintains soft tissue tension during the treatment period. Appropriate intravenous antibiotics are administered for 6–8 weeks and the patient is monitored for clinical signs of infection. If lab values normalize (white blood cell [WBC], erythrocyte sedimentation rate [ESR], C-reactive protein), the joint can be aspirated after antibiotics have been stopped for at least 2 weeks. If this is negative, the second-stage

reimplantation can be done. The success rate for this technique is often greater than 90%. If the pathologic organisms are highly virulent and resistant to antibiotic therapy, reimplantation can be delayed for more than 12 months.

Heterotopic ossification (HO) can form around a THR in 5–25% of cases. Heterotopic bone is histologically bone tissue. It forms within the muscle around the hip after arthroplasty. There is a metaplasia that occurs, forming a bone matrix that becomes calcified over the first 6–12 months after the surgery. Most commonly the presence of HO will not compromise the clinical result. Associated risk factors are patients with hypertrophic osteoarthritis, males, greater than age 65, HO formation after previous surgery, and ankylosing spondylitis.

Heterotopic ossification is graded according to the Brooker classification. Grade one consists of isolated islands of bone within the soft tissue between the femur and pelvis. Grade two is bone protruding from the proximal femur or pelvis with greater than 1 cm of separation. Grade three consists of bone protruding from the femur and/or pelvis with less than 1 cm between the bones. Grade four is radiographic ankylosis, with no visible space between the bone protruding from the femur and pelvis. Grades one and two are rarely symptomatic. Grade three patients usually have stiffness and mild pain. Patients with grade four usually have marked stiffness and can be very symptomatic (Fig. 13.20).

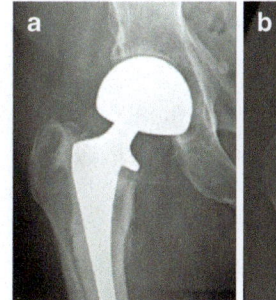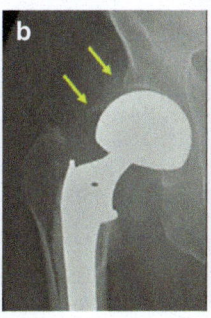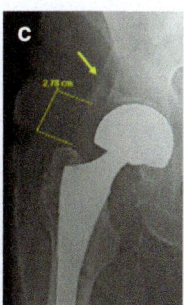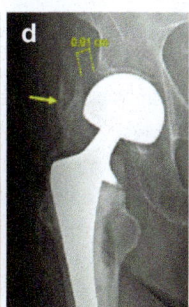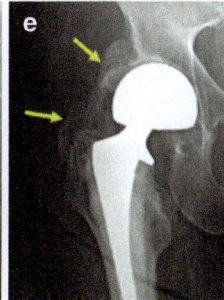

Fig. 13.20 The Brooker classification. (**a**) Immediate post-operative images. (**b, c, d, e**)—Grade 1 (**b**) through Grade 4 (**e**) progression. (From Hayashi D, Gould ES, Ho C, Caruana DL, Komatsu DE, Yang J, Zhu C, Mufti M, Nicholson J. Severity of heterotopic ossification in patients following surgery for hip fracture: a retrospective observational study. BMC Musculoskelet Disord. 2019 Jul 27;20(1):348. doi: 10.1186/s12891-019-2725-7. PMID: 31351447; PMCID: PMC6661104)

Patients who are at high risk for this complication can receive prophylaxis using indomethacin or low-dose radiation therapy. Once HO forms, the patients should be encouraged to maintain range of motion and activity, but passive stretching and passive range of motion should be avoided. Surgical intervention, in which the HO is excised, is indicated in patients with significant restriction of motion and pain. This occurs most commonly in patients with grade three and four HO. Surgery should be delayed until the HO is mature. Attempts to remove the bone prior to maturity have an increased rate of recurrence. After the bone is excised, the patient should receive prophylaxis to prevent recurrence with either indomethacin or radiation therapy. Radiation therapy is preferred in most patients as it is usually a one-dose regimen of 700–800 cGy and can be administered either immediately preoperatively or within the first 2 or 3 days postoperatively. The rate of recurrence after excision and prophylaxis is approximately 5–20%.

The limitations to the long-term fixation of a total hip arthroplasty are loosening and wear. As the implant, particularly the polyethylene liner, wears, the debris that is produced is released into the local tissues. The body has no mechanism to digest or eliminate the polyethylene debris. However, the local macrophages in the area recognize the material as a foreign substance and try to eliminate the debris. The macrophages ingest the material and try to digest it with catabolic enzymes and super-oxides, which fails to alter the material. As the debris accumulates within the cell, it breaks down, releasing the polyethylene, enzymes, and oxides into the local environment. This results in a local bone lysis that creates cysts in the bone and dissects along the fixation of the implant or cement and bone. If allowed to continue, the lysis leads to loosening.

Loosening can also result from mechanical failure of the implant bone or cement interface. The cement mantle can fragment or fracture, leaving the implant loose. In non-cemented fixation, the implant can also loosen. This can occur due to failed bony ingrowth resulting in a fibrous fixation. This fibrous tissue may not be sufficient to maintain stable fixation of the implant. The implant will then migrate slowly, best appreciated on serial radiographs. This will require revision to provide a stable implant.

Similar to the indications for primary arthroplasty, these are elective surgeries. However, in the revision setting, it is important to follow the patient closely with plain radiographs. If an accelerated pattern of bone loss is noted, revision surgery should be performed prior to the loss of an extensive amount of bone. The greater the loss of bone at the time of revision, the greater the difficulty in obtaining stable fixation for the revision components. This may also lead to a higher rate of repeated revision for aseptic loosening.

Summary

As noted initially, disorders involving the hip and femur are manifested by alteration in a patient's ability to ambulate. These can be diagnosed and treated by obtaining a careful history, thorough physical examination, and the appropriate use of radiographic studies. When proper diagnosis is made for most non-traumatic disorders, it is usually best to begin with non-operative treatment options. If the non-operative treatment alternatives are not successful, then operative intervention is considered and can result in an excellent outcome in the majority of patients.

Further Reading

Bauer TW, Parvizi J, Kobayashi N, Krebs V. Diagnosis of periprosthetic infection. J Bone Joint Surg Am. 2006;88:869–82.

Brooker AF, Bowerman JW, Robinson RA, Riley LH Jr. Ectopic ossification following total hip replacement. Incidence and a method of classification. J Bone Joint Surg Am. 1973;55(8):1629–32.

Byrd JW. Hip arthroscopy. J Am Acad Orthop Surg. 2006;14(7):433–44.

Callaghan JJ, Templeton JE, Liu SS, et al. Results of Charnley total hip arthroplasty at a minimum of 30 years. A concise follow-up of a previous report. J Bone Joint Surg Am. 2004;86-A(4):690–5.

Collier JP, Sutula LC, Currier BH, et al. Overview of polyethylene as a bearing material: comparison of sterilization methods. Clin Orthop Relat Res. 1996;333:76–86.

Evans BG. Late complications and their management. In: Callaghan JJ, Rosenberg AG, Rubash HE, editors. The adult hip. New York, NY: Lippincott-Raven; 1998. p. 1149–61.

Garvin KL, Evans BG, Salvati EA, Brause BD. Palacos gentamicin for the treatment of deep periprosthetic hip infections. Clin Orthop Relat Res. 1994;298:97–105.

Healy WL, Lo TC, DeSimone AA, Rask B, Pfeifer BA. Single-dose irradiation for the prevention of heterotopic ossification after total hip arthroplasty. A comparison of doses of five hundred and fifty and seven hundred centigray. J Bone Joint Surg Am. 1995;77(4):590–5.

Hoaglund FT, Steinbach LS. Primary osteoarthritis of the hip: etiology and epidemiology. J Am Acad Orthop Surg. 2001;9(5):320–7.

Jazrawi LM, Kummer FJ, DiCesare PE. Alternative bearing surfaces for total joint arthroplasty. J Am Acad Orthop Surg. 1998;6(4):198–203.

Meehan J, Jamali AA, Nguygen H. Prophylactic antibiotics in hip and knee arthroplasty. J Bone Joint Surg Am. 2009;91(10):2480–90.

Steinberg ME. Early diagnosis, evaluation, and staging of osteonecrosis. Instr Course Lect. 1994;43:513–8.

Trousdale RT, Ekkernkamp A, Ganz R, Wallrichs SL. Periacetabular and intertrochanteric osteotomy for the treatment of osteoarthrosis in dysplastic hips. J Bone Joint Surg Am. 1995;77(1):73–85.

Wiklund I, Romanus B. A comparison of quality of life before and after arthroplasty in patients who had arthrosis of the hip joint. J Bone Joint Surg Am. 1991;73(5):765–9.

Willert HG, Bertram H, Buchhorn GH. Osteolysis in allo-arthroplasty of the hip. The role of ultra-high molecular weight polyethylene wear particles. Clin Orthop Relat Res. 1990;258:95–107.

Woo RYG, Morrey BF. Dislocations after total hip arthroplasty. J Bone Joint Surg Am. 1982;64(9):1295–306.

Fernandez MA, Achten J, Parsons N, Griffin XL, Png ME, Gould J, McGibbon A, Costa ML, WHiTE 5 Investigators. Cemented or uncemented hemiarthroplasty for intracapsular hip fracture. N Engl J Med. 2022;386(6):521–30.

Parilla FW, Youngman TR, Layon DR, Ince DC, Pashos GE, Maloney WJ, Clohisy JC. Excellent 20-year results of Total hip arthroplasty with highly cross-linked polyethylene on cobalt-chromium femoral heads in patients ≤50 years. J Arthroplast. 2024;39(2):409–15.

Knee Osteoarthritis and Arthroplasty

14

Evan Jacquez, Brian G. Evans, and Kenneth M. Vaz

Introduction

This chapter will discuss the anatomy, biomechanics, and pathology of the knee as well as the pathophysiology and treatment of one of its most common ailments: osteoarthritis. The function of the knee is provided primarily by the soft tissue. Therefore, injury to these soft tissue structures will have a significant impact upon the stability of the knee.

Anatomy

The osseous anatomy of the knee consists of the proximal tibia, the distal femur, and the patella (Fig. 14.1). The distal femur consists of the medial and lateral condyles, the medial and lateral epicondyles, femoral trochlear groove, and the intercondylar notch. The medial condyle is larger and extends slightly distal compared to the lateral condyle. Both condyles are covered with articular cartilage. The trochlear groove lies on the anterior aspect of the distal femur between the medial and lateral femoral condyles. This surface is also covered by the articular cartilage and serves as the site of articulation of the patella. The lateral rim of the trochlear groove is frequently more prominent than the medial side to allow for proper patellar tracking along the femur.

The epicondyles serve as the site of insertion of several important structures. The deep and superficial medial collateral ligaments (MCL) attach to the medial epicondyle. The proximal margin of the medial epicondyle is enlarged and serves as the site of insertion of the adductor magnus (the adductor tubercle). The lateral or fibular collateral ligament (LCL) attaches to the lateral epicondyle. Inferior to the attachment of the LCL is the insertion of the popliteus muscle at the junction of the lateral condyle and epicondyle. The medial and lateral heads of the gastrocnemius muscle originate from the medial and lateral posterior femoral condyles. The intercondylar notch is the site of the femoral attachment of the cruciate ligaments. The anterior cruciate ligament (ACL) attaches in the posterior lateral aspect of the notch and the posterior cruciate ligament (PCL) attaches in the anterior medial aspect of the notch.

The proximal tibial surface is composed of the medial and lateral plateaus and the intercondylar eminence. The medial plateau is larger and extends further posterior compared to the lateral plateau. The surface of the medial plateau is slightly concave, whereas the lateral tibial pla-

E. Jacquez (✉) · B. G. Evans · K. M. Vaz
MedStar Georgetown Orthopedic Institute,
Georgetown University School of Medicine,
Washington, DC, USA

Department of Orthopedics, MedStar Georgetown
University Hospital, Washington, DC, USA
e-mail: Evan.A.Jacquez@medstar.net;
Kenneth.M.Vaz@medstar.net

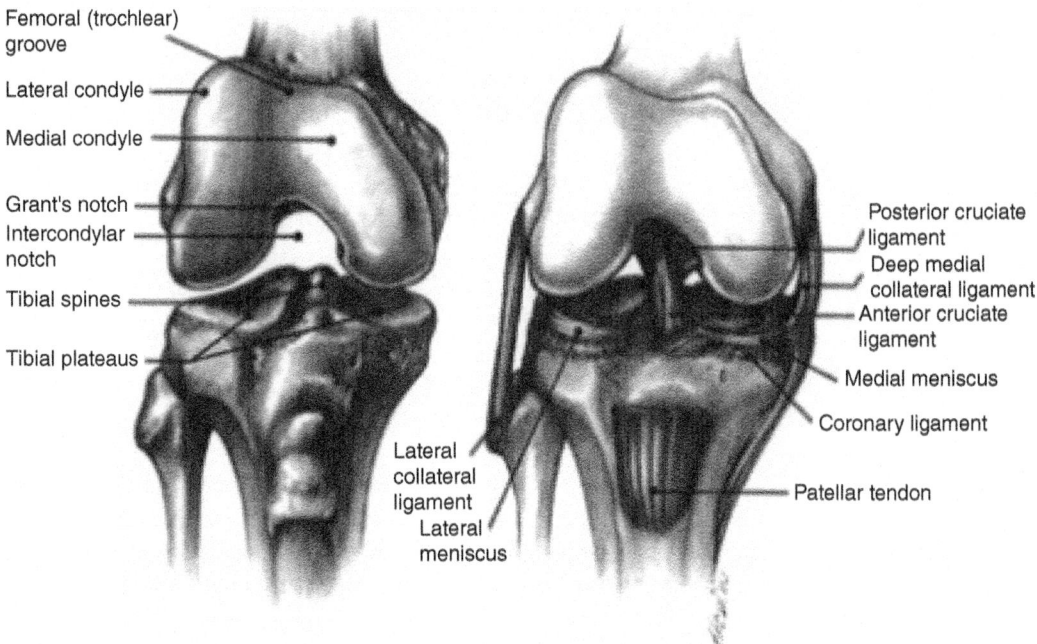

Femoral (trochlear) groove

Lateral condyle

Medial condyle

Grant's notch

Intercondylar notch

Tibial spines

Tibial plateaus

Posterior cruciate ligament

Deep medial collateral ligament

Anterior cruciate ligament

Medial meniscus

Coronary ligament

Patellar tendon

Lateral collateral ligament

Lateral meniscus

Fig. 14.1 Bony anatomy and major ligamentous structures of the flexed knee joint (anterior view)

teau is in fact slightly convex. Both of the tibial plateaus are covered with articular cartilage. The intercondylar eminence is the site of attachment of the menisci and the cruciate ligaments.

The patella is a sesamoid bone within the tendon of the quadriceps mechanism. There are two major facets on the patella, the medial and lateral facets. There is significant variability in the size and orientation of these facets. However, normally the lateral facet is broader and the medial facet is more acutely oriented to the femoral trochlea.

The osseous anatomy of the knee provides little to the stability of the knee. Stability and function are therefore provided by the complex soft tissue envelope around and in the knee (Figs. 14.2 and 14.3). The soft tissue components of the knee can be divided into several components: static restraints (ligaments), dynamic restraints (muscles and tendons), and the menisci. The static restraints are represented by the medial collateral ligament (MCL), lateral collateral ligament (LCL), anterior cruciate ligament (ACL), and posterior cruciate ligament (PCL). These structures resist valgus and varus stress as well as anterior and posterior translation of the tibia relative to the femur. The MCL consists of two layers.

The deep MCL spans from the medial epicondyle of the femur to the proximal tibial border, just below the medial tibial plateau. The superficial MCL has the same femoral origin; however, the ligament has a broad tibial insertion extending 6–10 cm below the tibial plateau along the posterior medial border of the tibia. The LCL is a more discrete band along the lateral aspect of the knee. It spans from its origin on the lateral femoral epicondyle and inserting not on the proximal tibia but instead on the fibular head.

The ACL resists the anterior translation of the tibia relative to the femur. The ligament runs from the anterior aspect of the tibial eminence to the posterior lateral aspect of the femoral notch. The PCL resists posterior translation of the tibia relative to the femur and resists hyperextension of the knee. The ligament extends from the posterior aspect of the intercondylar eminence and proximal tibia in the midline to the anterior medial aspect of the femoral intercondylar notch.

The dynamic restraints in the knee are the muscles and tendons which cross the knee joint. These are broadly divided into muscles which act to extend and those which act to flex the knee. The extensor muscles are the quadriceps femoris

Fig. 14.2 Cross section of the knee demonstrating the menisci and associated ligaments

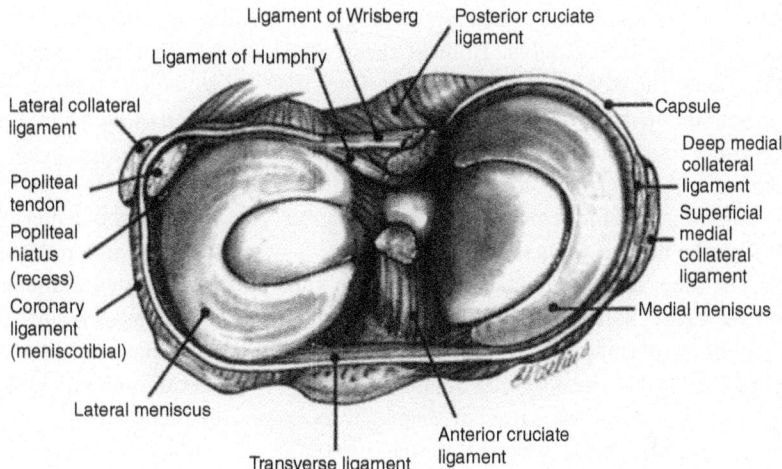

Fig. 14.3 Posterior aspect of the knee joint

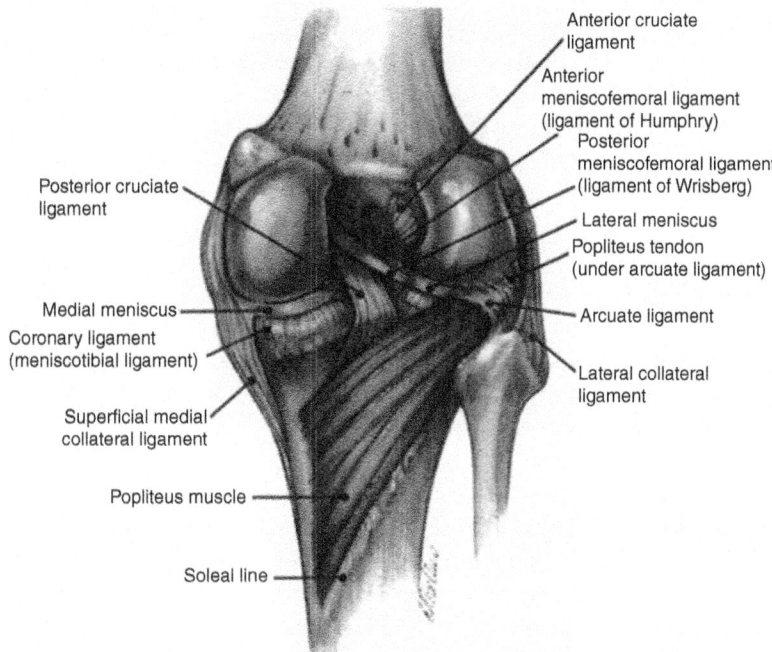

and the tensor fascia lata. The quadriceps is a group of four muscles all inserting onto the patella and patellar tendon, which in turn inserts upon the anterior tibial tubercle. The muscles that make up the quadriceps are the rectus femoris, vastus lateralis, vastus medialis, and vastus intermedius. These are all innervated by the femoral nerve. The tensor fascia lata originates upon the pelvic brim and inserts at Gerdy's tubercle on the proximal anterolateral tibia. The tensor fascia lata is innervated by the superior gluteal nerve.

The primary flexors of the knee are the hamstring muscles—semimembranosus, semitendinosus, and the biceps femoris—and the sartorius and gracilis. The hamstring muscles originate on the ischium and insert on the posterior medial and lateral proximal tibia. They receive their innervation from the sciatic nerve; all are innervated by the tibial division of the sciatic nerve except the short head of the biceps which is innervated by the peroneal division of the sciatic nerve. The sartorius originates from the anterior superior iliac spine and the gracilis originates from the pubis. Both of these muscles with the semitendinosus insert into the proximal medial tibia in the pes anserine (goose's foot, relating to the appearance of the three tendons inserting together). The sartorius is innervated by the femoral nerve and the gracilis by the obturator nerve.

The other muscles that serve to flex the knee are the gastrocnemius and popliteus which extend from the posterior aspect of the femoral condyles to the calcaneus and proximal tibia, respectively.

The menisci are two crescent-shaped fibrocartilaginous structures attached to the proximal tibial surface. They increase the surface area for weight-bearing, therefore, reducing the peak stress exerted upon the articular cartilage while also providing shock absorption. Additionally, they provide a small degree of stability to the knee by changing the relatively flat tibial articular surface to a cupped surface. The menisci are composed of dense organized cartilage tissue.

Biomechanics of the Knee

The mechanical axis of the lower extremity extends from the center of rotation of the hip to the center of the ankle joint. This normally crosses the knee joint in the lateral third of the medial tibial plateau. The normal anatomic alignment of the knee is 5–7° of valgus. When the knee is loaded, the medial compartment receives 60% of the weight-bearing stress and the lateral compartment receives 40% of the weight-bearing stress. This difference in the applied load in the normal knee is why the medial tibial plateau and medial femoral condyle are larger than the lateral side. Patients with significant angular deformity of the knee will have altered weight-bearing, resulting in increased stress in the medial (with varus or bow-legged deformity) or lateral (with valgus or knock-knee deformity) compartment. The increased stress will frequently result in early arthritis in the overused compartment of the knee.

The highest joint forces, however, are found in the patellofemoral articulation. Forces as high as three to five times the body weight across the patellofemoral articulation can be noted for activities such as stair climbing and jumping. The function of the patella is to provide a mechanical advantage to the quadriceps tendon. The patella moves the line of pull of the quadriceps further away from the center of rotation, thereby acting as a lever and reducing the force required to extend the knee. Patients who have had the patella removed as a result of arthritis or trauma are noted to have an approximately 30% reduction in the force in the quadriceps compared to patients with a patella.

Evaluation of the Painful Knee

History

The history should begin with the chief complaint and how long the patient has experienced the problem: the specific location of pain, any radiation, the nature of the pain (ache, burning, stabbing, etc.), and any exacerbating or ameliorating factors. The relationship of the pain with activity and rest is important to note in particular. Pain in the musculoskeletal system will commonly be relieved with rest. Severe pain that is present at rest can signal a septic process or neoplasm.

Frequently, knee problems begin with an injury. Detailed history describing the injury can be very helpful in determining the structures that are injured. The nature of any external force contacting the knee and the position of the knee at the time of injury should be elicited. Did an audible or palpable pop occur at the time of the injury? Shifting or abnormal movement of the knee may also have been noted at the time of injury. The degree and nature of any swelling around the knee are important to record. In addition to the description of injury, it is helpful to inquire about the patient's ability to use the knee after the injury: was the patient able to weight bear, was the onset of pain or swelling immediate or delayed, and could the patient flex or extend the knee after injury are important questions to ask the patient after knee injury.

In addition to pain, patients with knee problems will complain of mechanical problems in the knee. Patients may note an inability to fully bend or straighten the knee. This is referred to as locking of the knee. Locking can be a result of a loose body in the knee becoming lodged between the femoral condyle and tibial plateau, similar to a wedge "door stop." The patients who note intermittent locking of the knee will usually be able to relieve the locked knee by gently moving the knee without weight-bearing. This maneuver allows the loose fragment to be released from between the femur and tibia and motion will be restored. However, inability to fully flex and extend the knee can also be noted in patients with large effusions and ligament injuries.

Instability is another frequent complaint of patients with knee injuries. Patients will observe that their knee will shift or buckle with particular activities. Instability can result from two general etiologies. The first is ligamentous injuries. As noted previously, the stability of the knee is a result of the ligaments which cross from the tibia to the femur. Disruption of the ligaments will result in alteration of knee function; the knee may shift or subluxate with activity. The second common cause of a knee buckling or giving way is problems in the patellofemoral joint. Instability of the patella in the trochlear groove will result in a giving way sensation as the patella subluxates. Damage to the articular surfaces of the patella or the trochlear groove will result in pain as the patella tracks over the trochlea. This can occasionally lead to a sharp acute pain which will lead to the quadriceps releasing its contraction while the patient is weight-bearing on the leg as a result of a primitive reflex arc. The patient will note a giving way or buckling sensation in the knee and a few patients may actually fall as a result.

The majority of knee complaints are aggravated by activities. The specific problems the patient has encountered are important to note. Patients will commonly have difficulty ascending and descending stairs. Frequently descending stairs will be the most symptomatic as this places high stress across the patellofemoral joint. Bicycling can also aggravate the patellofemoral joint. Activities that involve quadriceps contrac-tion with the knee in flexion may result in subluxation in patients with patellar instability. Patients with meniscal tears will have difficulty squatting and may notice snapping or pain when rising from a chair or ascending stairs. Activities that involve stopping and turning or cutting will result in the knee shifting or giving way if there is insufficiency in the collateral or cruciate ligaments.

Physical Examination

Physical examination of the patient with a knee complaint begins with inspection. Observation of the alignment of the lower extremity should demonstrate a normal 5–7° valgus angle at the knee when a patient is standing. Deformity of the leg in varus or valgus beyond the normal 5–7° can be associated with either a ligamentous or osseous deficiency. Any swelling, bruising, or ecchymosis should be recorded. Next, the evaluation should focus on the patient's gait. Normal gait requires the range of motion from 0 to 65° of flexion. The gait should have a smooth cadence with the length of each step being equal on the left and right sides. The knee should not demonstrate any sudden shift to either the lateral or medial side. If abnormal lateral motion is noted, this is recorded as a medial or lateral thrust, respectively.

The knee should then be examined with the patient sitting with their legs over the edge of the examining table. The position of the patella should be anterior and symmetric. The patellar tracking can then be followed by asking the patient to flex and extend the knee with the examiner palpating the patella. There should be little lateral movement. Crepitus may also be noted as a grinding sensation between the patella and the femoral trochlear groove.

The knee should then be examined with the patient supine. For all aspects of the examination, the contralateral knee can be used as a normal control. Effusion or fluid within the knee can be assessed by placing both hands on the knee with one below the patella and one above the patella. Any fluid in the knee can then be displaced and palpated proximally and distally. The knee can be palpated to determine the specific site of maximum tenderness. The range of motion of the knee is measured with the knee in straight extension as 0° of flexion; normal full flexion is approximately 135°.

The collateral ligaments are then assessed by stabilizing the thigh with one hand and placing a varus or valgus stress on the knee with the other hand. A normal knee will have a small amount of medial and lateral laxity in the collateral ligaments. However, any laxity which is excessive or if pain is elicited should be noted. The cruciate ligaments can also be assessed. The anterior cruciate ligament is best assessed using the Lachman test. The examiner should stand by the patient's feet. The femur is stabilized with one hand holding the distal medial thigh. The tibia is then held with a thumb at the lateral joint line. The examiner then attempts to displace the tibia forward in relation to the femur. Translation less than 5 mm should be noted and the anterior cruciate ligament should be felt to "snap taut" in the normal knee. Injury to the posterior cruciate ligament can be demonstrated by noting the degree of recurvatum (back-knee) which can be obtained passively compared to the contralateral knee. Also, with both knees flexed 60–90° and the patient supine, the tibia on the deficient side will be noted to sag posteriorly compared to the uninjured leg when viewed from the side. A posterior drawer can be performed with the knee bent at 90° and exerting a posterior force on the tibia. There should be less than 5 mm of translation. Comparison to the contralateral knee is very important for examination of the collateral and cruciate ligaments.

The menisci are examined by palpation of their outer margin along the joint line at the proximal tibial articular surface. In addition, meniscal tears can be detected by the McMurray maneuver. This is done by flexing the knee internally and externally rotating the tibia and then extending the knee with a valgus force applied. If a reproducible snap is palpated or pain elicited at the joint line, this is suggestive of a tear. Patients with meniscal tears will also report pain when asked to squat down with the knees flexed. The most sensitive test for the meniscus is simple joint line tenderness.

Imaging

All of the available imaging techniques have been utilized in the evaluation of patients with knee problems. Plain radiographs are the most commonly obtained studies (Fig. 14.4). Plain radiographs are helpful in the evaluation of fractures and subluxation of the joint, and the condition of the articular surfaces can be investigated. The standard series of routine X-rays of the knee should include a standing anteroposterior (AP) radiograph of both knees, a lateral view and a merchant or "sunrise view." The sunrise view is a view taken with the knee in 45° of flexion with the beam directed inferiorly and parallel to the patellar articular surface. There should be a space of 5–10 mm between the ends of the femoral condyles and the tibial surface and beneath the patellar surface and the femoral trochlea. This "clear space" is in fact occupied by the articular cartilage.

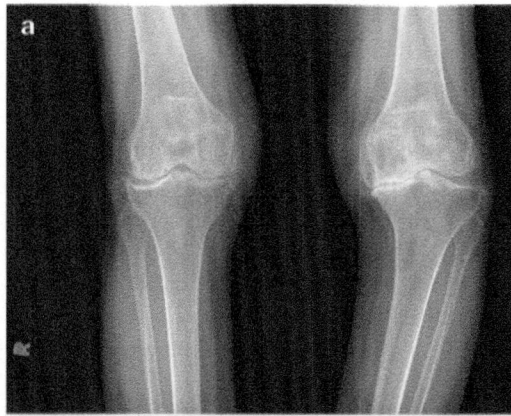
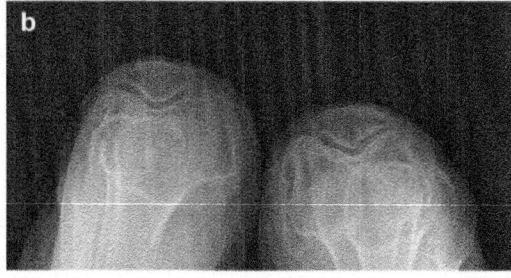

Fig. 14.4 (**a**) Standing, weight-bearing AP radiograph of both knees in an 87-year-old female with osteoarthritis of both knees with a windswept deformity (right knee valgus, left knee varus alignment). Note the asymmetric space between the medial and lateral femoral condyles and the tibial surface. (**b**) Sunrise view of the bilateral knees, useful in evaluating the patellofemoral joint space, reasonably well preserved in this patient

Routine radiography is an excellent tool for the evaluation of the knee for trauma, arthritis, and alignment. Plain radiographs, however, only demonstrate the osseous structures. As mentioned earlier, the soft tissues provide stability and allow the knee to function. Arthrography has been used in the past to evaluate the knee for meniscal pathology. However, this technique was inaccurate and invasive. The development of arthroscopy allows the direct visualization of the structures within the knee in a minor surgical procedure. However, this technique is also invasive and while arthroscopy is accurate, the procedure is relatively expensive compared to an imaging modality alone. Nuclear medicine studies are of limited use in the knee. These studies are sensitive; however, the specificity of these studies is limited. Magnetic resonance imaging (MRI) has provided a dramatic step forward in the ability to diagnose soft tissue injury to the knee. MRI provides accurate and non-invasive evaluation of all the soft tissue structures within the knee (Fig. 14.5). MRI is currently the study of choice for the evaluation of intra-articular pathology within the knee.

Computed tomography (CT) is another excellent imaging modality for cross-sectional evaluation of both the osseous and soft tissue structures of the knee. In the setting of periarticular trauma such as tibial plateau fractures, CT scans are invaluable to the treating surgeon as they characterize and evaluate fracture patterns and incongruity about the joint surface and significantly help with surgical planning. Additionally, CT can detect the presence of air or fluid within the joint and any bony or soft tissue masses or infectious processes about the knee.

Knee Pathology

Soft tissue injury is common in the knee. A knee with a bloody effusion after an injury has an incidence as high as 80% of significant soft tissue injury. The differential diagnosis of a post-traumatic bloody effusion in the absence of an intra-articular fracture includes most commonly a meniscal tear, an ACL tear, or a patellar dislocation.

Meniscal Tears

Tears of the meniscus can occur in two settings. One is the result of a specific injury. This usually involves a twisting injury with the knee in some flexion. Swelling and pain are noted immediately after the injury. There is increased pain with attempts at movement and there is a limitation in the range of motion. Pain with squatting down or arising from a chair is commonly reported. The torn meniscus can block regular joint motion. Occasionally, the knee can be gently manipulated to reduce the torn meniscal fragment and motion will be restored. However, the fragment will frequently re-displace and intermittent locking may occur. This form of tear is usually in younger patients with stout meniscal tissue.

In older individuals, the meniscal tissues soften and the edges become torn and frayed. As

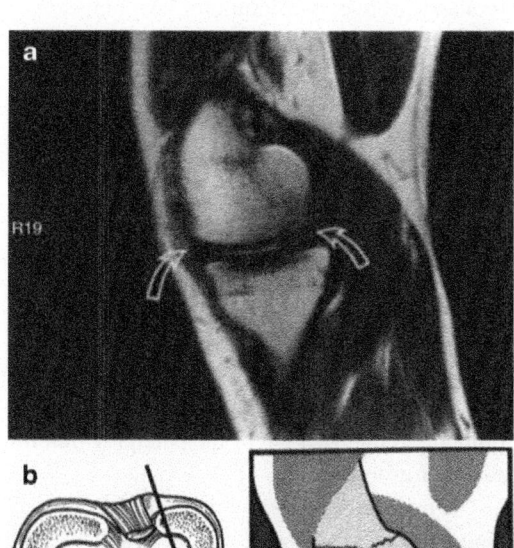

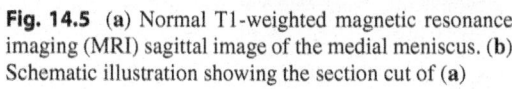

Fig. 14.5 (a) Normal T1-weighted magnetic resonance imaging (MRI) sagittal image of the medial meniscus. (b) Schematic illustration showing the section cut of (a)

this occurs, the frayed edges can become entrapped between the edges of the bone initiating a tear which can extend into the meniscal substance. This tear can occur with little or no trauma with minimal swelling and pain initially. The diagnosis is made by complaints of pain along the medial or lateral joint line, medial or lateral joint line tenderness, effusion, and, rarely, locking. Patients with locking will frequently require arthroscopic surgery to debride the torn portion of the meniscus. In older patients with meniscal tears, if the tear does not cause mechanical symptoms, it frequently can be treated with nonsteroidal anti-inflammatory medications and an intra-articular corticosteroid injection. These treatments will reduce the effusion and pain. With continued activity, the soft meniscal tissue can be worn down and a stable edge reestablished. However, for some persistently symptomatic cases, arthroscopic meniscectomy is curative (Fig. 14.6).

Ligament Injuries

Injury to the ligamentous structures manifest as instability in the knee. The four major ligaments of the knee are the medial collateral ligament, lateral collateral ligament, anterior cruciate ligament, and posterior cruciate ligament. Their location and function is described in detail in a previous section of this chapter. In addition to pain and swelling, patients will report a sense of the knee shifting or giving way. This may be with only specific activities, such as descending stairs

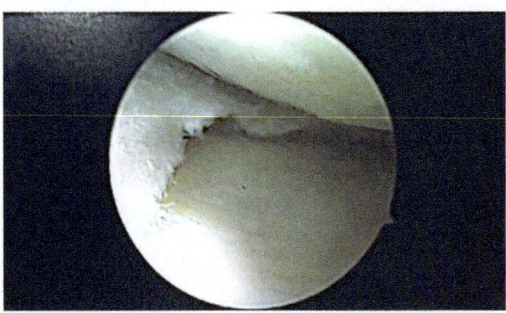

Fig. 14.6 Arthroscopic image of a frayed, torn medial meniscus in an active 69-year-old female

or when turning on the loaded extremity. The initial management of these injuries is rest, ice, and elevation. A splint or knee immobilizer can also be helpful to protect the knee. As the initial pain subsides, it is important to begin to work on restoring the range of motion using a brace to protect the injured ligament. As the pain further decreases, strengthening is begun. If the knee remains unstable after the strengthening program is completed, the patient may be a candidate for surgical reconstruction.

Patellofemoral Pathology

The patellofemoral joint is one of the most common areas of pain in the knee. Common complaints are anterior knee pain which is aggravated by activities involving high loads on a flexed knee, such as stair climbing, running, and bicycling. This pain can be the result of degenerative changes in the patellofemoral articulation or a result of maltracking of the patella within the trochlear groove. A grinding or snapping sensation may also be noted. Pain is usually relieved by rest; however, if the patient is sitting for a prolonged period of time with the knee flexed, such as in a theater, on a plane, or during a long car ride, anterior knee pain will result. Frequently, patients will try to change the position of the knee to relieve their discomfort. This symptom is referred to as "movie sign" and is indicative of stress in the patellofemoral joint. Softening of the articular surface is referred to as chondromalacia patella. This can be a primary problem or it may be secondary to excessive trauma to the joint due to maltracking of the patella within the trochlear groove.

The treatment of these conditions is primarily nonoperative. Improving the patellar tracking can be done through a series of exercises to retrain the quadriceps, abductor strengthening at the hip, and through patellar mobilization exercises. The exercise program needs to be maintained for a minimum of 6–8 weeks to demonstrate benefit. The symptoms can frequently be recurrent. If the symptoms are recurrent and do not respond to the nonoperative regimen and patellar maltracking is evident, operative intervention may be indicated. Operative intervention is directed at correcting the patellar tracking and to maximize the quadriceps function with postoperative physical therapy.

Arthritis

While numerous etiologies of arthritis in the knee exist, including rheumatoid and septic, this section will focus on the most commonly encountered form seen and managed by orthopedists: osteoarthritis. This progressive, degenerative, and debilitating condition affects over 250 million people worldwide and is likely to increase in prevalence with the continued upward shift of the mean population age. While it is now known that a cascade of inflammatory changes and both chondral and associated soft tissue remodeling is involved in the pathogenesis of osteoarthritis, it remains debated as to the exact sequence or predisposing conditions that initiate the degenerative pathways that cause this painful process to occur. Ultimately, the end result is cartilage wear, osteophyte formation, and potential imbalance of the normal alignment of the knee joint (Fig. 14.7).

The management of arthritic symptoms within the knee is similar to the management of arthritis elsewhere. The nonoperative management of arthritis within the knee consists of a five-modality approach. The first line of therapy is the use of nonsteroidal anti-inflammatory drugs (NSAIDs). These medications will reduce the pain and swelling associated with the knee. Although all of the NSAIDs function in a similar fashion, there is a wide variation in individual patient response. Therefore, minimally two or three different NSAIDs should be tried. The most common side effect of this course of treatment is gastritis and gastrointestinal (GI) intolerance.

The second line of treatment of arthritis is the selected use of intra-articular corticosteroid medication. This can be effective in patients who have an acute exacerbation of the arthritic pain. The injection can quiet their pain and restore them to a baseline level of discomfort. The injection should not be utilized for the control of baseline pain. If the injection is required at a frequency of greater than once every 3 months, some other course of treatment should be initiated, such as surgery. If the knee is injected more frequently three times per year, the corticosteroid may have a detrimental effect on the articular cartilage. Other forms of injections include hyaluronic acid derivatives and platelet-rich plasma. These injections do not have the detrimental effect of corticosteroids, although they are often not as effective.

Physical therapy can be very helpful in the treatment of arthritis of the knee. As the soft tissue sleeve is very important to the function of the knee, optimizing functions of the soft tissues can reduce the symptoms of arthritis. The physical therapy should be directed at maintaining the range of motion of the knee and optimizing the strength of the quadriceps and the hamstring

Fig. 14.7 Comparison illustration of healthy and arthritic knee joints

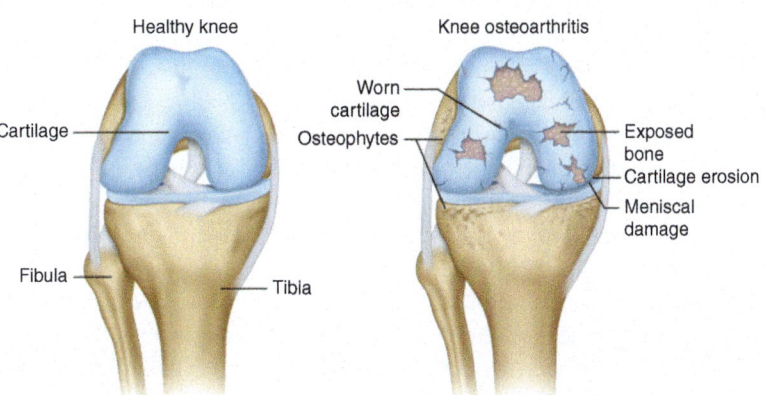

muscles. In the late stages of degenerative arthritis, physical therapy may worsen the patient's symptoms and should be limited to a program within the patient's tolerance.

Assistive devices such as a cane or crutch may aid in the management of arthritis of the knee. This can limit the stress across the painful knee and improve the patient's walking tolerance. The final approach to the management of arthritis of the knee is modification of activities. This includes alterations of the patient's activities such as sports, work environment, and possibly even assisting in arranging special parking for the patient. Frequently, patients with significant knee arthritis are also overweight. Weight loss in these patients can significantly reduce symptoms and the need for other treatment modalities. As the force across the knee joint may be three to five times the patient's body weight, weight loss can have a significant impact on a patient's knee symptoms.

Surgical Reconstruction for Arthritis

When all nonoperative measures have failed to relieve the symptoms of knee arthritis, surgical intervention should be contemplated. The surgical correction of knee arthritis can be separated into treatments which retain the patient's articular surfaces and knee replacement. Non-replacement options include the use of arthroscopy to "clean out" the knee; this procedure can remove the small cartilage fragments that accumulate in arthritic joints and debride any loose articular fragments and degenerative meniscal tears. This procedure should be reserved for patients with minimal arthritis only and is contraindicated for moderate to severe arthritis as it will frequently worsen the symptoms. In that setting, the patient is a candidate for knee replacement.

Patients with osteoarthritis of the knee will frequently develop angular deformities. The most common deformity is varus angulation of the knee. This results from erosion of the medial compartment of the knee. As the deformity progresses, a greater portion of the weight-bearing stress is concentrated in the medial compartment of the knee. Osteotomy is a procedure to realign the articulation. The proximal tibia is transected

and a wedge of bone is removed from the lateral aspect or a wedge can be inserted on the medial side. This will result in a correction of the alignment and the varus deformity. It also redistributes some of the weight-bearing stress to the lateral compartment and can result in improved symptoms in the knee. The result is generally successful for 5–10 years. Osteotomy is contraindicated in knees which are stiff or unstable. When the symptoms return, knee replacement surgery is indicated.

Arthrodesis or fusion of the knee is an option for the management of young active patients, particularly physical laborers. This will result in a stiff straight knee that will allow the patient to ambulate and stand for long periods of time without difficulty. However, significant limitations also exist. The gait pattern is significantly abnormal. In addition, patients will have difficulty sitting, particularly in confined spaces such as public transportation and theaters. Resection arthroplasty is a procedure where the articular surfaces are resected and a fibrous pseudoarthrosis forms within the joint space. Pain may be decreased; however, the knee is significantly unstable, requiring a brace for ambulation. Arthrodesis and resection arthroplasty are not commonly performed anymore as replacements are the mainstay of operative management of the arthritic knee. Currently, these procedures are reserved for the management of a failed total knee replacement.

Total knee replacement (TKR) is commonly utilized to relieve the symptoms of knee arthritis and restore function (Fig. 14.8). Approximately 250,000 arthroplasties are performed annually in the United States; the average age of patients receiving a TKR is 65–70 years. Successful results can be obtained in over 95% of patients with survivorship at 10–15 years of 90%. Components are typically fixed with polymethylmethacrylate (PMMA) bone cement. Non-cemented components, those used with porous ingrowth surfaces for bone ingrowth, have previously been associated with a higher incidence of loosening and pain, though advances continue to be made in this technique.

The proximal tibia is cut perpendicular to the long axis of the shaft, and the femoral articular

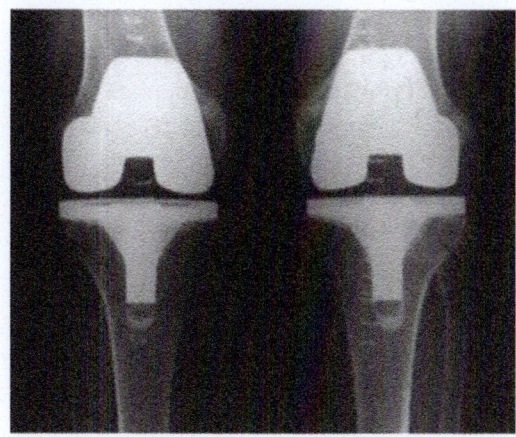

Fig. 14.8 Standing AP radiograph of both knees 2 weeks after one stage bilateral knee replacements

surface is cut using specific guides to remove the femoral trochlea, distal and posterior femoral condyles. The anterior cruciate ligament is removed; however, the posterior cruciate ligament can be resected or retained depending on the design of the implant chosen. For proper function of the arthroplasty, the MCL, LCL, and, if retained, PCL must be carefully balanced. The components are then fixed to the surfaces of the tibia and femur with bone cement. The patella is normally resurfaced as well after resecting the articular surface parallel to the anterior surface.

The patient is mobilized quickly following the procedure, and full weight-bearing may be allowed immediately. Perineural anesthesia, introduced as a single shot preoperatively or infused via catheter for patients remaining under observation postoperatively, has dramatically improved peri-procedural discomfort and enabled earlier mobilization. The critical element of postoperative therapy is the restoration of motion. If motion is not restored within the first 3–6 weeks, maturation of scar tissue may prevent major gains in motion after that point. Many total knee replacements are now performed as outpatient procedures, with patients returning home on postoperative day zero.

Frequently, however, these patients will require physical therapy after discharge to continue to work on the range of motion and ambulation in the first few weeks after surgery. While the total rehabilitation period after total knee replace-

ment is between 3 and 6 months, patients are functionally mobile after 2–3 weeks. Knee replacement can be performed bilaterally in one stage in medically healthy patients. The initial increase in debilitation postoperatively is offset by a reduction in the overall period of rehabilitation after sequential unilateral TKR.

Aseptic loosening of the implants after TKR occurs at a low rate. Several studies have documented a 15-year survivorship of greater than 90% and less than 0.5% per year rate of aseptic loosening after cemented TKR. If a TKR is noted to be loose prior to 5 years, it should be evaluated for deep infection. Deep sepsis is associated with early loosening after total knee replacement. Young age, marked obesity, and high demand will also negatively impact the long-term survival of the replacement. To date, the best data for non-cemented TKR is equal to the cemented replacement. Several studies suggest poorer results when cement is not used, particularly for fixation of the tibial component. Increased tibial loosening and pain have been noted with these devices. At present, due to the generally increased cost for non-cemented porous-coated implants and poorer clinical results, the use of these devices is difficult to justify.

The majority of complaints after cemented TKR are from the patellofemoral joint, which can be the result of poor soft tissue alignment at the time of arthroplasty. This may lead to painful subluxation or dislocation of the patellar component. If inadequate bone is resected from the patella at the time of resurfacing, a marked increase in the patellofemoral stress can be noted which may become painful. Some surgeons have advocated not resurfacing the patella; however, several studies now demonstrate a higher rate of patellofemoral complaints after TKR without patellar resurfacing. If significant patellofemoral arthritis exists at the time of arthroplasty, patients with weights greater than 60 kg and heights greater than 160 cm will have more pain postoperatively if the patella is not resurfaced.

The most common complication after TKR is thromboembolic disease (TED). The rate of asymptomatic deep venous thrombosis ranges from 25 to 50% of cases without prophylaxis in patients evaluated with venography or duplex

Doppler analysis. Similar to patients receiving total hip replacement (THR), it is currently recommended that all patients receive some form of prophylaxis against TED. Mechanical methods, such as the pneumatic compression stockings, appear to have a greater benefit after THR compared to TKR. Aspirin and low molecular weight heparin are two common medications used although there are several other anti-coagulant medications on the market as well. Some form of anti-coagulant medication is recommended and necessary.

Deep infection occurs at a rate of approximately 1% after TKR for osteoarthritis over the life of the implant. The most common organisms are skin flora, primarily *Staphylococcus aureus* and *S. epidermidis*. In particular to knee replacement, the relatively thin soft tissue envelope at the inferior aspect of the skin incision can lead to wound dehiscence and allow entry of the flora into the joint (Fig. 14.9). Any area of

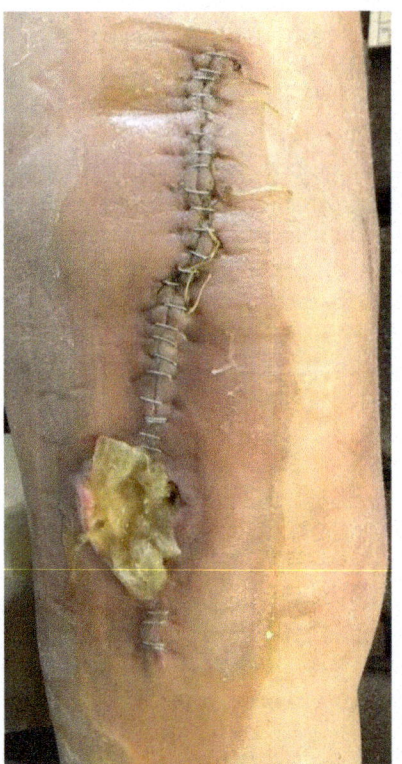

Fig. 14.9 Infection and surgical wound breakdown status post total knee replacement

skin breakdown after TKR should be treated aggressively to prevent deep infection. This is particularly true in patients with prior incisions and in those with diabetes or significant vascular disease.

If a deep infection is established, the only way to eradicate the infection is to remove the implants and all of the bone cement and thoroughly debride the joint. An antibiotic impregnated cement spacer is often placed into the joint space although single stage revisions can be performed. The patient should receive 6 weeks of intravenous (IV) antibiotics. After 6 weeks, the knee can be reimplanted if adequate soft tissue and bone remain. However, due to the inevitable scarring, the clinical result is compromised. There is some evidence suggestive that deep infections identified early enough can be managed without sacrificing initial implants, though results from this practice vary.

Occasionally after TKR, the range of motion of the knee does not progress well after surgery. If the patient is less than 2–6 weeks after surgery, a gentle manipulation of the knee in the operating room under anesthesia may be beneficial. If the motion cannot be restored, particularly if the patient is beyond 6 weeks after replacement, additional surgery may be necessary to restore functional range of motion.

Summary and Conclusions

The knee is a complex joint with function provided by the combination of osseous and soft tissue structures. The soft tissue envelope plays a significant role in the pathology of the knee and in the management of these conditions. With careful history, physical examination, and appropriate use of the available diagnostic modalities, knee pathology can be accurately diagnosed and successful treatment instituted. Successful management of knee pathology includes treatment of the specific etiology, but optimal management of the soft tissue envelope with directed physical therapy is essential to an optimal outcome.

Further Reading

Heck DA, Murray DG. Biomechanics in the knee. In: Evarts CM, editor. Surgery of the musculoskeletal system. 2nd ed. New York, NY: Churchill Livingston; 1990. p. 3243–54.

Katz JN, Arant KR, Thornhill TS. Knee osteoarthritis. In: Schoenfeld AJ, Blauwet CA, Katz JN, editors. Principles of orthopedic practice for primary care providers. Cham: Springer; 2021.

Mora JC, Przkora R, Cruz-Almeida Y. Knee osteoarthritis: pathophysiology and current treatment modalities. J Pain Res. 2018;11:2189–96.

Rand JA, Ilstrup DM. Survivorship analysis of total knee arthroplasty. Cumulative rates of survival of 9200 total knee arthroplasties. J Bone Joint Surg Am. 1991;73(3):397–409.

Ruiz-Pérez JS, Gómez-Cardero P, Rodríguez-Merchán EC. The infected total knee arthroplasty. In: Rodríguez-Merchán E, Gómez-Cardero P, editors. Comprehensive treatment of knee osteoarthritis. Cham: Springer; 2020.

Stavrakis A, Arshi A, Chiou D, Hsiue P, Horneff JG 3rd, Photopoulos C. Cemented versus noncemented total knee arthroplasty outcomes. J Am Acad Orthop Surg. 2022;30(6):273–80.

Stern SH, Insall JN. Posterior stabilized prosthesis. Results after follow-up of nine to twelve years. J Bone Joint Surg Am. 1992;74(7):980–6.

Windsor RE, Bono JV. Infected total knee replacements. J Am Acad Orthop Surg. 1994;2:44–53.

The Foot and Ankle

15

Paul S. Cooper, Nicholas D. Casscells,
and Julia A. McCann

Anatomy

The bony anatomy of the foot and ankle consists of the distal tibia and fibula in the leg and the 26 major bones that compose the foot, 28 if you include the sesamoids. The tibia distally terminates into the metaphyseal plafond with its medial malleolus. The lateral surface of the distal tibia has a sulcus to accommodate the adjacent fibula, forming the distal tibiofibular joint. The distal fibula which lies laterally and slightly posterior to the tibia is held there by the inferior tibiofibular ligaments. The fibula forms the lateral malleolus of the ankle joint. The relationship of the fibula to the tibia is not static. With ankle dorsiflexion, the fibula laterally translates, proximally migrates, and externally rotates.

The ankle is a diarthrodial joint (Figs. 15.1 and 15.2). It consists of an articulation between the talus and the mortise of the tibia and fibula. Dorsiflexion of the ankle joint is coupled with eversion of the foot, and plantar flexion is combined with inversion. The distal fibula provides a static buttress over the talus laterally and bears

1/6 of the transmitted weight during the stance phase of gait. The foot is composed of seven tarsals, five metatarsals, and 14 phalanges. Three anatomic groupings are defined for descriptive purposes: the hindfoot, the midfoot, and the forefoot (Fig. 15.3). The hindfoot consists of the talus and calcaneus bones. The talus consists of a body, neck, and head. Two-thirds of the talus is covered by articular cartilage. There is no muscle or tendon attachments on this bone. The talar dome is the superior portion of the body which articulates with the mortise of the tibia and fibula. The dome is wider anteriorly, which allows for stability in the mortise during dorsiflexion. Posteriorly, a sulcus is formed between the posterolateral and posteromedial tubercles to accommodate the flexor hallucis longus (FHL) tendon. If prominent, this structure is often referred to as the Stieda process or os trigonom if detached from the talus. The inferior surface of the talus articulates with the corresponding facet of the calcaneus to create a subtalar joint. The calcaneus is the largest bone in the foot, with its longitudinal axis directed dorsally and laterally. Its superior surface articulates with the talus and three facets—anterior, medial, and posterior—to form the subtalar joint (Fig. 15.4). The large posterior facet articulates with the corresponding articular facet on the inferior surface of the talus. The middle facet overlies the sustentaculum tali (a dense, medial projection of the calcaneus that contains a groove to accommodate the FHL tendon sheath)

P. S. Cooper · N. D. Casscells · J. A. McCann (✉)
MedStar Georgetown Orthopedic Institute,
Georgetown University School of Medicine,
Washington, DC, USA

Department of Orthopedics, MedStar Georgetown
University Hospital, Washington, DC, USA
e-mail: Nick.casscells@gunet.georgetown.edu;
Julia.A.McCann@medstar.net

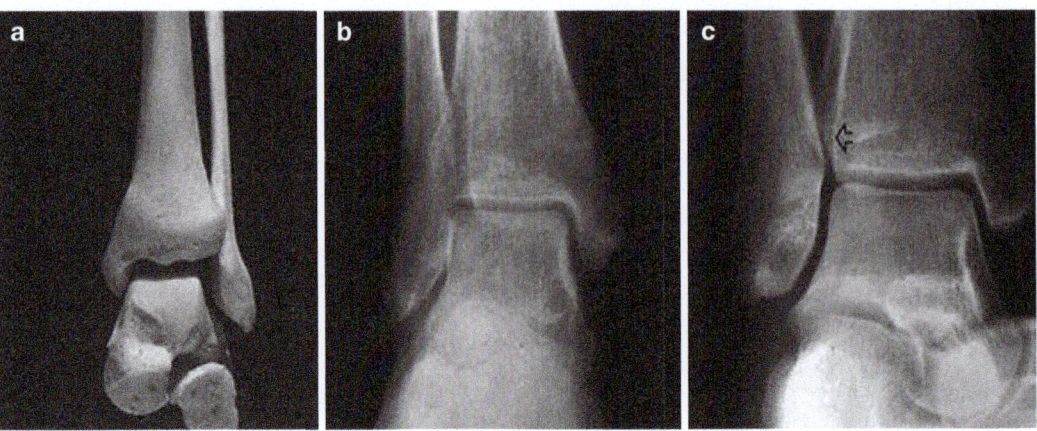

Fig. 15.1 (**a, b**) Photographic diagrammatic and radiologic anatomy of the normal ankle in anteroposterior views. (**c**) Note equal width of cartilage spaces and alignment of lateral talus with posterior cortex (*arrow*) on mortise view. (Reprinted from *Orthopedic Radiology*, Weissman BNW & Sledge CB, The Ankle, p. 590, Copyright Saunders (1985), with permission from Elsevier)

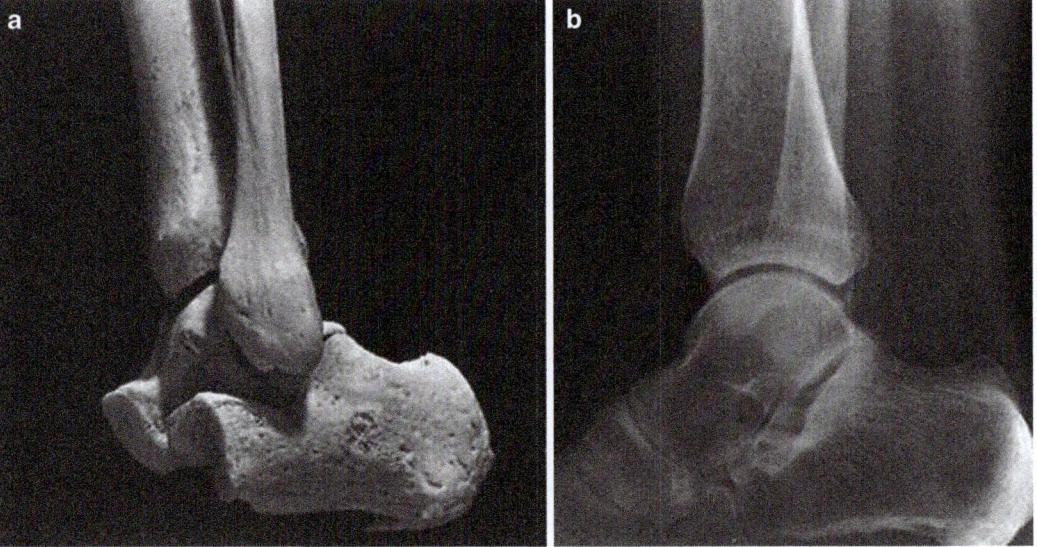

Fig. 15.2 Photographic (**a**) and radiologic (**b**) anatomy of the normal ankle in lateral projection. (Reprinted from *Orthopedic Radiology*, Weissman BNW & Sledge CB, The Ankle, p. 591, Copyright Saunders (1985), with permission from Elsevier)

and is often merged with the anterior facet. The middle facets and anterior facets articulate with the undersurface of the talar head.

The midfoot consists of the navicular, cuboid, and three cuneiform bones. The tarsonavicular bone articulates with the talar head and lies medially to the cuboid bone. It functions as a keystone for the medial longitudinal arch of the foot. The distal surface is composed of three facets that articulate with the medial, middle, and lateral

cuneiform bones, respectively. The medial pole of the navicular is also the primary insertion site for the posterior tibial tendon. In 10% of people, an unfused accessory navicular bone may be present, also known as an os navicular. The cuboid bone forms an articulation with the calcaneus proximally and the fourth and fifth metatarsals distally. Laterally, a groove within the cuboid accommodates the peroneus longus tendon as it courses plantarly. It is not uncommon to have a

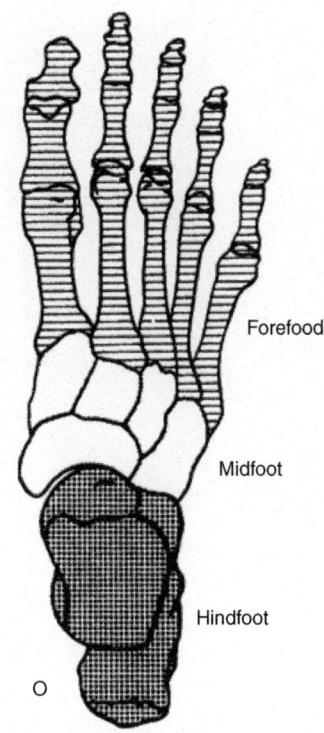

Fig. 15.3 Anatomic regions of the foot. (Reprinted from *Orthopedic Radiology*, Weissman BNW & Sledge CB, The Foot, p. 628, Copyright Saunders (1985), with permission from Elsevier)

sesamoid bone within the peroneus longus at this location referred to as an os peroneum. Three cuneiform bones have distal articulations with the first, second, and third metatarsals and contribute to the formation of part of the tarsometatarsal or Lisfranc's joint (Fig. 15.5). The middle cuneiform bone is shorter axially, adding to greater stability in the second tarsometatarsal joint. This is also known as the keystone.

The forefoot consists of the metatarsal and phalangeal bones. Five metatarsals terminate distally with articulations to the proximal phalanges creating metatarsal phalangeal (MTP) joints. The fifth metatarsal has a prominent styloid process proximally to which the peroneus brevis attaches dorsally, and the lateral band of the plantar fascia attaches on the plantar aspect. Each of the lesser toes, two through five, has three phalanges—a proximal, middle, and distal phalanx—and the hallux has only two phalanges, proximal and distal. Each distal phalanx terminates in a tuft of bone and serves as an anchor for the toe pad. Underlying the first MTP joint are the two sesamoid bones. Tibial (medial) and fibular (lateral) sesamoid bones are encased by the flexor hallucis

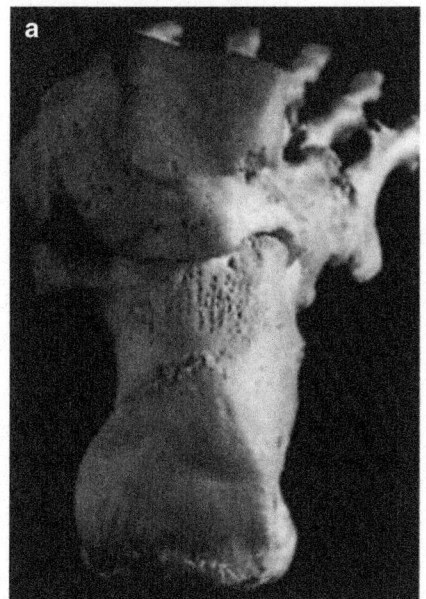

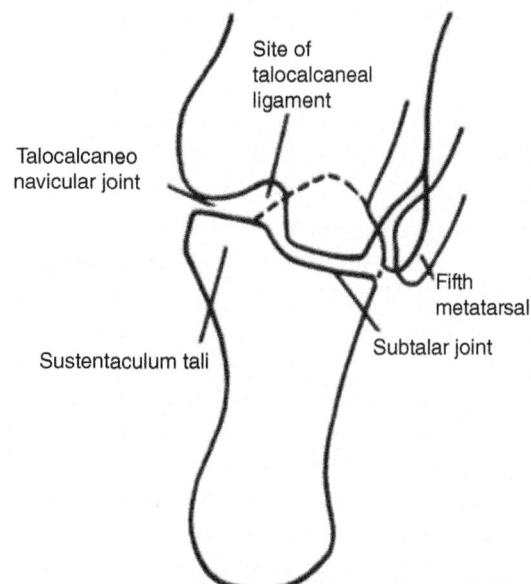

Fig. 15.4 Photographic (**a**) and diagrammatic (**b**) anatomy of the normal ankle in tangential calcaneal (Harris) projection. (Reprinted from *Orthopedic Radiology*, Weissman BNW & Sledge CB, The Foot, p. 628, Copyright Saunders (1985), with permission from Elsevier)

Fig. 15.5 Photographic, diagrammatic, and radiologic anatomy of the normal foot in posteroanterior (**a**, **b**) and internal oblique (**c**, **d**) projections. (Reprinted from *Orthopedic Radiology*, Weissman BNW & Sledge CB, <u>The Foot</u>, p. 626, Copyright Saunders (1985), with permission from Elsevier)

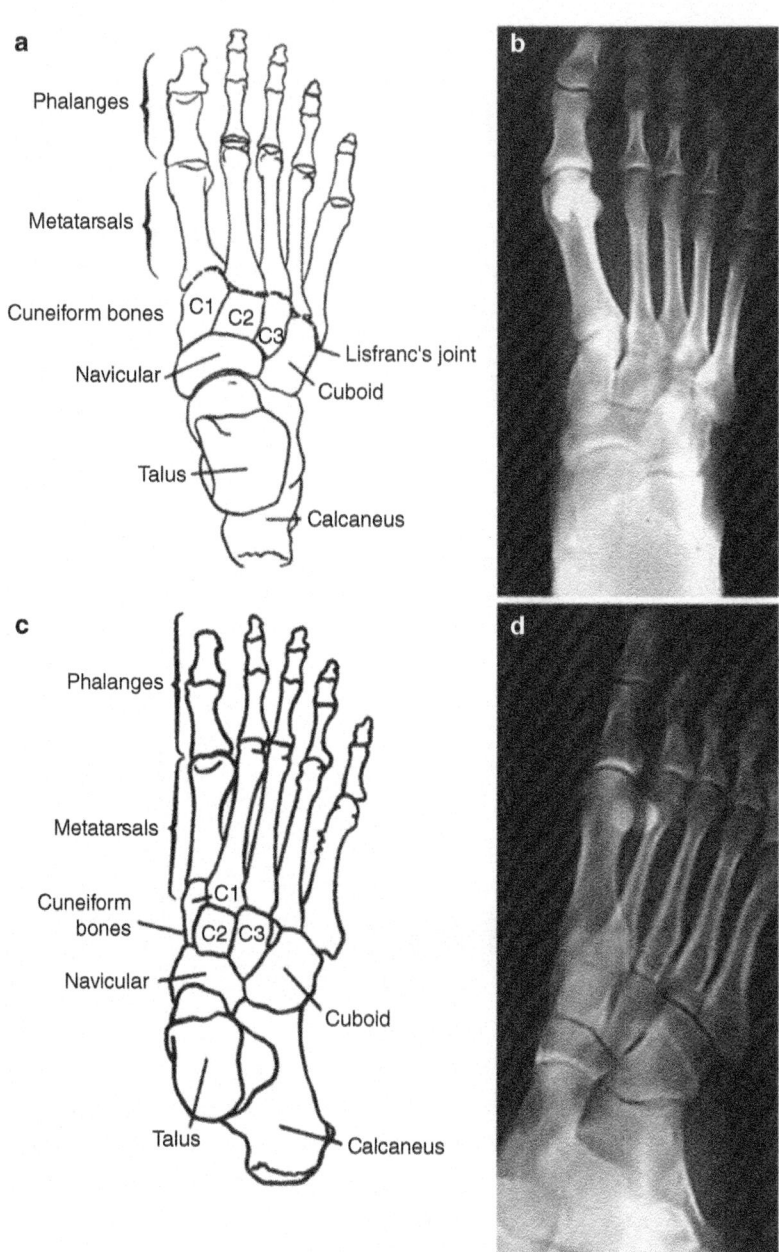

brevis tendon (FHB) which inserts at the base of the proximal phalanx and comprise the plantar plate of the great toe.

Ligaments

The ligamentous structures of the ankle joint (Fig. 15.6) include the medial deltoid ligament complex and the lateral ankle ligament complex. The deltoid ligament medially has both superficial and deep components and is the primary contributor to medial stability of the ankle joint. The superficial component is responsible for the majority of the strength of the deltoid ligament. The lateral ligament complex consists of three major ligaments including the anterior talofibular ligament (ATFL), the calcaneofibular ligament (CFL), and the posterior talofibular ligament (PTFL). These contribute to lateral stability of the ankle joint.

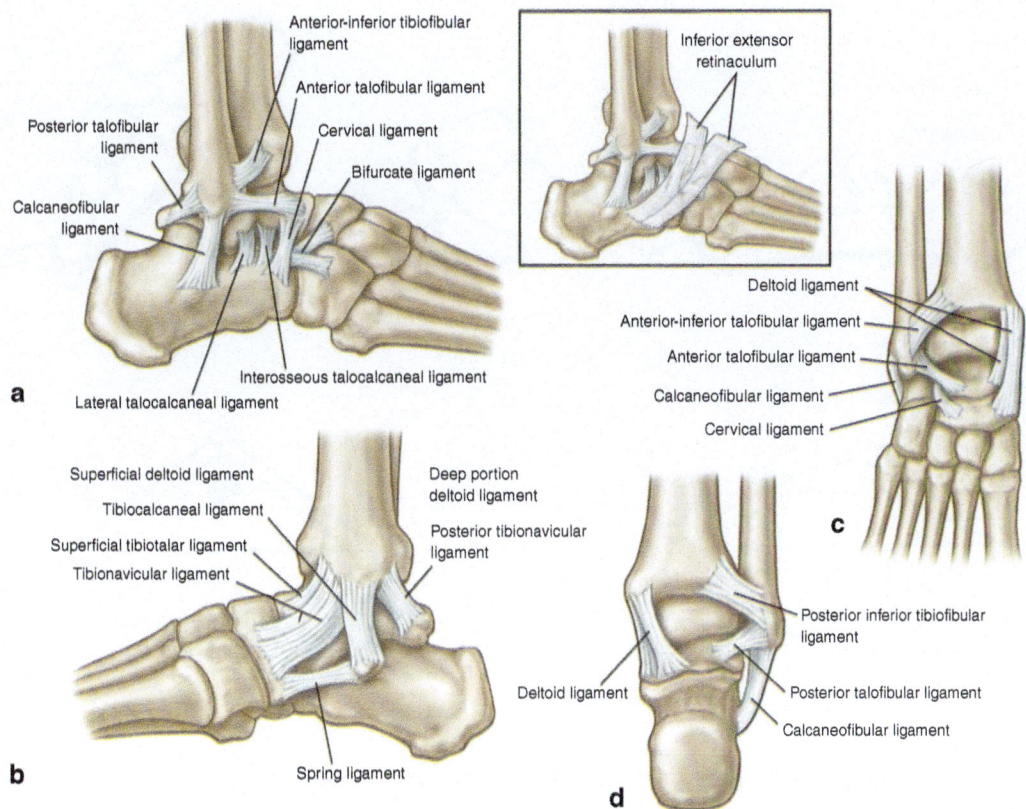

Fig. 15.6 Ligaments of the foot and ankle seen from the (**a**) lateral view of the foot and ankle, (**b**) medial view of the foot and ankle, (**c**) anterior view of the ankle and hindfoot, and (**d**) posterior view of the ankle and hindfoot. Not pictured are two components of the syndesmosis: the interosseous membrane which runs between the fibula and tibia, and the inferior transverse ligament which is a posterior structure running from the lateral malleolus across the posterior border of the tibial plafond. (Reprinted from *DeLee, Drez & Miller's Orthopaedic Sports Medicine*, Miller MD & Thompson SR, Ligamentous Injuries of the Foot and Ankle, Rothenberg P, Swanton E, Molloy A, Aiyer AA, Kaplan JR, p. 1445, Copyright Elsevier (2020), with permission from Elsevier)

Ligaments of the ankle syndesmosis include the anterior tibiofibular, posterior tibiofibular, and interosseous ligaments. Injuries to these ligaments may occur with hyperdorsiflexion and external rotation, creating a "high-ankle sprain" which is seen especially in athletes. Ligamentous support of the subtalar joint is contributed by the CFL, the ligaments of the anterior capsule, the posterior subtalar joint capsule, the interosseous talocalcaneal ligaments, and the ligaments of the tarsal canal. The midfoot joints are stabilized by multiple ligaments as well as the intrinsic bony architecture of the wedge-shaped cuneiform bones. Little motion occurs through the midfoot. Stabilizing ligaments include the bifurcate ligament and a V-shaped structure composed of the lateral calcaneonavicular and medial calcaneocuboid ligaments. They insert on the anterior process of the calcaneus, navicular, and cuboid bones, respectively. Superficial and deep plantar ligaments span from the calcaneus to the cuboid bone and metatarsals. These serve as static stabilizers of the longitudinal arch. Another important structure is the plantar aponeurosis (or plantar fascia). This thick fibrous structure runs from the plantar surface of the calcaneus to distally insert into the metatarsals. It stabilizes the arch during gait (Fig. 15.7). There is no true transverse interosseous ligament between the first and second metatarsal bases. Instead, there is an oblique plantar ligament that connects the first cuneiform bone to the second metatarsal. It is known as

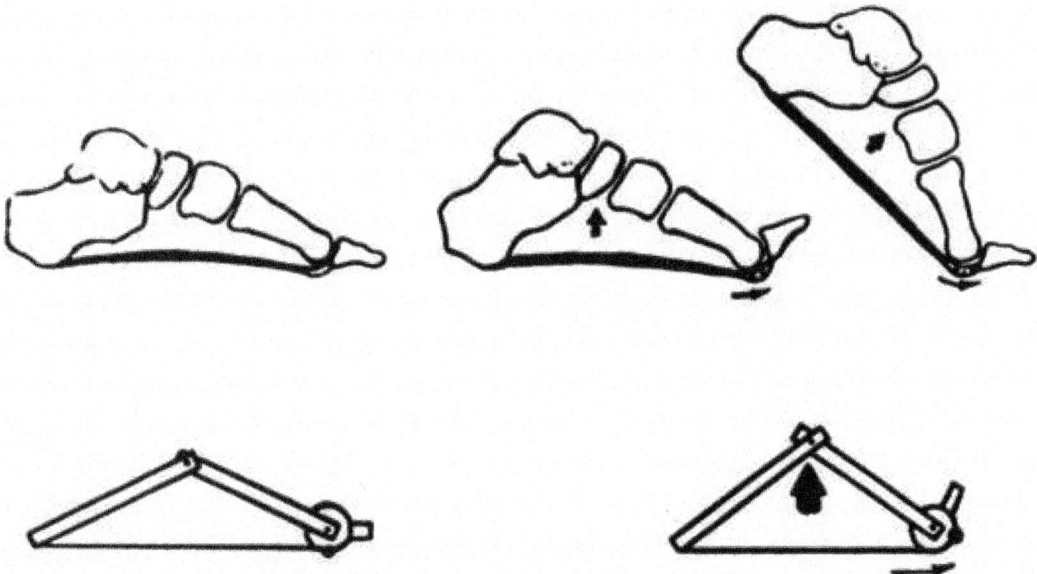

Fig. 15.7 Plantar aponeurosis and windlass mechanism provide stability to the longitudinal arch of the foot when the first metatarsophalangeal joint is forced into dorsiflexion and it secondarily plantar flexes the first metatarsal.

(Reprinted from *Orthopedic Clinics of North America*, 20(4), Mann RA, The Great Toe, p. 524, Copyright (1989), with permission from Elsevier)

Lisfranc's ligament. Stabilizing the MTP joints is a deep transverse metatarsal ligament as well as medial and lateral collateral ligaments.

Muscles

The muscles of the leg are encased in four leg compartments: the superficial and deep posterior compartments, the lateral compartment, and the anterior compartment. The superficial posterior compartment includes the gastrocnemius, the plantaris, and the soleus muscles. This compartment houses the main plantar flexors of the ankle (Fig. 15.8) that are innervated by the tibial nerve. The tendon fibers of the soleus merge with the gastrocnemius tendon fibers to form the tendo calcaneus or Achilles tendon. The Achilles tendon rotates 90° to insert on the posterior-superior tuberosity of the calcaneus. The deep posterior compartment contains three muscles which invert the foot and serve as secondary plantar flexors. These muscles are the tibialis posterior muscle, the flexor digitorum longus (FDL) muscle, and the flexor hallucis longus muscle. The lateral compartment, innervated by the superficial peroneal nerve, contains the peroneus longus and

peroneus brevis muscles, the main evertors of the foot. The deep peroneus longus muscle courses distally underneath the cuboid to insert on the base of the first metatarsal and medial cuneiform bone. The peroneus brevis inserts on the base of the fifth metatarsal. The anterior leg compartment contains the tibialis anterior, the extensor hallucis longus (EHL), and the extensor digitorum longus (EDL) muscles. These muscles serve as the primary dorsiflexors of the ankle and foot. These muscles are innervated by the deep peroneal nerve.

The intrinsic muscles of the foot are arranged in four plantar layers and there is a single dorsal muscle, the extensor digitorum brevis (EDB). The EDB is innervated by the deep peroneal nerve. The first superficial layer of the intrinsic plantar muscles includes the flexor digitorum brevis (FDB), the abductor hallucis, and the abductor digiti minimi (ADM) muscles. The second layer contains the muscles for toe motion and includes the quadratus plantae and lumbrical muscles as well as the tendons of the FHL and FDL. The third layer includes the flexor hallucis brevis, abductor hallucis, and the adductor hallu-

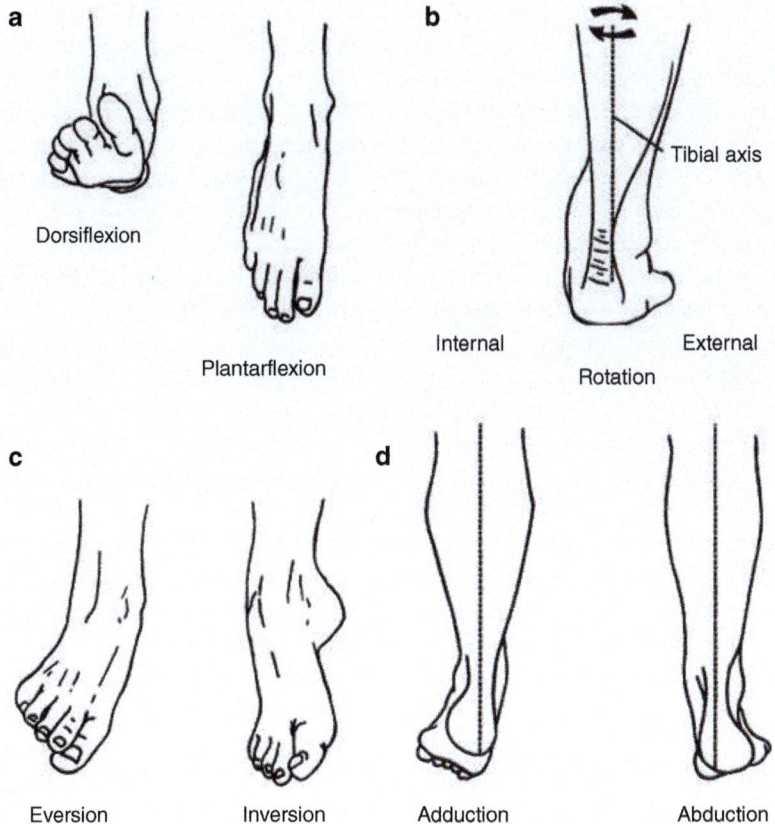

Fig. 15.8 Motions of the foot and ankle. (**a**) *Plantar flexion* and *dorsiflexion* refer to movement of the foot downward or upward. *Supination* and *pronation* refer to rotation of the foot internally or externally around the longitudinal axis of the foot. (**b**) *Internal rotation* and *external rotation* of the foot refer to motion around the vertical axis of the tibia. (**c**) *Eversion* directs the sole laterally, whereas *inver-sion* refers to rotation of the foot until the sole is directed medially. (**d**) *Adduction* and *abduction* describe motion of the forefoot toward or away from the midline. (Reprinted from *Orthopedic Radiology*, Weissman BNW & Sledge CB, <u>The Ankle</u>, p. 606, Copyright Saunders (1985), with permission from Elsevier)

cis (ADH) tendon. These muscles assist in first and fifth toe function. The fourth and deepest layer of intrinsic muscles contains the seven interosseous muscles and the insertions of the peroneus longus and anterior and posterior tibial tendons. The interossei are divided into two groups with four dorsal interossei and three plantar interossei. The dorsal interossei are involved in toe adduction, and the plantar interossei are involved in toe abduction.

Nerves and Vessels

The neurovascular structures of the foot and ankle include five major nerve branches and three arteries. The tibial and common peroneal nerves are terminal branches of the sciatic nerve which arises from the lumbosacral plexus. The common peroneal nerve from L5 branches into the superficial peroneal nerve and deep peroneal nerve. The superficial peroneal nerve courses through the lateral compartment and exits the lateral compartment approximately 10–15 cm above the lateral malleolus through a fascial defect and continues subcutaneously to provide sensory innervation of the dorsal aspect of the foot and toes. The deep peroneal nerve courses through the anterior compartment with the anterior tibial artery, continues into the foot with the dorsalis pedis artery to provide innervation to the intrinsic foot muscles including the EDB and EHB muscles, and terminates as a cutaneous nerve in the first web space. The tibial nerve, a branch of S1, travels through the popliteal fossa into the deep posterior compartment. It courses medial to the Achilles tendon, enters the tarsal tunnel just posterior to the medial malleolus, and divides into the median and lateral plantar nerves. The medial and lateral plantar nerves supply motor and sensory function to the plantar aspect of the foot. The sural nerve is a sensory branch of the tibial nerve and provides sensation to the posterolateral hindfoot and lateral border of the foot. The saphenous nerve courses along the anteromedial aspect of the lower limb posterior to the greater saphenous vein and provides sensation to the medial side of the ankle.

Vascular supply to the foot and ankle is derived from the anterior and posterior tibial arteries and peroneal arteries. The anterior tibial artery becomes the dorsalis pedis in the foot. The posterior tibial artery divides into the medial plantar artery and lateral plantar artery to supply the plantar structures in the foot. The peroneal artery branches from the posterior tibial artery and travels posterior to the interosseous membrane, deep to the FHL muscle, terminating at the distal tibiofibular joint.

The major structures of the venous system of the leg include the greater saphenous vein and the lesser saphenous vein. The greater saphenous vein courses anteromedial to end in the femoral vein. It drains the dorsum of the foot. The lesser saphenous vein runs posterior to the fibula and drains the lateral foot and arch.

Gait Cycle

The gait cycle consists of one heel strike to the next heel strike of the same foot. It is traditionally divided into a *stance phase* that makes 62% of the cycle and the *swing phase* that makes the remaining 38% of the cycle. At initial heel strike, the lower extremity is in internal rotation. The ankle joint is plantar flexed, and the subtalar joint is everted. The transverse tarsal joint is unlocked to allow shock absorption. Anterior compartment muscles are active in helping decelerate the limb. At foot flat, the lower extremity externally rotates, the ankle joint dorsiflexes, and the subtalar joint begins to

invert. This increases stability throughout the midfoot in anticipation of push-off. Anterior compartment muscles become inactive. Intrinsic muscles of the foot become active, and the posterior compartment calf muscles are contracting. At pre-swing, the ankle joint is in plantar flexion.

Clinical Evaluation of the Foot and the Ankle

History and Physical Examination

A complete medical and surgical history, the mechanism of injury, and the duration of the symptoms should be elicited. The location and quality of pain should be documented. Existing systemic disorders should be ruled out with an emphasis on diabetes and gout. Musculoskeletal history involving the spine and lower extremities is helpful. A physical examination should be done with both stockings and shoes removed. Gait patterns should be determined, with the patient walking both toward and away from the examiner. The stance phase or station should be examined with emphasis placed on the relationship of the hindfoot with the forefoot and longitudinal arch. Once inspection has been completed, examination of the bony and soft tissue structures follows. The area should be examined for the presence of edema, effusion, skin temperature changes, and previous sites of surgery or trauma. Systemic examination can be divided into the ankle, hindfoot, midfoot, and forefoot subgroups. When examining the ankle, note any effusion. Range of motion of the ankle is normally 20° of dorsiflexion and 40–50° of plantar flexion. Loss of ankle dorsiflexion may be associated with a tight Achilles tendon, posterior capsular contracture, or bony impingement. Limitation of dorsiflexion with the knee in full extension that improves passively with the knee flexed to 90° indicates a contracture of the gastrocnemius muscle. This is diagnosed clinically with the Silfverskiöld test, where the examiner compares ankle dorsiflexion in knee full extension and 90° flexion. Ligamentous laxity should be evaluated in comparison with the contralateral ankle joint and palpation of the tendons should be performed to note evidence of subluxation or dislocation. Midfoot examination involves selective palpation of the bony anatomy to isolate specific joint or joint involvement. Forefoot examination should include MTP joint motion with any documentation of subluxation and pain.

Pulses and sensation are vital to the evaluation. Both the dorsalis pedis and posterior tibial artery should be documented for strength and quality. Sensation evaluation should document intact levels in all nerve distributions around the foot, for pin, light touch, and vibratory. In addition, the Semmes–Weinstein monofilament test is applied in the diabetic patient to quantitate protective sensation. A failed test at the 5.07 level indicates a loss of sensation and signifies a risk for skin ulceration.

Radiology of the Foot and Ankle

Radiographic studies of the foot and ankle require weight-bearing X-rays when possible. Important views involve the anteroposterior (AP), lateral, and oblique views of the foot and AP, lateral, and mortise views of the ankle. The AP view of the foot can be used to assess forefoot and midfoot pathology. The lateral view of the foot shows the relationship of the talus and calcaneus to that of the midfoot, forefoot, and ankle joint. The medial oblique view is used to evaluate the lateral tarsometatarsal joints. Other studies are available to assess the sesamoids, the calcaneus, or the subtalar joint. The sesamoid view involves the X-ray beam directed tangential to the plantar surface of the sesamoid region, while the patient's toes are in hyperextension. Harris axial heel view is used to assess the calcaneal tuberosity and is important in calcaneus fractures or tarsal coalitions. Ancillary radiographic studies include computed tomography (CT) (Fig. 15.9), magnetic resonance imaging (MRI), and radionuclide studies. MRI can be used to assess soft tissue structures such as soft tissue tumors, osteomyelitis, avascular necrosis, bone tumors, chondral lesions, ligamentous injuries, and tendon abnormalities. CT is best to assess bone abnormalities including

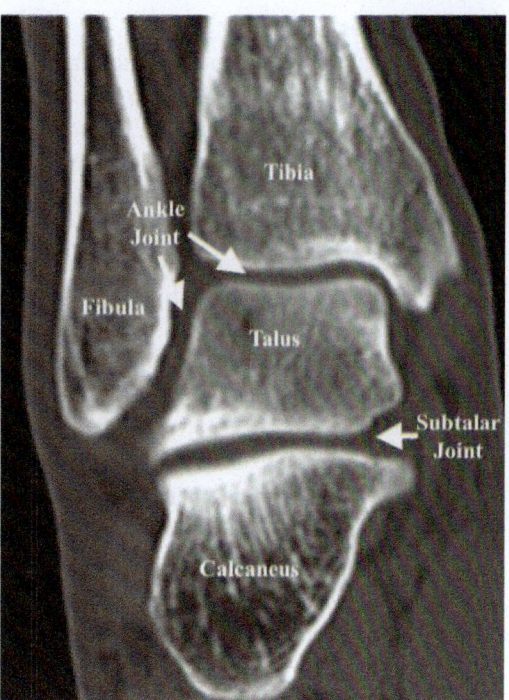

Fig. 15.9 Normal hindfoot and ankle anatomy seen on computed tomography (CT) scan

sequestrum and nonunions. Weight-bearing CT scanners now allow evaluation of complex pathology of the bones and joints of the foot and ankle in three dimensions with the foot in a position of function.

Diseases of the Foot and Ankle

This overview of the pathologic states that affect the foot and the ankle is discussed by diagnostic category. This is not meant to be an exhaustive catalog of every affliction but rather a representative sampling of the more common disease states that mandate medical care.

Trauma

Ankle

Injuries of the ankle mortise include pilon fractures, ankle fractures, and syndesmotic injuries.

Pilon Fractures

Pilon fractures involve the intraarticular fractures of the tibial metaphysis which extend to the weight-bearing portion of the tibia (Fig. 15.10). There is often extensive comminution. Nondisplaced pilon fractures may be treated nonoperatively with immobilization in a cast; however, since these are often displaced injuries, treatment consists of some type of operative fixation. Initially and temporarily, an ankle-spanning external fixator may be applied to maintain length and ankle joint reduction until soft tissue swelling subsides within 1–2 weeks. At that point, open reduction and internal fixation using screws and a plate can be done. In high-energy injuries with soft tissue compromise, external fixation may be the definitive treatment.

Ankle Fractures

Ankle fractures are discussed in the trauma chapter.

Syndesmosis Injuries

With disruption of the syndesmotic ligaments, a diastasis, or separation, of the distal tibia and fibula can occur (Fig. 15.11). This injury is often associated with higher grades of ankle fractures when medial stability is compromised by a medial malleolar fracture or a deltoid tear. Definitive diagnosis of a syndesmotic injury can be made with stress X-rays which show a diastasis at the distal tibial and fibular joint. If this exists, reduction and stabilization of the syndesmosis are achieved with screw placement, or flexible fixation, across the tibial and fibular joint or tibial and fibular syndesmosis. The transsyndesmotic screw should remain in place for a minimum of 12–16 weeks and is then removed, most flexible fixation techniques no longer require subsequent removal.

Fractures to the Hindfoot

Fractures of the hindfoot involve the calcaneus, talus, and navicular bones.

Talus Fractures

The talus articulates with the ankle, calcaneus, and navicular bones and is covered by articular cartilage on 60% of its surface (Fig. 15.12). Since the majority of the talus is covered by articular

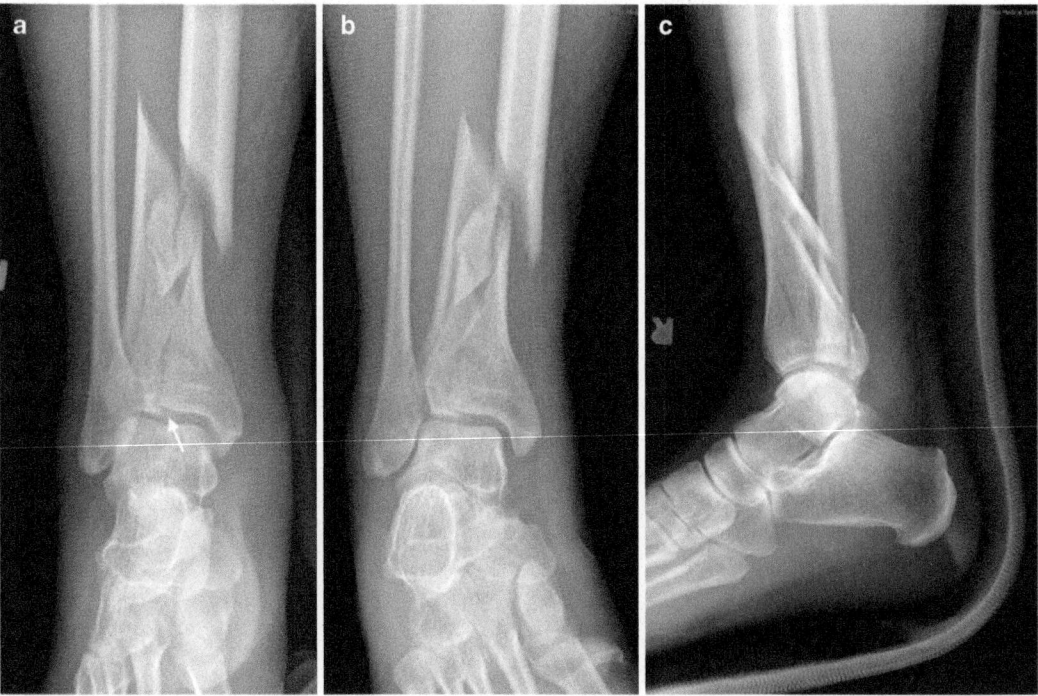

Fig. 15.10 (**a**) AP, (**b**) mortise, and (**c**) lateral radiographs showing a pilon fracture with involvement of the distal third tibial shaft. The fracture line extends into the tibial plafond (arrow) making it a pilon fracture

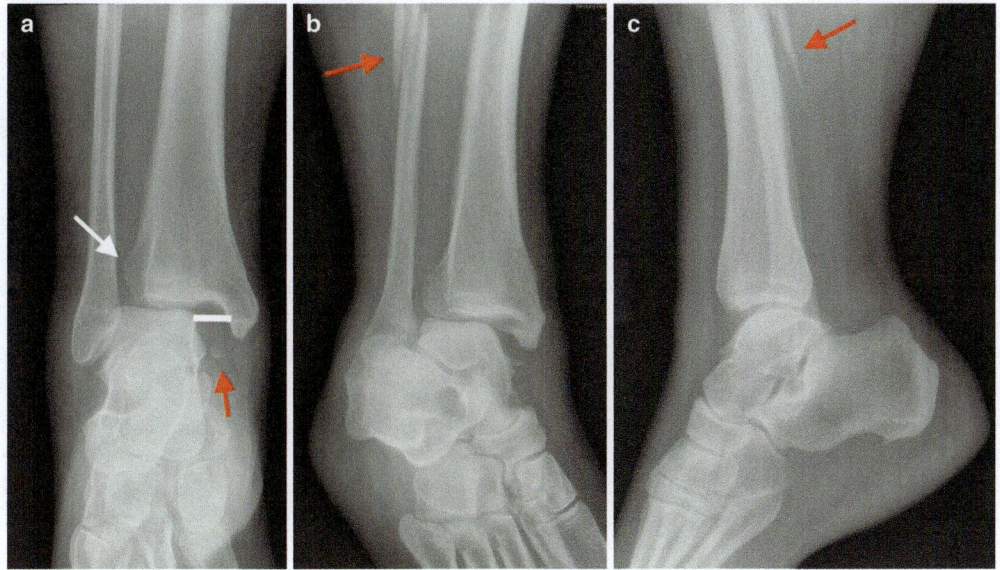

Fig. 15.11 (**a**) AP, (**b**) mortise, and (**c**) lateral radiographs showing syndesmotic injury with a mid-shaft fibula and medial malleolus avulsion fractures (red arrows). Notice the increased medial clear space widening (white line) and decreased tibia-fibula overlap (white arrow) on the (**a**) AP and (**b**) mortise radiographs

Fig. 15.12 Important anatomic structures of the talus. (Reprinted from *Orthopedic Clinics of North America*, 20(4), Adelaar RS, The treatment of complex fractures of the talus, p. 692, Copyright Saunders (1989), with permission from Elsevier)

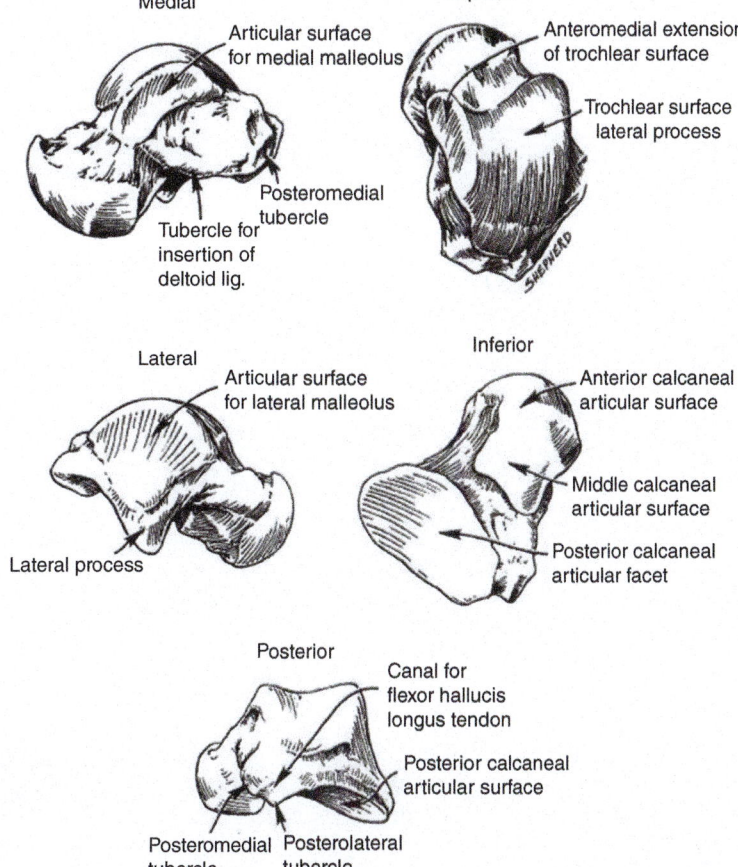

cartilage and there are no muscle or tendinous attachments, there is limited space for blood vessels to enter this bone, making the blood supply tenuous. The blood supply enters the talus at the neck and travels retrograde into the body and the dome (Fig. 15.13). Fractures of the talus, depending upon the severity, can often disrupt this blood supply. Fractures of the talus typically occur through the neck and result from an acute dorsiflexion injury. Standard radiographs with CT scans are usually adequate to demonstrate the nature of the fracture. Treatment is tailored to restore normal talar anatomy. If nondisplaced, conservative nonsurgical treatment with cast immobilization can be used. If displaced, often anatomic reduction and rigid fixation is the best

approach. This is done in an effort to prevent avascular necrosis which can result as a disruption of the tenuous blood supply. Hawkins' classification of talar neck fractures categorizes these fractures into three patterns (Fig. 15.14): Type I is a nondisplaced fracture of the neck, type II is a displacement of the neck fracture with subluxation or dislocation of the talar body from the subtalar joint, and type III is a neck displacement fracture with subluxation or dislocation of the body from both the ankle and the subtalar joints. A fourth pattern, which has been described, involves a displaced neck fracture which includes dislocation of the talonavicular joint. The incidence of avascular necrosis increases significantly with each increase in type. Radiographic signs of intact vascularity of the talus are demonstrated by the crescent or "Hawkins" sign at 8–10 weeks out from injury.

Calcaneus Fractures

The calcaneus is the most commonly fractured tarsal bone. Fractures are classified as intraarticular or extraarticular (Figs. 15.15 and 15.16). Calcaneus fractures are often seen when an axial load is applied to the foot, resulting from falls or motor vehicle accidents. Patients typically present with severe pain and swelling. Radiographs including the axial heel view in addition to CT scanning can fully define the injury. Closed treat-

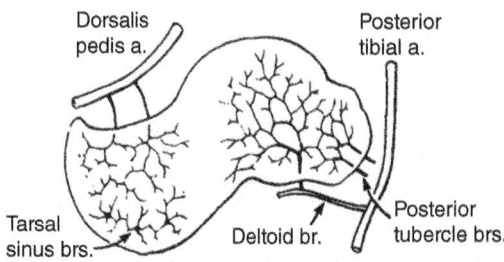

Fig. 15.13 Extraosseous and intraosseous circulation of the talus. (Reprinted from *Orthopedic Clinics of North America*, 20(4), Adelaar RS, The treatment of complex fractures of the talus, p. 693, Copyright Saunders (1989), with permission from Elsevier)

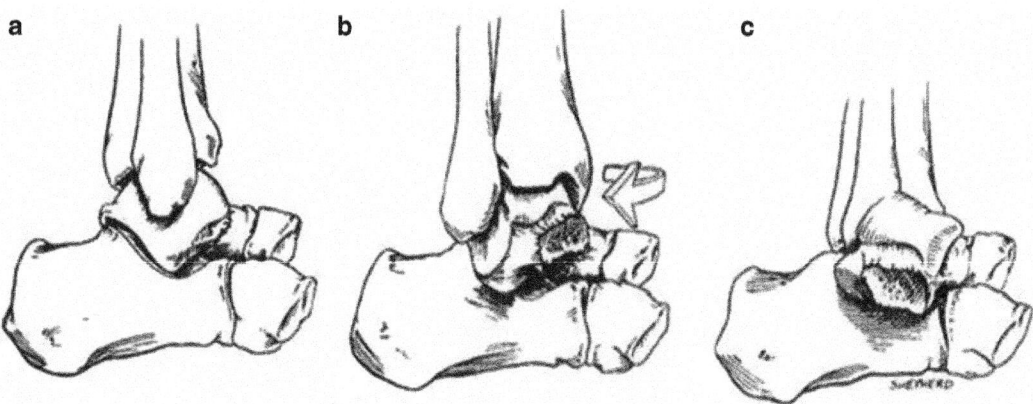

Fig. 15.14 Classification of talus neck fractures: (**a**) Class I, (**b**) class II, (**c**) class III. (Modified from *Journal of Bone and Joint* Surgery, 52A, Fractures of the neck of the talus, Hawkins LG, p. 991–1002, 1970; and reprinted

from *Orthopedic Clinics of North America*, 20(4), Adelaar RS, The treatment of complex fractures of the talus, p. 696, Copyright Saunders (1989), with permission from Elsevier)

Fig. 15.15 Lateral radiographs of the calcaneus demonstrating Böhler angle (blue star/solid line) and angle of Gissane (red star/dashed line). These are important measurements determining the need for operative intervention of a calcaneus fracture. A normal Böhler angle is 20–40° with values <20° indicating a calcaneus fracture due to a collapse of the posterior facet. A normal angle of Gissane is 120–145°, with an increased angle representing a collapse of the posterior facet diagnostic of a calcaneus fracture

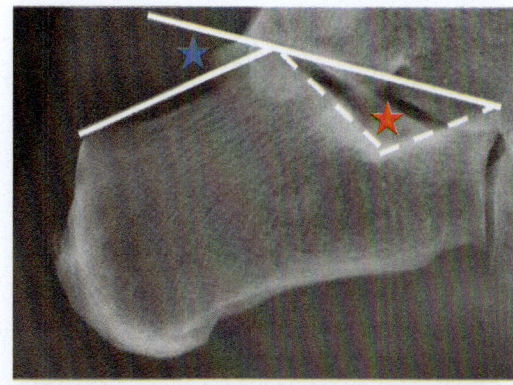

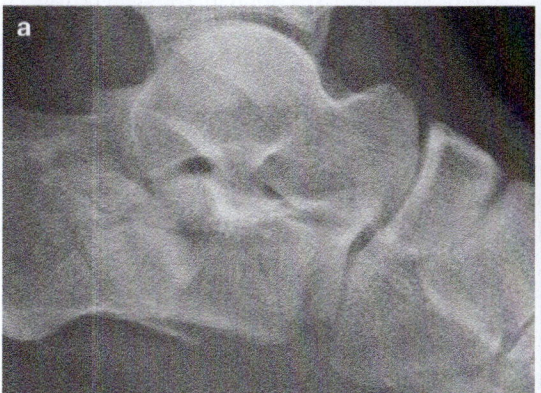

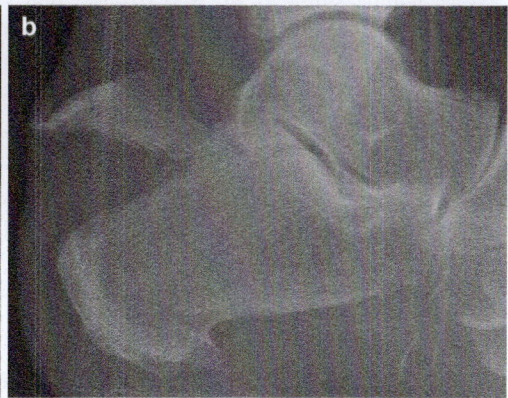

Fig. 15.16 Two examples of calcaneus fractures comprising the Essex-Lopresti classification of calcaneus fractures. (**a**) Joint-depression-type fracture, an intraarticular fracture with significant comminution that demonstrates a decreased Böhler angle and angle of Gissane. (**b**) Tongue-type fracture, an extraarticular fracture which is an avulsion due to contraction of the gastric-soleus complex. Tongue-type fractures have a high rate of skin compromise and require urgent surgical intervention

ment of these fractures is reserved for nondisplaced fractures or poor surgical candidates with severe soft tissue compromise or complicated medical conditions. Open reduction and internal fixation is indicated for displaced intraarticular fractures and significantly displaced extraarticular fractures. Surgical intervention should not proceed until the soft tissues and excessive swelling have stabilized. Assessment of this can be done by observation of wrinkling of the lateral hindfoot soft tissues. If soft tissues are not amenable to open reduction and internal fixation, other techniques including percutaneous fixation and external fixation may be utilized. Despite anatomic reduction and adequate treatment, these patients often develop subtalar stiffness and symptomatic osteoarthritis. Salvage would con-

sist of a subtalar fusion without bone loss or an intercalary tricortical graft to restore axial height.

Injury to the Midfoot

The midfoot injuries include those of the tarsonavicular, cuboid, cuneiform, and tarsometatarsal joints. Injuries to the Lisfranc (tarsometatarsal) joints include subtle sprains to frank fracture dislocations. Bony architecture is similar to that of a Roman arch and designed for stability. The keystone of the arch is the second metatarsal, which has a wedge-shaped base that is recessed between the medial and lateral cuneiform bones. Strong plantar interosseous ligaments provide the main support for the tarsometatarsal joints. There is an absence of an intermetatarsal ligament between the first and second metatarsal joint which makes this area susceptible to injury. The "Lisfranc liga-ment" spans the plantar lateral aspect of the medial cuneiform bone and the medial base of the second metatarsal and resists lateral transla-tion of the lesser metatarsals. Mechanisms of Lisfranc injury include a direct crush injury to the midfoot and an indirect twisting-type injury when an axial load is applied to the heel with the foot in fixed equinus, as in motor vehicle acci-dents or sporting activities. Up to 20% of these injuries are missed on initial evaluation because of their potential subtle nature. Plantar ecchymo-sis is pathognomonic of a Lisfranc injury (Fig. 15.17c). It is important to obtain standard three-view radiographs of the injured foot and look for the appropriate signs of injury. Subtle injuries can often be elucidated with weight-bearing AP foot radiographs including the con-tralateral foot for comparison. Lisfranc injuries can be bony (e.g., fractures of the metatarsal bases) or ligamentous in nature (Fig. 15.17a, b). Treatment involves anatomic reduction of the

involved joints with rigid fixation via percutane-ous method or open reduction internal fixation. Over 80% of patients develop posttraumatic arthrosis and stiffness, necessitating a fusion of the involved joints in the most refractory cases.

Ankle Sprains

Ligamentous disruptions, partial and complete, are common about the ankle. The most common ligament to be injured is the anterior talofibular ligament (Fig. 15.18). Inversion stress testing can elicit pain and demonstrate instability on radio-graphs (Fig. 15.19). Partial injuries can be treated with either a fracture boot or a brace with pro-gression as tolerated back to activity. A complete ligament disruption (grade III) can be similarly managed with nonoperative treatment the vast majority of the time. In the case of severe recur-rent instability, operative intervention consisting of repair may be necessary. Repairs are divided into anatomic and non-anatomic. Anatomic repairs involve repairing the ligaments primarily

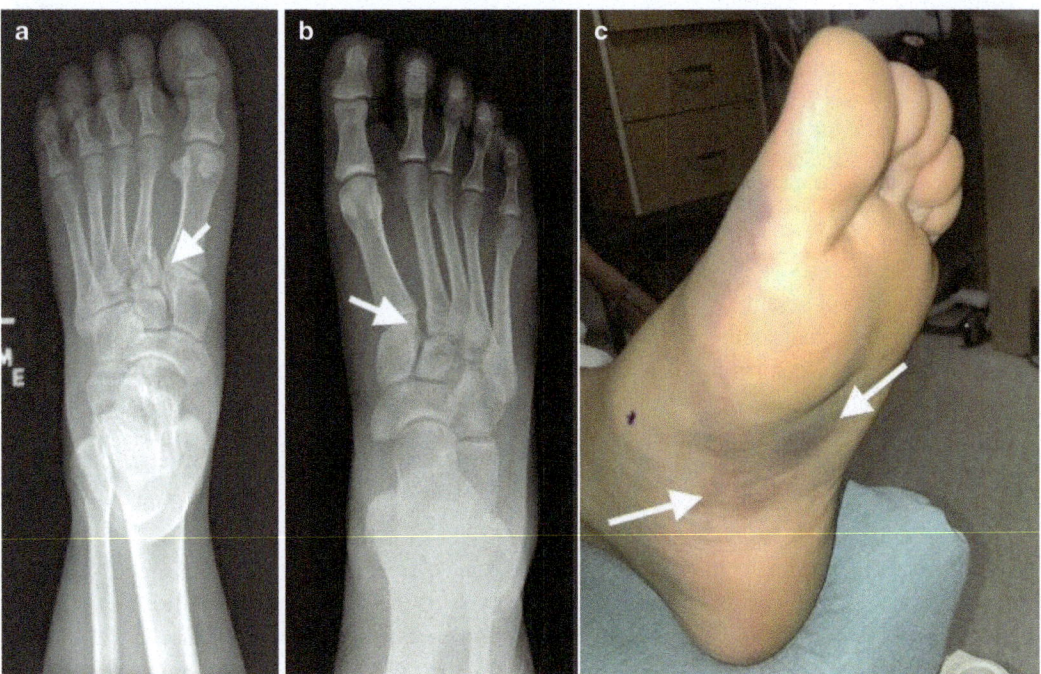

Fig. 15.17 (**a**) AP foot radiographs of a bony Lisfranc injury at the second and third metatarsal bases. (**b**) AP foot radiograph of a ligamentous Lisfranc injury. Notice the separation of the bases of the first and second metatar-sal bases. (**c**) An example of plantar ecchymosis, pathog-nomonic for a Lisfranc injury. This patient also has ecchymosis extending dorsally over the hallux

Fig. 15.18 Anatomic specimen of right ankle showing lateral ligament structures from anterolateral view. (**a**) Anterior inferior tibiofibular ligament with three bands. (**b**) Anterior talofibular ligament, somewhat atrophic. (**c**) Calcaneofibular ligament. (**d**) Cervical ligament. (Reprinted from *Coughlin and Mann's Surgery of the Foot and Ankle,* 10th edition, Haskell A & Coughlin MJ, <u>Athletic Soft Tissue Injuries of the Foot and Ankle,</u> Waldrop III NE, p. 1463, Copyright Elsevier (2024), with permission from Elsevier)

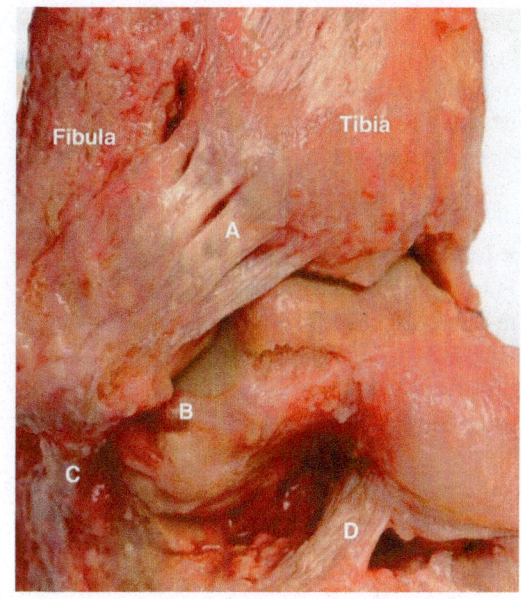

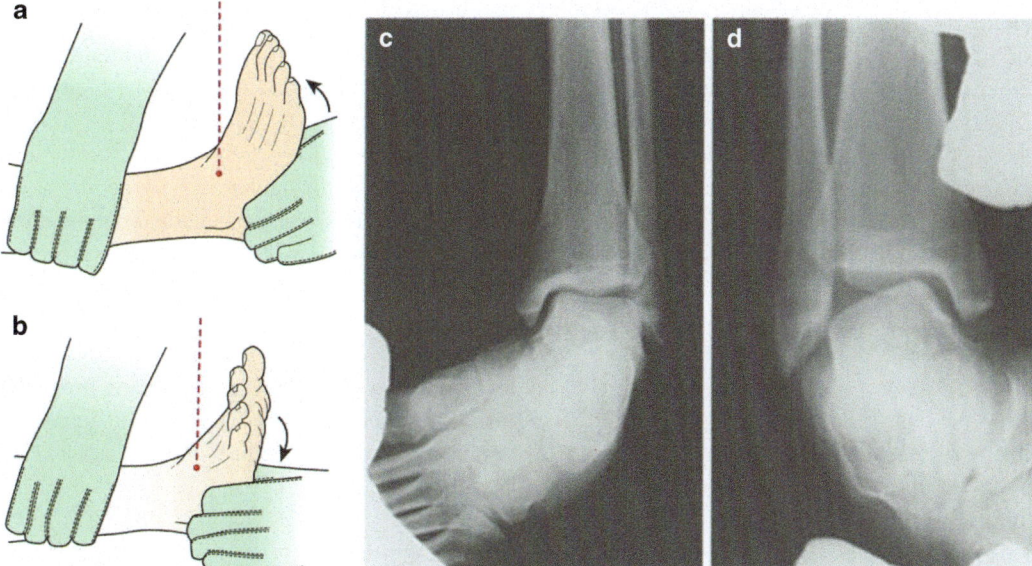

Fig. 15.19 Varus and valgus stress views of the ankle. Positioning for varus (**a**) and valgus (**b**) stress views of the ankle is illustrated. Varus stress in ankle plantar flexion tests for anterior talofibular and calcaneofibular ligament insufficiency. Valgus stress tests for deltoid ligament insufficiency. The use of stress radiography remains controversial because reliability may be compromised by the large range of normal variation in joint laxity. In the acute trauma setting, local analgesia probably increases accuracy. An abnormal varus or valgus stress examination is regarded as demonstrating either (a) talar tilt greater than or equal to 10° more than the normal side or (b) greater than or equal to 3 mm discrepancy in lateral ankle joint opening distance between the injured and normal side, as measured from the most lateral aspect of the talar dome to the adjacent tibial articular surface. In the example here, an abnormal varus stress radiograph (**d**) is shown relative to the normal side (**c**). (Reprinted from *Coughlin and Mann's Surgery of the Foot and Ankle,* 10th edition, Haskell A & Coughlin MJ, <u>Imaging of the Foot and Ankle,</u> Linklater JM, Read JW, Sofka CM, Hayter CL & Dimmick SJ, p. 62, Copyright Elsevier (2024), with permission from Elsevier)

and reinforcing the injured tissues with a second layer utilizing the inferior extensor retinaculum (modified Broström). Non-anatomic repairs require reconstructing the ligaments with a "cable" using either local tissue (spitting the peroneus brevis) or allograft.

Injuries of the Forefoot

Fractures of the sesamoid bones occur relative to direct trauma or use or both injuries associated with hyperdorsiflexion of the first metatarsal phalangeal joint. Bipartite sesamoid bones (congenital separation of the two poles of the sesamoid) occur in approximately 25% of individuals, the majority involving the tibial sesamoid bone. If the sum of the parts is greater than the adjacent sesamoid, then a congenital condition is more likely. Management is mostly conservative. However, a severe turf toe injury with complete transection of the plantar plate frequently requires operative repair, particularly in the elite athlete. Phalangeal fractures may be either displaced or nondisplaced and angulated. Closed manipulation is often needed under local anesthetic; then taping the affected toe to the adjacent toe as a splint mechanism or "buddy taping" is done with wearing of a stiff-soled shoe or sandal.

Acquired Deformities of the Foot and Ankle

Deformities of the Forefoot

Hallux Valgus

This is a condition of medial prominence of the first MTP joint with lateral drifting of the big toe (Fig. 15.20). It is almost exclusively related to shoe wear. Radiographically, it is defined as an MTP joint angle of more than 15° (the hallux valgus angle or HVA) and an angle between the first and second metatarsals that is more than 9° (intermetatarsal angle, or IMA). Symptoms include pain, swelling, and inflammation over the medial first MTP joint related to shoe wear. Range of motion of the first MTP joint should be assessed, and AP and lateral radiographs are taken to determine the degree of hallux valgus deformity, the associated metatarsus primus varus, joint congruity, and degenerative changes, as well as position of the sesamoids. Treatment of hallux valgus deformity in the early stages is conservative and includes shoe modification to a high, wide toe box and a soft leather upper portion of the shoe. Orthotic devices can be helpful. When conservative measures are not successful, surgical procedures are recommended. These include a simple exostectomy, soft tissue repair, proximal metatarsal osteotomy, distal metatarsal osteotomy, resection arthroplasty, proximal phalangeal osteotomy, and arthrodesis. Rarely is a simple exostectomy or soft tissue procedure performed in isolation. In cases of mild to moderate hallux valgus angles (<30°) where the joint is congruous, a distal type of procedure like the chevron osteotomy is indicated. In more severe angled bunions with incongruous joints, a proximal osteotomy in conjunction with a distal soft tissue release is best suited.

Hallux Varus

This is a medial deviation of the great toe at the MTP joint. The causes include complications from overcorrection of hallux valgus surgery or rupture of the conjoined tendon as seen in rheumatic conditions. Treatment in early or flexible cases consists of an abductor hallucis release with transfer of the extensor hallucis brevis. In more advanced cases, salvage with fusion of the metatarsophalangeal joint will leave satisfactory results.

Hallux Rigidus

Hallux rigidus is degenerative arthritis at the first MTP joint (Fig. 15.21). Patients present with an enlarged, warm, and swollen first MTP joint, with a decreased range of motion, predominantly in dorsiflexion. Shoes with elevated heels tend to increase pain. Initial treatment is conservative with orthotic devices and shoe modifications to reduce the stress across the first MTP joint. Surgical intervention includes resection arthroplasty, cheilectomy, metatarsal or phalangeal osteotomy, or arthrodesis.

Fig. 15.20 (**a**) Classic abnormalities in a bunion: 1, hallux valgus; 2, the exostosis; and 3, metatarsus primus varus. (Reprinted from *Orthopedic Clinics of North America*, 20(4), Mann RA, The Great Toe, p. 524, Copyright Saunders (1989), with permission from Elsevier) (**b**) Clinical photo of a bunion deformity. (**c**) Diagram of the intermetatarsal angle (IMA), hallux valgus angle (HVA) and (**d**) distal metatarsal articular angle (DMAA). Normal values: IMA is <9°, HVA <15° and DMAA <10°. In this patient, there is a severe hallux valgus deformity with a HVA of 55°, IMA of 16°, and DMAA of 41°

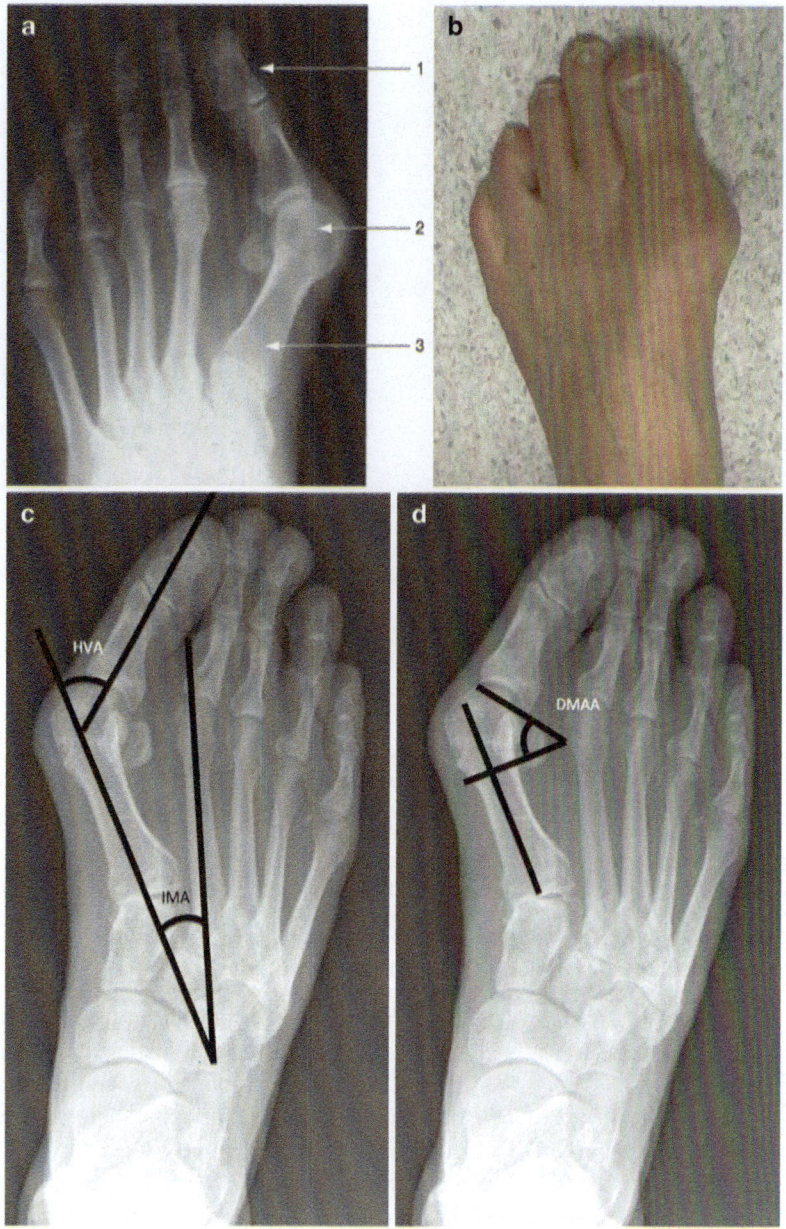

Lesser Toe Deformities

There are three common lesser toe deformities: claw, hammer, and mallet (Fig. 15.22). In contrast to the hallux, the lesser toes have proximal, middle, and distal phalanges, and they have two flexor tendons (FDB and FDL) and a complex extensor mechanism for each toe. Over time, imbalances in the tendons, muscles, and collateral ligaments can cause deformity. High heels and ill-fitting shoes are often implicated.

The deformities differ by their angulation at the metatarsophalangeal (MTPJ), proximal interphalangeal joint (PIPJ), and distal interphalangeal joint (DIPJ). Claw toes are characterized by hyperextension of the MTPJ and flexion of the DIPJ. This is resultant from hyperextension of the MTPJ causing stretched intrinsic muscles. This stretches the plantar flexor tendons and results in hyperflexion of the distal two joints. Hammer toes have normal or hyperex-

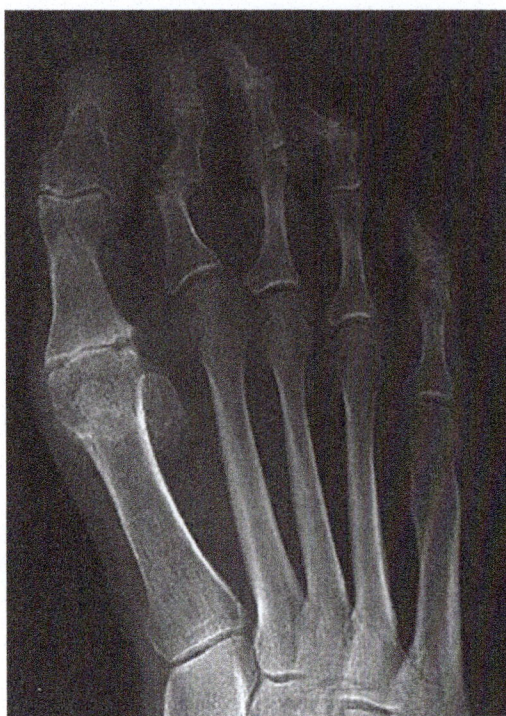

Fig. 15.21 AP radiograph of severe hallux rigidus evident by joint space narrowing, loss of cartilage, subchondral sclerosis, and osteophytes causing loss of motion at the first metatarsal phalangeal joint. This patient also has metatarso-sesamoid arthritic changes with osteophytes off the fibular sesamoid. (Reprinted from *Reconstructive Foot and Ankle Surgery: Management of Complications,* 3rd edition, Myerson MS & Kadakia AR, Arthrodesis of the Hallux Metatarsophalangeal and Interphalangeal Joints, p. 417, Copyright Elsevier (2019), with permission from Elsevier)

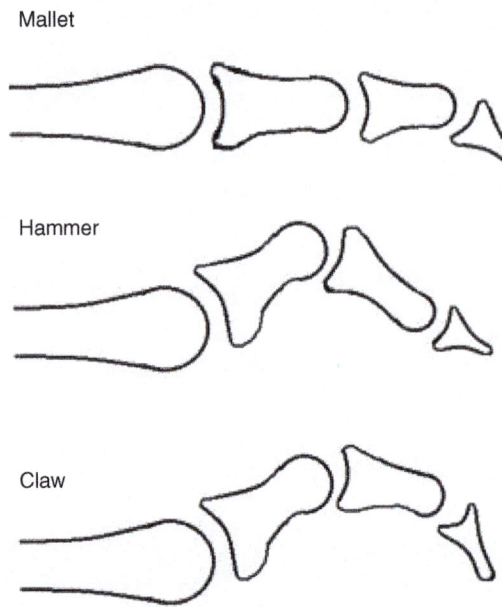

Fig. 15.22 Diagram of lesser toe deformities. (Reprinted from *Surgery (Oxford),* 34:9, Montgomery HC & Davies MB, Common disorders of the adult foot and ankle, p. 477, Copyright Elsevier (2016), with permission from Elsevier)

Injuries of the Tendons of the Foot and Ankle

Tendinitis is a nonspecific term for a variety of pathological conditions of tendons. Tendinitis is the inflammatory process of the structures of the connective tissue structure surrounding a tendon. Tendinosis is characterized by intratendinous degeneration commonly manifesting as longitudinal vertical cleavage tears or splits within a tendon.

Management is often conservative with rest and immobilization with anti-inflammatory medications. Common disorders of tendons are those involving the peroneal tendon complex, the anterior tibial tendon, the Achilles tendon, the posterior tibial tendon, and the FHL tendon.

Peroneal Tendon Pathology

Peroneal tendon disorders include injury and degeneration of the peroneus brevis or longus and instability of the peroneal tendon complex.

tended MTPJ, flexion of the PIPJ, and neutral or hyperextension of the DIPJ. The starting deformity is at the PIPJ, which can occur with poor shoe wear pushing the PIPJ into flexion. The extensors then are unable to fix the PIPJ abnormality and cause DIPJ hyperextension. Mallet toes are flexed at the DIPJ and normal at the MTPJ and DIPJ. This can also occur due to poor fitting shoe wear.

The abnormal joints can cause painful calluses in shoes. Treatment is either symptomatic management with shoe wear modification or surgical with soft tissue releases or fusions.

Peroneus brevis tendon injuries may manifest as tenosynovitis, a longitudinal split in the tendon, and subluxation or frank dislocation of the tendon. The patient may have a history of an inversion supination sprain and/or a foot with a high arch. Radiographic studies are often normal. Indications for operative treatment are persistent pain and failure of conservative treatment with cast/boot immobilization for 2–3 weeks and physical therapy. Goals of surgery are to reconstruct the superior peroneal retinaculum, perform a tenosynovectomy when applicable, and repair any longitudinal splits in the tendon. If a cavus deformity is present, consideration may be made to simultaneously surgically correct the bony deformity.

Cavovarus Foot Deformity

Cavovarus foot is a complex deformity characterized by plantar flexion of the first ray, hindfoot varus, and equinus (Fig. 15.23c). It can present in pediatric or adult years and results from several etiologies, including hereditary and motor and sensory neuropathies (e.g., polio, Charcot–Marie–Tooth), arthrogryposis, cerebral palsy, cerebrovascular accidents causing cerebral injury, posttraumatic from compartment syndrome or talar neck malunion. This subsequently causes an imbalance of the muscular forces on the foot depending on the affected weak muscles, most often a strong tibialis posterior and a strong peroneus longus overpowering a weak tibialis anterior and a weak peroneus brevis, The imbalances of foot during stance often lead to abnormal loading of the lateral border of the foot and the first or lateral metatarsal heads, leading to ulcers, stress fractures, and secondary osteoarthritis of overloaded joints due to the abnormal forces.

The Coleman block test is an important tool to determine if the deformity is driven (Fig. 15.23a, b). In this test, the patient stands with a block under the lateral forefoot: if the hindfoot varus corrects, then the deformity is flexible and is forefoot-driven. If the deformity does not correct, it is either rigid or hindfoot-driven. With a flexible varus deformity, the varus positioning of the hindfoot is secondary to the abnormal plantar

flexion of the first ray. Management is often surgical, aimed at tendon rebalancing with transfers and releases, osteotomies to correct hindfoot varus and equinus before the deformity becomes rigid. Once a rigid deformity exists, fusions are generally required to correct the deformity.

Anterior Tibial Tendon Pathology

Injuries of the anterior tibial tendon are rare. Tenosynovitis may result from irritation by shoe wear but is often attributed to an underlying rheumatic condition. Full rupture is due to wear associated from the superior border of the extensor retinaculum. Often when the tendon ruptures, proximal retraction results in a mass above the ankle joint, the so-called pseudotumor. Surgery is indicated for a young, active individual with an acute rupture. Neglect will result in a profound foot drop requiring an ankle–foot orthosis (AFO) long term or a tendon transfer.

Achilles Tendon Disorders

Disorders of the Achilles tendon include peritendinitis, tendinosis, partial and complete rupture, and insertional tendinitis with retrocalcaneal bursitis. Achilles tendinitis is painful inflammation and degeneration of either the surrounding peritenon (peritendinitis) or tendon (tendinosis) or both that occur proximal to the insertion site of the Achilles in the calcaneus. This is often seen in runners with tight Achilles tendons and poor flexibility. Treatment is often conservative with a period of immobilization to allow inflammation to subside and followed by physical therapy, stretching, and eccentric strengthening of the Achilles tendons daily, except in advanced cases of tendinopathy. When conservative measures fail, debridement of the Achilles tendon can be done surgically where the tendon is approached medially, split longitudinally to debride, and repaired side to side. When tendinitis occurs at the Achilles tendon insertion onto the posterior aspect of the calcaneus, it is called "insertional Achilles tendinitis." The insertion site typically calcifies forming a posterior enthesophyte that can be visualized on a lateral radiograph. Often, there is also an enlarged posterior-superior calcaneal process called a Haglund's deformity (Fig. 15.24). This

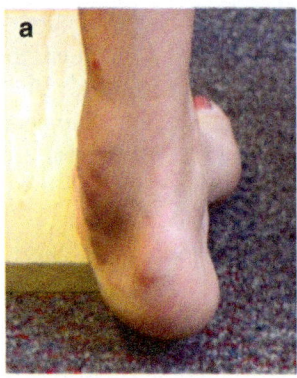
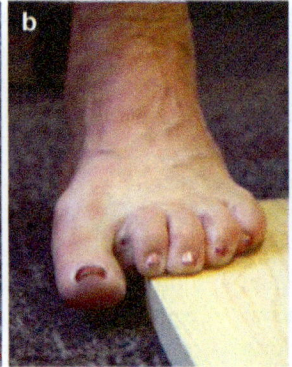
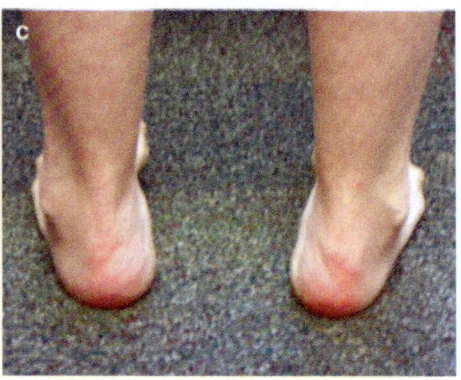

Fig. 15.23 The Coleman block test is performed by placing a block under the lateral foot and allowing the first metatarsal to come to the ground. (**a**) and (**b**) In these photographs, the foot is quite rigid, and no correction of the heel varus took place. (**c**) This patient was an adolescent. The heel corrected into neutral with the test, suggesting more of a forefoot-driven varus deformity. (Reprinted from *Reconstructive Foot and Ankle Surgery: Management of Complications,* 3rd edition, Myerson MS & Kadakia AR, Cavus Foot Correction, p. 142, Copyright Elsevier (2019), with permission from Elsevier)

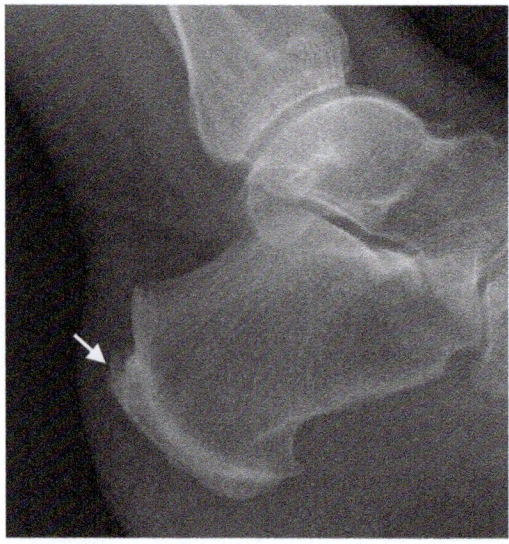

Fig. 15.24 A lateral radiograph of the calcaneus showing a Haglund's deformity, an enlargement of the posterior-superior calcaneal process

tendinitis is also associated with a retrocalcaneal bursitis which is inflammation of the bursa directly anterior to the Achilles tendon at its insertion. Conservative treatment includes a period of immobilization, heel lifts to shorten the Achilles tendon and take the pressure off the insertion, stretching and eccentric strengthening exercises through physical therapy, and modification of shoe wear. When conservative measures fail, surgery consists of debridement of the calcified insertion Achilles tendon, and resection of the calcaneal posterior-superior tuberosity, in addition to reattachment of the Achilles tendon.

Ruptures of the Achilles tendon can be acute or chronic. They commonly occur in middle-aged men at the hypovascular zone of the Achilles tendon approximately 3–5 cm above the insertion site due to the "watershed" of the proximal and distal blood supply. Ruptures occur because of forceful eccentric contraction of the elongating tendon. They rarely result from direct trauma. Symptoms include severe pain at the back of the calf. Patients often describe being hit in the back of the leg and an audible "pop." Palpating a defect above the Achilles insertion with the patient in a prone position confirms the diagnosis. Two findings are consistent with complete rupture of the tendon. The first is loss of passive resting tension in comparison to the opposite extremity which causes the foot to be at right angle to the remainder of the lower extremity (Fig. 15.25). Normal tone with the tendon intact is approximately 25° of plantar flexion passive. The second finding is performing the Thompson test, which is done with the patient's foot hanging over the edge of the examination table in a prone position (Fig. 15.25). The midcalf is squeezed. If the tendon is intact, the ankle passively plantar flexes. If the tendon is ruptured, no plantar flexion occurs.

Fig. 15.25 Clinical exam findings of an Achilles tendon rupture. *Top*: Example of resting tension in normal (left) and injured (right) extremities. Notice the slight plantar flexion of the normal foot, while the injured side is in neutral to dorsiflexed position. *Bottom*: The Thompson squeeze test. On the normal (left) side, the Achilles mechanism is squeezed which contracts the mechanism and causes the foot to plantarflex. The foot does not move with the Thompson squeeze on the injured (right) side since there is no longer tension of the heel cord

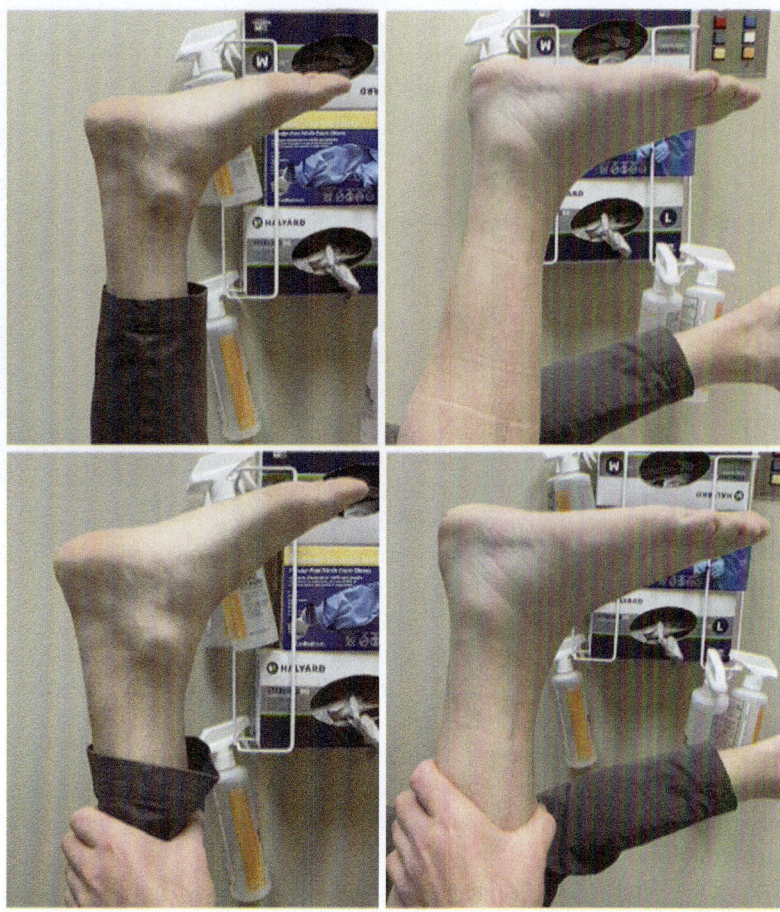

In difficult cases, MRI or ultrasound can confirm the diagnosis.

Treatment of an acute rupture of the Achilles tendon can be conservative or surgical. Nonoperative management includes immobilization in a plantar flexed position for 4–6 weeks followed by progressive weight-bearing and aggressive physical therapy. Disadvantages of conservative management include a higher re-rupture rate. Some postulate that nonoperative treatment results in weaker push-off strength, but this has not been proven. Surgical repair includes direct repair of the ends of the Achilles tendon. Potential complications involve wound complications, infection, and sural nerve injury. Treatment of chronic neglected ruptures includes bracing with an ankle–foot orthosis or complex surgical reconstruction including flexor hallucis longus tendon transfer to fill the defect.

Posterior Tibial Tendon

The posterior tibial tendon is the primary dynamic arch support to the medial arch of the foot. It functions as a hindfoot inverter and ankle plantar flexor, and when the muscle contracts, it locks the transverse tarsal joint to allow a rigid lever arm for the toe-off phase of the gait cycle. Overuse of the posterior tibial tendon causes conditions that range from mild tendonitis to complete rupture and asymmetrical flatfoot deformity. Posterior tibial tendon dysfunction etiologies include trauma, inflammatory arthropathies, or nutritional degenerative conditions. Predisposing factors include hypertension, obesity, diabetes, steroid exposure, and prior surgery or trauma. Early stages include pain, swelling, and fullness localized to the posterior and medial hindfoot. As the tendon continues to deteriorate and becomes dysfunctional, a progressive asymmetrical flatfoot deformity develops with lateral hindfoot impingement and peroneal tendonitis. Clinical exam may show tenderness and swelling over the posterior medial hindfoot, a secondary Achilles tendon contracture, and weakness with resisted plantar flexion and inversion. Patients are unable to perform a single stance heel rise and often show a "too-many-toes sign" when visualizing the foot from behind in a standing position. Too-many-toes sign refers to an advanced collapse of the arch with the heel in significant valgus. The toes are abducted more on the affected foot than the unaffected foot and show more prominently on exam. Weight-bearing X-rays may show uncovering or "sag" of the talar head by the navicular on both AP and lateral views (Fig. 15.26); the normal angle is close to zero. The forefoot and midfoot are abducted in relation to the hindfoot. MRI can confirm tenosynovitis versus tendinosis. Treatment options are determined by the stage of dysfunction and presentation. Stage I, which is very mild tendon weakness and pain without flatfoot deformity, can be addressed with orthotics, anti-inflammatory medicines, and physical therapy. A period of immobilization is often helpful to decrease the inflammation. Stage II, which involves posterior tibial tendon elongation or partial disruption and the presence of a flexible flatfoot deformity, can be treated conservatively with orthotics or surgically, which involves repair of the posterior tibial tendon. In advanced cases, reconstruction is accomplished by using the adjacent flexor digitorum longus tendon as a transfer. Alone, tendon repair or reconstruction will yield a 50% failure within 2 years post-reconstruction unless a bone procedure is added to correct the deformity. Options include a medial displacement calcaneal osteotomy, a lateral column lengthening at the anterior one-third calcaneus, or a plantar flexion osteotomy through the medial cuneiform. Stage III, which involves a rigid foot or advanced arthritis, can be treated conservatively with orthotics or surgically with the appropriate joint fusions. Typically, a triple arthrodesis involving fusions of the subtalar, talonavicular, and calcaneocuboid joints is recommended.

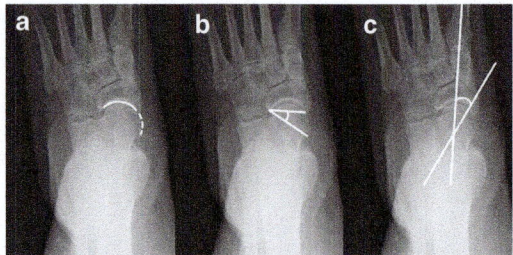

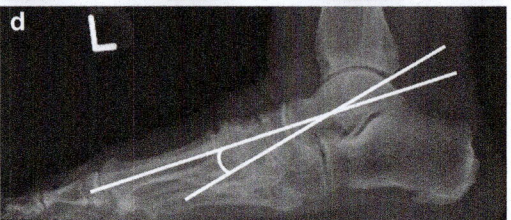

Fig. 15.26 Weight-bearing AP (*top*) and lateral (*bottom*) foot radiographs showing a flatfoot deformity, also known as pes planus. The AP weight-bearing radiograph can show (**a**) talonavicular joint uncoverage percentage—the percentage of the talar articular surface that is uncovered by the navicular, pes planus values >30% and normal considered <30% coverage, (**b**) talonavicular coverage angle—the angle between the articular surface of the navicular and articular surface of the talus, pes planus is >7° and normal is 7°, and (**c**) talo-first metatarsal angle, also called the AP Meary's angle—the angle between the axis of the first metatarsal and axis of the talus, pes planus >16 and normal <16. The lateral weight-bearing radiograph can be used to measure the (**d**) lateral Meary's angle, also called the talo-first metatarsal angle measured with a line bisecting the first metatarsal shaft and the axis of the talus. Normal is zero degrees and values greater than 4° indicate pes planus, with <15 mild, 15–30 moderate, and >30 severe pes planus

Heel Pain

Plantar heel pain is one of the most common and most disabling conditions of the foot. There are many causes including tumors, infection, stress fractures, inflammatory arthropathies, and neuropathies. The most common cause of plantar heel pain is associated with chronic injury of the plantar fascial origin. This heel pain syndrome is also known as heel spur syndrome and plantar fasciitis. Typical pain occurs at the plantar medial aspect of the heel. Onset is insidious and often patients recall no trauma. Classic pain and stiffness occur when arising from bed and taking the first step on the floor in the morning. Symptoms often decrease after prolonged walking. High-heeled shoes typically alleviate symptoms, whereas barefoot walking and wearing flat shoes may increase symptoms. Physical examination shows point tenderness on the plantar medial heel. Often, there is a tight Achilles tendon complex with limited ankle dorsiflexion. Occasionally, fat pad or heel pad atrophy is present. Radiographs include a lateral X-ray which may show a plantar heel spur (Fig. 15.27). This is often associated with a flexor digitorum brevis origin and can signify a chronic condition. It is important to rule out a calcaneal stress fracture and tumor via X-rays and a calcaneus "squeeze test" which should not generate pain in plantar fasciitis. Treatment is almost always conservative consisting of rest, anti-inflammatory medication, orthotic devices, and aggressive stretching. Isolated stretching of the gastrocsoleus complex and plantar fascia is important. Surgery is typically reserved for chronic conditions that have lasted over 6 months to a year and involves partial release of the plantar fascial origin in addition to tarsal tunnel decompression.

Arthritic Conditions of the Foot and Ankle

Osteoarthritis

Ankle

The causes of ankle joint degeneration include primary osteoarthritis, posttraumatic arthritis, avascular necrosis, osteochondritis dissecans, synovial chondromatosis, and rheumatologic conditions. By far, the most common cause of ankle arthritis is posttraumatic, unlike the hip or knee joint. Conservative management includes anti-inflammatory medications, bracing, and intraarticular cortisone injections. Surgical management is dependent on the extent and location of the arthrosis. Options are split between reconstruction and salvage. For early to intermediate stage or focal involvement, options include joint debridement either arthroscopically or open, low tibial osteotomy, osteochondral auto or allograft replacement, and distraction arthroplasty. Salvage procedures

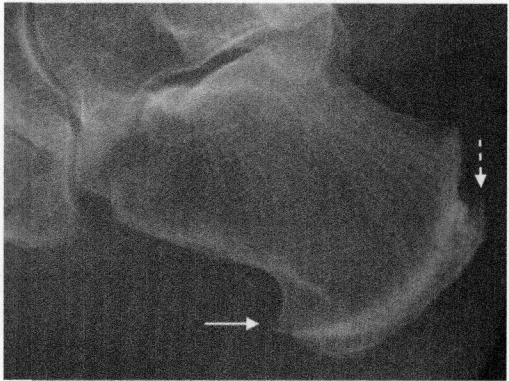

Fig. 15.27 Bone spurs of the calcaneus. The plantar heel spur (solid arrow) can be present in cases of plantar fasciitis. This patient also has a Haglund deformity (dashed arrow)

include ankle arthrodesis (fusion) or a total ankle replacement (Fig. 15.28). While the main advantage with fusion is permanency, the downside is that stress transference into adjacent joints leading to osteoarthritis can occur. Ankle replacement avoids this problem by maintaining ankle motion; however, longevity of the implant may require revision surgery over a lifetime. Recent advances in implants have resulted in custom implant printing when necessary.

Foot (Hindfoot, Midfoot, and Forefoot)

Arthritis of the foot is very common and can affect all joints. It can be secondary to all the causes listed above for ankle arthritis. Forefoot arthritis is very common, with hallux rigidus being the most frequent subset. This is discussed in more detail in an earlier section. Isolated midfoot arthritis is the least common and is commonly attributed to posttraumatic, inflammatory, or neuropathic arthritis. Lisfranc injuries and midfoot fractures are common causes of posttraumatic arthritis in the midfoot. It is also worth noting that hindfoot fusion will cause transfer of stresses to the midfoot joints and cause secondary osteoarthritis. Hindfoot arthritis is most commonly posttraumatic but can be secondary to flatfoot, cavovarus foot deformities, or inflammatory arthropathies. It includes degeneration of the subtalar, talonavicular, and calcaneocuboid joints.

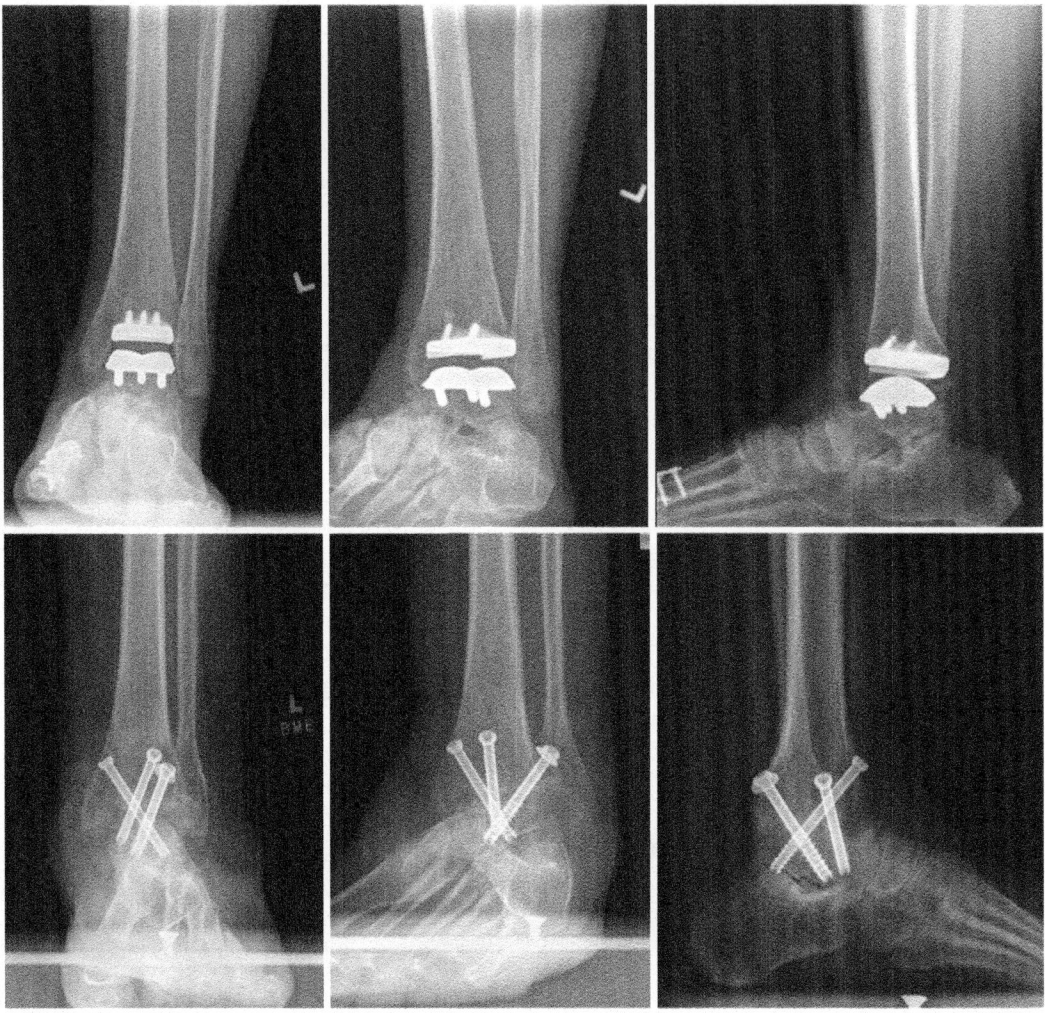

Fig. 15.28 *Top*: AP, mortise, and lateral radiographs demonstrating a total ankle arthroplasty for ankle arthritis. *Bottom*: AP, lateral, and oblique foot radiographs of an ankle fusion. The former allows for retention of ankle range of motion

Management begins with conservative treatment as noted above. Surgical options aim to reduce pain and include osteophyte resection in early stages and fusion as the gold standard in late stages.

Rheumatoid Arthritis

Rheumatoid arthritis is a systemic disease that commonly involves the foot as there are many joints lined with synovium (Fig. 15.29). It affects both the synovial lining of the joint and the surrounding tendons. These problems are less often encountered in the present day due to advances in medical management, particularly the newer bio-logic medications. Physical examination shows an antalgic gait, generalized swelling, and decreased motion in the joints of the foot. Weight-bearing radiographs of the foot and ankle are essential for showing deformity and often show a valgus angulation of either the ankle or subtalar joint.

Treatment options include conservative management such as patient education, activity modification, intermittent steroid injections, optimizing medical management, shoe modifications, and the use of an ankle–foot orthosis. Surgical options include simple synovectomy, arthrodesis, and total ankle arthroplasty.

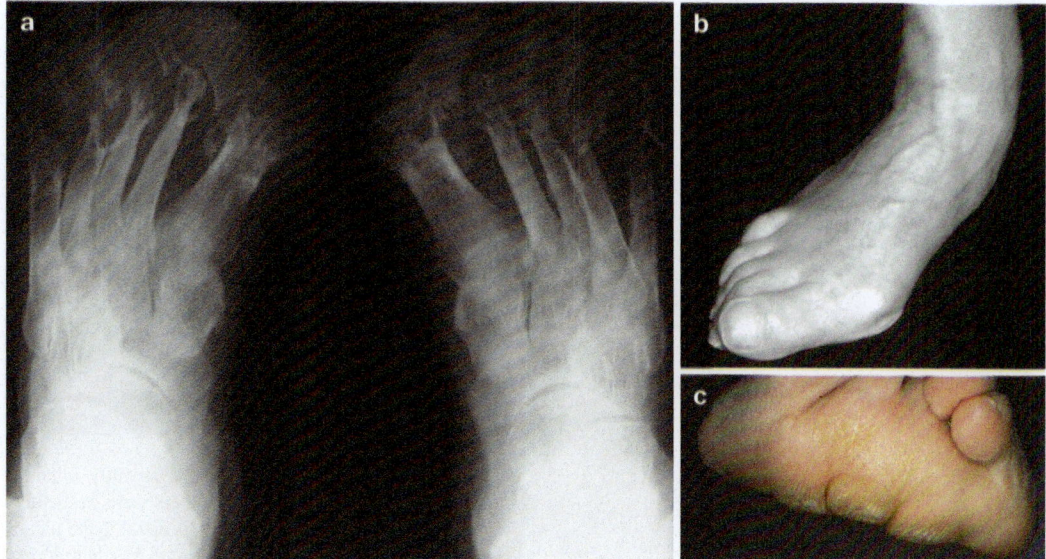

Fig. 15.29 The rheumatoid foot. (**a**) Plain radiograph of severe forefoot deformity in rheumatoid arthritis. (**b**) The clinical appearance of the typical forefoot deformity. (**c**) Prominent plantar bursae in established rheumatoid arthri- tis. (Reprinted from *Neale's Disorders of the Foot and Ankle*, 9th ed., Burrow JG, Rome K & Padhiar N, Rheumatic Diseases, Rome K & Stewart S, p. 222–260, Copyright Elsevier (2020), with permission from Elsevier)

Infections

Both the bones and joints of the foot can be involved in musculoskeletal septic processes such as osteomyelitis and septic arthritis.

Puncture Wounds

Puncture wounds in the foot can be caused by many objects including glass, nail, and plant and animal parts. Typically, the puncture occurs through the sole of the sneaker and enters the foot. Since the insole of a sneaker can be colonized with the *Pseudomonas* organism, care should be taken to treat the patient with an infection from a puncture wound for this organism. Patients frequently present late with a swollen cellulitic foot. Standard radiographs and a bone scan can confirm the diagnosis. When bone or joint involvement is extensive, aggressive surgical debridement is mandatory for satisfactory resolution. Appropriate antibiotic coverage is required until the infection has resolved.

Paronychia

A paronychia is an infection of the medial or lateral nail fold, often seen in the great toe (Fig. 15.30). Paronychiae are often seen in an abnormally growing nail or "in-grown toenail," which penetrates the skin of the lateral nail fold, introducing bacteria.

A soft tissue abscess forms and a paronychia develops. Decompression of the abscess is done under local anesthesia and removing the lateral portion of the nail often allows temporary relief. With more chronic paronychial infections, more aggressive nail procedures including either partial or total nail ablation may be required.

Diabetic Foot Infections

People with diabetes can develop a sensory neuropathy which prevents them from protective sensation. Because of abnormal pressures unremitting for 20 min or more, ulcerations which allow bacterial inoculation and infection to develop may result. Typical scenarios in which this can happen is after a pedicure or from the abrasions of a poorly

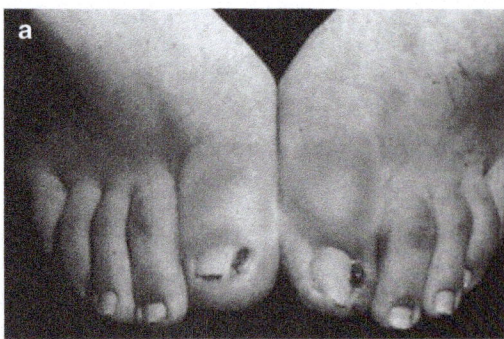

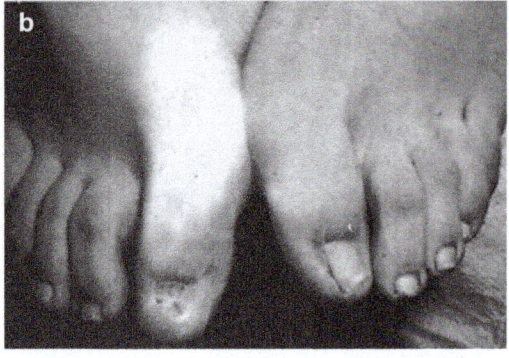

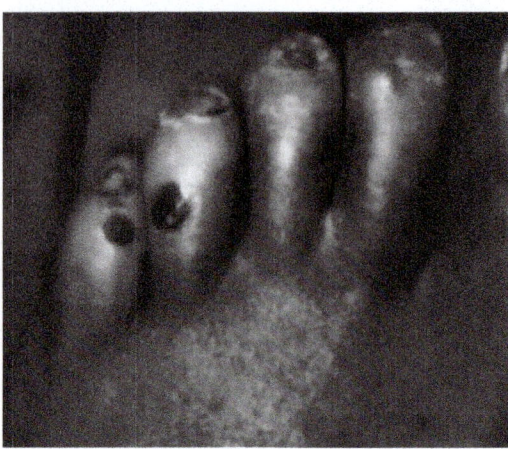

Fig. 15.31 This diabetic patient had recently obtained new shoes. The two small, dorsal ulcers were exquisitely painful. Note the blanching of the toes distal to the ulcers. (Reprinted from *Orthopedic Clinics of North America,* 20(4), Harrelson JM, Management of the diabetic foot, p. 606, Copyright Saunders (1989), with permission from Elsevier)

Fig. 15.30 (**a**) Bilateral infected ingrowing of both edges of the big toenails. The toenail of the right big toe was practically completely separated from its bed and was avulsed. The operation, which was performed under a local anesthetic, consisted of bilateral resection of all ony-chogenic tissue in the longitudinal grooves. (**b**) Sixteen months after surgery. (Reprinted from *Disorders of the Foot*, Vol II, Jahss MH, The toenails, Lapidus PW, p. 1589, Copyright Saunders (1991), with permission from Elsevier)

fitting shoe (Figs. 15.31 and 15.32). With abscesses and ulcers, both acute and chronic septic arthritis and osteomyelitis are frequently the end result. Aggressive treatment of any infection in the dia-betic foot is mandatory for salvage. Medical man-agement of diabetes is crucial and the patient must be under strict diabetic control. Intravenous antibi-otics are almost always necessary in the acute sce-nario. Antibiotics are often broad spectrum due to the polymicrobial nature of these infections. It is important to distinguish between infection and Charcot arthropathy, discussed below.

Charcot Arthropathy

Charcot arthropathy, a noninfectious degrada-tion of joints, can be confused with infection or inflammatory arthropathies. It was named by

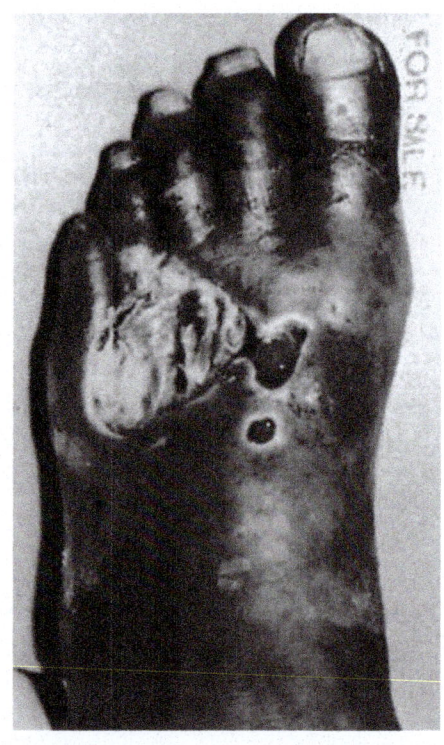

Fig. 15.32 One day of new shoe wear produced the ulcers seen over the fifth metatarsal head and lateral sides of the fourth and fifth toes. (Reprinted from *Orthopedic Clinics of North America,* 20(4), Harrelson JM, Management of the diabetic foot, p. 606, Copyright Saunders (1989), with permission from Elsevier)

Jean-Martin Charcot for joint destruction associated with tertiary syphilis, but other causes include neuropathies caused by diabetes, Charcot-Marie-tooth, alcoholic peripheral neuropathy, leprosy, Caisson's disease (the bends). The pathophysiology is unclear at this time but leading theories are (1) autonomic dysregulation from the underlying neuropathy leading to alterations in vascularity and (2) repetitive microtrauma in an insane extremity triggering an inflammatory cascade resulting in the collapse of the joint. There are three clinical stages classified by Eikenholz: (1) development, (2) coalescence, and (3) reconstruction and reconstitution. Physical exam is characterized by erythema, edema, and elevated temperature that is resolved with elevation of the affected joint, termed "dependent rubor." Plain radiographs demonstrate complete destruction of the joint, extreme to that of other inflammatory arthropathies or infections. Nonoperative treatment with total contact casting is first line treatment. Surgical therapies are utilized when nonoperative management has failed or is not feasible in a patient, with the goal to offload the affected part of the foot to prevent ulceration and allow for weight-bearing through fusions and tendon releases.

Tumors

A complete discussion of soft tissue and bone tumors is beyond the scope of this chapter; however, a few specific lesions are mentioned here.

Soft Tissue Lesions

The anterolateral ankle is the common site for the development of a ganglion cyst as well as soft tissue lipomas. These are both benign lesions and excision can be performed if symptoms warrant. Thickening of the plantar fascia on the plantar surface of the foot can be palpated on some patients. Sometimes these thickenings are large, firm nodules known as plantar fibromas. They are benign and should be treated conservatively at all costs.

Bone Tumors

Common bone tumors include enchondroma, a benign cartilage tumor that can occur in the short tubular bones such as the phalanges. The chondromyxoid fibroma (Fig. 15.33) is another benign cartilage tumor that can affect the bones of the foot. It is usually managed by curettage of the lesion. Occasionally, a bone cyst can form in the calcaneus. Pathologic fracture through this can occur and may, in fact, be the chief complaint at a patient's presentation. Treatment usually requires curettage and bone grafting. It is uncommon to have metastatic disease to the small bones of the foot. When seen, one should suspect the lung as the primary site of the patient's disease.

Complex Regional Pain Syndrome

This disabling disorder of unknown pathophysiology has a variable symptom complex with many hypothesized causes and mechanisms. Renamed from the limited descriptive term reflex sympathetic dystrophy, complex regional pain syndrome (CRPS) is more common in women than men, and more common in adults than children. It can occur after a minor injury or surgery with no nerve involvement, or after a significant injury with nerve involvement. Patients present with disproportionate extremity pain, swelling, autonomic symptoms (i.e., changes in sweating, skin discoloration), and motor symptoms (i.e., weakness). Diagnosis of any obvious, treatable causes of pain should be done prior to definitively selecting CRPS as the diagnosis. Treatment involves extensive therapy and pain relief with desensitization through medication or nerve blockade.

Fig. 15.33 Chondro-myxoid fibroma of the first metatarsal. (**a**) Preoperative radiograph revealing first metatarsal lesion; (**b**) radiograph 3 months after treatment with curettage and bone grafting. (Reprinted from *International Orthopedics*, 30(3), Sharma H, Jane M & Reid R, <u>Chondromyxoid fibroma of the foot and ankle: 40 years' Scottish bone tumour registry experience</u>, p. 206, Copyright Springer Nature (2006), with permission from Springer Nature)

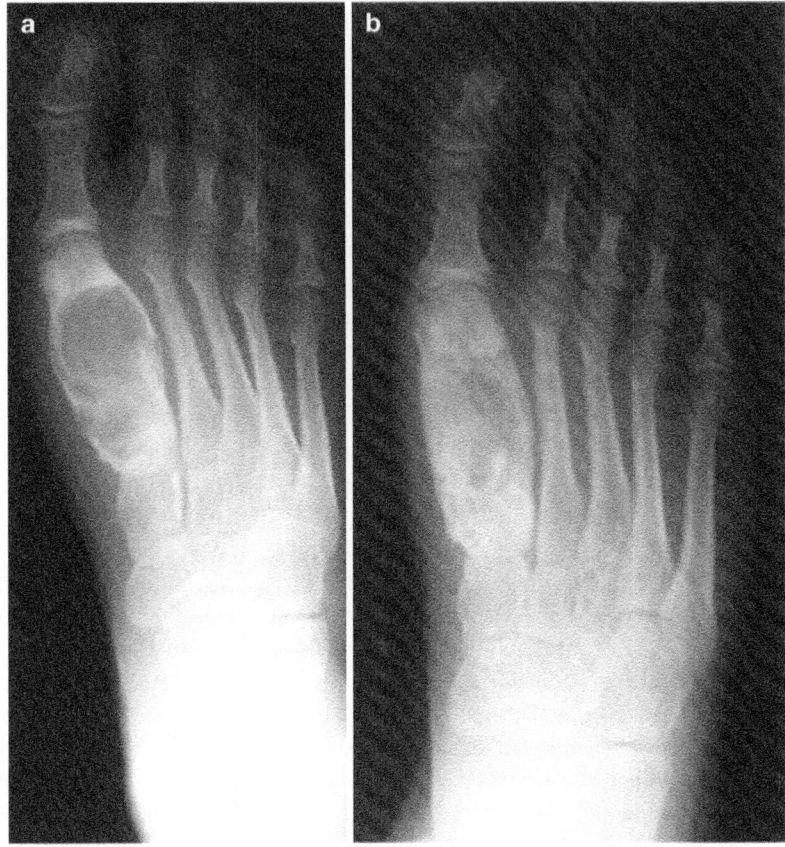

Summary and Conclusions

Numerous conditions affect the foot and ankle, and foot pain remains a very common presenting complaint. A knowledge of anatomy and common foot and ankle problems can provide the diagnostician adequate tools to treat patients. The last figures in this chapter provide algorithms that can assist in the diagnosis and treatment of foot and ankle pain. Figure 15.34 can assist in the diagnosis and treatment of patients with foot and ankle complaints resulting from an acute injury. Figure 15.35 provides steps to evaluate and treat patients that have foot and ankle pain without a history of an acute injury but with radiographic evidence of deformity or pathology. Figure 15.36 should provide some structure to the diagnosis and treatment of patients with foot and ankle complaints without injury and no radiographic evidence of deformity or pathology. These are not comprehensive algorithms but should provide some guidance when encountering patients with foot and ankle complaints.

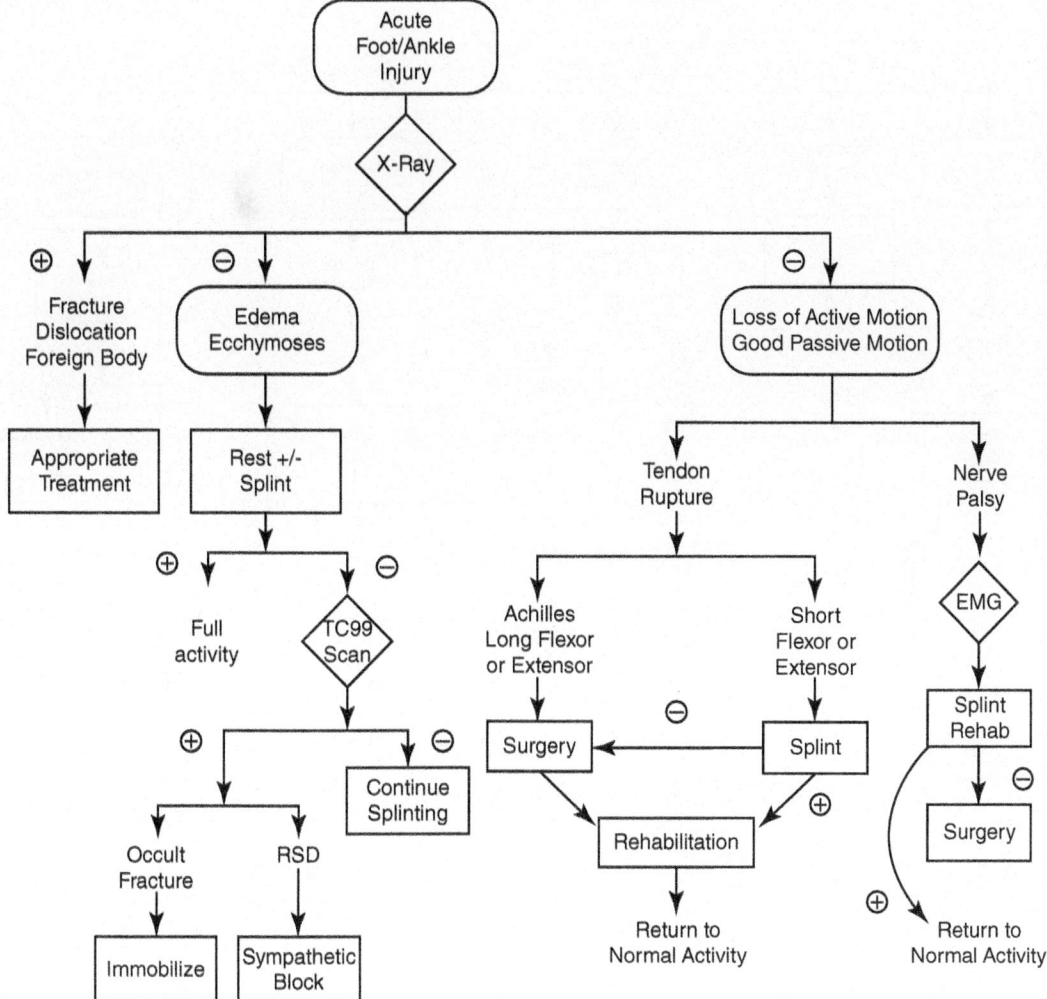

Fig. 15.34 Algorithm for diagnosis and treatment of foot and ankle pain with acute injury

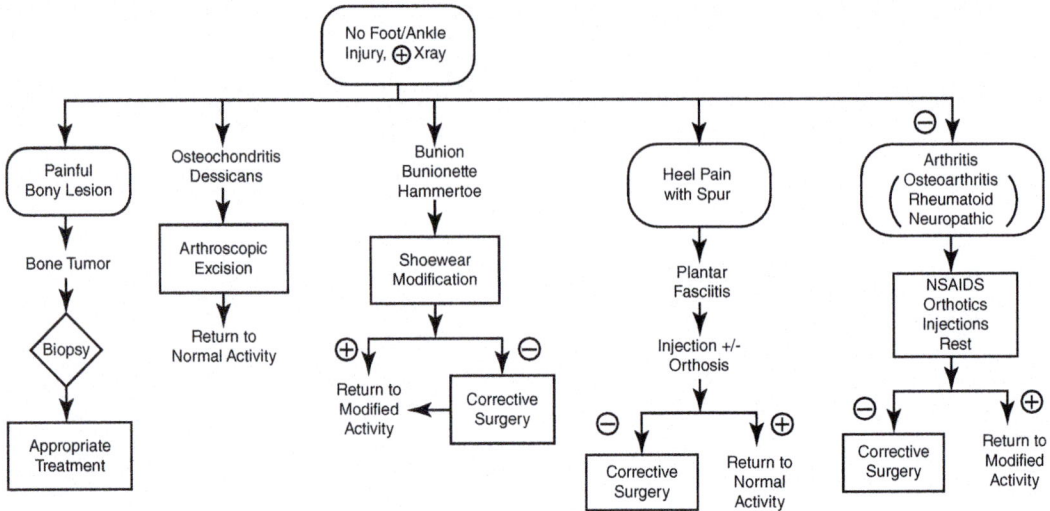

Fig. 15.35 Algorithm for diagnosis and treatment of foot and ankle pain with no injury and positive radiograph

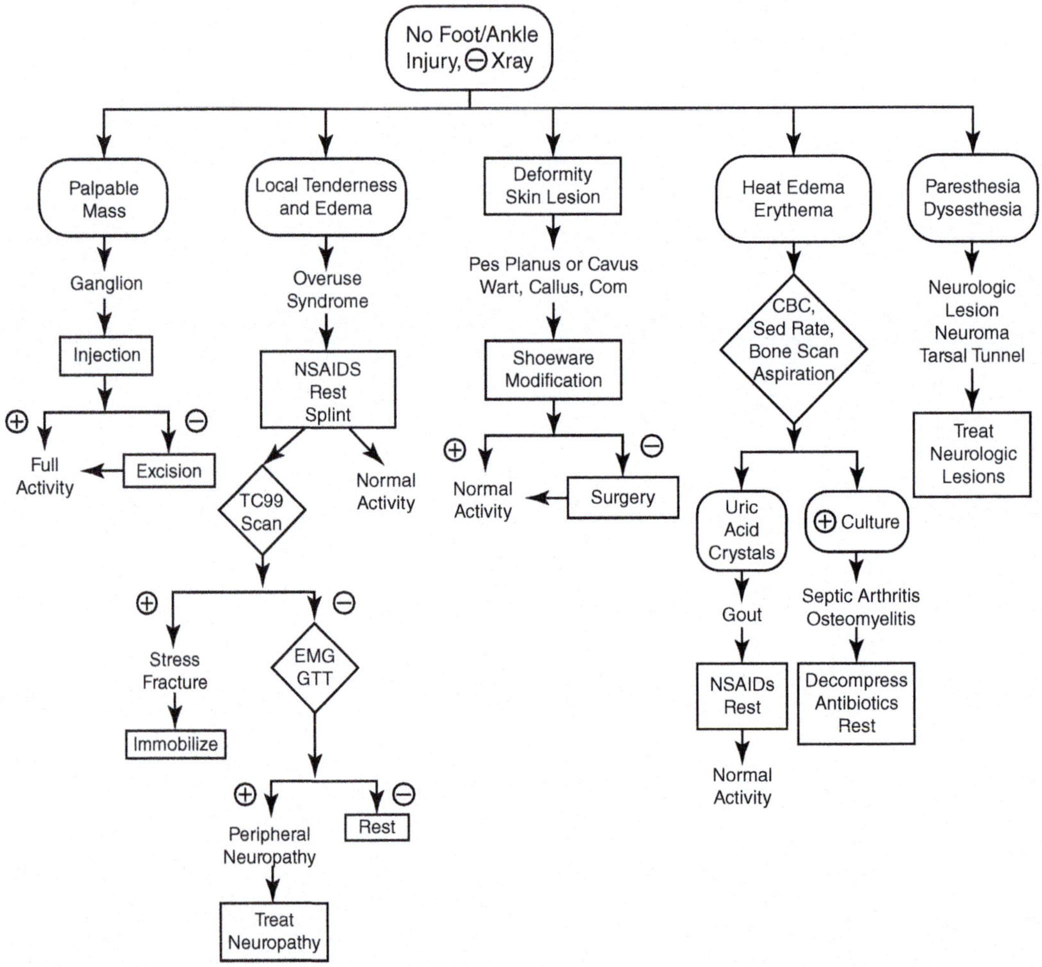

No Foot/Ankle Injury, ⊖ Xray

Palpable Mass
↓
Ganglion
↓
Injection
⊕ ↓ ⊖
Full Activity — Excision

Local Tenderness and Edema
↓
Overuse Syndrome
↓
NSAIDS Rest Splint
↓ ↘
TC99 Scan   Normal Activity
⊕ ↓ ⊖
Stress Fracture   EMG GTT
↓
Immobilize
⊕ ↓ ⊖
Peripheral Neuropathy   Rest
↓
Treat Neuropathy

Deformity Skin Lesion
↓
Pes Planus or Cavus Wart, Callus, Com
↓
Shoeware Modification
⊕ ↓ ⊖
Normal Activity — Surgery

Heat Edema Erythema
↓
CBC, Sed Rate, Bone Scan Aspiration
↓ ↘
Uric Acid Crystals   ⊕ Culture
↓
Gout   Septic Arthritis Osteomyelitis
↓   ↓
NSAIDs Rest   Decompress Antibiotics Rest
↓
Normal Activity

Paresthesia Dysesthesia
↓
Neurologic Lesion Neuroma Tarsal Tunnel
↓
Treat Neurologic Lesions

Fig. 15.36 Algorithm for diagnosis and treatment of foot and ankle pain with no injury and negative radiograph

Further Reading

Adelaar RS. The treatment of complex fractures of the talus. Orthop Clin N Am. 1989;20(4):692–3, 991–1200.

Harrelson JM. Management of the diabetic foot. Orthop Clin N Am. 1989;20(4):606.

Hawkins LG. Fractures of the neck of the talus. J Bone Joint Surg. 1970;52A:991–1002.

Lapidus PW. Chapter 53: the toenails. In: Jahss MH, editor. Disorders of the foot, vol. 2. Philadelphia, PA: Saunders; 1991. p. 1589.

Linklater JM, Read JW, Sofka CM, Hayter CL, Dimmick SJ. Chapter 3: Imaging of the foot and ankle. In: Haskell A, Coughlin MJ, editors. Coughlin and Mann's surgery of the foot and ankle. 10th ed. Amsterdam: Elsevier; 2024. p. 62.

Mann RA. The great toe. Orthop Clin N Am. 1989;20(4):524.

Montgomery HC, Davies MB. Common disorders of the adult foot and ankle. Surgery (Oxford). 2016;34(9):477.

Myerson MS, Kadakia AR. Chapter 11. Arthrodesis of the hallux metatarsophalangeal and interphalangeal joints. In: Myerson MS, Kadakia AR, editors. Reconstructive foot and ankle surgery: management of complications. 3rd ed. Amsterdam: Elsevier; 2019. p. 142.

Myerson MS, Kadakia AR. Chapter 27. Arthrodesis of the hallux metatarsophalangeal and interphalangeal joints. In: Myerson MS, Kadakia AR, editors. Reconstructive foot and ankle surgery: management of complications. 3rd ed. Amsterdam: Elsevier; 2019. p. 417.

Rome K, Stewart S. Chapter 9. Rheumatic diseases. In: Burrow JG, Rome K, Padhiar N, editors. Neale's disorders of the foot and ankle. 9th ed. Amsterdam: Elsevier; 2020. p. 222–60.

Rothenberg P, Swanton E, Molloy A, Aiyer AA, Kaplan JR. Chapter 117. Ligamentous injuries of the foot and ankle. In: Miller MD, Thompson SR, editors. DeLee, Drez & Miller's orthopaedic sports medicine. Amsterdam: Elsevier; 2020. p. 1445.

Sharma H, Jane M, Reid R. Chondromyxoid fibroma of the foot and ankle: 40 years' Scottish bone tumour registry experience. Int Orthop. 2006;30(3):206.

Waldrop NE III. Chapter 36. Athletic soft tissue injuries of the foot and ankle. In: Haskell A, Coughlin MJ, editors. Coughlin and Mann's surgery of the foot and ankle. 10th ed. Amsterdam: Elsevier; 2024. p. 1463.

Weissman BNW, Sledge CB. Chapter 10. The ankle. In: Weissman BNW, Sledge CB, editors. Orthopedic radiology. Philadelphia, PA: Saunders; 1985.

Weissman BNW, Sledge CB. Chapter 11. The foot. In: Weissman BNW, Sledge CB, editors. Orthopedic radiology. Philadelphia, PA: Saunders; 1985.

Index

The manufacturer's authorised representative in the EU is Springer
Nature Customer Service Centre GmbH, Europaplatz 3, 69115 Heidelberg,
Germany. If you have any concerns regarding our products, please
contact ProductSafety@springernature.com

Printed and bound by CPI Group (UK) Ltd, Croydon, CR0 4YY

08/06/2026

02131539-0002